# Maternal Child
# Health Nursing

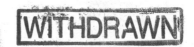

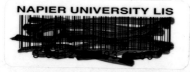

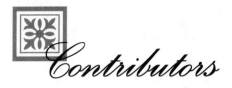
# Contributors

**Maryann Foley, RN, BSN**
Independent Clinical Consultant
Flourtown, Pennsylvania

**Susan Galea, RN, MSN, CCRN**
Independent Nurse Consultant
Blue Bell, Pennsylvania
Critical Care Nurse
University of Pennsylvania
Philadelphia, Pennsylvania

**Mary Gyetvan, RN, BSEd, MSN**
Independent Clinical Consultant
Levittown, Pennsylvania

**Beverly Tscheschlog, RN**
Staff Per Diem
Grand View Hospital
Sellersville, Pennsylvania
Independent Clinical Consultant
Ottsville, Pennsylvania

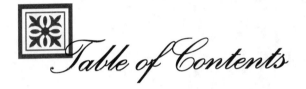

# Table of Contents

# Section 1

# Overview of Maternal–Newborn Care

▨ ▨ ▨

# REPRODUCTIVE ANATOMY AND PHYSIOLOGY

Flushing
Increased Muscle Tension

MALE RESPONSE

Penile Erection
Congested Scrotal Skin
Testicular Elevation
Nipple Erection
Flushing
Increased Heart Rate and Blood Pressure
Increased Muscle Tension

## Plateau Phase

FEMALE RESPONSE

Outer Vaginal Wall Engorgement
Engorged, Darkened, and Swollen Labia
Minora
Retracted Clitoris
Nipple Engorgement
Flushing
Increased Muscle Tension

MALE RESPONSE

Increased Penile Size
Continued Testicular Elevation
Increased Heart Rate and Blood Pressure
Increased Respiratory Rate
Increased Muscle Tension

## Orgasmic Phase

FEMALE RESPONSE

Strong Vaginal Muscle Contraction
Uterine Muscle Contraction
Peaking of Flushing
Strong Voluntary and Involuntary Muscle
Contraction
Increased Respiratory Rate
Doubling of Heart Rate
Increased Blood Pressure

MALE RESPONSE

Rhythmic Contraction
Semen Expulsion
Peaking of Heart Rate
Loss of Voluntary Muscle Control
Onset of Refractory Period

## Resolution Phase

FEMALE RESPONSE

Decreased Vaginal Engorgement
Vaginal Shrinking

▩ ▩ ▩

# FAMILY PLANNING AND CONTRACEPTION

▨ ▨ ▨

# FETAL GROWTH AND DEVELOPMENT

▨ ▨ ▨

# BIOPHYSICAL CHANGES OF PREGNANCY

▨ ▨ ▨

# ANTEPARTAL CARE

&#9672; &#9672; &#9672;

# COMMON DISCOMFORTS OF PREGNANCY

⌘ ⌘ ⌘

# NUTRITION DURING PREGNANCY

⌘ ⌘ ⌘

# HIGH-RISK PREGNANCY

WOMAN WITH SPECIAL NEEDS
  Pregnant Adolescent
  Mature Woman (Over Age 35)
  Drug-Dependent Woman

🖼 🖼 🖼

# LABOR PROCESS

THEORIES OF LABOR ONSET
  Progesterone Deprivation
  Oxytocin Stimulation
  Uterine Stretching
  Prostaglandin Cascade
COMPONENTS OF LABOR
  Passage
  Passenger
    FETAL SKULL
      Structure
      Diameter
    MOLDING
    *PRESENTATION*     *114*
      Attitude
        vertex
        sinciput
        face
        brow

▓ ▓ ▓

# FIRST STAGE OF LABOR

IMMEDIATE ASSESSMENT OF WOMAN
IN LABOR
Initial Interview

▩ ▩ ▩

# SECOND STAGE OF LABOR

BIRTH
**Postoperative Follow-Up**
PAIN CONTROL
FLUID BALANCE
UTERINE ASSESSMENT
VITAL SIGNS
VOIDING
BOWEL MANAGEMENT
INCISIONAL CARE
MOBILITY

⌘ ⌘ ⌘

## THIRD STAGE OF LABOR

PLACENTAL SEPARATION
PLACENTAL EXPULSION
IMMEDIATE POSTPARTAL ASSESSMENT
Perineal Repair
Vital Signs
Perineal Care

⌘ ⌘ ⌘

## DANGER SIGNS OF LABOR

⌘ ⌘ ⌘

## COMFORT DURING LABOR

▨ ▨ ▨

# COMPLICATIONS DURING LABOR AND DELIVERY

▨ ▨ ▨

## POSTPARTAL COMPLICATIONS

✖ ✖ ✖

# NEWBORN CARE

⊠ ⊠ ⊠

# NEWBORN NUTRITION

⊠ ⊠ ⊠

# HIGH-RISK NEWBORN

*Section*
**2**

# Maternal–Newborn
# Care Topics

# ABORTION, ELECTIVE

## DESCRIPTION

- Elective abortion is a procedure performed deliberately to end a pregnancy before fetal viability; also referred to as therapeutic, medical, or induced abortion.
- It may be performed for a number of reasons, including to end a pregnancy that threatens a woman's life or involves a fetus found on amniocentesis to have a chromosomal defect, to end a pregnancy that is unwanted because it is the result of rape or incest, or to end a pregnancy of a woman who chooses not to have a child at this time.
- Elective abortion may be accomplished by a variety of techniques, including menstrual extraction, dilatation and curettage (D&C), dilatation and vacuum extraction (D&E), saline induction, hysterotomy, or RU486 medication.

## NURSING IMPLICATIONS

- Be aware of personal feelings regarding elective abortion.
- Allow the client to make the decision to terminate the pregnancy on her own; offer answers to questions in a nonjudgmental manner.
- Obtain necessary laboratory studies before the procedure, including pregnancy test, complete blood count, blood typing including Rh factor, gonococcal smear, serologic test for syphilis, urinalysis, and Papanicolaou (Pap) smear.
- Have the client void before the procedure.
- Following the procedure, have the client remain supine for about 15 minutes until uterine cramping quiets and to prevent hypotension on standing.
- Anticipate use of oral oxytocin to ensure full uterine contraction.
- Monitor vital signs closely for changes indicating problems.
- Instruct the client that vaginal bleeding similar to her normal menstrual flow will continue for about 1 week, with occasional spotting for up to 2 to possibly 3 weeks.
- Advise the client, following a D&E, that cramping may continue for up to 24 to 48 hours and to use a mild analgesic for discomfort.

- Encourage the client to refrain from douching, using tampons, or engaging in coitus until after her return visit.
- Instruct the client to return in 2 weeks for follow-up visit and pelvic examination.
- Instruct the client in danger signs of hemorrhage (heavy vaginal bleeding or passing clots) and infection (abdominal pain or tenderness, fever over 100.4°F) to report to physician.
- Closely monitor the client undergoing a saline induction for signs of hypernatremia and water intoxication.
- Assist the client with contraceptive counseling as necessary.
- If the client is Rh-negative, administer $Rh_o$ (D) immunoglobulin.
- Offer explanations throughout the procedure to minimize the client's fears and anxieties.
- Offer emotional support to make the termination as untraumatic as possible; refer the client to counseling if appropriate.

### Following a saline induction
- Examine the products of conception to ensure that the entire conceptus has been delivered.
- Assess the client closely for signs of hemorrhage, especially if the delivery was unusually prolonged, placing the client at risk for *disseminated intravascular coagulation (DIC)*.
- Allow the client to view the fetus if she wishes; swaddle the fetus as if it were a full-term infant.
- Arrange for a follow-up examination in 2 to 4 weeks.
- Instruct the client to refrain from douching and coitus until after the follow-up visit.
- Advise the client that vaginal spotting may occur for as long as 2 weeks and that menstrual flow will return in 2 to 8 weeks.

## ABORTION, SPONTANEOUS

### DESCRIPTION
- Abortion is defined as any interruption of pregnancy before the fetus is viable, usually 20 to 24 weeks' gestation or weighing 500 g.
- A spontaneous abortion, also called a miscarriage, occurs from natural causes; it is termed early if it occurs

before week 16 of pregnancy, late if it occurs between weeks 16 and 24.

- Spontaneous abortion is one of the most common causes of bleeding during the first trimester of pregnancy, most commonly caused by abnormal fetal formation either from a teratogenic factor or chromosomal aberration or by implantation abnormalities.
- Types of spontaneous abortion include threatened, imminent (inevitable), complete, incomplete, missed, and recurrent.

### ASSESSMENT FINDINGS

- *Vaginal bleeding* (all types)

**For threatened abortion**
- Moderate bright red *vaginal bleeding*
- No cramping
- No *cervical dilation*

**For imminent abortion**
- Moderate bright red *vaginal bleeding*
- *Uterine contractions*
- *Cervical dilation*
- Possible passage of tissue fragments

**For complete abortion**
- Moderate bright red *vaginal bleeding*
- *Uterine contractions*
- *Cervical dilation*
- Spontaneous expulsion of entire products of conception (fetus, membranes, and placenta)

**For incomplete abortion**
- Moderate bright red *vaginal bleeding*
- *Uterine contractions*
- *Cervical dilation*
- Spontaneous expulsion of part of the products of conception (usually fetus only)

**For missed abortion**
- No increase in fundal height measurement
- Inaudible fetal heart sounds (previously present)
- Painless; *vaginal bleeding* or no symptoms at all

**For recurrent abortion**
- History of three spontaneous abortions occurring at the same gestational age in three pregnancies

### NURSING IMPLICATIONS

- Obtain a thorough history and physical examination to establish a baseline; include *estimating date of birth*.

- Assess the client's complaints of *vaginal bleeding,* including onset, duration, frequency, intensity, amount, color, and any associated symptoms.
- Ascertain if anything happened that may have started the bleeding and what, if anything, the client has done to control the bleeding.
- Obtain *ultrasonograraphy* to confirm pregnancy.
- Weigh perineal pads to determine accurately amount of vaginal blood loss.
- Monitor vital signs frequently for signs of hemorrhage.
- Recommend iron supplement and increases in dietary iron as indicated.
- Prepare for RhoGAM administration to an Rh-negative mother, as prescribed.
- Monitor fluid balance, including intravenous fluids and laboratory studies, especially in the presence of heavy *vaginal bleeding* to prevent shock.
- Offer support to the client and partner; reassure client that abortions happen spontaneously and not because of anything that she did.
- Offer emotional support and anticipatory guidance related to expected recovery, need for rest, and delaying another pregnancy until the client is fully recovered.
- Provide support to help the client accept the reality of the fetus' death; anticipate counseling for anxiety about future pregnancies.

### For a threatened abortion

- Obtain serum *HCG* levels at the start of bleeding and again in 48 hours.
- Anticipate obtaining serum progesterone level to evaluate any disruption in pregnancy.
- Instruct the client to limit activities for 24 to 48 hours.
- Instruct the client that if spotting is going to stop, it usually does so within 24 to 48 hours after reducing activity.
- If bleeding stops, advise the client to resume normal activities gradually, restricting coitus for approximately 2 weeks following the bleeding episode to prevent the possibility of infection and to avoid possibly inducing further bleeding.
- If bleeding does not stop, prepare the client for an imminent abortion.

### For an imminent abortion

- Instruct the client to save and bring any tissue fragments passed to the hospital.

- If no fetal heart sounds are detected, prepare the client for dilatation and curettage (D&C).
- Explain to the client that the pregnancy was already lost and all procedures are to clean and ready the uterus for another pregnancy.
- Save any tissue fragments passed in the labor room so they can be examined for abnormalities and for assurance that all the products of conception have been removed from the uterus.

### For a complete abortion

- Observe tissue fragments for passage of the complete products of conception.
- Instruct the client that *vaginal bleeding* will be minimal and self-limiting.

### For an incomplete abortion

- Save any tissue fragments to determine the amount of products of conception expelled.
- Prepare the client for D&C or suction curettage to evacuate the remainder of the pregnancy from the uterus.
- Be certain that the client is informed of what is happening and that she knows the pregnancy is already lost and the procedure is being done to prevent hemorrhage and infection.

### For a missed abortion

- Anticipate *ultrasonography* to confirm *fetal death*.
- Prepare the client for induced abortion.

## ABRUPTIO PLACENTAE

### DESCRIPTION

- Abruptio placentae, a complication of pregnancy, refers to a premature separation of the placenta.
- This usually occurs after the 20th to 24th week of pregnancy; it also may occur as late as during the first or second stage of labor.
- Abruptio placentae may occur during an otherwise normal labor.
- The primary cause is unknown, but predisposing factors include high parity, chronic hypertensive disease, *pregnancy-induced hypertension,* direct trauma, and vasoconstriction from cocaine use.
- Pressure on the vena cava from an enlarging uterus also may contribute, putting tension on the uterus from back pressure.

- Premature separation may follow a rapid decrease in uterine volume, such as that occurring with the sudden release of amniotic fluid.
- Degrees of placental separation are graded and are as follows:

> Grade 0—No symptoms apparent; diagnosis made after delivery
>
> Grade 1—Minimal separation enough to cause vaginal bleeding and changes in maternal vital signs; no fetal distress or hemorrhagic shock
>
> Grade 2—Moderate separation; evidence of fetal distress; uterus tender and painful on palpation
>
> Grade 3—Extreme separation; without immediate intervention, maternal shock and fetal death result

## ASSESSMENT FINDINGS

- Sharp stabbing pain high in uterine fundus as initial separation occurs
- Uterine outline possibly enlarged or changing shape
- Pain over and above the pain of contractions if labor begins with separation
- Tenderness on uterine palpation with contractions
- Heavy bleeding (may not be readily apparent)
- External bleeding if placenta separates first at the edges and blood escapes freely from the cervix
- Hard, boardlike uterus with minimal or no apparent bleeding (especially if center of placenta separates first)

## NURSING IMPLICATIONS

- Assess the time bleeding began and whether it was accompanied by pain.
- Evaluate the amount and type of bleeding.
- Anticipate laboratory analysis, including hemoglobin, type and crossmatch, fibrinogen level, and fibrin breakdown products.
- Administer oxygen by mask to minimize fetal anoxia.
- Monitor *fetal heart rate* and maternal vital signs.
- Position the client in the lateral position to prevent pressure on vena cava, further compromising *fetal circulation*.
- Avoid vaginal or pelvic examinations and enemas to prevent further placental disruption.
- Anticipate immediate delivery.

- Assess the client for *disseminated intravascular coagulation (DIC),* and treat as necessary.
- Assess for signs and symptoms of infection in the postpartum period.

## ALCOHOL USE IN PREGNANCY

### DESCRIPTION

- Alcohol has been isolated as a fetal teratogen.
- Fetuses cannot remove the breakdown products of alcohol from their body, leading to vitamin $B_6$ deficiency and accompanying neurologic damage.
- Infants born to mothers who use alcohol are at risk for *fetal alcohol syndrome* manifested by size *small for gestational age,* mental retardation, and characteristic craniofacial deformity (short palpebral fissures, thin upper lip, and upturned nose).

### NURSING IMPLICATIONS

- Be aware that it is impossible to define a safe level of alcohol consumption because of individual variations in metabolism.
- Advise the client to abstain from alcohol completely or at least limit intake to less than 1 ounce per day.
- Refer the client to an alcohol treatment program early in pregnancy, if indicated.

## AMNIOCENTESIS

### DESCRIPTION

- Amniocentesis is the aspiration of amniotic fluid from the pregnant uterus for examination.
- It may be done as early as the 12th or 13th week of pregnancy.
- Amniocentesis may be performed for chromosomal determination (approximately 14 to 16 weeks), Rh isoimmunization (20 to 28 weeks), maturity determination (34 to 42 weeks), and *evaluation of fetal well-being* (34 to 42 weeks).

### NURSING IMPLICATIONS

- Explain the events of the procedure, including skin preparation, positioning, use of ultrasound, use of local anesthetic, needle insertion, and aspiration.
- Have the client void before procedure.
- Obtain maternal blood pressure and *fetal heart rate* for baseline levels and continue to monitor throughout and after the procedure for changes.

- Keep in mind that although amniocentesis is an easy procedure technically, it poses some risks to the fetus and may be frightening to the client.
- Although they are rare, anticipate for the following complications: *hemorrhage* from placental perforation, infection, puncture of the fetus, and irritation of the uterus leading to *premature labor.*

# AMNIOTIC FLUID EMBOLISM

## DESCRIPTION

- Amniotic fluid embolism occurs when the amniotic fluid is forced into an open maternal uterine blood sinus through some defect in the membranes or after membrane rupture or partial premature separation of the placenta. Solid particles in the amniotic fluid enter the maternal circulation and reach the lungs as small emboli.
- A pulmonary embolism, the severity of which is out of proportion to the size of the particles, results.
- Amniotic fluid embolism may occur during labor or in the postpartum period.
- Amniotic fluid embolism is associated with the following risk factors: oxytocin administration, *abruptio placentae,* and polyhydramnios.

## ASSESSMENT FINDINGS

- Sudden sitting up and grasping of chest
- Sudden inability to breathe
- Sharp chest pain
- Tachypnea
- Pallor
- Coughing with pink, frothy sputum
- Cyanosis
- Severe drop in maternal blood pressure
- Increasing restlessness and anxiety

## NURSING IMPLICATIONS

- Institute emergency resuscitation measures, including cardiopulmonary resuscitation, intubation, and oxygen administration.
- Plan for immediate delivery of fetus by cesarean birth.
- Assess for possible complication of *disseminated intravascular coagulation (DIC).*
- Administer fibrinogen therapy to counteract *DIC.*
- Transfer to intensive care unit.

# AMNIOTOMY

### DESCRIPTION

- Amniotomy is the artificial rupture of membranes.
- Rupturing the membranes if they do not rupture spontaneously allows the fetal head to contact the cervix more directly and may improve the efficiency of contractions.

### NURSING IMPLICATIONS

- Place the client in the dorsal recumbent position.
- Monitor *fetal heart rate* immediately following rupture of membranes to determine that a loop of cord has not escaped with the fluid.

## ANALGESIA, NARCOTIC

### DESCRIPTION

- Narcotics are often given in labor because of their potent analgesic effect.
- All narcotics cause fetal central nervous system depression.
- Drugs commonly used for narcotic analgesia include meperidine hydrochloride (Demerol), morphine sulfate, nalbuphine (Nubain), fetanyl (Sublimaze), and butorphanol tartrate (Stadol).
- Meperidine is advantageous as an analgesic during labor because it has additional sedative and antispasmodic actions, effective in relieving pain, helping to relax the cervix, and giving a feeling of euphoria and well-being.
- Meperidine crosses the placenta within minutes of being administered, possibly causing respiratory depression in the fetus 2 to 3 hours after administration.
- Other narcotic analgesics, such as nalbuphine, butorphanol tartrate, and synthetic narcotic analgesics, also leave a degree of respiratory depression in the neonate.

### NURSING IMPLICATIONS

- Assess the client's complaints of pain, including onset, location, duration, intensity, and character.
- Administer narcotics as prescribed; keep in mind that the smallest dose effective is used.
- Monitor the client's vital signs and *fetal heart rate* closely for changes.

- Assess the client and fetus for possible side effects, including respiratory depression.
- Keep in mind that the fetal liver takes 2 to 3 hours to activate the drug into the fetal system.
- Administer meperidine when the client is more than 3 hours away from birth to allow the peak action time of the drug in the fetus to have passed by the time of birth.
- Monitor the neonate for 4 hours following the administration of meperidine within 1 hour of birth.
- Keep a narcotic antagonist, such as naloxone (Narcan), immediately available for administration to the infant at birth, if needed.
- If severe respiratory depression is suspected, administer naloxone to the client just before birth, increasing the chance for spontaneous respiratory activity.
- Observe the neonate who receives naloxone in the immediate birth period because when naloxone wears off the neonate's respirations may become severely depressed again.
- Institute comfort measures, such as position changes, back rubs, and relaxation techniques, to help with pain control.

## ANALGESIA, SEDATIVE-HYPNOTIC

### DESCRIPTION

- Sedative and hypnotic agents can be used for pain relief during labor.
- Agents, such as secobarbital sodium (Seconal), may be administered to encourage rest in a woman who is becoming exhausted by labor.
- These agents cause maternal sedation and relaxation.
- Adverse effects include nausea, vomiting, hypotension, restlessness, and vertigo.
- These agents also affect the fetus because they readily cross the placenta, causing central nervous system depression, prolonged drowsiness, and delayed establishment of feeding (due to poor sucking reflex or poor sucking pressure).

### NURSING IMPLICATIONS

- Assess the client's complaints of pain, including onset, location, duration, intensity, and character.
- Administer sedative-hypnotic as prescribed.

- Monitor the client's vital signs and *fetal heart rate* closely for changes.
- Assess the client and fetus for possible adverse effects, including central nervous system depression.
- Keep in mind that because of the rapid transfer across the placenta and lack of antagonist, these agents are generally inappropriate during active labor.
- Provide comfort measures, such as position changes, back rubs, and relaxation techniques, to assist with pain control.

# ANEMIA, IRON DEFICIENCY

### DESCRIPTION

- Iron deficiency anemia is a preexisting disorder or newly acquired illness that places the pregnant woman at high risk for complications.
- Iron deficiency anemia complicates as many as 15% to 25% of all pregnancies, occurring in as many as 40% of pregnant African-American women.
- Many women enter pregnancy with an iron deficiency anemia resulting from poor diet, heavy menstrual periods, or unwise weight reduction programs.
- As a rule, the average woman depends on iron stores to supply enough iron for pregnancy.
- Iron deficiency anemia is associated with low fetal birth weight and preterm birth.

### ASSESSMENT FINDINGS

- Microcytic, hypochromic red blood cells
- Hematocrit below 33%
- Hemoglobin below 11 g/dl
- Serum ferritin below 10 $\mu$g/L
- Serum transferrin saturation level below 16%
- Serum iron level below 10 $\mu$g/dl
- Mean corpuscular hemoglobin concentration (MCHC) below 30
- Iron binding capacity over 400 $\mu$g/L
- Fatigue
- Poor exercise tolerance

### NURSING IMPLICATIONS

- Obtain a thorough history and physical examination to establish a baseline and ongoing levels for changes.

- Prepare the client for serum blood studies; evaluate results and notify physician of abnormal values.
- Keep in mind that some women develop pica, or the eating of substances, such as ice or starch.
- Instruct the client in use of prenatal vitamins containing an iron supplement as prophylactic therapy against iron deficiency anemia.
- Encourage the client to take the supplement with orange juice to enhance absorption.
- Instruct the client in foods that are high in vitamins and iron.
- Develop a medication teaching plan, discussing the rationale for, action of, possible adverse effects of, and need for compliance.
- Instruct the client that stools may turn black and tarry; encourage client to eat foods high in fiber and drink plenty of fluids to prevent constipation.
- If iron deficiency is severe, anticipate administering iron supplement intramuscularly or intravenously.

## ANESTHESIA, GENERAL

### DESCRIPTION

- General anesthesia is never preferred for childbirth because it carries the dangers of hypoxia and possible inhalation of vomitus during administration, which can be fatal.
- Pregnant women are particularly prone to gastric reflux because of increased stomach pressure from the pressure of the full uterus beneath it; the gastro-esophageal valve may be displaced and may not be functioning properly.
- General anesthesia may be necessary in emergency situations, such as *abruptio placentae,* requiring an immediate *cesarean birth.*
- Thiopental sodium (Pentothal), a short-acting barbiturate, is the drug of choice for general anesthesia; it causes rapid induction of anesthesia and minimal postpartal bleeding.
- After induction, the client is intubated and maintained by nitrous oxide and oxygen.
- Thiopental sodium crosses the placenta rapidly; therefore, neonates may be slow to respond at birth and need resuscitation.

### NURSING IMPLICATIONS

- Check the delivery or birthing room to be certain that adequate equipment, such as additional drugs, laryngoscope, endotracheal tube, 100% oxygen source, and suction equipment, is available for safe administration.
- Prepare the client physically and emotionally for anesthesia as much as possible; include all aspects of preoperative and postoperative care.
- Obtain a thorough history and physical examination before administering anesthesia to establish a baseline.
- Anticipate administering cimetidine (Tagamet), ranitidine (Zantac), or an antacid before anesthesia to reduce the level of acid in stomach contents; be aware that metoclopramide (Reglan) may also be prescribed to increase gastric emptying.
- Position the client on her back with a wedge under her right hip to displace the uterus from the vena cava.
- Begin an intravenous infusion to prevent the occurrence of hypotension and establish a line for emergency medications.
- Perform a thorough review of all systems, including vital signs, neurologic status, cardiopulmonary status, and gastrointestinal and urinary elimination, following general anesthesia.
- Assess the client for complaints of sore throat following general anesthesia; offer cold liquid or ice cubes as soon as this is safe to relieve the discomfort.
- Closely assess the client in the postpartum period for signs of *uterine atony* and *hemorrhage* because most gases used cause uterine relaxation, thereby reducing effective contractions and hemostasis postpartum.
- Assess the neonate for effects of general anesthesia, such as slowness in responding and circulatory and respiratory depression.
- If aspiration occurs in the delivery room, assist the anesthesiologist with tracheal suctioning; administering 100% oxygen; administering medications, such as isoproterenol to decrease bronchospasm and a corticosteroid to reduce inflammation; mechanical ventilation; diagnostic studies, such as chest x-ray and blood gases; and transfer to the critical care unit.

# ANESTHESIA, LOCAL

### DESCRIPTION

- Local anesthesia refers to the injection of an anesthetic into a specific area to block the nerves in that area.
- Pudendal nerve block is the injection of a local anesthetic just before delivery into the right and left pudendal nerves at the level of the ischial spine.
- Local infiltration is the injection of an anesthetic, such as lidocaine, into the superficial nerves of the perineum just before delivery by placing the anesthetic along the borders of the vulva; it is commonly used for episiotomy incision and repair.
- Either route provides rapid anesthesia of the perineum with no apparent effects on labor progress, the fetus, or neonate.

### NURSING IMPLICATIONS

- Place the client in the lithotomy or dorsal recumbent position.
- Keep in mind that anesthesia achieved with a pudendal nerve block is sufficiently deep to allow the use of low forceps during birth and episiotomy repair.
- Assess the *fetal heart rate* and maternal blood pressure immediately after the injection in case maternal hypotension occurs.
- Instruct the client that the effects of a pudendal nerve block last approximately 60 minutes.

# ANESTHESIA, REGIONAL

### DESCRIPTION

- Regional anesthesia refers to the injection of a local anesthetic to block specific nerve pathways, achieving pain relief by blocking sodium and potassium flux in the nerve membrane, thereby stabilizing the nerve in a polarized resting state so it is unable to conduct sensations.
- Effects on the fetus are minimal compared with those of systemic anesthetic agents.
- Regional anesthesia allows the woman to be completely awake and aware of what is happening during birth.
- They leave the uterus capable of optimal contraction after birth, and important concern in preventing *postpartum hemorrhage*.

- Epidural anesthesia (peridural block) is placed into the epidural space and blocks not only spinal nerve roots in the space, but also the sympathetic nerve fibers that travel with them.
- Epidural anesthesia provides pain relief for both labor and birth.
- Such a block may actually increase contraction strength and blood flow to the uterus, but because the woman no longer experiences pain, the release of catecholamines with a beta-blocking effect from a pain response is decreased.
- Epidural blocks are commonly used for many women in labor; they are advantageous for women with heart disease, pulmonary disease, *diabetes mellitus,* and sometimes severe *pregnancy-induced hypertension,* making labor virtually pain free and minimizing the stress from the discomfort of labor; because the woman does not feel contractions, her physical energy is preserved.
- Epidural blocks are acceptable for use in preterm labor because the drug has scant effect on the fetus allowing for a controlled and gentle birth with less trauma to an immature fetal skull; because the woman receives no systemic medication, the neonate responds more quickly after birth than if *narcotic analgesia* is used.
- The chief problem with epidural blocks is their tendency to induce hypotension.
- Other problems include the prolongation of the *second stage of labor* (because the woman, unaware of contractions, does not push with them, and fetal descent slows leading to a greater need for *vacuum extraction* or *cesarean birth*) and relaxation of levator ani muscle (impedes internal rotation of fetal head, further slowing labor or making it necessary for forceps).

### Nursing Implications

- Assess client's complaints of pain, including onset, duration, location, intensity, frequency, and character.
- Be aware that lumbar epidural anesthesia is begun when the cervix is dilated 4 to 6 cm.
- Explain the procedure to the client and her partner, ensuring informed consent.
- Position the client on her side or sitting upright.

- Establish an intravenous fluid line and administer a fluid bolus of 500 to 1000 ml of intravenous fluid, such as Ringer's lactate, as prescribed to decrease the possibility of hypotension.
- Keep in mind that Ringer's lactate is preferred to a glucose solution because too much maternal glucose can cause hyperglycemia with rebound hypoglycemia in the neonate.
- Attach a continuous blood pressure monitoring cuff to detect hypotension.
- Assist the anesthesiologist with injection of local anesthetic, providing support to the client as she undergoes a potentially frightening procedure.
- Assist the anesthesiologist with evaluating whether the catheter is placed appropriately by using a test dose to produce lower extremity flushing and feeling of warmth.
- Be aware that if the catheter is inadvertently placed below the dura, paralysis of lower extremities will occur; if it is in the blood stream, extreme symptoms of confusion will occur.
- Evaluate the client for pain relief, which should occur in 10 to 15 minutes.
- Keep the client positioned on the left side to prevent supine hypotension syndrome.
- If hypotension occurs, raise the client's legs and administer oxygen, intravenous fluids, and drugs, such as ephedrine, to elevate blood pressure and stabilize cardiovascular status.
- If convulsions occur (rare), administer small amounts of short-acting barbiturates or diazepam (Valium) as prescribed to control them.
- Assist the client to see that labor is progressing despite her loss of pain sensation.
- Assess the client's bladder for filling and distention because the client will have decreased ability to detect bladder filling; a full bladder can interfere with fetal descent.
- Help the client with effective second stage pushing, which may be difficult because of the loss of sensation.
- Provide support and guidance to the client and partner regarding all events and procedures to ensure a safe, satisfactory labor and delivery.

# ANESTHESIA, SPINAL

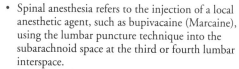

### DESCRIPTION

- Spinal anesthesia refers to the injection of a local anesthetic agent, such as bupivacaine (Marcaine), using the lumbar puncture technique into the subarachnoid space at the third or fourth lumbar interspace.
- Spinal anesthesia is rarely used today in preference to lumbar epidural blocks; it may be used in an emergency because the administration technique is simpler than that of an epidural block and can be accomplished more rapidly.
- The major complication that can occur immediately after administration is hypotension from sympathetic blockage in the lower extremities, leading to vasodilation and a falling central blood pressure, thereby compromising placental perfusion.
- A late complication is a spinal headache occurring because of a leakage of spinal fluid from the needle insertion and possibly from the irritation of a small amount of air that enters at the injection site, shifting the pressure of the cerebrospinal fluid on the cerebral meninges causing pain.

### NURSING IMPLICATIONS

- Assess the client's complaints of pain, including onset, duration, intensity, frequency, and character.
- Position the client in a sitting position with the head bent forward so that the back curves and the intravertebral spaces are open.
- Support the client in this position because she is "front-heavy" by her pregnancy and could easily fall forward if not well supported.
- Assist the anesthesiologist with injection of the local anesthetic.
- Be aware that the anesthetic normally reaches the level of T-10 with anesthesia up to the umbilicus, including both legs.
- Keep in mind that the anesthetic agent may be loaded or weighted with glucose to make it heavier than the cerebrospinal fluid, preventing it from rising too high in the spinal canal and interfering with the motor control of the uterus or with respiratory muscles.

- Administer intravenous fluid, such as lactated Ringer's, before injection to ensure good hydration and prevent the possibility of hypotension.
- Following the injection, have the client lie down with a pillow under her head to allow the drug to rise high enough in the canal to achieve pain relief without allowing it to rise too high.
- Attach a continuous blood pressure monitoring cuff to detect hypotension.
- If hypotension occurs, turn the client to her left side to reduce vena cava compression and increase the rate of intravenous fluids as prescribed.
- Anticipate administering a vasopressor to increase blood pressure and oxygen to increase tissue perfusion, as prescribed.
- Have the client remain flat in bed for 8 to 12 hours after giving birth to prevent air from rising to the cerebral meninges causing a spinal headache.
- Encourage a high fluid intake (about 3000 ml/day) to replace spinal fluid lost, preventing spinal headache.
- Make sure that the client understands the need for lying flat and drinking plenty of fluids.
- If headache occurs, have the client lie flat again and administer analgesic as prescribed.
- Offer comfort measures, such as cool compresses.
- If the headache is incapacitating, anticipate a blood patch technique in which 10 ml of blood is withdrawn from the client's arm and then immediately injected into the epidural space over the spinal injection site, thereby clotting and sealing off any further leakage of cerebrospinal fluid.
- Offer support and guidance to the client and partner throughout to alleviate anxiety and fears.

# ANTEPARTAL HISTORY AND PHYSICAL EXAMINATION

### DESCRIPTION

- Antepartal history and physical examination is a major component of antepartal care involving the physical, emotional, and social needs of the woman, unborn child, partner, and other family members.
- Antepartal history and physical examination begins with the first prenatal consultation, establishing a baseline of information, and continues throughout

pregnancy, helping to ensure a positive outcome of pregnancy.

- Antepartal history includes information about demographic data, chief complaints, past medical history, family history, family and social profile, gynecologic and obstetric history, and review of systems.
- Antepartal physical examination includes height, weight, vital signs, system examination, fundal height measurement, fetal heart sound auscultation, pelvic examination, pelvic size estimation, and laboratory testing.
- Information also is gathered about *estimated date of birth,* assessment of gestational age, *evaluation of fetal well-being,* self-care needs, childbirth education, prevention of fetal exposure to teratogens, nutritional needs of pregnancy, and any discomforts the client may be experiencing.
- Information gathered from the antepartal history and physical examination helps to identify any potential factors that may place the mother and baby at risk for problems during pregnancy.

### Assessment Findings

Assessment findings vary with the client; any deviation from normal should be reported.

### Nursing Implications

- Perform a thorough health history, investigating any complaints that the client may be experiencing.
- Be certain to evaluate the client's understanding of her status and changes associated with pregnancy at each visit.
- Be aware of cultural influences on the client's pregnancy.
- Be alert to possible risk factors, such as inadequate or excessive weight gain, history of diabetes or heart disease, infections, substance use and abuse, and abnormal laboratory tests.
- Ask the client about the date of her last menstrual period (LMP).
- Obtain baseline height and weight at the first visit and at each visit thereafter.
- Measure *fundal height.*
- Assist with pelvic examination and pelvic size estimation.

- Coordinate laboratory testing, including blood and urine specimens, *ultrasonography,* and *amniocentesis.*
- Assess client for *presumptive, probable,* and *positive signs* of pregnancy.
- Assess for fetal movement and audible fetal heart sounds.
- Provide client counseling and instructions regarding childbirth education; self-care measures, such as exercise, pain management, breathing techniques, birthing methods, hygiene, *breast care,* physical and sexual activity, sleep, *dental care,* and *immunizations;* prevention of fetal exposure to teratogens; and management of common discomforts of pregnancy, such as heartburn, *constipation,* nausea and vomiting, breast tenderness, palmar erythema, fatigue, hemorrhoids, varicosities, urinary frequency, palpitations, leukorrhea, backache, headache, *dyspnea, ankle edema,* leg cramps, and *Braxton-Hicks contractions.*

- Evaluate the client's nutritional intake; provide instructions about appropriate food and fluid choices to meet nutritional needs of pregnancy.
- Offer support and guidance to the client and family; allow time for questions and answers.
- Prepare the client for labor and delivery; instruct in signs of *true,* and *false labor.*

## ANTEPARTAL SYSTEMIC CHANGES, CARDIOVASCULAR

### Description
- During pregnancy, the cardiovascular system undergoes changes.
- These changes are extremely significant to the health of the fetus because they are important for adequate placental and *fetal circulation.*

### Assessment Findings
- Increased blood volume
- Decreased hemoglobin and erythrocyte concentration (as plasma volume first increases)
- Increased cardiac output
- Increased heart rate (approximately 10 beats/minute)
- Shifting of heart to transverse position in the chest cavity

- Impaired blood flow to lower extremities, leading to edema and varicosities of the vulva, rectum, and legs
- Palpitations
- Blood pressure changes
- Increased levels of fibrinogen and clotting factors (VII, VIII, IX, and X)
- Increased platelet count
- Elevated white blood cell count
- Decreased total protein level
- Increased blood lipid levels

### NURSING IMPLICATIONS

- Obtain a thorough health history and physical examination to establish a baseline.
- Perform ongoing data collection and follow-up regarding the client's complaints.
- Monitor routine diagnostic tests for changes and possible problems.
- Provide instructions to help minimize the effects of the cardiovascular changes.
- Be aware of the impact of cardiovascular changes on maternal status.
- Assist the client in voicing concerns about the effects of cardiovascular changes.

## ANTEPARTAL SYSTEMIC CHANGES, ENDOCRINE

### DESCRIPTION

- During pregnancy, the endocrine system undergoes changes.
- The most striking change is the addition of the placenta as an endocrine organ, producing large amounts of progesterone and estrogen.

### ASSESSMENT FINDINGS

- Increased levels of estrogen
- Increased levels of progesterone
- Halt in the production of follicle-stimulating hormone and luteinizing hormone
- Increased production of growth hormone and melanocyte-stimulating hormone
- Oxytocin production (late in pregnancy)
- Increased prolactin production
- Thyroid vascularization and hyperplasia

- Increased parathyroid size
- Increased glucocorticoid levels
- Increased insulin production
- Increased adrenal gland activity
- Elevated levels of corticosteroids
- Elevated levels of aldosterone

### Nursing Implications

- Obtain a thorough health history and physical examination to establish a baseline.
- Perform ongoing data collection and follow-up regarding the client's complaints.
- Monitor routine diagnostic tests for changes and possible problems.
- Provide instructions to help minimize the effects of the endocrine changes.
- Be aware of the impact of endocrine changes on maternal status.
- Assist the client in voicing concerns about the effects of endocrine changes.

## ANTEPARTAL SYSTEMIC CHANGES, GASTROINTESTINAL

### Description

- During pregnancy, the gastrointestinal system undergoes changes.
- These changes often result in many of the common discomforts of pregnancy.

### Assessment Findings

- Nausea
- Vomiting
- Increased gastric acidity
- Delayed gastric emptying
- Decreased intestinal motility
- Stomach and intestinal displacement toward the back and sides of abdomen
- Gum hypertrophy
- Gingival bleeding

### Nursing Implications

- Obtain a thorough health history and physical examination to establish a baseline.
- Perform ongoing data collection and follow-up regarding the client's complaints.

- Assist the client with measures to relieve discomforts.
- Monitor routine diagnostic tests for changes and possible problems.
- Provide instructions to help minimize the effects of the gastrointestinal changes.
- Be aware of the impact of gastrointestinal changes on maternal status.
- Assist the client in voicing concerns about the effects of gastrointestinal changes.

## ANTEPARTAL SYSTEMIC CHANGES, INTEGUMENTARY

### DESCRIPTION
- During pregnancy, the integumentary system undergoes changes.
- These changes are the result of the growing fetus and hormonal secretion.

### ASSESSMENT FINDINGS
- Abdominal striae
- Linea nigra
- Melasma
- Vascular spiders on thighs
- Increased sweat and sebaceous gland activity

### NURSING IMPLICATIONS
- Obtain a thorough health history and physical examination to establish a baseline.
- Perform ongoing data collection and follow-up regarding the client's complaints.
- Provide instructions to help minimize the effects of the integumentary changes.
- Be aware of the impact of the integumentary changes on maternal status.
- Assist the client in voicing concerns about the effects of integumentary changes.
- Inform client that striae will become barely noticeable after pregnancy and that melasma and linea nigra will lighten and disappear with the decrease in hormones after pregnancy.

## ANTEPARTAL SYSTEMIC CHANGES, METABOLIC

### DESCRIPTION
- During pregnancy, the body's metabolic processes undergo changes.

- These changes often result in some of the common discomforts of pregnancy.

### ASSESSMENT FINDINGS
- Increased metabolism
- Weight gain
- Water retention
- Increased maternal glucose level

### NURSING IMPLICATIONS
- Obtain a thorough health history and physical examination to establish a baseline.
- Perform ongoing data collection and follow-up regarding the client's complaints.
- Monitor routine diagnostic tests for changes and possible problems.
- Provide instructions to help minimize the effects of the metabolic changes.
- Be aware of the impact of metabolic changes on maternal status.
- Assist the client in voicing concerns about the effects of metabolic changes.

## ANTEPARTAL SYSTEMIC CHANGES, MUSCULOSKELETAL

### DESCRIPTION
- During pregnancy, the musculoskeletal system undergoes changes.
- Because the fetal skeleton must be built, calcium and phosphorus needs are increased.

### ASSESSMENT FINDINGS
- Softening of pelvic ligaments and joints
- Joint relaxation
- Symphysis pubis separation
- Increased lumbodorsal spinal curve
- Backache

### NURSING IMPLICATIONS
- Obtain a thorough health history and physical examination to establish a baseline.
- Perform ongoing data collection and follow-up regarding the client's complaints.
- Monitor routine diagnostic tests for changes and possible problems.
- Provide instructions to help minimize the effects of the musculoskeletal changes.

- Be aware of the impact of musculoskeletal changes on maternal status.
- Assist the client in voicing concerns about the effects of musculoskeletal changes.

## ANTEPARTAL CHANGES, REPRODUCTIVE

### DESCRIPTION

- Antepartal reproductive changes include those physiologic changes involving the uterus, ovaries, vagina, and breasts.
- Typically, antepartal reproductive changes that occur during pregnancy are categorized as local changes.
- Some *presumptive, probable,* and *positive signs of pregnancy* are a result of antepartal reproductive changes.

### ASSESSMENT FINDINGS

- Uterine growth and enlargement
- Uterine tissue hyperplasia
- Uterine inversion
- Reproductive tract displacement
- Cervical vascularization and softening
- Vaginal vascularization, thickening, and discharge
- Breast hypertrophy and hyperplasia
- Amenorrhea

### NURSING IMPLICATIONS

- Obtain a thorough health history and physical examination at the first visit.
- Perform ongoing data collection and follow-up regarding the client's complaints.
- Monitor routine diagnostic tests for changes and possible problems.
- Plan time for questions and teaching regarding the changes associated with pregnancy.
- Develop a teaching plan for self-care measures related to the changes.
- Be aware of the impact of reproductive physiologic changes on maternal status.
- Assist the client in voicing concerns about the effects of reproductive changes associated with pregnancy.

# ANTEPARTAL SYSTEMIC CHANGES, RESPIRATORY

### DESCRIPTION

- During pregnancy, the respiratory system undergoes changes.
- These changes can affect fetal well-being and often result in some of the common discomforts of pregnancy.

### ASSESSMENT FINDINGS

- Diaphragm elevation and displacement
- Shortness of breath
- Decreased residual volume
- Increased tidal volume
- Increased total oxygen consumption
- Increased plasma pH
- Increased $PO_2$ levels
- Decreased $PCO_2$ levels
- Mild hyperventilation
- Nasal stuffiness
- Epistaxis

### NURSING IMPLICATIONS

- Obtain a thorough health history and physical examination to establish a baseline.
- Perform ongoing data collection and follow-up regarding the client's complaints.
- Monitor routine diagnostic tests for changes and possible problems.
- Provide instructions to help minimize the effects of the respiratory changes.
- Be aware of the impact of respiratory changes on maternal status.
- Assist the client in voicing concerns about the effects of respiratory changes.

# ANTEPARTAL SYSTEMIC CHANGES, URINARY

### DESCRIPTION

- During pregnancy, the urinary system undergoes changes.
- The kidneys must excrete not only the waste products of the woman's body, but also those of the growing fetus.
- These changes often result in some of the common discomforts of pregnancy.

## ASSESSMENT FINDINGS

- Increased urinary output
- Decreased specific gravity
- Increased total body water
- Increased glomerular filtration rate
- Increased bladder capacity
- Urethral and kidney dilatation
- Frequency

## NURSING IMPLICATIONS

- Obtain a thorough health history and physical examination to establish a baseline.
- Perform ongoing data collection and follow-up regarding the client's complaints.
- Monitor routine diagnostic tests for changes and possible problems.
- Provide instructions to help minimize the effects of the urinary changes.
- Be aware of the impact of urinary changes on maternal status.
- Assist the client in voicing concerns about the effects of urinary changes.

# APGAR SCORING

## DESCRIPTION

- Apgar scoring is a rating method used to assess a neonate's well-being 1 minute and 5 minutes after birth.
- It standardizes neonatal evaluation and serves as a baseline for future evaluations.
- Apgar scoring involves 5 categories: heart rate, respiratory effort, muscle tone, reflex irritability, and color.
- Each category is scored as 0, 1, or 2; all 5 scores are added, with 10 being the highest possible score.
- A score of 7 to 10 is considered good.
- A score of 4 to 6 means that the neonate's condition is guarded and the neonate may need airway clearing and supplemental oxygen.
- A score under 4 means that the neonate is in serious danger and needs resuscitation.

# APNEA IN THE NEWBORN

*see also page 245*

### DESCRIPTION

- Apnea is a pause in respiration longer than 20 seconds with accompanying bradycardia and beginning cyanosis.
- Many *preterm infants* have periods of apnea as a result of fatigue or immaturity of their respiratory mechanisms.
- Infants with secondary stress, such as infection, hyperbilirubinemia, hypoglycemia, or hypothermia, tend to have a high incidence of apnea.

### ASSESSMENT FINDINGS

- Pause in respirations greater than 20 seconds
- Bradycardia
- Early cyanosis

### NURSING IMPLICATIONS

- Closely observe the neonate for changes in respiratory status.
- Gently shake an infant or flick the sole of the foot to stimulate breathing.
- If the infant does not respond, administer oxygen and be prepared to begin resuscitation.
- Attach neonate to an apnea monitor for early detection of failing respiration.
- Anticipate the need for ventilator assistance if the neonate has frequent or difficult-to-correct episodes.
- Maintain a neutral thermal environment to minimize oxygen requirements.
- Gently handle the neonate to avoid excessive fatigue.
- Suction gently to minimize nasopharyngeal irritation.
- Consider using indwelling nasogastric tubes rather than intermittent ones to reduce the amount of vagal stimulation.
- Observe the neonate carefully after feeding because a full stomach puts pressure on the diaphragm; burp the neonate frequently to minimize the pressure.
- Avoid rectal temperatures to reduce vagal stimulation.
- Be prepared to administer theophylline or caffeine sodium benzoate to stimulate respirations.

- Counsel the parents regarding the increased risk of *sudden infant death syndrome (SIDS)* in neonates with apnea.
- Instruct parents in use of home apnea monitoring equipment.
- Teach parents how to stimulate respirations and perform cardiopulmonary resuscitation.

## APPENDICITIS

### DESCRIPTION
- Appendicitis is the inflammation of the appendix.
- It has a high incidence in young adults, occurring in about 1 in 1500 to 2000 pregnancies.
- If the appendix ruptures, maternal and fetal risks increase dramatically.

### ASSESSMENT FINDINGS
- Abrupt onset of nausea over a few hours
- Generalized abdominal discomfort
- Vomiting
- Sharp, peristaltic lower right quadrant pain (pain may be so high, because of the displacement of the appendix, that it resembles the pain of gallbladder disease)
- Leukocytosis
- Elevated temperature
- Ketonuria
- Ultrasound revealing inflamed appendix

### NURSING IMPLICATIONS
- Assess the client's complaints of pain, including type, location, and duration.
- Monitor maternal vital signs and *fetal heart rate* for changes.
- If the client is past 36 weeks, and the fetus is believed to be mature, prepare the client for a *cesarean birth.*
- If appendicitis occurs early in the pregnancy, prepare the client for surgery to remove the inflamed appendix.
- Do not allow the client to have food, fluids, or laxatives while waiting to see the physician because increased peristalsis can cause an inflamed appendix to rupture.

- If appendix ruptures, institute emergency measures.

# BATTERED WOMAN

### DESCRIPTION

- Battered woman refers to any client who is abused by a spouse.
- The battered woman may be pregnant because she was unable to resist sexual advances from her abusive partner.
- Beatings may increase during pregnancy because stress is often a "trigger" to beatings, and pregnancy increases stress.
- The battered woman may desire the pregnancy because she thinks that having a child will change the partner and make him a better person.

### ASSESSMENT FINDINGS

- Late prenatal care
- Avoidance of diagnostic tests
- Noncompliance with recommendations about nutrition and health promotion
- Anxiety
- Fear
- Frequent calls or appointment cancellations
- Visible trauma, such as bruises, lacerations
- Low self-esteem
- Depression
- Inability to make simple decisions
- Feelings of powerlessness and social isolation

### NURSING IMPLICATIONS

- Thoroughly assess client and support systems for problems and risk factors.
- Assist with decision making and offer support for decisions made.
- Be familiar with shelters for battered women in the community.
- Discuss with the client about notifying the police at any time with any problem.
- Refer the client to social services for assistance with obtaining a restraining order, if client agrees and situation necessitates it.
- After the child's birth, try to caution the client that the newborn does love her but that the child needs time to grow.

- Instruct the client about the child and assist with helping her develop realistic expectations about the child.
- Ensure that a support system is available for the client.
- Arrange for follow-up community resources, such as home care or shelters, for ongoing support.

## BIPARIETAL DIAMETER

### DESCRIPTION

- Biparietal diameter refers to the side-to-side measurement of the fetal head.
- It is the narrowest diameter, measuring approximately 9.25 cm.
- At the pelvic inlet, the biparietal diameter must be presented to the anteroposterior diameter of the pelvis.
- Biparietal diameter, when measured by *ultrasonography,* may also be used to predict the maturity of the fetus.

  When the biparietal diameter of the fetal head is 8.5 cm or more, in 90% of pregnancies, the infant will weigh more than 2500 g (5 1/2 lb).

  A biparietal diameter of 9.5 cm indicates a fetus of 40 weeks' gestation.

## BRAXTON-HICKS CONTRACTIONS

*see also page 225*

### DESCRIPTION

- Braxton-Hicks contractions are considered a *probable sign of pregnancy.*
- They refer to periodic uterine tightening, beginning as early as the 12th week of pregnancy, and are often not noticeable.
- Braxton-Hicks contractions also are considered a discomfort of middle to late pregnancy; at this time, the contractions become stronger, and the client who tenses at the sensation may even experience some minimal pain similar to a menstrual cramp.
- Strong Braxton-Hicks contractions occur in the last week or days before labor begins and are considered one of the *preliminary signs of labor;* however, they are not *signs of true labor.*

### ASSESSMENT FINDINGS

- Periodic but irregular abdominal tightening
- Complaints of discomfort or pain

### NURSING IMPLICATIONS

- Evaluate the client's complaints of contractions, including location, duration, frequency, and intensity.
- Reassure the client that the contractions are normal and not a *sign of true labor.*
- Be certain that the client understands the difference between Braxton-Hicks contractions, *false labor,* and *true labor* contractions.
- Offer support to the client experiencing strong Braxton-Hicks contractions and not in *true labor;* reassure client that misinterpreting Braxton-Hicks contractions for *true labor* is natural.

## BREAST CARE

### DESCRIPTION

- Breast care is a self-care need for health promotion.
- It is a key component of childbirth education, helping to dispel any misconceptions or inappropriate information.
- Specific precautions during pregnancy help to prevent loss of breast tone, which can result in painful, pendulous breasts in later life.

### NURSING IMPLICATIONS

- Instruct the client to wear a firm, supportive bra with wide straps.
- Advise the client that she may have to buy a larger-sized bra halfway through the pregnancy to accommodate increasing breast size.
- Warn the client that fluid leakage (colostrum) may occur about the 16th week of pregnancy.
- Instruct the client to wash breasts with clear water, using no soap, daily, to remove the colostrum and minimize the risk of infection.
- If colostrum is profuse, suggest the client place gauze pads or breast pads inside the bra, changing them frequently to maintain dryness and prevent nipple excoriation, pain, and fissures.

## BREAST-FEEDING

### DESCRIPTION

- Breast-feeding is generally considered to be the superior source of nutrition for infants through the first year of life.

- Breast milk provides numerous health benefits to both the mother and the infant.
- Breast milk is formed in the acinar or alveolar cells of the mammary glands.

    With delivery of the placenta, the level of progesterone in the mother's body falls dramatically, stimulating the production of prolactin, an anterior pituitary hormone, which acts on the acinar cells to stimulate breast milk production.

    When an infant sucks at the breast, nerve impulses travel from the nipple to the hypothalamus to stimulate the production of prolactin-releasing factor, which then passes to the pituitary, stimulating further active production of prolactin.

    Other anterior pituitary hormones, such as adreno-corticosteroid hormone, thyroid-stimulating hormone, and growth hormone, probably also play a role in growth of the mammary glands and their ability to secrete milk.

    Milk flows from alveolar cells through small tubules to reservoirs for milk behind the nipple; this constantly forming milk is called foremilk.

    For the first 3 to 4 days after birth, the milk cells produce colostrum, a thin, watery, high-protein fluid.

    As the infant sucks at the breast, oxytocin is released from the posterior pituitary, causing the collecting sinuses of the mammary glands to contract, forcing milk forward through the nipples, making it available for the infant; this action is called the let-down reflex; new milk, called hind milk, is formed after the let-down reflex.

    Oxytocin causes smooth muscle contraction, so when it is produced, the uterus also contracts.

- Breast-feeding involves both physical and psychological preparation.

    Physical preparation includes breast massage, manual expression, and breast care.

    Psychological preparation involves making an informed decision to breast-feed involving the partner in the decision-making process, and feeling comfortable with the decision and the process.

- Breast-feeding should begin as soon after birth as possible, ideally, while the client is still in the birthing room and the neonate is in the first reactivity period.
- Breast-feeding at this time releases oxytocin, which begins breast milk production and stimulates *uterine contractions.*
- The neonate must grasp the areola and the nipple itself when sucking to allow for effective sucking action and to help empty the collecting sinuses completely.
- Milk forms in response to being used; if the breasts are completely emptied, they completely fill again.

### NURSING IMPLICATIONS
- Discuss with the client and partner early on in pregnancy their choice of feeding to allow them to make an informed choice.
- Involve the partner in the decision-making process to minimize feelings of jealousy.
- Instruct the client in breast massage techniques to help move the milk forward into the milk ducts.
- Encourage the client to handle her breasts to grow accustomed to touching them, thus enabling milk production in the first few days after birth.
- Instruct the client to avoid using soap on breasts because soaps tend to dry and crack the nipples.
- Advise the client to refrain from using creams and lotions other than A&D OINTMENT on her breasts because their use may lead to nipple fissures and soreness.
- Provide information about lactation and proper positioning techniques.
- Instruct the client to wash her hands before breast-feeding to prevent infection.
- Assure the client that the breast milk's thin, almost blue-tinged appearance is normal.
- Suggest that the client lie on her side with a pillow under her head when first attempting breast-feeding.
- Instruct the mother to brush the neonate's cheek with her nipple to stimulate the rooting reflex.
- Encourage frequent breast-feeding to ensure adequate nutrition and complete emptying of the breasts.

- Instruct the client in appropriate technique for helping the neonate break away from the breast when finished feeding.
- Teach the client to make sure that the neonate is fully awake before feeding.
- Suggest the client use breast massage after feeding to empty her breast manually if the neonate is not sucking well.
- Provide anticipatory guidance for potential problems.
- Instruct the client in proper methods for burping the neonate.
- Provide instructions for measures to relieve engorgement and sore nipples.
- Encourage the client to obtain adequate rest and fluid intake, for example, at least 4 8-oz glasses of fluid per day to maintain an adequate milk supply.
- Provide information about the use of supplemental feedings, such as manual expression of breast milk into a bottle if client will not be home or use of prepared formulas.
- Instruct the client about weaning the infant and to discontinue breast-feeding gradually to prevent engorgement and pain.

## CAPUT SUCCEDANEUM

### DESCRIPTION

- Caput succedaneum is edema of the scalp at the presenting part of the head.
- It may involve wide areas of the head, or it may be the size of a goose egg.
- The swelling can cross the suture lines.
- The edema is gradually absorbed and disappears about the 3rd day of life.
- Observing for caput succedaneum is part of the *newborn physical assessment.*

### ASSESSMENT FINDINGS

- Localized swelling, not restricted by the suture lines, at the presenting part

### NURSING IMPLICATIONS

- Obtain a thorough labor and delivery history to identify any problems.

- Inspect the newborn closely during the initial *newborn physical assessment* for any signs of swelling.
- Instruct the parents that the edema will gradually be absorbed and disappear about the 3rd day of life.

# CEPHALHEMATOMA

### DESCRIPTION
- Cephalhematoma refers to a collection of blood under the periosteum of the skull bone.
- It is caused by rupture of a periosteum capillary as a result of the pressure of birth.
- It does not cross the suture lines.
- Observing for cephalhematoma is part of assessing the skin during the *newborn physical assessment.*
- It takes weeks for a cephalhematoma to be absorbed.

### ASSESSMENT FINDINGS
- Well-outlined, severe, egg-shaped swelling
- Fluid collection restricted to one area, not crossing the suture line
- Bruising

### NURSING IMPLICATIONS
- Obtain a thorough labor and delivery history to identify any problems.
- Inspect the newborn closely during the initial *newborn physical assessment* for any signs of fluid collection of the skull.
- Instruct the partners that it may take weeks for the cephalhematoma to be absorbed.
- Be aware that jaundice may occur as the blood captured in the space is broken down, releasing a large amount of indirect bilirubin.

# CERVICAL CAP

### DESCRIPTION
- Cervical cap is a barrier method of contraception.
- It has only recently been approved for use in the United States.
- A cervical cap is made of soft rubber and is shaped like a thimble, fitting snugly over the uterine cervix.
- Before insertion, it is filled with a spermicidal jelly.
- Many women are unable to use a cervical cap because their cervix is too short for the cap to fit properly.

- The cervical cap also may dislodge more readily than a diaphragm during coitus.
- It can be left in place for up to 48 hours.

### NURSING IMPLICATIONS

- Obtain a thorough history and physical examination to establish a baseline.
- Discuss with the client and partner barrier methods of contraception.
- Instruct the client that she must be fitted for the device.
- Educate the client about the use and care of the cervical cap, including the need for spermicidal jelly.
- Be aware that although the cervical cap may increase the risk of cervical irritation, in contrast to the diaphragm, it does not put pressure on the walls of the vagina or urethra, which could possibly interfere with vaginal blood supply or urine flow.
- Encourage client follow-up for reevaluation and compliance.

## CERVICAL DILATION

### DESCRIPTION

- Cervical dilation refers to the enlargement of the cervical canal from an opening a few millimeters to one large enough (approximately 10 cm) to permit passage of the fetus.
- It occurs for two reasons: *Uterine contractions* gradually increase the diameter of the cervical canal lumen by pulling the cervix up over the presenting part of the fetus; the fluid-filled membranes press against the cervix.
- There is an increase in the amount of vaginal secretions as cervical dilation begins because the mucus plug in the cervix is dislodged, and minute capillaries in the cervix rupture.
- Cervical dilation begins in the *first stage of labor* and continues through the *second stage of labor*.

## CERVICAL EFFACEMENT

### DESCRIPTION

- Effacement refers to one of the cervical changes occurring during labor associated with the power component of labor.

- It also is one of the *signs of true labor.*
- Effacement is the shortening and thinning of the cervical canal from its normal length of 1 to 2 cm to a structure with paper-thin edges in which no canal distinct from the uterus appears to exist.
- It occurs because of longitudinal traction from the contracting uterine fundus.
- In primiparas, effacement is accomplished before *dilation* begins; once it is complete, *cervical dilation* progresses rapidly.
- In multiparas, *cervical dilation* may proceed before effacement is complete.
- Effacement must occur at the end of *cervical dilation,* before the fetus can be safely pushed through the cervical canal; otherwise, cervical tearing can result.

## CESAREAN BIRTH

### DESCRIPTION

- Cesarean birth refers to a surgical procedure in which the neonate is delivered through an incision made in the maternal abdomen.
- It may be planned (elective) or arise from an unanticipated problem (emergency).
- It was previously termed C-section.
- In a classic cesarean delivery, a vertical midline incision is made in the skin and body of the uterus, allowing easier access to the fetus, and thus indicated in emergency situations; typically, it is done when the fetus is in a transverse lie and when adhesions from previous cesarean deliveries are present and with an anteriorly implanted *placenta;* the blood loss is increased because large blood vessels of the myometrium are involved; there is also a greater possibility of rupture of the scar in subsequent pregnancies because the uterine musculature is weakened.
- In a low segment cesarean delivery, the most common type, the skin incision is made low ("bikini" or Pfannenstiel incision), and the uterine incision is horizontal in the lower uterine segment; blood loss is minimal with fewer postdelivery complications; the incision is easy to repair with less chance of rupture of the uterine scar during future deliveries; the procedure takes longer to perform than the classic incision, and, therefore, it is not useful in emergencies.

- The type of *anesthesia* varies, either *general* or *spinal,* and the preoperative and postoperative care depends on the type used.

## ASSESSMENT FINDINGS
- Cephalopelvic disproportion
- Uterine dysfunction
- Malposition or malpresentation
- Previous uterine surgery
- Complete or partial *placenta previa*
- Preexisting medical conditions, such as *diabetes* or cardiac disease
- *Prolapsed umbilical cord*
- Fetal distress

## NURSING IMPLICATIONS
- Obtain a thorough history and physical examination to establish a baseline and identify any possible pre-existing conditions that might indicate a need for cesarean birth.
- Assess the client's progress through labor, including frequency, duration, and intensity of contractions; *evaluation of fetal status;* and physical and emotional responses to events.
- Develop a preoperative teaching plan and modify it to meet the needs of the client having a planned or emergency cesarean birth; depth and breadth of instructions given depend on the circumstances and time available.
- Promote a "family-centered" birth experience by including the partner and other members in preparation for, during, and after delivery.
- Provide preoperative preparation for major abdominal surgery, such as skin preparation, preoperative laboratory results, informed consent, intravenous fluids, and urinary catheter insertion.
- Provide intraoperative care for the mother and neonate, including timing and documentation of events and immediate neonate care.
- Provide immediate postoperative care following the delivery, including meeting the client's physiologic and psychosocial needs after delivery, surgery, and anesthesia.
- If the neonate is compromised, provide immediate care as needed.

- Allow parents to talk about and relive the experience to minimize feelings of failure resulting from not having a "normal birth."
- Refer to home care for follow-up, if necessary, to assist with transition.
- Provide discharge teaching and assist family in planning for care of mother and infant at home, taking into consideration the mother's need for increased rest and fluids, length of labor, type of incision, and inability to climb stairs or drive a car.

# CHORIONIC VILLI SAMPLING (CVS)

## DESCRIPTION
- CVS is a method for *evaluation of fetal well-being.*
- CVS is the retrieval and analysis of chorionic villi for chromosome analysis.
- It may be done as early as the 5th week of pregnancy; it is more commonly done at 8 to 10 weeks.
- With this technique, the chorion cells are located by *ultrasonography.*
- A thin catheter is inserted vaginally or a biopsy needle is inserted abdominally or intravaginally, and a number of chorionic cells are removed for analysis.
- CVS carries a small risk of causing labor contractions and excessive bleeding; there is some evidence of children born with missing limbs following the procedure, but the risk is apparently small.
- The cells removed are karyotyped or submitted for DNA analysis to reveal whether or not the fetus has a genetic disorder.
- Because chorionic villi cells are dividing rapidly, results are available rapidly, sometimes as soon as the following day.
- If a twin or *multiple gestation* is present, with two or more separate placentas, it is important that cells be removed separately from each placenta.

## ASSESSMENT FINDINGS
- Family history of genetic disorder
- Increased maternal age
- High-risk ethnic group

## NURSING IMPLICATIONS
- Obtain a thorough maternal history and physical examination to establish a baseline.

- Explain all aspects of the procedure, including the risks, benefits, potential complications, and posttest decision making about the pregnancy.
- Remember that not all inherited disorders can be detected by CVS, only those that involve abnormal chromosomes or whose gene location or specific DNA disorder is known.
- Assist the client and partner in decision making about having the test.
- Check to make sure that an informed consent has been obtained.
- Provide support before, during, and after the test.
- Support the client and partner in the decision to terminate or continue with the pregnancy.
- Instruct the client to report any complaints of chills or fever, suggesting an infection, or to report any complaints of *uterine contractions* or *vaginal bleeding,* suggesting an abortion.
- Be aware that clients with an Rh-negative blood type need Rh immune globulin administration to guard against isoimmunization of the fetus.

## CIRCUMCISION

### DESCRIPTION

- Circumcision refers to the surgical removal of the penis foreskin.
- In only a few males, the foreskin is so constricted that it obstructs the urinary meatal opening; otherwise there is no valid medical indication for circumcision of the newborn male.
- Circumcision is performed on Jewish males on the 8th day of life as a part of a religious requirement.
- Reasons supporting circumcision (from the 1920s to 1960s) were easier hygiene because the foreskin does not have to be retracted during bathing and possibly fewer urinary tract infections; there may be an increased incidence of cervical cancer in the sexual partners of an uncircumcised male and increased incidence of penile cancer in the male.
- This procedure does carry some risk.
- Some contraindications include congenital abnormalities, such as hypospadias or epispadias, because the prepuce may be needed when a plastic surgeon repairs the defect. Another reason not to circumcise an infant would be a history of a bleeding tendency in the family.

### Nursing Implications

- Keep in mind that the procedure should not be done immediately after birth because the infant's vitamin K level is low, predisposing the infant to hemorrhage, and the infant should not be exposed to unnecessary cold.
- Restrain the infant in a supine position for the procedure.
- After the procedure, wrap the penis with a strip of petroleum gauze to keep the diaper from adhering to the denuded glans and to ensure blood coagulation.
- Check the infant every 15 minutes for the first hour for bleeding.
- Observe and record the first voiding after the circumcision.
- Observe the infant closely for about 2 hours after the circumcision for signs of hemorrhage, infection, or urethral fistula formation.
- Teach the parents to remove the petroleum gauze with each diaper change. If the penis becomes soiled, it should be washed gently with water and covered with petroleum gauze or ointment.
- Instruct the parents that the site will appear red but should not have a strong odor or discharge.
- Teach the parents to keep the area clean and covered with petroleum for approximately 3 days until healing is complete.
- Instruct the parents to notify the physician if they see any redness or tenderness or if the baby cries as if in constant pain.

## CONDOM, FEMALE

### Description

- A female condom, a barrier method of contraception, is a latex sheath made of polyurethane and lubricated with nonoxynol 9.
- A female condom covers the vulva as well as lines the vagina and cervix.
- Similar to male condoms, they are intended for one time use only and offer protection from conception and *sexually transmitted diseases.*
- Female condoms have received provisional approval by the Food and Drug Administration.

- The failure rate in preliminary studies was somewhat greater than the failure rate for male condoms, about 15%; most of these pregnancies occurred because of incorrect or inconsistent use.

### NURSING IMPLICATIONS

- Be aware of personal feelings and values about contraception and sexuality.
- Perform a thorough history and physical examination to establish a baseline.
- Be sensitive to the client's personal, religious, cultural, and social beliefs about birth control.
- Answer the client's questions honestly and openly.
- Provide education for the client and partner about family planning methods.
- Be aware that to be effective, a female condom must be inserted any time before sexual activity and must be removed after ejaculation occurs.
- Instruct the client how to insert and remove the condom properly.

## CONDOM, MALE

### DESCRIPTION

- A male condom, a barrier method of contraception, is a latex rubber or synthetic sheath that is placed over the erect penis before coitus.
- A condom prevents pregnancy because spermatozoa are deposited not in the vagina, but in the tip of the condom.
- The condom has an ideal failure rate of 2% and a typical failure rate of about 12%.
- Condoms have the additional potential of preventing the spread of *sexually transmitted diseases.*
- There are no contraindications except for a rare sensitivity to rubber.

### NURSING IMPLICATIONS

- Be aware of personal feelings and values about contraception and sexuality.
- Perform a thorough history and physical examination to establish a baseline.
- Be sensitive to the client's personal, religious, cultural, and social beliefs about birth control.
- Answer the client's questions honestly and openly.
- Provide education for the client and partner about family planning methods.

- Be aware that to be effective, condoms must be applied before any penile-vulvar contact.
- Instruct the client to position the condom loosely enough at the penis to collect the ejaculate without putting undue pressure on the condom.
- Encourage the client to withdraw the penis while holding the condom carefully in place, before the penis becomes flaccid after ejaculation.
- Encourage the use of condoms as a means to prevent the spread of *sexually transmitted diseases.*

## CONSTIPATION

### DESCRIPTION

- Constipation is a common discomfort of the first trimester of pregnancy.
- It is also a common nutritional problem of pregnancy.
- Constipation tends to occur in pregnancy as a result of the pressure of the growing uterus against the bowel slowing peristalsis, the effects of the placental hormone relaxin, or possibly progesterone levels.
- Constipation leads to a feeling of bloating or fullness and lack of appetite.

### ASSESSMENT FINDINGS

- Complaints of bloating or feeling full
- Lack of appetite
- Change in bowel elimination patterns

### NURSING IMPLICATIONS

- Assess the client's nutritional and bowel elimination patterns for possible contributing factors.
- Encourage the client to evacuate her bowels regularly.
- Instruct the client to increase the amount of fiber foods in her diet by eating raw fruits and vegetables, and to drink extra amounts of water each day.
- If the client is taking oral iron supplements, assist her to relieve or prevent constipation through other measures than avoiding to take the iron supplement, which is necessary for building fetal iron stores.
- Caution the client against using home medications to prevent constipation, especially mineral oil, which interferes with the absorption of fat-soluble vitamins needed for good fetal growth and maternal health.
- Instruct the client to avoid using enemas because their action might initiate labor.

- Encourage the client to avoid using any over-the-counter (OTC) drugs during pregnancy unless prescribed or sanctioned by the physician.
- Administer stool softeners, mild laxatives, and evacuation suppositories as ordered.
- Advise the client to avoid gas-forming foods, such as cabbage or beans, which helps to control *flatulence*.

## CONTRACEPTION, NATURAL METHODS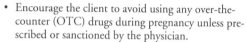

### DESCRIPTION

- Natural methods of contraception, also known as natural family planning or fertility awareness, refer to methods used for contraception that rely on periods of temporary abstinence or temporary contraceptive use.
- These methods require an understanding of the changes that occur in the woman's ovulatory cycle and the woman's fertile period.
- Five commonly used methods include calendar (rhythm) method, basal body temperature method, cervical mucus (symptothermal) method, coitus interruptus, and abstinence.

    Calendar method relies on periods of temporary abstinence during the woman's ovulatory cycle, requiring the couple to abstain from coitus on the days of a menstrual cycle when the woman is most apt to conceive, usually 3 to 4 days before and after ovulation.

    Basal body temperature uses a woman's basal body temperature to determine her fertile period; just before the day of ovulation, a woman's basal body temperature falls about a half degree. At the time of ovulation, the temperature rises a full degree because of the influence of progesterone.

    Cervical mucus (symptothermal) method uses changes in cervical mucus that naturally occur with ovulation each month to predict ovulation; before ovulation, cervical mucus is thick and does not stretch when pulled between the thumb and finger; just before ovulation, mucus secretion becomes copious; with ovulation, on the peak day, the mucus becomes thin, watery, and transparent; it feels slippery and stretches a distance of at least 1 inch before the strand breaks (property known as spinnbarkeit);

all the days the mucus is copious and the 3 days after the peak day are considered to be fertile days; sexual abstinence is required to avoid conception.

Coitus interruptus, one of the oldest known and least effective methods, involves the couple proceeding with coitus until the moment of ejaculation, when the man withdraws and spermatozoa are emitted outside the vagina; unfortunately, ejaculation may occur before withdrawal is complete, and, despite care used, some spermatozoa may be deposited in the vagina; because there may be a few spermatozoa in preejaculation fluid, even though withdrawal seems controlled, fertilization may occur.

Abstinence involves refraining from sexual intercourse; it is the most effective way to protect from conception, with a 0% failure rate, and it also is the most effective way to prevent *sexually transmitted diseases.*

### Nursing Implications
- Be aware of personal feelings and values about contraception and sexuality.
- Perform a thorough history and physical examination to establish a baseline.
- Be sensitive to the client's personal, religious, cultural, and social beliefs about birth control.
- Answer the client's questions honestly and openly.
- Provide education for the client and partner about natural family planning methods.

### For calendar method
- Instruct the client to keep a diary of 6 menstrual cycles.
- Assist with calculating client's "safe days":
  Subtract 18 days from the shortest cycle documented (represents her first fertile day).
  Subtract 11 from the longest cycle documented (represents her last fertile day).
- Instruct the client to avoid coitus during this fertile period.

### For basal body temperature method
- Instruct the woman to take and chart her temperature each morning immediately on awakening, before any activity.

- Inform the woman that as soon as she notices a slight drop in temperature followed by a rise, ovulation has occurred.
- Tell the woman to abstain from sexual intercourse from this point until after the 3rd day of the sustained high temperature (the combined life of ova and sperm).

### For cervical mucus method

- Instruct the client to be conscientious about assessing vaginal secretions daily to avoid the possibility of missing the phenomenon of changing cervical secretions.
- Teach the client and partner to abstain from coitus for the days that the mucus is copious and for 3 days after the peak.
- Remind the client that the feel of vaginal secretions following coitus is unreliable because seminal fluid has a watery, postovulatory consistency and can be confused with ovulatory mucus.

## CONTRACTION STRESS TEST (CST)

### DESCRIPTION

- CST is a method for *evaluation of fetal well-being* that measures the response of the *fetal heart rate* in relation to *uterine contractions.*
- When this test was first developed, oxytocin was administered to initiate *contractions;* this caused problems because of the difficulty in stopping *uterine contractions* leading to *premature labor.*
- Today, CST uses gentle nipple stimulation, which releases oxytocin, to stimulate *uterine contractions.*
- After a baseline *fetal heart rate* is obtained, nipple stimulation is performed until *uterine contractions* begin; the *contractions* are recorded by a uterine monitor.
- Three contractions with a duration of 40 seconds or more must be present in a 10-minute window before the test can be interpreted.
- The test is negative (normal) when no *fetal heart rate* decelerations are present with *uterine contractions.*
- It is positive (abnormal) when 50% or more of *contractions* cause a late deceleration (a dip in the *fetal heart rate* that occurs toward the end of a *uterine contraction* and continues after the contraction).

**NURSING IMPLICATIONS**
- Obtain a thorough history and physical examination to establish a baseline.
- Obtain a baseline *fetal heart rate.*
- Attach the client to a uterine monitor.
- Instruct the client to roll a nipple between her finger and thumb gently until *uterine contractions* begin.
- Monitor the client and fetus for signs of problems, such as changes in vital signs or *fetal heart rate* or continuation of *uterine contractions.*
- Following a CST, encourage the client to remain in the health care facility for approximately 30 minutes to be certain that *uterine contractions* have quieted and *premature labor* is not a risk.

# CONTRACTIONS, INADEQUATE OR PROLONGED

**DESCRIPTION**
- Inadequate or prolonged contractions are a *maternal labor danger sign.*
- Normally, *uterine contractions* become more frequent, intense, and longer as labor progresses.
- If they become less frequent, less intense, or shorter in duration, this may indicate uterine exhaustion (inertia).
- This problem must be corrected or else a *cesarean birth* may be necessary.
- A period of relaxation must be present between contractions so that the intervillous spaces can fill and maintain an adequate supply of oxygen and nutrients to the fetus.

**NURSING IMPLICATIONS**
- Obtain a thorough history and physical examination to establish a baseline.
- Assess the client's *uterine contractions,* noting frequency, intensity, and duration; report any changes.
- As a rule, report *uterine contractions* lasting longer than 70 seconds because they may begin to compromise fetal well-being by not allowing adequate uterine artery filling.
- Monitor *fetal heart rate* for changes indicating hypoxia.
- Provide support and education to the client and partner regarding all events and procedures.

- Anticipate the need for *cesarean birth* if the client's inadequate or prolonged contractions cannot be corrected.

# CONTRACTIONS, UTERINE

### DESCRIPTION

- Uterine contractions refer to the involuntary tightening of the uterine muscle.
- For most women, labor begins with uterine contractions.
- Uterine contractions can be a sign of *true labor* or *false labor.*
- True labor contractions usually start in the back and sweep forward across the abdomen similar to the tightening of a band, gradually increasing in frequency, duration, and intensity.
- Typically, they are irregular but become regular and predictable, continuing no matter what the woman's level of activity.
- False labor contractions are first felt abdominally and remain confined to the abdomen, beginning and remaining irregular.
- They typically do not increase in duration, frequency, or intensity and often disappear when the woman ambulates.
- Uterine contractions begin at a pacemaker point located in the myometrium of the uterus near one or the other uterotubal junctions.
- Each contraction begins at that point and then sweeps down over the uterus as a wave; after a short rest period, another contraction is initiated, and the downward wave begins again.
- A uterine contraction consists of three phases: the increment (intensity of the contraction increases); the acme (the contraction is at its strongest); and the decrement (intensity decreases).
- As labor progresses, the relaxation intervals increase from 10 minutes early in labor to 2 to 3 minutes; the duration of contractions also changes, increasing from 20 to 30 seconds, to a range of 60 to 90 seconds.
- The frequency of a contraction is the interval time from the beginning of one contraction to the beginning of the next contraction.

**NURSING IMPLICATIONS**

- Obtain a thorough history and physical examination to establish a baseline.
- Teach the client about the type of contractions felt during *true labor* and *false labor;* instruct the client to contact the physician when contractions occur.
- Advise the client to telephone the health care facility when contractions begin to alert the health care personnel that she is in labor; reinforce instructions about when to come to the health care facility.
- Be aware that because contractions are involuntary and come without warning, they can be frightening in early labor until the client realizes that she can predict their pattern and control the degree of discomfort if she uses the breathing exercises learned.
- Assess the client's contractions, including onset, frequency, duration, and intensity; instruct the client how to monitor the frequency, duration, and intensity of the contractions.
- Institute uterine and *fetal monitoring* to evaluate contractions and fetal responses to labor.
- Reinforce breathing techniques and comfort measures to minimize discomfort.
- Provide support and guidance to the client and partner to alleviate anxiety.

## CORD, ANOMALIES OF THE

**DESCRIPTION**

- Anomalies of the cord include a two-vessel cord and unusual cord length.
- Normally, the umbilical cord contains one vein and two arteries; absence of the umbilical arteries is associated with congenital heart and kidney defects because the insult that caused the loss of the vessel probably led to other mesoderm germ layer structures as well.
- An unusually short umbilical cord can result in premature separation of the placenta or abnormal fetal lie; an unusually long cord can be compromised more easily because of its tendency to twist or knot; however, the umbilical cord rarely varies to these extremes.

**NURSING IMPLICATIONS**

- Inspect the cord immediately at birth for the number of vessels.

- Document prominently on the neonate's chart if only two vessels are present.
- Assess the neonate for other anomalies.
- Keep in mind that occasionally a cord actually forms a knot, but the natural pulsations of blood through the vessels and muscle in the vessel walls keep blood flow adequate.
- Remember that it is not unusual for a cord to wrap once around the fetal neck, without any interference to *fetal circulation.*

## CYTOMEGALOVIRUS (CMV)

### DESCRIPTION

- CMV is a member of the herpes family of viruses.
- It is a maternal infection which is a fetal teratogen that can cause extensive damage to a fetus.
- It is transmitted by droplet infection from person to person.
- If a woman acquires CMV during a pregnancy, transplacental transmission of the virus may result in congenital CMV infection.
- The virus also can be passed from the cervix to the neonate at delivery.
- The mother has almost no symptoms and so is unaware that she has contracted the infection.
- Diagnosis in the mother or infant can be established by isolating CMV antibodies in the serum.
- No treatment for the infection exists even if it presents with enough symptoms to allow it to be detected in the mother.
- Similar to herpes simplex, a primary CMV infection may become latent and then reactive periodically; these recurrences are not thought to have teratogenic effects on the fetus, but they can cause infection in the newborn during birth from genital secretions or postpartum from exposure to CMV-infected breast milk.

### NURSING IMPLICATIONS

- Obtain a thorough history and physical examination to establish a baseline.
- Be aware that because there is no treatment or vaccine, routine screening is not recommended.
- If the mother is known to have CMV infection, anticipate the delivery of a neonate with problems, such

as severe brain damage including hydrocephalus, microcephaly, or spasticity; eye damage including optic atrophy or chorioretinitis; deafness; or chronic liver disease.
- Assess the neonate's skin for large petechiae (blueberry muffin lesions) characteristic of infection.
- Provide emotional support to the client and partner.

# DATE OF BIRTH, ESTIMATING

### DESCRIPTION
- Estimated date of birth (EDB) refers to the predicted date of birth of a child.
- Previously termed estimated date of confinement (EDC), it is more commonly called EDB or expected date of delivery (EDD).
- It is impossible to predict accurately the date of birth of a child because of the variations in the menstrual cycle and the timing of ovulation and fertilization.
- Nägele's rule is a standard method used to predict the length of pregnancy.

### NURSING IMPLICATIONS
- Obtain a thorough history and physical examination to establish a baseline and provide information about menstrual cycle, ovulation, and possible fertilization.
- Assess the client for *presumptive, probable,* and *positive signs of pregnancy.*
- Obtain a serum pregnancy test to confirm pregnancy.
- Use Nägele's rule to estimate date of birth: Count backward 3 calendar months from the first day of the last menstrual period and add 7 days.

# DENTAL CARE IN PREGNANCY

### DESCRIPTION
- Dental care is a self-care need for health promotion.
- It is important for women to continue good dental care habits throughout pregnancy.
- Gingival tissue tends to hypertrophy during pregnancy.
- Tooth decay occurs from the action of bacteria on sugar, lowering the pH of the mouth, resulting in an acid medium that leads to etching of teeth.
- Dental care is a key component of health teaching, helping to dispel misconceptions and prevent future problems.

NURSING IMPLICATIONS

NURSING IMPLICATIONS
- Obtain a thorough history and physical examination to establish a baseline and identify any dental problems.
- Encourage thorough brushing and flossing to prevent pockets of placque from forming between the enlarged gum line and teeth.
- Suggest the client eat snacks that dissolve easily in the mouth to keep sugar levels to a minimum.
- Encourage the client to snack on health foods, such as apples and carrots.
- Instruct the client in proper dental hygiene measures, including regular visits to the dentist, especially one early in pregnancy.

## DIABETES MELLITUS (DM) IN PREGNANCY

DESCRIPTION
- DM is a preexisting condition that places the client at high risk during pregnancy.
- DM is an endocrine disorder in which the pancreas is unable to produce adequate insulin to regulate body glucose.
- It affects approximately 1% to 5% of women during pregnancy.
- Even a woman who has successful regulation of glucose-insulin metabolism before pregnancy is apt to develop less than optimum control during pregnancy because of the changes occurring in the glucose-insulin regulatory system as pregnancy progresses.
    Glomerular filtration of glucose is increased.
    Rate of insulin secretion is increased.
    Insulin resistance develops.
    Continued use of glucose by the fetus leads to hypoglycemia.
- The primary problem is control of the balance between insulin and blood glucose to prevent acidosis, a threat to the fetus.
- DM has been categorized to predict the outcome of pregnancy; the outcome becomes less successful with more diabetic involvement in the mother.
- The categories include class A, B, C, D (with subcategories 1, 2, 3, 4, and 5), E, F, H, R, T.
- In class A, fetal survival is high; infants of mothers in classes D and E may have a perinatal mortality as high

as 25%; class F and R women may have a perinatal mortality close to 100% (usually advised not to become pregnant); women in class T can complete a pregnancy successfully.

- Approximately 2% to 3% of all women who do not begin a pregnancy with DM become diabetic during pregnancy, usually at the midpoint of the pregnancy, when insulin resistance becomes most noticeable; this is called gestational diabetes.

- DM places the mother and fetus at risk for problems, including fetal growth retardation; asphyxia; abortion; stillbirth; maternal *pregnancy-induced hypertension;* infection; *large-for-gestational-age* infants; delivery problems (if the fetus' large size causes cephalopelvic disproportion); infants prone to congenital anomalies, hypoglycemia, *respiratory distress syndrome,* hypocalcemia, and hyperbilirubinemia; and *hydramnios.*

## ASSESSMENT FINDINGS
- Glycosuria
- Thirst
- Polyuria
- Ketonuria
- Dizziness (if hypoglycemic)
- Confusion (if hyperglycemic)
- Possible monilial infection
- Serum glucose greater than 140 mg/dl with 1-hour glucose screening test
- Fasting serum glucose of 105 mg/dl or greater with 3-hour glucose tolerance test; 1-hour serum glucose level of 190 mg/dl or greater with 3-hour glucose tolerance test; 2-hour serum glucose level of 165 mg/dl or greater with 3-hour glucose tolerance test; 3-hour serum glucose level of 145 mg/dl or greater with 3-hour glucose tolerance test

## NURSING IMPLICATIONS
- Obtain a thorough history and physical examination to establish a baseline and identify any diabetic history.
- Instruct the client with diabetes to see her obstetrician before becoming pregnant to assist in regulating her condition so that no hyperglycemia occurs during the early weeks of pregnancy (when the tendency for congenital anomalies is the highest). Assist with arranging glycosylated hemoglobin levels as necessary.

- Prepare the client for glucose screening test at 24 to 28 weeks of pregnancy.
- Keep in mind that women with a history of large babies, unexplained fetal loss, or congenital anomalies in previous pregnancies; who are obese; or who have a family history of DM should be screened earlier in the pregnancy because they represent a high-risk group for developing DM.
- Be aware that resistance to insulin during pregnancy requires the client to increase her insulin dosage at about 24 weeks of pregnancy to prevent hyperglycemia.
- Warn the client that because of the continued use of glucose by the fetus, she may experience hypoglycemia between meals or overnight, especially common in the second and third trimesters of pregnancy.
- Arrange for ophthalmic examination during each trimester to detect retinal changes.
- Educate the client about necessary dietary changes, including the adherence to an 1800- to 2200-calorie diet (or one calculated at 35 Kcal/kg of ideal weight) divided into 3 meals with 3 snacks; urge the client to make her final snack of the day one of protein and complex carbohydrate to prevent hypoglycemia at night.
- Instruct the client about an appropriate exercise program, including the effect of exercise on insulin requirements.
- Teach the client about changes in insulin, including the types and preparations.
- Reinforce instructions about insulin administration and blood glucose monitoring.
    If hypoglycemia is present, instruct the client to drink a glass of milk and eat some crackers; use of a less concentrated fluid such as milk, rather than orange juice, and including a complex carbohydrate helps prevent a rebound phenomenon in which high glucose is created that then becomes even more pronounced hypoglycemia.
    If hyperglycemia is present, instruct the client to check her urine for acetone and report the findings to the health care professional.
- Assist with arranging diagnostic tests for *evaluation of fetal well-being,* such as serum alpha-fetoprotein

levels, *ultrasonography,* nonstress test, and biophysical profile.
- Teach the client how to monitor and record fetal movement; a healthy fetus has approximately 10 movements per hour.
- Encourage the client and partner to discuss fears and concerns about the pregnancy, complications, and birth.
- Anticipate the care for an infant of a diabetic mother; provide the client and her partner with information about the infant, offering emotional support and guidance, when needed.
- If the client is to receive an epidural anesthetic, be certain that an intravenous glucose solution is not used for a plasma volume expander (or its presence is accounted for by additional insulin administration).
- Monitor the client's blood glucose levels closely following delivery; obtain 1- or 2-hour postprandial blood glucose levels to determine insulin requirements.
- Keep in mind that following delivery, with insulin resistance gone, the client often needs no insulin during the immediate postpartum period.
- Provide information about contraceptives, as appropriate, to encourage the client planning another pregnancy to be certain that the disease is stabilized and in good control.

## DIAPER AREA CARE

### DESCRIPTION
- Diaper area care is a crucial aspect of normal newborn care.
- It is essential for the newborn's safety.

### NURSING IMPLICATIONS
- Wash the area with clear water and dry thoroughly with each diaper change to prevent ammonia in the urine from irritating the infant's skin and causing a diaper rash.
- Apply an ointment, such as petroleum jelly or A & D ointment, to the buttocks to keep the ammonia away from the skin and facilitate the removal of meconium.
- Use gloves when performing diaper care as part of universal precautions.

- Instruct the client and partner in diaper area care, reviewing the infant's normal bladder and bowel elimination patterns (usually 6 to 8 wet diapers per day; usually 2 to 3 stools per day, more frequently if the infant is breast-fed).

## DIAPHRAGM

### DESCRIPTION

- Diaphragm is a barrier method of contraception.
- A diaphragm is a circular rubber disk that fits over the cervix and forms a barricade against the entrance of spermatozoa.
- When combined with a *spermicide,* it is considered a barrier and chemical method of contraception.
- Clients using a diaphragm may experience a higher number of urinary tract infections than nonusers probably because of the pressure on the urethra.
- Diaphragms may not be competent if the uterus is prolapsed, retroflexed, or anteflexed to such a degree that the cervix is also displaced in relation to the vagina.
- Intrusion of the vagina by a cystocele or rectocele may make inserting a diaphragm difficult.
- Diaphragms should not be used in the presence of acute cervicitis because the close contact of the rubber may cause additional irritation.
- Failure rate may be as low as 5% to 6% if the woman checks it periodically, uses spermicidal jelly, and checks for proper insertion.
- Using a diaphragm allows for sexual relations during menstrual flow without the flow of menstrual blood interfering with enjoyment.
- If a woman should become pregnant while using a diaphragm, there is no risk or harm to the fetus.

### NURSING IMPLICATIONS

- Be aware of personal feelings and values about contraception and sexuality.
- Perform a thorough history and physical examination to establish a baseline.
- Be sensitive to the client's personal, religious, cultural, and social beliefs about birth control.
- Answer the client's questions honestly and openly.

- Provide education for the client and partner about family planning methods.
- Instruct the client that a diaphragm must be fitted by a health care professional.
- Instruct the client to be refitted after pregnancy, miscarriage, cervical surgery, therapeutic abortion, or gaining or losing more than 15 pounds because of the possible change in the shape of the cervix.
- Teach the client how to insert the diaphragm properly:
    After applying spermicidal jelly or cream, pinch the diaphragm between the fingers and thumb, gently inserting it into the vagina, pushing backward as far as it will go.
    Feel the cervix to check for proper positioning.
- Advise the client that the diaphragm can be inserted up to 2 hours before coitus but that it should remain in place for at least 6 hours following coitus; it may remain in place for as long as 24 hours, but if longer, cervical inflammation may result from the stasis of fluid.
- Teach the client that if coitus is repeated before 6 hours, the diaphragm should not be removed and replaced; instruct the client to add more spermicidal jelly.
- Instruct the client how to remove the diaphragm properly:
    After inserting the finger into the vagina, loosen the diaphragm by pressing against the anterior rim and withdrawing it carefully.
  Teach the client how to care for the diaphragm properly:
    Wash in mild soap and water, drying gently and storing it in its protective case.
    Inspect the diaphragm periodically to see that the rubber is not deteriorating.

## DISSEMINATED INTRAVASCULAR COAGULATION (DIC)

### Description

- DIC is an acquired disorder of blood clotting that results from excessive trauma or some similar underlying stimulus.
- It can develop during pregnancy, placing the client at high risk for problems; it also is a postpartal complica-

tion, one of the major causes of *postpartal hemorrhage.*
- Situations associated with DIC and childbirth include *pregnancy-induced hypertension, amniotic fluid embolism,* placental retention, septic abortion, retention of a dead fetus, and saline abortion.
- DIC occurs when there is extreme bleeding and so many platelets and fibrin from the general circulation are used that there are not enough left for clotting.
- This situation results in a paradox: At one point in the circulatory system, the person has increased coagulation; throughout the rest of the system, a bleeding defect exists.
- DIC is an emergency situation. Maternal death can result if hypofibrinogenemia does not reverse; the fetus is at risk from hypoxia, maternal sepsis, acidosis, and hypotension.

### Assessment Findings
- Vaginal bleeding continues despite usual measures to induce *uterine contractions*
- Oozing from an intravenous or blood-drawing site
- Thrombocytopenia
- Decreased fibrinogen levels
- Increased prothrombin time (PT)
- Increased partial thromboplastin time (PTT)

### Nursing Implications
- Obtain a thorough history and physical examination to establish a baseline and identify any possible conditions associated with DIC.
- Be aware that if DIC is a complication of pregnancy, ending the pregnancy by delivering the fetus helps to stop the process of DIC.
- Assess the mother and fetus closely for changes; have emergency equipment available.
- Prepare to administer heparin, intravenously, to release the coagulation factors in the one part of the system aiding coagulation throughout the rest of the body.
- Keep in mind that heparin does not cross the placenta.
- Anticipate administering blood and blood factors after administering heparin to prevent the consumption of these new blood factors by the coagulation process.
- Monitor the client's coagulation studies for return to normal levels.

- Assess the fetus for signs of placental insufficiency and *fetal danger signs;* following birth, assess the newborn for signs that placental circulation remained sufficient.
- Provide the client and partner with explanations about what is happening and measures to treat the problem.
- Offer support to alleviate fears; allow the client and partner to verbalize concerns.

## DRUG USE

### DESCRIPTION

- Drug use during pregnancy is possibly teratogenic to the fetus.
- Many women assume that the rule of being cautious with drugs during pregnancy applies only to prescription drugs and take over-the-counter drugs freely.
- Not all drugs cross the placenta, but most do.
- The Food and Drug Administration has established five categories of safety, identifying drugs that are unsafe for ingestion during pregnancy.
- These categories include: A (studies have failed to show no risk to fetus in first trimester, with no evidence of risk in later trimesters); B (studies have failed to show an adverse effect on fetus, but no adequate clinical studies are available for pregnant women); C (pregnancy risk unknown); D (evidence of risk to fetus, but potential benefits may outweigh the risks); and X (risk outweighs potential benefits).
- Two principles underly the use of drugs during pregnancy:

    Any drug under certain circumstances may be detrimental to fetal welfare; therefore, during pregnancy, the woman should not take any drug not specifically prescribed or approved by the health care professional.

    A woman of childbearing age and ability should take no drugs other than those prescribed because a fetus is endangered at the beginning of a pregnancy as well as when the pregnancy is further along.

- Recreational drug use during pregnancy places the fetus at risk in two ways:

    The drug itself may have a direct teratogenic effect.

Intravenous drug use also risks exposure to diseases, such as *human immunodeficiency virus (HIV) infection* and hepatitis B.

- Narcotics such as meperidine (Demerol) have been implicated in causing intrauterine growth retardation. Cocaine, which causes maternal vasoconstriction, compromising the fetus' blood and nutrient supply, has been associated with *spontaneous abortion, preterm labor, meconium staining,* intrauterine growth retardation, limb defects, and long-term effects.

### NURSING IMPLICATIONS

- Obtain a thorough history, especially medication history, to establish a baseline and identify potential for drug use.
- Encourage the client to check with the health care provider before taking any medications.
- Teach the client about the potential teratogenic effects of drug use.
- Advise the recreational drug user to stop using the drugs; if necessary, assist with referral to drug dependency and detoxification programs.
- Anticipate the care for the woman with a drug dependency and an infant of a *drug-dependent mother.*

## DYSPNEA

### DESCRIPTION

- Dyspnea is a common discomfort of middle to late pregnancy.
- It occurs as the expanding uterus puts pressure on the diaphragm, causing some lung compression.
- Dyspnea leads to a feeling of shortness of breath.

### ASSESSMENT FINDINGS

- Complaints of shortness of breath, commonly at night, when lying flat and on exertion
- Sleeping on two or more pillows at night as the pregnancy progresses

### NURSING IMPLICATIONS

- Obtain a thorough history and physical examination to establish a baseline and rule out any pathologic causes.
- Encourage the client to sit upright to allow the weight of the uterus to fall away from the diaphragm.

- Caution the client to limit activities before becoming short of breath.
- Tell the client that anxiety adds to the sensation of breathlessness.
- Instruct the client and partner in distraction and relaxation techniques to draw attention away from the discomfort.

## ECTOPIC PREGNANCY

### DESCRIPTION

- Ectopic pregnancy is a complication of pregnancy, placing the client at a high risk for problems.
- It is a pregnancy in which implantation occurs outside the uterine cavity, such as on the ovary or in the cervix or most commonly in the fallopian tube.
- Ectopic pregnancy is the second most frequent cause of *vaginal bleeding* early in pregnancy.
- Ectopic pregnancy is associated with the use of *intrauterine devices,* pelvic inflammatory disease, progestin-only oral contraceptives, postconceptual estrogen, or ovarian induction drugs.
- At about 6 to 12 weeks of pregnancy, the growing zygote ruptures the slender tube with resultant invasion and destruction of the blood vessel in the tube; a ruptured ectopic pregnancy is a serious condition.

### ASSESSMENT FINDINGS

- *HCG* pregnancy test positive
- Amenorrhea
- *Vaginal bleeding* (extent depends on the number and size of the ruptured vessels)
- Sharp stabbing pain on one of the lower abdominal quadrants
- Light-headedness
- Rapid, thready pulse
- Rapid respirations
- Falling blood pressure
- *Ultrasonography* positive for ruptured tube and collecting pelvic fluid
- Rigid abdomen
- Positive Cullen's sign (bluish discoloration around the umbilicus)
- Referred shoulder pain
- Palpable tender mass in Douglas' cul de sac

### Nursing Implications

- Immediately assess the client's hemodynamic status to determine extent of blood loss.
- Obtain hemoglobin level, type, and crossmatch.
- Obtain serum *HCG* level to confirm pregnancy.
- Administer fluid volume replacement intravenously.
- Prepare for abdominal laparotomy to ligate bleeding vessels and remove or repair damaged tube.
- Administer $Rh_o(D)$ immune globulin (RHIG) for isoimmunization protection for the client with Rh-negative blood.
- If the tube has not ruptured, anticipate using oral methotrexate followed by leucovorin until a negative *HCG* titer is achieved.
- Offer emotional support to the client and partner; allow them to grieve over the loss of pregnancy and possible loss of fallopian tube; allow the client to verbalize concerns about losses and future childbearing.

## EDEMA, ANKLE

### Description

- Ankle edema, swelling of the ankles, occurs most commonly at the end of the day during late pregnancy.
- It is thought to be caused by reduced blood circulation in the lower extremities as a result of uterine pressure and general fluid retention.
- It is a normal occurrence of pregnancy unless accompanied by proteinuria and hypertension, which may indicate *pregnancy-induced hypertension.*

### Nursing Assessment

- Complaints of difficulty putting shoes on after taking them off in the evening.
- Swelling of ankles and feet, especially later in the day.

### Nursing Implications

- Evaluate for signs of *pregnancy-induced hypertension,* such as proteinuria, edema of other nondependent parts, and sudden weight gain.
- Encourage resting in side-lying position.
- Advise the client to sit for 1/2 hour in afternoon and evening with legs elevated.

- Caution against wearing constricting clothing, such as panty girdles, knee-high stockings, and garters.
- Reassure the client that ankle edema is normal.

# ENDOMETRITIS

## DESCRIPTION

- Endometritis, an infection of the endometrium, is a postpartal complication, usually occurring 48 to 72 hours after delivery.
- Bacteria gain access to the uterus through the vagina and enter the uterus either at the time of birth or during the postpartal period.
- If the infection is limited to the endometrium, the course is about 7 to 10 days.
- Endometritis can lead to tubal scarring and interfere with future fertility.

## ASSESSMENT FINDINGS

- Fever above 100.4°F (38°C) for 2 consecutive 24-hour periods (usually the 3rd or 4th post-partum day), excluding the first 24-hour period after birth
- Chills
- Loss of appetite
- General malaise
- Large, tender, poorly contracted uterus
- Severe postpartum cramping
- Brownish red, foul-smelling *lochia* (increased in amount, but if infection accompanied by high fever, may be scant or absent)

## NURSING IMPLICATIONS

- Inspect the perineum at least twice daily for redness, edema, ecchymosis, and discharge.
- Assess fundal size, consistency, and tenderness for changes indicating poor involution.
- Evaluate for abdominal pain, fever, and malaise.
- Assess *lochia* for color, quantity, and odor; report any foul-smelling *lochia.*
- Obtain culture and sensitivity of *lochia.*
- Administer appropriate antibiotic as prescribed.
- Provide additional fluids to combat fever.
- Administer an analgesic as ordered to relieve severe cramping and discomfort.

- Urge the client to use Fowler's position and ambulation to encourage lochia drainage by gravity and prevent pooling of infected secretions.
- Instruct the client in proper handwashing techniques to prevent infection transmission.
- Instruct the client in self-care measures, including perineal hygiene.
- Educate the client about the antibiotic therapy regimen, including drug, dosage, adverse effects, need for compliance, and follow-up.
- Instruct the client about signs and symptoms to report to physician following discharge.

## ENGAGEMENT

### DESCRIPTION

- Engagement is a term used to describe *fetal presentation.*
- Engagement has occurred when the presenting part of the fetus has settled far enough into the pelvis to be at the level of the ischial spines, a midpoint of the pelvis.
- The fetal presenting part is at 0 station.
- Descent to this point means that the widest part of the fetus (the biparietal diameter in a cephalic presentation or intertrochanteric diameter in a breech presentation) has passed through the pelvis intact or the pelvic inlet is adequate for birth.
- Another term for engagement is *lightening.*
- In primiparas, nonengagement of the head at the beginning of labor indicates a possible complication: abnormal *fetal presentation* or *position,* abnormality of the fetal head, or cephalopelvic disproportion.
- In multiparas, engagement may or may not be present at the beginning of labor.

### NURSING IMPLICATIONS

- Obtain a thorough antepartal and labor history to establish a baseline.
- Assist with vaginal and cervical examination to determine fetal presenting part and *station.*

## ENVIRONMENTAL EXPOSURE HAZARDS

### DESCRIPTION

- Exposure to environmental hazards during pregnancy can be teratogenic to the fetus.

- It can be as lethal as those that are directly or deliberately ingested.
- Environmental hazards include metal and chemical hazards, such as exposure to pesticides and carbon monoxide and lead ingestion; radiation exposure, such as from x-rays and possibly from computers and word processors; and temperature extremes, including hyperthermia, such as from saunas, hot tubs, tanning beds, or working next to a furnace, and hypothermia.

### NURSING IMPLICATIONS

- Obtain a thorough history and physical examination to establish a baseline and identify any possible exposure to environmental hazards, such as in the workplace.
- Educate the client about environmental hazards and the teratogenic effects of these on the fetus.
- Encourage the client to evaluate the workplace for possible hazards and instruct her to avoid them.
- Allow women of childbearing age to be exposed to pelvic radiation only in the first 10 days of the menstrual cycle (a time when pregnancy is unlikely because ovulation has not yet occurred), unless an emergency exists.
- Perform a rapid serum assay pregnancy test on all women who have reason to believe that they might be pregnant before using diagnostic tests involving x-rays.
- Avoid radiation of the pelvis during pregnancy; use other methods for *evaluation of fetal well-being* if possible; use pelvic x-rays only at term and only if the data revealed cannot be obtained by any other means.
- Shield the pelvis with a lead apron if the woman needs nonpelvic radiation during pregnancy.
- Shield self with a lead apron if asked to assist with a client undergoing x-rays.
- Encourage the client to avoid temperature extremes to prevent effects of hyperthermia and hypothermia.

## EPISIOTOMY

### DESCRIPTION

- An episiotomy is a surgical incision of the perineum made to prevent tearing of the perineum with birth and to release pressure on the fetal head with birth.

- An episiotomy incision is made with blunt-tipped scissors in the midline of the perineum (midline episiotomy) or begun in the midline but directed laterally away from the rectum (mediolateral episiotomy).
- Midline episiotomies have the advantage over mediolateral ones in that, if tearing occurs beyond the incision, it will be away from the rectum with less danger of complication from rectal mucosal tears.
- Midline episiotomies appear to heal more easily, cause less blood loss, and result in less discomfort to a woman in the postpartal period.
- There is a slight loss of blood at the time of the incision, but the pressure of the presenting part serves to tamp the cut edges and keep the bleeding to a minimum; the fetal head generally moves forward considerably once the tension on the perineum is relieved.
- Once considered a routine part of a normal birth, episiotomies now are used less frequently.

### Nursing Implications
- Anticipate the possibility of an episiotomy during labor and delivery; instruct the client about the possibility and explain all events to alleviate her anxieties.
- Inspect the client's perineum postpartally and evaluate the suture line for signs and symptoms of infection and bleeding.
- Keep in mind that the perineum is an extremely tender area with the muscles of that area involved with many activities, such as sitting, walking, stooping, bending, urinating, and defecating.
- Assess the client postpartally for complaints of perineal discomfort and any interference with rest, sleeping, eating, and being able to sit and hold the baby comfortably.
- Assure the client that the discomfort is normal and does not usually last more than 5 or 6 days.
- Apply ice, soothing cream, or anesthetic spray as prescribed to relieve the discomfort.
- Instruct the client to use sitz baths or cortisone-based cream as prescribed to decrease inflammation and therefore decrease tension on the suture line.
- Encourage the client to use witch hazel preparations to help relieve the discomfort.
- Explain to the client that the sutures are made of absorbable material and usually dissolve within 10 days.

- Instruct the client in proper perineal care, including cleansing the area, wiping from front to back, and changing perineal pads frequently.
- Instruct the client in signs and symptoms of infection, such as elevated temperature, foul-smelling *lochia,* or increased tenderness or discomfort in the area, and the need to notify the physician immediately.

# EXTERNAL CEPHALIC VERSION

### DESCRIPTION

- External cephalic version refers to the turning of a fetus from a breech to a cephalic *fetal position.*
- It is used for the client who develops a complication during labor and birth, specifically a problem with the passage.
- The breech and vertex of the fetus are located and grasped transabdominally; gentle pressure is applied to rotate the fetus in a forward direction.
- Use of external version can decrease the number of *cesarean births* necessary.
- Contraindications to the procedure are *multiple gestation,* severe oligohydramnios, nuchal cord, and unexplained third-trimester bleeding.

### ASSESSMENT FINDINGS

- Breech position
- Failure to progress in labor

### NURSING IMPLICATIONS

- Obtain a thorough history to identify any possible contraindications for the procedure.
- Inform the client about the procedure, including its purpose and what to expect during it.
- Assist with performing a thorough physical examination to determine *fetal position.*
- Assess the client's progress in labor.
- Continuously record *fetal heart rate* and possibly *ultrasonography* throughout the procedure for changes.
- Offer support to the client and partner throughout the procedure to minimize anxieties and fears.

# FETAL ACIDOSIS

### DESCRIPTION

- Fetal acidosis is a *fetal danger sign* of labor.
- It is a certain sign that fetal well-being is becoming compromised.

### ASSESSMENT FINDINGS
- Fetal scalp blood pH below 7.2

### NURSING IMPLICATIONS
- Perform a thorough assessment of fetal status to identify problems.
- Obtain fetal scalp blood pH levels to determine the degree of acidosis.
- Institute measures to correct the underlying cause of the acidosis.
- Explain all events, treatments, and procedures to the client and partner; offer emotional support to minimize client's and partner's fears and anxieties.

## FETAL ALCOHOL SYNDROME (FAS)

### DESCRIPTION
- FAS refers to a disorder found in newborns of women who ingested varying amounts of alcohol during pregnancy.
- Alcohol is teratogenic to the fetus because alcohol crosses the placenta in the same concentration as is present in the maternal blood stream; newborns with FAS are considered high risk.
- FAS appears in 2 per 1000 newborns.

### ASSESSMENT FINDINGS
- Prenatal and postnatal growth retardation
- Central nervous system involvement, such as mental retardation, microcephaly, and cerebral palsy
- Facial anomalies, such as short palpebral fissures and thin upper lip
- Tremulousness, irritability
- Weak sucking reflex
- Sleep disturbances (either always awake or always asleep depending on the mother's alcohol level close to birth)

### NURSING IMPLICATIONS
- Obtain a thorough maternal history to establish a baseline and identify *alcohol use.*
- Educate all clients about the effects of *alcohol use* on the fetus and advise them to avoid alcohol intake during pregnancy to prevent any teratogenic effects on the fetus; refer to alcohol treatment center, if necessary.

- Keep in mind that there is no safe threshold of alcohol ingestion during pregnancy.
- Provide an environment free from excessive stimuli; darken the room if possible to minimize stimuli.
- Anticipate the need for gavage feeding if the newborn has difficulty sucking.
- Explain to the client about the newborn's need for quiet and avoidance of excessive stimulation.

## FETAL CIRCULATION

### DESCRIPTION
- Fetal circulation differs from extrauterine circulation.
- As early as the 3rd week of intrauterine life, fetal blood has begun to exchange nutrients with the maternal circulation across the chorionic villi.
- During intrauterine life, the fetus derives its oxygen and excretes carbon dioxide not from oxygen exchange in the lungs, but from the placenta; blood does enter lung vessels while in utero, but this blood flow is to supply the cells of the lungs themselves, not for oxygen exchange.

  Blood arriving at the fetus from the placenta (highly oxygenated blood) enters the fetus through the umbilical vein and into an accessory vein, the ductus venosus.

  The ductus venosus supplies blood to the fetal liver and then empties into the inferior vena cava, through which blood flows to the right side of the heart.

  As the blood enters the right atrium, the bulk of it is shunted into the left atrium through an opening in the atrial septum, the foramen ovale.

  From the left atrium, it follows the course of normal circulation into the left ventricle and into the aorta.

  Blood returning from the superior vena cava enters the right atrium and leaves it by the normal circulatory route (through the tricuspid valve into the right ventricle).

  This blood leaves the right ventricle through the pulmonary artery in the normal manner.

  A small portion of this blood flow services the lung tissue; the larger portion is shunted away from

the lungs, through an additional vessel, the
ductus arteriosus, directly into the aorta.

Two umbilical arteries transport most of the blood
flow from the descending aorta back through the
umbilical cord to the placental villi, where new
oxygen exchange takes place.

- The shunts of fetal circulation are necessary to supply
the most important organs of the fetus: the brain,
liver, heart, and kidneys.
- The ductus venosus supplies the liver, and the foramen ovale allows oxygenated blood to move directly
to the left side of the heart and the aorta, the vessel
from which the arteries arise that supply the brain,
heart, and kidneys.

## FETAL DEATH

### DESCRIPTION

- Fetal death is one of the most severe complications of
pregnancy.
- The most likely causes include chromosomal abnormalities, congenital malformations, infections such as
hepatitis B, immunologic causes, and complications of
maternal disease.
- If fetal death occurs before quickening, the woman
will not be aware that the fetus has died because
she was not able to feel fetal movements; this is usually discovered at a routine prenatal visit when no
fetal heartbeat can be heard; delivery occurs naturally but may not occur for 4 to 5 weeks after
death; a dead fetus in utero for this long a time
can initiate *disseminated intravascular coagulation
(DIC)*.
- If a fetus dies in utero past the point of quickening,
the woman becomes aware that fetal movements are
suddenly absent.

### ASSESSMENT FINDINGS

- Absence of fetal movement
- No fetal heartbeat on *ultrasonography*
- Painless spotting, gradually accompanied by *uter-
ine contractions* with *cervical effacement*
- Fetus born lifeless and emaciated

### NURSING IMPLICATIONS

- Obtain a thorough history and physical examination
to establish a baseline.

- Assess for presence of fetal heartbeat and fetal movement.
- If labor does not begin spontaneously, anticipate induction with prostaglandin gel (to effect ripening of the cervix) and oxytocin (to begin *uterine contractions*).
- Obtain blood studies to detect possible DIC.
- Allow the client opportunities to express how she feels about the loss; if older children are involved, help the client explore how to explain the fetal death to them.
- Encourage a support person to remain with the client during labor; it makes the birth real, ends the pregnancy, and allows the client and partner to begin active grieving.
- Ask the couple if they want to see the baby; if so, wash away obvious blood, swaddle the baby as if he or she were a newborn, and bring the baby to them; point out particularly endearing features that may provide a focus for memories.
- If the child had a congenital anomaly that led to the death, prepare them for this before bringing the child to them and explain how the anomaly affected the child.
- Explain hospital procedures such as when the body will be released or what additional permission for autopsy is needed.
- Advise the client and partner to check with the health care provider regarding future pregnancies.
- Prepare the couple for the possibility that they may feel sad on the day the infant would have been born if the pregnancy had been carried to term or they visit a friend's child of the age their child would have been.
- Be certain before the client is discharged that she has a support person she can rely on during the following week or month when the full impact of the fetal loss registers.
- Ensure that the client has a return appointment for follow-up so that both her physical and psychological health can be evaluated at that time.

## FETAL DEVELOPMENTAL MILESTONES— 4 WEEKS

### DESCRIPTION

- Developmental milestones refer to the key areas of development occurring in the fetus throughout the pregnancy.

- The life of the fetus is generally measured from the time of ovulation or fertilization (ovulation age), but the length of pregnancy is generally measured from the first day of the last menstrual period (gestation age).
- It is helpful when talking to expectant parents to be able to correlate fetal development to the way they measure pregnancy, from the first day of the last menstrual period.
- By the end of 4 weeks' gestation, the human embryo is a rapidly growing formation of cells but does not resemble a human being as yet.
- Developmental milestones for 4 weeks' gestation include the following:
    Length—0.75 to 1 cm
    Weight—400 mg
    Spinal cord formation and fusing at midpoint
    Back bent (head touches tail)
    Rudimentary heart, appearing as a bulge on the anterior surface
    Budlike arms and legs
    Rudimentary eyes, ears, and nose

## FETAL DEVELOPMENTAL MILESTONES— 8 WEEKS

### DESCRIPTION

- Developmental milestones refer to the key areas of development occurring in the fetus throughout the pregnancy.
- The life of the fetus is generally measured from the time of ovulation or fertilization (ovulation age), but the length of pregnancy is generally measured from the first day of the last menstrual period (gestation age).
- It is helpful when talking to expectant parents to be able to correlate fetal development to the way they measure pregnancy, from the first day of the last menstrual period.
- By the end of 8 weeks' gestation, organogenesis is complete.
- Developmental milestones for 8 weeks' gestation include the following:
    Length—2.5 cm
    Weight—20 g

Beating heart with septum and valves
Discernible facial features
Extremities (legs, arms, fingers, toes, elbows, and
knees) developed
Tail retrogression
Large abdomen
Gestational sac
External genitalia present but not distinguishable

# FETAL DEVELOPMENTAL MILESTONES— 12 WEEKS

### DESCRIPTION

- Developmental milestones refer to the key areas of
  development occurring in the fetus throughout the
  pregnancy.
- The life of the fetus is generally measured from the
  time of ovulation or fertilization (ovulation age),
  but the length of pregnancy is generally measured
  from the first day of the last menstrual period (gesta-
  tion age).
- It is helpful when talking to expectant parents to be
  able to correlate fetal development to the way they
  measure pregnancy, from the first day of the last men-
  strual period.
- Developmental milestones for 12 weeks' gestation in-
  clude the following:
  Length—7 to 9 cm
  Weight—45 g
  Nail beds
  Spontaneous fetal movement
  Positive Babinski reflex
  Formation of ossification plates
  Sex distinguishable by outward appearance
  Beginning kidney secretion; urine not yet evident
  in amniotic fluid
  Audible heartbeat with Doppler

# FETAL DEVELOPMENTAL MILESTONES— 16 WEEKS

### DESCRIPTION

- Developmental milestones refer to the key areas of
  development occurring in the fetus throughout the
  pregnancy.

- The life of the fetus is generally measured from the time of ovulation or fertilization (ovulation age), but the length of pregnancy is generally measured from the first day of the last menstrual period (gestation age).
- It is helpful when talking to expectant parents to be able to correlate fetal development to the way they measure pregnancy, from the first day of the last menstrual period.
- By the end of 16 weeks, the fetus actively swallows amniotic fluid.
- Developmental milestones for 16 weeks' gestation include the following:
  > Length—10 to 17 cm
  > Weight—55 to 120 g
  > Audible fetal heart tones with stethoscope
  > Lanugo formation
  > Pancreatic and liver functioning
  > Intact swallowing reflex

## FETAL DEVELOPMENTAL MILESTONES—20 WEEKS

### DESCRIPTION

- Developmental milestones refer to the key areas of development occurring in the fetus throughout the pregnancy.
- The life of the fetus is generally measured from the time of ovulation or fertilization (ovulation age), but the length of pregnancy is generally measured from the first day of the last menstrual period (gestation age).
- It is helpful when talking to expectant parents to be able to correlate fetal development to the way they measure pregnancy, from the first day of the last menstrual period.
- By the end of 20 weeks' gestation, the spontaneous fetal movements have become strong enough for the mother to feel.
- Developmental milestones for 20 weeks' gestation include the following:
  > Length—25 cm
  > Weight—223 g
  > Quickening
  > Antibody production

Hair formation
Meconium in upper intestines
Brown fat formation
Distinguishable sleep and activity patterns

# FETAL DEVELOPMENTAL MILESTONES—24 WEEKS

## DESCRIPTION

- Developmental milestones refer to the key areas of development occurring in the fetus throughout the pregnancy.
- The life of the fetus is generally measured from the time of ovulation or fertilization (ovulation age), but the length of pregnancy is generally measured from the first day of the last menstrual period (gestation age).
- It is helpful when talking to expectant parents to be able to correlate fetal development to the way they measure pregnancy, from the first day of the last menstrual period.
- When fetuses reach 24 weeks, or 601 g, they have achieved a practical low-end age of viability if they are cared for after birth in a modern intensive care facility.
- Developmental milestones for 24 weeks' gestation include the following:
    Length—28 to 36 cm
    Weight—550 g
    Passive antibody transfer from mother to fetus
    Vernix caseosa
    Meconium in rectum
    Active surfactant production
    Well-defined eyelids and eyelashes
    Open eyelids, reactive pupils

# FETAL DEVELOPMENTAL MILESTONES—28 WEEKS

## DESCRIPTION

- Developmental milestones refer to the key areas of development occurring in the fetus throughout the pregnancy.
- The life of the fetus is generally measured from the time of ovulation or fertilization (ovulation age), but the length of pregnancy is generally measured

from the first day of the last menstrual period (gestation age).

- It is helpful when talking to expectant parents to be able to correlate fetal development to the way they measure pregnancy, from the first day of the last menstrual period.
- The blood vessels of the retina are extremely sensitive to damage from high oxygen concentrations, an important consideration when caring for low-birth-weight infants who need oxygen).
- Developmental milestones for 28 weeks' gestation include the following:
    Length—35 to 38 cm
    Weight—1200 g
    Lung alveoli maturation
    Surfactant in amniotic fluid
    Testicular descent (in males)

# FETAL DEVELOPMENTAL MILESTONES—32 WEEKS

### DESCRIPTION

- Developmental milestones refer to the key areas of development occurring in the fetus throughout the pregnancy.
- The life of the fetus is generally measured from the time of ovulation or fertilization (ovulation age), but the length of pregnancy is generally measured from the first day of the last menstrual period (gestation age).
- It is helpful when talking to expectant parents to be able to correlate fetal development to the way they measure pregnancy, from the first day of the last menstrual period.
- By the end of 32 weeks, the fetus may have already assumed delivery position.
- Developmental milestones for 32 weeks' gestation include the following:
    Length—38 to 43 cm
    Weight—1600 g
    Subcutaneous fat deposition
    Active Moro reflex
    Iron stores development
    Fetal awareness of sounds outside the mother
    Fingernails reach end of fingertips

# FETAL DEVELOPMENTAL MILESTONES— 36 WEEKS

### DESCRIPTION

- Developmental milestones refer to the key areas of development occurring in the fetus throughout the pregnancy.
- The life of the fetus is generally measured from the time of ovulation or fertilization (ovulation age), but the length of pregnancy is generally measured from the first day of the last menstrual period (gestation age).
- It is helpful when talking to expectant parents to be able to correlate fetal development to the way they measure pregnancy, from the first day of the last menstrual period.
- By the end of 36 weeks, many babies turn in utero into a vertex or head-down *fetal position.*
- Developmental milestones for 36 weeks' gestation include the following:

    Length—42 to 49 cm
    Weight—1900 to 2700 g (5 to 6 lb)
    Augmented stores of glycogen, iron, carbohydrates, and calcium
    Increased subcutaneous fat deposits
    1 to 2 plantar creases
    Diminished lanugo
    Usually vertex *fetal position*

# FETAL DEVELOPMENTAL MILESTONES— 40 WEEKS

### DESCRIPTION

- Developmental milestones refer to the key areas of development occurring in the fetus throughout the pregnancy.
- The life of the fetus is generally measured from the time of ovulation or fertilization (ovulation age), but the length of pregnancy is generally measured from the first day of the last menstrual period (gestation age).
- It is helpful when talking to expectant parents to be able to correlate fetal development to the way they measure pregnancy, from the first day of the last menstrual period.

- In primiparas, the fetus often sinks into the birth canal during these last 2 weeks, giving the mother the feeling that her load is being lightened. It is a fetal announcement that the third trimester of pregnancy has ended and birth is at hand.
- Developmental milestones for 40 weeks' gestation include the following:
    Length—48 to 52 cm
    Weight—3000 g (7 to 7 1/2 lb)
    Active fetal kidneys
    Fully formed vernix caseosa
    Plantar creases
    Fingernails extend over fingertips

## FETAL HEART RATE (FHR)

### DESCRIPTION

- FHR, as determined by fetal heart sounds, can be determined as early as the 11th week of pregnancy by using an ultrasonic Doppler technique.
- Normal FHR ranges from 120 to 160 beats/minute.
- The pattern of the FHR is important for the *evaluation of fetal well-being* during the antepartal and intrapartal periods.
- Antepartally, FHR can be evaluated by rhythm strip testing (assesses baseline and long-term and short-term variability), nonstress testing (evaluates FHR in response to movement), vibroacoustic stimulation (evaluates FHR in response to movement that is stimulated by a sharp sound), and *contraction stress testing* (analyzes FHR in response to contractions).
- During labor, three important parameters of FHR patterns are evaluated: the baseline FHR, variabilities (long-term and short-term), and periodic changes in rate (accelerations and decelerations).
- Baseline FHR is determined by analyzing a range of fetal heartbeats recorded on a 10-minute tracing obtained between contractions; the rate fluctuates slightly when the fetus moves or is asleep; abnormal patterns include fetal bradycardia (FHR below 120 beats/minute for a 10-minute period), which if severe (below 100 beats/minute) indicates hypoxia, and fetal tachycardia (FHR above 160 beats/minute for a 10-minute period), which, if marked, indicates fetal distress.

- Variability, considered one of the most reliable indicators of fetal well-being, refers to the variation in the FHR over time and is reflected on the FHR tracing as a slight irregularity or "jitter" to the wave; baseline variability increases when the fetus is stimulated and slows when the fetus sleeps.

    Long-term variability refers to fluctuations in FHR of 6 to 10 beats occurring 3 to 10 times per minute.

    Short-term variability or beat-to-beat variability refers to the difference between successive heartbeats, usually about 2 to 3 beats per minute.

- Decreasing variability indicates the development of fetal distress; absent variability is considered a severe sign, indicating serious fetal compromise.

- Periodic changes occur in response to contractions and fetal movements and include accelerations, early deceleration, late deceleration, and variable deceleration.

    Accelerations are temporary increases in FHR resulting from fetal movement or compression of the umbilical vein during contraction.

    Early decelerations are periodic decreases in FHR resulting from pressure on the fetal head during contraction following the pattern of the contraction; they are normal if they occur late in labor when the head has descended but are abnormal if they occur early in labor before the head has fully descended.

    Late decelerations are those that are delayed until 30 to 40 seconds after the onset of the contraction and continue beyond the end of the contraction; they are an ominous pattern in labor suggesting uteroplacental insufficiency or decreased blood flow through the intervillous spaces of the uterus during *uterine contractions*.

    Variable decelerations occur at unpredictable times during contractions and indicate compression of the cord, which is an ominous sign in terms of fetal well-being.

## NURSING IMPLICATIONS

- Assess FHR at every antepartal visit and report any changes.

- Instruct the client about methods used for monitoring the fetus and FHR antepartally and during labor.
- Prepare the client physically and emotionally for antepartal evaluations of FHR.
- Evaluate the FHR for changes in rate, such as fetal bradycardia or fetal tachycardia, and variability.
- During labor, obtain a baseline FHR; be aware that if an increase or decrease occurs and is sustained for a 10-minute period, a new baseline is established.
- Monitor FHR tracing for periodic changes.
- Assess the degree of fetal descent during labor; be aware that early decelerations occurring before the head has fully descended could be the result of head compression from cephalopelvic disproportion; notify the physician if this occurs.
- Monitor the FHR tracing for late decelerations; if they occur:

    Stop or slow the rate of oxytocin administration if being used.

    Change the client's position from supine to lateral to relieve pressure on the aorta and vena cava.

    Administer oxygen and intravenous fluid as ordered.

    Prepare for possible delivery of infant if the occurrence of late decelerations persists and if FHR variability becomes abnormal.

Monitor the FHR tracing for variable decelerations; if they occur:

    Change the client's position from supine to lateral or to a Trendelenburg position to relieve pressure on the cord.

    Administer oxygen as ordered.

    Anticipate cesarean birth if measures do not correct the problem.

- Explain all aspects of monitoring the FHR tracing to the client and partner; provide reassurance if complications arise and prepare client and partner for interventions to correct the problem.
- Provide emotional support throughout the labor process.

## FETAL LIE

### Description

- Fetal lie refers to the relationship between the long (cephalocaudal) axis of the fetal body and the long axis of the mother's body.

- It describes whether the fetus is lying in a horizontal (transverse) or vertical (longitudinal) position.
- Approximately 99% of fetuses assume a longitudinal lie (with their long axis parallel with the long axis of the mother).
- Longitudinal lies are further classified as cephalic (the head is the presenting part) or breech (the breech, or buttocks, is the portion to contact the cervix first).

# FETAL MONITORING, EXTERNAL ELECTRONIC

## DESCRIPTION

- Electronic external monitoring is a noninvasive, easily applied technique used for *evaluation of fetal well-being*.
- It can be used to monitor both *uterine contractions* and *fetal heart rate* on a continuous or intermittent basis from sensors attached to the client's abdomen.
- *Uterine contractions* are monitored by means of a pressure transducer or tocodynamometer placed against the abdomen over the uterine fundus (to register the area of greatest contractility) and held in place by an adjustable strap; the transducer converts the pressure registered into an electronic signal that is recorded on graph paper.
- *Fetal heart rate* is monitored through an ultrasonic sensor or monitor strapped against the woman's abdomen with an adhesive closure; the small Doppler unit converts fetal heart movements into audible beeping sounds and prints out a permanent graph paper recording.
- Electronic external fetal monitoring can be introduced early in labor because it does not depend on *cervical dilation* or on the fetus being well descended.

## NURSING IMPLICATIONS

- Assure both the client and partner that monitoring is a routine procedure and that it provides more accurate information about the progress in labor than manual palpation.
- Keep in mind that some clients find the device confining and limiting, whereas the client who is worried that something will happen to her child during labor will find it reassuring to listen to the regular beeping sound of the undistressed fetal heart from an accompanying fetal heart transducer.

- Apply talcum powder to the strap holding the unit in place to make it more comfortable.
- Remove the sensor periodically and allow the client to change position.
- Remember that if the client changes her position herself, reposition the sensor.
- Remind the client that if she changes position, the accompanying fetal heart signal may stop.
- Continue to assess the client thoroughly even with the monitor in place.
- Provide emotional support and communication to the client and partner.

## FETAL MONITORING, INTERNAL ELECTRONIC

### DESCRIPTION

- Internal electronic fetal monitoring is the most precise method for assessing *fetal heart rate* and *uterine contractions.*
- Contractions are monitored via a pressure-sensing catheter that is passed through the vagina, alongside the fetus, into the uterine cavity.
- The catheter extending from the vagina is attached to a pressure recorder.
- As each contraction puts pressure on the uterine contents, the relation can then be made between the *fetal heart rate* and uterine pressure from contractions.
- The *fetal heart rate* recording is obtained from a fetal scalp electrode.
- When the fetal head is engaged, the electrode is inserted vaginally and attached to the fetal scalp; a fetal electrocardiograph signal is obtained and amplified and then fed into a cardiotachometer whose output is recorded on permanent graph paper.
- When the *uterine contractions* are monitored by an internal pressure gauge, the frequency, duration, baseline strength, and peak strength of contractions can be evaluated.
- Because this method is intrusive and carries the risk of uterine infection, internal electronic fetal monitoring usually is reserved for women who are considered as high risk during labor.

### Nursing Implications

- Obtain a thorough history and physical examination to obtain a baseline.
- Assess the client's complaints of *uterine contractions* for onset, frequency, duration, and intensity.
- Assess the *fetal heart rate* and notify physician of any changes.

- Explain all aspects of internal electronic monitoring to the client and partner.
- Assess the client for *rupture of membranes* and *cervical dilation;* keep in mind that membranes must have ruptured and the cervix must be dilated to at least 3 cm for internal electronic monitoring to be used.
- Provide support and comfort to the client during insertion of uterine catheter and fetal scalp electrode.
- Assess the strength of contractions by evaluating the size of the peak of the contraction on the tracing.
- Evaluate the return of uterine tone to baseline strength between contractions to ensure adequate placental filling between contractions.
- Be aware that if baseline readings do not return to 20 mm Hg or below, uterine hypotonia and fetal compromise are indicated.

## FETAL POSITION

### Description

- Fetal position refers to the relationship of the presenting part to a specific quadrant of the woman's pelvis.
- For convenience, the woman's pelvis is divided into four quadrants according to the woman's right and left: right anterior, left anterior, right posterior, and left posterior.
- Four parts of the fetus have been chosen as points of direction to describe the relationship of the presenting part to one of the pelvic quadrants.

  In vertex presentation, the occiput is the chosen point.

  In face presentation, the chin is the chosen point.

  In a breech presentation, the sacrum is the chosen point.

  In a shoulder presentation, the scapula or acromion process is the chosen point.

- A position is marked by an abbreviation of three letters: The middle letter denotes the fetal landmark

(O for occiput, M for mentum, Sa for sacrum, and A for acromion process). The first letter denotes where the landmark is pointing to the mother's right (R) or left (L); the last letter defines where the landmark points anteriorly (A), posteriorly (P), or transversely (T).

- Fetal position is important because it influences the process and efficiency of labor; a fetus delivers fastest from a right or left ocippitoanterior position; labor is considerably extended if the position is posterior, and it may be more painful for the client because the rotation of the fetal head puts pressure on the sacral nerves, causing sharp back pains.

## FETAL PRESENTATION

### DESCRIPTION

- Fetal presentation denotes the body part that first contacts the cervix or delivers first.
- This is determined by *fetal lie* (the relationship between the long [cephalocaudal] axis of the fetal body and the long axis of the mother's body; describes whether the fetus is lying in a horizontal [transverse] or vertical [longitudinal] position) and attitude (the degree of fetal flexion or the relation of the fetal parts to each other).
- There are three types of fetal presentation: cephalic presentation (vertex, brow, face, and mentum), breech presentation, and shoulder presentation.
- Cephalic presentation is the most frequent type of presentation, denoting the head as the presenting body part that first contacts the cervix or delivers first.
- Four types of cephalic presentation include vertex presentation, brow presentation, face presentation, and mentum presentation.

    In vertex presentation (the most common), the head is sharply flexed, making the parietal bones or the space between the fontanelles (the vertex) the presenting part; fetal lie is longitudinal and fetal attitude is good (full flexion).

    In brow presentation, the head is only moderately flexed so the brow (or sinciput) becomes the presenting part; fetal lie is longitudinal, and fetal attitude is moderate; the area of the fetal skull that contacts the cervix often becomes edematous during labor owing to continual pressure against it (called *caput succedaneum*); in the newborn, the point of presentation can be analyzed from the location of the caput.

In face presentation, the fetus has extended his or her head to make the face the presenting part; fetal lie is longitudinal and fetal attitude is poor; from this position, extreme edema and distortion of the face may occur; the present diameter (occipitomental) is so wide, delivery may be impossible.

In mentum presentation, the fetus has completely hyperextended the head to present the chin with the widest diameter (occipitomental); fetal lie is longitudinal, and fetal attitude is poor; as a rule, the fetus cannot enter the pelvis in this presentation.

- Breech presentation, affected by fetal attitude, denotes the buttocks or lower extremities as the presenting body part; breech presentations are difficult deliveries and occur in only a small percentage of births.
- Three types of breech presentations include complete, frank, and footling.

In a complete breech presentation, the fetus' legs are tightly flexed on the abdomen; both the buttocks and the tightly flexed feet present to the cervix; the fetal lie is longitudinal, and fetal attitude is good (full flexion).

In a frank breech presentation, the fetus' hips are flexed, but the knees are extended to rest on the chest; the buttocks alone present to the cervix; the fetal lie is longitudinal, and the fetal attitude is moderate.

In a footling breech presentation, neither the thighs nor lower legs are flexed; if one foot presents to the cervix, it is a single footling breech; if both present, it is a double footling breech.

- Shoulder presentation denotes one of the shoulders (acromion process), iliac crest, hand, or elbow as the presenting part; the fetus is in a transverse lie, lying horizontally in the pelvis so that its long axis is perpendicular to that of the mother.
- Fewer than 1% of fetuses lie transversely; if so, the fetus must be delivered by *cesarean birth* because the

fetus is unable to deliver normally from this wedged position.

- The presentation of a body part other than the vertex puts the fetus at a risk because there is apt to be a proportional difference between the fetus and pelvis, making a *cesarean birth* necessary and the membranes more apt to rupture early, increasing the possibility of infection; the fetus is more apt to suffer anoxia and *meconium staining,* complications that lead to *respiratory distress* at birth.

## FETAL RESPONSES TO LABOR

### DESCRIPTION

- Although the fetus is basically a passive participant in labor, the effect of pressure and circulatory changes occurring with contractions causes detectable physiologic differences.
- Fetal responses to labor affect the neurologic, cardiovascular, integumentary, musculoskeletal, and respiratory systems.

### ASSESSMENT FINDINGS

- Increased intracranial pressure
- Slight slowing of *fetal heart rate* returning to baseline
- Minimal petechiae and edema of presenting part
- Full fetal flexion
- Maturation of surfactant production with clearing of lung fluid

### NURSING IMPLICATIONS

- Obtain a thorough *antepartal* and *intrapartal history and physical examination* to establish a baseline.
- Continually monitor the client and fetus for changes, both normal and abnormal responses to labor and danger signs.
- Provide emotional support, guidance, and instructions throughout the labor process.

## FETAL WELL-BEING, EVALUATION OF

### DESCRIPTION

- Evaluation of fetal well-being involves methods used to determine the status of the fetus and the progression of the pregnancy.
- It is a component of the *antepartal history and physical examination.*

- A variety of assessment techniques can be used to gather information about the size and health of the fetus; these techniques include:
    *Fetal heart rate* monitoring
    *Ultrasonography*
    *Fundal height* measurement
    Fetal movement measurement
    *Electronic fetal monitoring*
    *Contraction stress test*
    *Amniocentesis*
    *Chorionic villi sampling*
    *Maternal serum assay*
    *Percutaneous umbilical cord sampling*
    Biophysical profile
    Fetal blood flow studies

### NURSING IMPLICATIONS

- Assist with scheduling the procedure(s).
- Explain the procedure(s) to the client and partner; answer any questions and concerns that they might have.
- Provide proper physical and psychological preparation for the upcoming procedure.
- Support the client during the procedure if possible.
- Provide follow-up care after the procedure, including the client, equipment used, and any specimens collected.
- Check to make sure that an informed consent has been obtained before the procedure; ensure that, if the procedure carries any risk that would not be present if it were not performed, the client is fully aware of what the procedure consists of and what risk (to herself and the fetus) is present by having or not having the procedure performed.

## FORCEPS DELIVERY

### DESCRIPTION

- A forceps delivery refers to a method of delivery involving steel instruments constructed of two blades that slide together at their shaft to form a handle.
- Forceps are applied first by one blade being slipped into a woman's vagina next to the fetal head and then the other side being slipped into place; the shafts are brought together in the midline to form the handle.
- Forceps may be necessary to deliver the baby if a woman is unable to push with contractions in the

pelvic division of labor, such as after *regional anesthesia;* if progress ceases in the *second stage of labor;* or if the fetus is in an abnormal *fetal position.*

- A fetus in distress from a complication such as *prolapsed cord* can be delivered more quickly by the use of forceps.
- Forceps are designed to prevent pressure from being exerted on the fetal head and also may be used to reduce pressure and avoid subdural hemorrhage in the fetus as the fetal head reaches the perineum.
- A forceps birth is an outlet procedure when the forceps are applied after the fetal head reaches the perineum.
- A low forceps birth may be used to indicate the fetal head is at a +2 station; if the fetal head is still at the level of the ischial spines (0 station), this is a midforceps birth (although rarely seen today).
- Some anesthesia, at least a pudendal block, is necessary for forceps application to achieve pelvic relaxation and reduce pain.

### Nursing Implications

- Prepare the client physically and emotionally for forceps application.
- Provide emotional support and guidance throughout the procedure to alleviate anxieties and fears; allow the client and partner to verbalize feelings and concerns.
- Assess the client's membranes for rupture, which must be present before forceps are applied.
- Be aware that no cephalopelvic disproportion can be present before forceps are applied.
- Assess the client for complete *cervical dilation* before using forceps.
- Assist the client to empty her bladder before using forceps.
- Monitor the *fetal heart rate* before applying the forceps and immediately after applying them, because a danger of forceps use is that the cord could be compressed between the blade and the head.
- Anticipate an *episiotomy* to prevent perineal tearing owing to pressure on the perineum.
- Assess the client's cervix after a forceps birth to be certain that no laceration has occurred.

- Record the time and amount of the client's first voiding to rule out bladder injury.
- Assess the neonate for facial palsy or subdural hematoma, possible complications of a forceps birth.
- Inform the client and partner that the neonate may have a transient erythematous mark on the cheek; assure them that this will fade in 1 to 2 days.

## FORMULA FEEDING

### DESCRIPTION

- Formula feeding is an acceptable alternative to *breast-feeding* for infant nutrition.
- Commercial formulas are available that closely resemble human milk.
- The contents of commercial formulas are supervised by the federal Food and Drug Administration and are available in three types: milk-based, soy-based, and elemental.
- Milk-based formulas are used for the average infant; soy-based formulas are used for infants with lactose intolerance or galactosemia; elemental formulas are used with infants with protein allergies and fat malnutrition.
- Both milk-based and soy-based formulas, designed to simulate breast milk as closely as possible in terms of protein, fat, and minerals, contain 20 calories per ounce when diluted according to directions.
- Four separate forms of commercial formulas are available: powder that is combined with water; a condensed liquid that is diluted with an equal amount of water; a ready-to-pour type, which requires no dilution; and individually prepackaged and prepared bottles of formula.

### NURSING IMPLICATIONS

- Discuss with the client early in pregnancy about the types of infant feeding methods and the advantages and disadvantages of each.
- Instruct the client about necessary supplies, proper methods for formula and bottle preparation and storage, and administering the formula.
- Provide education about appropriate feeding techniques, including proper infant and bottle holding and infant burping.

- Encourage the client to allow adequate time for the feeding and not to rush the infant.
- Instruct the client how to test flow of milk from the nipple, with a flow rate of about 1 drop per second.
- Encourage the client to avoid propping bottle to prevent aspiration.
- Assist the client with interpreting infant's cues regarding feeding.
- Provide support and guidance to minimize anxiety and fears.

## FUNDAL HEIGHT

### DESCRIPTION
- Fundal height, the measurement of uterine height, is a method for estimating fetal growth.
- McDonald's rule is the method used to measure fundal height: The fundus-to-symphysis distance in centimeters is equal to the week of gestation between the 20th and 31st weeks of pregnancy.
- McDonald's rule becomes inaccurate during the 3rd trimester because the fetus is growing more in weight than height at this time.

### NURSING IMPLICATIONS
- Obtain a thorough history and physical examination to establish a baseline and ongoing to detect changes.
- Measure the client's fundal height at each antepartal visit.
  Palpate the fundus location.
  Measure from the notch above the symphysis pubis to the superior aspect of the uterine fundus.
- Keep in mind that research suggests that fundal height measurements be obtained by the use of calipers and by the same clinician throughout the pregnancy.
- Record all measurements on a graph, including typical milestones, such as over the symphysis pubis at 12 weeks, at the umbilicus at 20 weeks, and at the xiphoid process at 36 weeks.
- If any abnormalities are detected, anticipate further investigation with *ultrasonography*.
- Be aware that:

A fundal height much greater than the standard suggests *gestation pregnancy,* miscalculated due date, *large-for-gestational-age* infant, *hydramnios,* or *gestational trophoblastic disease* mole.

A fundal height much less than standard suggests that the fetus is failing to thrive (*small for gestational age*), the pregnancy length is miscalculated, or an anomaly such as anencephaly is developing.

## GENETIC DISORDERS, AUTOSOMAL

### Description

- Autosomal disorders refer to a group of genetic disorders involving an aberration of the autosome.
- Autosomal disorders can be dominant or recessive.
- Autosomal dominant disorders are caused by an abnormal dominant gene on an autosome; the disease trait is heterozygous; there is a corresponding healthy recessive gene for that trait.
- Examples of autosomal dominant disorders include Marfan's syndrome, osteogenesis imperfecta, and Huntington's disease.
- Autosomal recessive disorders are caused by an abnormality of both autosomes; the disease is homozygous.
- In autosomal recessive disorders, the normal gene is dominant, so the person must have two abnormal genes to be affected.
- Examples of autosomal recessive disorders include cystic fibrosis, adrenogenital syndrome, albinism, Tay-Sachs disease, galactosemia, phenylketonuria, limb-girdle muscular dystrophy, and Rh factor incompatibility.

### Nursing Implications

- Obtain a thorough health history, including a detailed family history; physical examination; and laboratory analysis of blood, chorionic villi, and amniotic fluid.
- Assist couples to arrange further follow-up.
- Assist couples in setting realistic goals.
- Encourage the client and partner to make informed reproductive choices.
- Plan for genetic counseling and screening.

- Assist with identifying support people who can be helpful to the couple.

## GENETIC DISORDERS, SEX-LINKED

### DESCRIPTION

- Sex-linked genetic disorders refer to those disorders or diseases that are passed from one generation to another by the gene for the disorder that is located on the female sex chromosome, the X chromosome.
- This is called X-linked inheritance.
- X-linked inheritance can be dominant or recessive.
- If the gene is dominant, it need be present on only one of the X chromosomes for symptoms of the disorder to be manifested.

   All individuals with the gene are affected.

   Female children of affected males are all affected; male children of affected males are unaffected.

   It appears in every generation.

   All children of homozygous affected females are affected;

   50% of heterozygous affected females are affected.

- If the gene is recessive, the mother will be the carrier for the disorder; any time a normal gene also is present, such as in female children, the expression of the disease will be blocked; if the gene is not paired, such as in male children, the disorder will be manifested.

   Only males in the family will have the disorder.

   A history of females dying at birth for unknown reasons often exists.

   Sons of an affected male are unaffected.

   The parents of affected children do not have the disorder.

- The majority of X-linked disorders are recessive, such as hemophilia A, Christmas disease, color blindness, and Duchenne's muscular dystrophy; X-linked dominant disorders are rare.

### NURSING IMPLICATIONS

- Obtain a thorough health history, including a detailed family history; physical examination; and laboratory analysis of blood, chorionic villi, and amniotic fluid.
- Assist couples to arrange further follow-up.
- Assist couples in setting realistic goals.

- Encourage the client and partner to make informed reproductive choices.
- Plan for genetic counseling and screening.
- Assist with identifying support people who can be helpful to the couple.

# GESTATIONAL TROPHOBLASTIC DISEASE (GTD)

### DESCRIPTION

- GTD, hydatiform mole, is the proliferation and degeneration of the trophoblast villi.
- As the cells degenerate, they become filled with fluid, appearing as fluid-filled, grape-sized vesicles.
- In this condition, the embryo fails to develop beyond a primitive start.
- Such structures are associated with choriocarcinoma, a rapidly metastasizing malignancy.
- GTD is one of the main causes of *vaginal bleeding* during the second trimester.

### ASSESSMENT FINDINGS

- Greater than standard *fundal height* measurements for week of pregnancy.
- Absence of fetal heart sounds.
- Strongly positive serum or urine HCG test.
- Continuous strongly positive *HCG* levels after day 100 of pregnancy.
- Marked nausea and vomiting.
- Hypertension, edema, and proteinuria present before 20th week of pregnancy.
- Dense growth (snowflake-like pattern) on *ultrasonography*.
- Dark brown or profuse *vaginal bleeding* accompanied by clear fluid–filled vesicle discharge (if not identified earlier by ultrasonography).

### NURSING IMPLICATIONS

- Obtain a thorough history and physical examination to establish a baseline.
- Inspect *vaginal bleeding* for passage of clear fluid–filled vesicles.
- Prepare the client for diagnostic evaluation including serum or urine *HCG* levels and *ultrasonography*.
- Prepare the client for suction and curettage to evacuate the mole.

- Monitor serum *HCG* levels at regular intervals following suction and curettage.
- Instruct the client about the need for follow-up visits, serum *HCG* levels, and chest x-ray every 2 to 4 weeks until levels are normal, then every month for a full year.
- Be aware that if the *HCG* level is gradually declining, this is suggestive that no complications are developing; if it plateaus for three times or increases in amount, it suggests malignant transformation.
- Instruct the client to use a reliable contraceptive method during the year so that a positive pregnancy test resulting from a new pregnancy will not be confused with a developing malignancy.
- Keep in mind that some physicians prescribe a prophylactic course of methotrexate, the drug of choice for choriocarcinoma; monitor the client for possible side effects, including leukopenia.
- Advise the client to postpone a second pregnancy until after the first year, when if *HCG* levels are still negative, the risk of malignancy is theoretically gone.
- Offer emotional support to the client and partner; allow them to grieve the loss and verbalize fears and anxieties over the possibility of a malignancy.
- Allow the client to express anger, sense of unfairness, feelings of inadequacies, and fear of recurrence over this event.
- Keep in mind that women who have had one incidence of GTD have a four to five times increased risk of a second molar pregnancy; provide early screening and follow-up.

## HEART FAILURE, MATERNAL

### DESCRIPTION
- Maternal heart failure is a preexisting condition that places the pregnant woman at risk during pregnancy.
- Heart failure can be left-sided or right-sided.
- Left-sided heart failure occurs with conditions such as mitral stenosis, mitral insufficiency, and aortic coarctation.
  Left-sided heart failure occurs when the left ventricle is unable to move forward the volume of blood received by the left atrium from the pulmonary circulation; the reason is often at the level of the mitral valve.

The normal physiologic tachycardia of pregnancy shortens diastole and decreases the time available for blood to flow across this valve, causing back pressure on the pulmonary circulation resulting in distention and interference with gas exchange at the alveoli.

If mitral stenosis is present, it is so difficult for blood to leave the left atrium that a secondary problem of thrombus formation can occur.

If coarctation is causing the difficulty, dissection of the aorta and thrombus formation can be secondary problems.

- Right-sided heart failure may result from congenital heart defects, such as pulmonary valve stenosis and atrial and ventricular septal defects.

    Right-sided heart failure occurs when the output of the right ventricle is less than the blood volume the heart receives at the right atrium from the vena cava or venous circulation.

    Back pressure results in congestion of the systemic venous circulation and decreases cardiac output to the lungs.

    The congenital anomaly that is most apt to cause right-sided heart failure in women of reproductive age is Eisenmenger's syndrome (a right-to-left atrial or ventricular septal defect with an accompanying pulmonary stenosis).

    These women, if the anomaly is not corrected, have a 50% chance of dying during pregnancy.

- Regardless of the type of heart failure, the fetus is at risk because of decreased placental perfusion leading to intrauterine growth retardation, fetal distress, or prematurity.

### Assessment Findings
#### *Left-sided heart failure*
- Decreased cardiac output
- Pulmonary hypertension
- Pulmonary edema
- Productive cough with blood-speckled sputum (if pulmonary capillaries rupture)
- Increased respiratory rate
- Fatigue
- Weakness
- Dizziness

- Increased heart rate
- Increased blood pressure
- Sodium and water retention
- Difficulty sleeping in any position (if pulmonary edema is severe)
- Paroxysmal nocturnal *dyspnea*

**Right-sided heart failure**
- Decreased cardiac output
- Jugular venous distention
- Enlarged liver and spleen
- Ascites
- Peripheral edema
- *Dyspnea* and pain (from enlarged liver)

### NURSING IMPLICATIONS

- Obtain a thorough *antepartal history and physical examination* to establish a baseline and ongoing to identify changes.
- Classify the client's heart failure based on her symptoms according to the criteria from the New York State Heart Association to predict pregnancy outcome.
- Continually assess the client for signs and symptoms indicating a worsening of her condition.
- Provide education regarding the need for close follow-up throughout pregnancy to prevent possible complications.
- Encourage the client to take frequent rest periods to minimize oxygen demands, lessen the strain of the increased burden on her heart, and prevent fatigue.
- Instruct the client to rest in the left lateral recumbent position to prevent hypotension and increase heart effort.
- Discuss activity level and instruct the client in specific activities that are allowed and that are to be avoided.
- Suggest that the client sleep with her head and chest elevated to aid in her breathing.
- Be aware that many physicians prefer that women with heart disease remain on complete bed rest after week 30 of the pregnancy to ensure that the pregnancy will be carried to term or at least past week 36 so that fetal maturity can be assured.
- Develop a sound nutritional program with the client to ensure adequate weight gain without excessive

weight gain that could overburden the heart and circulatory system.

- If the client was following a sodium-restricted diet before pregnancy, encourage her to continue it during pregnancy.
- Instruct the client in the need for prenatal vitamins and evaluate compliance.
- Warn the client taking cardiac medications before pregnancy that she may need to increase their maintenance dose because of the expanded blood volume during pregnancy.
- Instruct the client in any newly prescribed medications, such as cardiac glycosides or prophylactic antibiotics.
- Be aware that some physicians prescribe a course of prophylactic antibiotics for the client with valvular or congenital heart disease close to the anticipated date of birth to prevent possible postpartum subacute bacterial endocarditis.
- Educate the client regarding the need to avoid infection to prevent increased oxygen and cardiac demands.
- Assist the client with methods to reduce psychological stress; offer support and guidance throughout the pregnancy.
- Keep in mind that a client with heart disease should not push with contractions; anticipate the use of *epidural anesthesia* and low *forceps delivery.*
- During labor, closely monitor the client's *uterine contractions, fetal heart rate,* and vital signs; report any significant findings to the physician.
- Encourage the client to remain in the side-lying position during labor to reduce the possibility of supine hypotension syndrome.
- Anticipate the need for decreased activity and possibly anticoagulant and digitalis therapy following the birth to compensate for the dramatic rise in blood volume.
- Ambulate the client as soon as possible after birth and apply antiembolism stockings to prevent the formation of emboli.
- Be aware that if the client was not on prophylactic antibiotic therapy before birth, she will be started on them immediately postpartly to discourage

subacute bacterial endocarditis caused by introduction of microorganisms from the denuded uterus.

- Allow the client to see the baby immediately after birth to allay her fears and anxieties about possible fetal problems.
- Be sure to point out that acrocyanosis is normal in newborns so that the client does not interpret this as a cardiac inadequacy.
- Postpartally, administer a stool softener as prescribed to decrease straining.
- Provide education regarding the need for follow-up both for gynecologic health and cardiac status.

## HELLP SYNDROME

### DESCRIPTION

- HELLP syndrome refers to a variation of *pregnancy-induced hypertension (PIH)* named for the common symptoms that occur: hemolysis, elevated liver enzymes, and low platelets.
- It occurs in 4% to 12% of clients with *PIH,* or affects approximately 1 every 150 births.
- It is a complication of pregnancy that places the mother and fetus at high risk because it results in a maternal mortality rate as high as 20%.
- The cause of the syndrome is unknown, occurring in primigravidas and multigravidas, accompanying mild or severe preeclampsia, and occurring either in late pregnancy or immediately following birth.
- Complications associated with this syndrome include subcapsular liver hematoma, hyponatremia, and hypoglycemia.

### ASSESSMENT FINDINGS

- Nausea
- Epigastric pain
- General malaise
- Right upper quadrant tenderness
- Red blood cell hemolysis
- Thrombocytopenia (below 1000,000/mm³)
- Elevated alanine aminotransferase (ALT)
- Elevated serum aspartate aminotransferase (AST)

#### NURSING IMPLICATIONS

- Obtain a thorough *antepartal history and physical examination* to establish a baseline and ongoing to identify changes.
- Monitor complete blood cell count and serum liver enzyme studies for changes.
- During labor, closely monitor the client's *uterine contractions* and *fetal heart rate,* reporting any significant changes to the physician.
- Institute measures to prevent and control bleeding.
- Be aware that *epidural anesthesia* may not be possible because of the low platelet count and the high possibility of bleeding at the epidural site.
- Anticipate transfusion of fresh frozen plasm or platelets to improve the platelet count.
- If hypoglycemia is present, administer intravenous dextrose infusion as prescribed.
- Keep in mind that the infant is delivered as soon as feasible by either vaginal or *cesarean birth.*
- Provide comfort and support to the client and partner throughout to help minimize their anxieties and fears.

## HEMATOMA, PERINEAL

### DESCRIPTION

- Perineal hematoma is a collection of blood in the subcutaneous layer of tissue of the perineum.
- As a rule, the overlying skin is intact with no noticeable trauma.
- Such collections may be caused by injury to blood vessels in the perineum during birth; they are most likely to occur following rapid spontaneous deliveries and in women who have perineal varicosities.
- It may occur at an *episiotomy* or laceration repair site if a vein was pricked during repair.
- They can cause the woman acute discomfort and concern, but, fortunately, they usually represent only minor bleeding.

### ASSESSMENT FINDINGS

- Severe pain in perineal area
- Complaints of pressure between the legs
- Purplish discoloration

- Obvious swelling (ranging from 2 cm to as much as 8 cm in diameter)
- Tender, fluctuant area on palpation (may progress to firm globular area)

**NURSING IMPLICATIONS**

- Inspect the perineal area closely for presence of hematoma.
- Assess its size and degree of discomfort and notify the physician.
- Administer a mild analgesic as prescribed for pain relief.
- Apply an ice pack to help prevent further bleeding.
- Be aware that if the hematoma is large when discovered or continues to increase in size, the client may have to be returned to the delivery room to have the site incised and the bleeding vessel ligated.
- Reassure the client that even though the hematoma is causing her discomfort, her hospital stay probably will not be lengthened (unless it is extremely extensive).
- Advise the client that the hematoma should be absorbed over the next 6 weeks.
- If the episiotomy line is open to drain the hematoma, anticipate the line being left open and packed with gauze; prepare for packing removal in 24 to 48 hours.
- Provide clear instructions to the client before discharge regarding any measures needed to be performed at home.

# HEMOLYTIC DISEASE OF THE NEWBORN

**DESCRIPTION**

- Hemolytic disease of the newborn refers to a disorder most often caused by an ABO incompatibility.
- In the past, hemolytic disease of the newborn was most often caused by an *Rh incompatibility*. This has changed, however, because of the availability of prevention of Rh antibody formation.
- With this disease, the mother builds antibodies against the infant's red blood cells, leading to hemolysis of the cells causing severe anemia and hyperbilirubinemia.
- In most instances of ABO incompatibility, the maternal blood type is O and the fetal blood type is A; it may also occur when the fetus has type B or AB

blood. A reaction in an infant with type B blood is often the most serious.

- Hemolysis can be a problem in the first pregnancy because the antibodies to A and B cell types are naturally occurring and present from birth in individuals whose red cells lack these antigens; these antibodies are large and do not cross the placenta; therefore, the newborn is not born anemic, and hemolysis begins with birth when blood and antibodies are exchanged during the mixing of maternal and fetal blood as the placenta is loosened.

- In the case of *Rh incompatibility,* if the mother's blood type is Rh(D) negative and the fetal blood type is Rh positive (containing the D antigen), the introduction of fetal blood causes sensitization to occur, and the mother begins to form antibodies against the D antigen; after this sensitization, in a second pregnancy, there will be a high level of antibody D circulating in the mother's blood stream, which acts to destroy the fetal red blood cells early in the pregnancy as they cross the placenta and severely compromise the fetus by the end of the pregnancy.

## ASSESSMENT FINDINGS

### Rh incompatibility
- Rising maternal anti-Rh titer or rising level of antibodies (indirect Coombs' test) during pregnancy
- Positive direct Coombs' test (via umbilical cord blood sampling or testing of the newborn at birth)
- Maternal Rh-negative blood type
- Progressive jaundice within first 24 hours of birth
- Rapidly rising indirect bilirubin level (newborn)
- Enlarged liver and spleen (newborn)
- Extreme edema (newborn)
- Severe edema (newborn)
- Congestive heart failure (newborn)

### ABO incompatibility
- No anemia at birth
- Progressive jaundice within first 24 hours of birth
- Rapidly rising indirect bilirubin level

## NURSING IMPLICATIONS
- Keep in mind that most preterm newborns do not seem to be affected by ABO incompatibility.

- Antepartally, screen the mother for blood type and Rh factor.
- Obtain a thorough maternal history and physical examination and newborn assessment to establish a baseline and identify contributing factors.
- Obtain indirect bilirubin levels on the newborn and evaluate for changes; keep in mind that an increasing indirect bilirubin level rising above 20 mg/dl in a term newborn or above 12 mg/dl in a preterm newborn can result in brain damage from kernicterus.
- Be aware that infants with severe hemolytic disease tend to have a continuing drop in the hemoglobin concentration during the first 6 months of life, or their bone marrow fails to increase its production of erythrocytes in response to continuing hemolysis; anticipate the need for additional blood transfusions to correct this late anemia or treatment with erythropoietin to stimulate red blood cell production.
- Encourage early feeding to stimulate bowel peristalsis and remove bilirubin from the body.
- Advise the mother to suspend breast-feeding temporarily for 24 hours to reduce an accumulating indirect bilirubin level; suggest that the mother express her milk manually to maintain milk supply.
- Anticipate the use of phototherapy to stimulate the newborn's liver to process bilirubin.

    Cover the newborn's eyes to prevent damage to the retina; check frequently to be certain that the dressings have not slipped off or are causing corneal irritation.

    Assess the newborn's skin turgor and fluid balance status because stools are frequently loose, irritating the skin and placing the newborn at risk for dehydration.

    Assess the newborn's temperature to prevent overheating from the phototherapy lights.

    Offer glucose water every 2 hours as indicated to prevent dehydration.

    Remove the newborn from the lights and remove the eye patches for feeding to promote interaction with the mother and provide visual stimulation.

- If bilirubin levels are rising rapidly (if indirect bilirubin level exceeds 5 mg/100 ml at birth, 10 mg/100 ml at age 8 hours, 12 mg/100 ml at age 16 hours, and

15 mg/100 ml at age 24 hours or if serum bilirubin is rising more than 0.5 mg/hour in infants with Rh incompatibility or 1.0 mg/hour in infants with ABO incompatibility), prepare for an exchange transfusion to clear bilirubin.
- Keep the newborn warm during the procedure to minimize energy expenditure.
- Administer the blood at room temperature, warming only with a commercial blood warmer unit if necessary.
- Administer albumin 1 to 2 hours as prescribed before the procedure to increase the number of bilirubin binding sites and increase the efficiency of the transfusion.
- If the newborn is transferred to a regional center, ensure that a sample of the mother's blood accompany the newborn so that crossmatching on the mother's serum can be done there.
- Monitor the heart rate, respirations, and venous pressure throughout the procedure.
- After the procedure, monitor the newborn closely for umbilical vessel bleeding, redness, or inflammation of the cord suggesting infection.
- Assess glucose levels for approximately 2 hours after the procedure to prevent hypoglycemia resulting from the hyperglycemia from the preservative used during the transfusion and the newborn's response of insulin overproduction and subsequent hypoglycemia.
- Assess bilirubin levels for 2 to 3 days afterward to ensure that the level of bilirubin is not rising again and that no further transfusion is necessary.
- Administer erythropoietin as prescribed to increase new blood cell growth and prevent extended anemia.
- Provide teaching and emotional support to the parents throughout to help alleviate their anxieties and fears.
- If the newborn is transferred to another facility, assist the parents with contacting that facility to get updates on the newborn's condition.

## HEMORRHAGE, POSTPARTUM

### DESCRIPTION
- Hemorrhage is one of the most important causes of maternal mortality associated with childbearing.

- It is a possibility throughout pregnancy, but it is a major danger in the immediate postpartal period.
- With a normal birth, the average blood loss is 300 to 500 ml.
- Postpartal hemorrhage has been traditionally defined as any blood loss from the uterus greater than 500 ml within a 24-hour period.
- Hemorrhage may occur either immediately, within the first 24 hours, or late, during the remaining days of the 6-week puerperium.
- The greatest danger of bleeding is in the first 24 hours because of the grossly denuded and unprotected area left after detachment of the placenta.
- There are four main reasons for postpartal hemorrhage: *uterine atony, perineal lacerations, retained placental fragments,* and *disseminated intravascular coagulation (DIC).*

## ASSESSMENT FINDINGS

- Vaginal blood loss greater than 500 ml within the first 24 hours
- Signs of shock
- *Uterine atony*
- *Perineal lacerations*
- *Retained placental fragments*
- Low fibrinogen level (with *DIC*)

## NURSING IMPLICATIONS

- Perform a thorough postpartal examination immediately following delivery to establish a baseline and ongoing to detect changes.
- Obtain a history of labor and delivery to identify any contributing factors associated with postpartal hemorrhage.
- Assess the fundus for involution.
- Monitor *lochia,* including amount and color.
- Assess vital signs, including pulse and blood pressure, frequently for changes.
- Instruct the client about the need to report any changes in *vaginal bleeding.*
- Provide emotional support to help alleviate the client's fears and anxieties.
- Prepare to institute measures to treat the cause of the hemorrhage.

# HEMORRHAGIC DISEASE OF THE NEWBORN

## DESCRIPTION
- Hemorrhagic disease of the newborn is a disorder resulting from a deficiency of vitamin K, essential for the formation of prothrombin by the liver.
- A deficiency of vitamin K causes decreased prothrombin function and poor blood coagulation.
- Because the intestinal tract of a newborn is sterile, the newborn forms minimal vitamin K (formed by the action of bacteria in the intestine) until normal intestinal tract flora are established at about 24 hours of age.
- Newborns born to mothers taking anticonvulsive medication are at high risk for the condition because many of these medications interfere with vitamin K formation.

## ASSESSMENT FINDINGS
- Petechiae (from superficial bleeding into the skin)
- Conjunctival, mucous membrane, or retinal hemorrhage
- Vomiting fresh blood
- Black tarry stools
- Prolonged prothrombin time (usually day 2 to 5 of life)
- Prolonged or normal coagulation time

## NURSING IMPLICATIONS
- Obtain a thorough maternal medication history, specifically checking for the use of any anticonvulsive medications.
- Administer vitamin K to mothers taking anticonvulsants before delivery to help protect the newborn.
- Assess newborn's stools; keep in mind that distinguishing tarry stools from normal meconium stools is difficult in the first 1 to 2 days of life; however, if the newborn's stool does not change as it should from greenish black to the yellow color, or if the stool color changes normally then becomes black again, gastrointestinal bleeding should be suspected.
- Check stools for blood using guaiac or dipstick test.
- Administer 1 mg vitamin K intramuscularly to all newborns immediately after birth.

- Treat the newborn who develops hemorrhagic disease with vitamin K, intravenously or intramuscularly as prescribed.
- If bleeding is severe, anticipate the need for a transfusion of fresh, whole blood to increase the prothrombin level immediately.
- Handle the newborn gently to prevent further bleeding.
- Provide teaching and emotional support to the parents about the disease and treatment to help alleviate their fears and anxieties.

## HERPES SIMPLEX VIRUS (TYPE 2) (HSV) IN PREGNANCY

### DESCRIPTION

- HSV refers to genital herpes infection, a *sexually transmitted disease.*
- During pregnancy, it places the mother and fetus at high risk for complications.
- Herpes can be transmitted across the placenta to cause congenital infection in the newborn, or it can be transmitted at birth if lesions are present at the time in the vagina or on the vulva.
- Congenital herpes in the newborn results in a severe systemic infection that is often fatal.

### ASSESSMENT FINDINGS

- Painful, small, pinpoint vesicles surrounded by erythema on the vulva or in the vagina 3 to 7 days following exposure
- Positive enzyme-linked immunosorbent assay (ELISA)

### NURSING IMPLICATIONS

- Obtain a thorough history and physical examination to establish a baseline and ongoing to identify changes.
- Screen the pregnant client for exposure to the virus.
- Be aware that acyclovir, the drug of choice for treating HSV, is contraindicated in pregnancy because its effects on fetal growth are not yet documented.
- Encourage the client to use sitz baths to reduce the pain of infection.
- Instruct the client to have yearly Papanicolaou smears for the remainder of her life since the HSV type 2 infection is associated with the development of cervical cancer, even after one episode of infection.

- Anticipate *cesarean birth* for the client with active lesions.
- Provide teaching and support for the client throughout the pregnancy to alleviate anxieties and fears.

# HUMAN CHORIONIC GONADOTROPIN (HCG)

### DESCRIPTION
- HCG is the first hormone produced during pregnancy.
- It can be demonstrated in maternal blood serum and urine as early as the time of the first missed menstrual period (shortly after implantation has occurred) through about the 100th day of pregnancy.
- The mother's serum is completely negative for HCG within 1 to 2 weeks after delivery.
- Testing for HCG after delivery can be used as proof that all of the placental tissues has been delivered.
- HCG acts as a fail-safe measure to ensure that the corpus luteum of the ovary continues to produce estrogen and progesterone; if the corpus luteum should fail, falling levels of progesterone would cause endometrial sloughing, with loss of the pregnancy followed by a rise of pituitary gonadotropins to induce a new menstrual cycle.
- HCG also may play a role in suppressing the maternal immunologic response so that placental invasion will not be rejection.
- Because its structure is similar to luteinizing hormone of the pituitary gland, HCG exerts an effect on the fetal testes to begin testosterone production, causing maturation of the male reproductive tract.
- At about the 8th week of pregnancy, the outer layer of cells of the developing placenta begins to produce progesterone; the corpus luteum is no longer needed, so the production of HCG begins to decrease.
- Continually rising HCG levels after day 100 are used to diagnose *gestational trophoblastic disease.*

# HUMAN IMMUNODEFICIENCY VIRUS (HIV) INFECTION

### DESCRIPTION
- HIV infection in pregnancy places the woman and fetus as high risk for problems.

- HIV, which leads to acquired immunodeficiency syndrome (AIDS), is the most serious of the *sexually transmitted diseases* because it may be fatal to both the mother and the child.
- About 1.5 out of every 1000 women giving birth is HIV positive.
- The disease is caused by a retrovirus that infects T lymphocytes, disabling the body's ability to fight infection through either T cell or B cell activity.
- HIV may be contracted through sexual intercourse, by exposure to infected blood, by vertical transmission across the placenta to the fetus at birth, or by breast milk to the newborn.
- Women at greatest risk are those who have multiple sexual partners or a sexual partner who has multiple partners, use intravenous drugs, have a sexual partner who is a drug user, or engage in prostitution.
- Women are contracting this disease at much faster rates than formerly, and in many areas they are the fastest-growing category of HIV-infected persons.
- Early symptoms are more subtle and often difficult to differentiate from other diseases or even from the symptoms of early pregnancy.
- HIV infection progresses through various states from the initial invasion of the virus (perhaps accompanied by mild flu-like symptoms), seroconversion (converts from HIV serum negative to HIV serum positive 6 to 12 weeks after exposure), an asymptomatic latency period in which the woman appears to be disease free except for symptoms such as weight loss and fatigue, and finally a symptomatic period in which the woman develops opportunistic infections and malignancies.
- HIV is associated with low-birth-weight infant and *preterm infant.*
- The more serious the mother's disease symptoms, the more apt placental transmission is likely to occur.

### Assessment Findings

- Positive history for high-risk behavior
- Wasting syndrome (weight loss and fatigue)
- Positive enzyme-linked immunosorbent assay (ELISA) and Western blot analysis
- Presence of opportunistic infection(s)
- CD4 cell count below 300 cells/mm$^3$

### Nursing Implications

- Obtain a thorough history and physical examination to establish a baseline.
- Provide information about and discuss safer sex practices, testing of sexual contacts, and continuation or termination of pregnancy.
- Advise the client who is HIV positive not to become pregnant until more is learned about how to prevent transmission to the fetus.
- Ask the client who practices high-risk behavior if she wishes to be screened for the infection.
- Be aware that the client with HIV may also have contracted other *sexually transmitted diseases,* such as syphilis, gonorrhea, chlamydia, and hepatitis B, and should be screened as well for these.
- Question the client about cat ownership and mild flu-like symptoms because clients are also high risk for the development of toxoplasmosis and *cytomegalovirus* infections.
- Screen the client for *tuberculosis* because it occurs at a high rate in clients with HIV.
- If the client is already pregnant and HIV positive, anticipate the use of stronger than usual antibiotics because the woman does not have the usual response to antibiotics as a result of low lymphocyte levels.
- If the client's CD4 cell count is below 200 cells/mm$^3$, administer zidovudine (AZT) to prevent opportunistic infections, especially *Pneumocystis carinii* pneumonia (PCP).
- Monitor the client receiving AZT for thrombocytopenia and granulocytopenia from suppression of bone marrow function; anticipate the need for blood transfusion to help restore the levels; assess the neonate at birth for similar suppression.
- If pneumocystis develops, anticipate treating with trimethoprim/sulfamethoxazole; keep in mind that trimethoprim may be teratogenic in early pregnancy and that sulfamethoxazole may lead to increased bilirubin in the newborn if it is administered late in the pregnancy.
- Be aware that pentamidine, the drug of choice for PCP in nonpregnant clients, may be administered by aerosol.

- If the client has Kaposi's sarcoma, keep in mind that chemotherapy, although contraindicated in early pregnancy because of its potential for fetal injury, may be used later in pregnancy to halt the malignant growth.
- Use universal precautions when caring for the client and neonate to protect against the spread of HIV.
- Institute measures to reduce the possibility that the fetus may be exposed to maternal blood.
- Determine fetal age by *ultrasonography,* if possible, to prevent the risk of fetal exposure to maternal blood.
- Avoid use of *internal electronic fetal monitoring,* scalp blood sampling, *forceps delivery,* and *vacuum extraction* to prevent an open lesion of the fetal scalp.
- Be aware that because the client is at an increased risk for infection if membranes rupture early, membranes are usually not ruptured artificially.
- Anticipate the possibility of *cesarean birth* if the client is too fatigued to be able to push with the *second stage of labor* or if fetal distress occurs.
- Assess the client postpartally for endometritis because she is at risk for contracting any type of infection; also assess the client for anemia.
- Advise the HIV-positive client not to breast-feed her infant to prevent possible transmission.
- Offer support and guidance to the client throughout her pregnancy, encouraging her to continue with prenatal care in the hope that prenatal transmission to the fetus will not occur.
- Arrange for consultation with social services to assist the client during pregnancy.
- Instruct the client about signs and symptoms of infection and labor, including *rupture of membranes,* and need to notify the health care facility promptly should they occur.
- Encourage the client to keep follow-up appointments for herself and the neonate for further evaluation.

## HYDRAMNIOS

### Description
- Hydramnios refers to excessive amniotic fluid formation, usually an amount greater than 2000 ml or an amniotic fluid index above 24 cm.
- It is a complication of pregnancy that places the mother and fetus at high risk for problems.

- It can cause fetal malpresentation because of the extra uterine space it provides.
- It can lead to *premature rupture of membranes,* which adds the additional risks of infection and *prolapsed cord,* and *premature labor* because of the increased intrauterine pressure.
- Accumulation of amniotic fluid suggests difficulty with the fetus' ability to swallow, such as in anencephaly, tracheoesophageal fistula, or intestinal obstruction; absorb amniotic fluid; or excessive urine production, such as in fetuses of diabetic women.

## Assessment Findings
- Unusually rapid uterine enlargement
- Difficulty palpating small fetal parts
- Difficulty auscultating *fetal heart rate*
- Extreme shortness of breath
- Lower extremity varicosities
- Increased weight gain
- Positive *ultrasonography* for excess amniotic fluid

## Nursing Implications
- Obtain a thorough history and physical examination to establish a baseline.
- If the hydramnios is severe, anticipate admission to the hospital for bed rest and further evaluation.
- Advise the client to maintain bed rest to increase uteroplacental circulation and reduce pressure on the cervix preventing *premature labor.*
- Educate the client to report any sign of ruptured membranes or *uterine contractions.*
- Help the client avoid *constipation* by increasing fiber in the diet or using a stool softener as prescribed because there is a possibility that straining on defecation could increase uterine pressure and cause rupture of membranes.
- Assess vital signs and lower extremities for edema every 4 hours because the extremely tense uterus puts unusual pressure on the diaphragm and pelvic vessels.
- Anticipate the possibility of *amniocentesis* to remove some of the extra fluid, giving the client some relief from the increasing pressure.
- Be aware that a nonsteroidal anti-inflammatory agent such as indomethacin may be effective in reducing the amount of fluid formed.

- Be prepared for tocolysis with magnesium sulfate to prevent or halt *premature labor.*
- Keep in mind that in most instances of hydramnios, there is *premature rupture of the membranes* owing to excessive pressure followed by *premature labor;* anticipate the use of a thin needle inserted vaginally to pierce the membranes to allow for slow, continued release of fluid rather than a sudden loss of fluid and an accompanying *prolapsed cord.*
- Assess the newborn carefully for factors that made him or her unable to swallow in utero.
- Provide emotional support and teaching throughout the pregnancy to alleviate the client's fears and anxieties and ensure compliance with instructions.

## HYPERCHOLESTEROLEMIA IN PREGNANCY

### DESCRIPTION
- Hypercholesterolemia in pregnancy may occur in women who have an inherited tendency toward elevated cholesterol levels.
- During pregnancy, increasing progesterone levels cause a further elevation of cholesterol, which can result in an increased tendency to form gallstones and an increased risk of cardiovascular disease.
- Hypercholesterolemia is a common nutritional problem affecting pregnancy.
- Preventing these complications during pregnancy is important because an attack of gallstones causes extremely sharp pain, and surgery to remove them during pregnancy can be a threat to the fetus because of the necessary anesthesia.

### ASSESSMENT FINDINGS
- Elevated serum cholesterol levels
- Family history of elevated cholesterol levels

### NURSING IMPLICATIONS
- Obtain a thorough history and physical examination to establish a baseline.
- Screen the pregnant client for elevated cholesterol levels.
- Keep in mind that a woman who has had difficulty with hypercholesterolemia before pregnancy may need to continue to reduce her intake of fat during pregnancy to prevent any further increases.

- Encourage daily exercise.
- Teach the client about methods to reduce cholesterol, such as broiling meats rather than frying, using a minimum of salad oils, removing the skin from poultry, avoiding lunch meats, and substituting margarine for butter.
- Advise the client with a family history of high cholesterol levels to limit intake of eggs to one per week.
- Advise the client to check with the physician about continuing cholesterol-lowering drugs during pregnancy because they may be teratogenic to the fetus.
- Assess the client for adequate weight gain.
- Evaluate the client's diet and make sure that she does include some oil daily to provide a source of linoleic acid.

# HYPEREMESIS GRAVIDARUM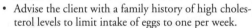

### DESCRIPTION
- Hyperemesis gravidarum, sometimes called pernicious vomiting, is nausea and vomiting of pregnancy that is prolonged past week 12 of pregnancy or is so severe that dehydration, ketonuria, and significant weight loss occur within the first 12 weeks.
- Women with this disorder tend to have increased thyroid function owing to thyroid-stimulating properties of *HCG* hormone.
- It occurs at an incidence of 1 in 200 to 300 women.
- It is associated with intrauterine growth retardation.

### ASSESSMENT FINDINGS
- Severe nausea and vomiting interfering with nutrition
- Elevated hematocrit (from hemoconcentration)
- Reduced serum levels of sodium, potassium, and chloride
- Hypokalemic acidosis
- Polyneuritis (from deficiency of vitamin B)
- Weight loss
- Urine positive for ketones

### NURSING IMPLICATIONS
- Obtain a thorough history and physical examination to establish a baseline.
- Determine the extent of the client's nausea and vomiting, including how much, when it occurs,

how long it lasts and how many times, and amount of food eaten.

- Allow the client nothing by mouth (NPO) for the first 24 hours after hospitalization.
- Administer intravenous solutions, such as Ringer's lactate with added vitamin B.
- Anticipate administering a sedative, such as phenobarbital, to encourage rest and an antiemetic, such as chlorpromazine.
- Assess intake and output closely for changes.
- Advance the client's diet as tolerated.
- Anticipate the need for total parenteral nutrition if dietary measures are unsuccessful.
- Assist the client with measures to minimize stress.
- Encourage the client to use small food servings with foods at appropriate temperatures to minimize the effects of cooking food on the client.
- Store the emesis basin out of sight but within easy reach of the client.
- Allow the client to express how she feels about this problem and about how it feels to be pregnant and live with the ever-present nausea.
- If necessary, refer the client for counseling.

# HYPERTENSIVE VASCULAR DISEASE, CHRONIC

### DESCRIPTION

- Chronic hypertensive vascular disease is a preexisting condition that places the client at high risk during pregnancy.
- Women with chronic hypertensive disease come into pregnancy with an elevated blood pressure of 140/90 mm Hg or above.
- Hypertension of this kind is usually associated with arteriosclerosis or renal disease.
- It tends to be a problem with the older pregnant woman.
- Chronic hypertensive disease can compromise fetal well-being resulting from poor placental perfusion during the pregnancy.

### ASSESSMENT FINDINGS

- Blood pressure readings of 140/90 mm Hg or above

- Retinal changes
- Chronic proteinuria
- Edema

## NURSING IMPLICATIONS

- Obtain a thorough history and physical examination to establish a baseline and ongoing for changes.
- Encourage follow-up with the client's medical physician, in addition to the client's obstetrician, throughout pregnancy.
- Assist with scheduling of *ultrasonography* for *evaluation of fetal well-being* at 16 to 24 weeks.
- Obtain baseline renal function studies, such as creatinine clearance and a 24-hour urine protein early in pregnancy and ongoing about every 8 weeks throughout the pregnancy.
- Evaluate the client's medication regimen before pregnancy; assist client with any changes in medication therapy, such as using methyldopa, pregnancy risk category B, as an antihypertensive agent instead of thiazide or loop diuretics, which are pregnancy risk category D.
- Avoid using calcium channel blockers because they may decrease uterine blood flow.
- If blood pressure becomes extremely elevated as pregnancy progresses, encourage complete bed rest, on the left side to promote diuresis.
- Be sure that pregnancy may have to be terminated to prevent the risk of cerebral vascular accident in some clients.
- Keep in mind that the infants of women with chronic hypertensive disease tend to have retarded fetal growth or can be stillborn or register fetal distress during labor from poor placental perfusion.
- Anticipate the possibility of *abruptio placentae* during pregnancy because of the increased vascular tension leading to rupture of the capillaries supplying the placenta.
- Provide emotional support and teaching to the client and partner throughout pregnancy to help alleviate fears and anxieties.
- Discuss alternative contraceptive measures because women with chronic hypertensive vascular disease are advised not to take *oral contraceptives.*

# HYPERTENSION, PREGNANCY-INDUCED (PIH)

## DESCRIPTION

- PIH, a systemic disorder affecting almost all organs, is a complication of pregnancy that places the mother and fetus at high risk for problems.
- It is a condition unique to pregnancy that occurs in 5% to 10% of pregnancies in the United States.
- Originally, it was called toxemia because researchers pictured a toxin of some kind being released by the woman in response to the foreign protein of the growing fetus with the toxin leading to the typical symptoms. Its cause, however, is still unknown.
- In PIH, the symptoms result from peripheral vascular spasm, but why this vascular spasm occurs is difficult to establish.
- With PIH, there is a loss in the reduced responsiveness to blood pressure changes, resulting in vasoconstriction and dramatic increases in blood pressure.
- The vascular effects of vasospasm include vasoconstriction and poor organ perfusion which leads to increased blood pressure.
- The kidney effects of vasospasm include decreased glomeruli filtration rate, increased permiability of glomeruli membrane, increased serum blood urea nitrogen, uric acid creatine which leads to decreased urine output and proteinuria.
- The interstitial effects include diffusion of fluid from the blood stream into interstitial tissue which leads to edema.
- Blood supply to organs is reduced; this is followed by tissue hypoxia in the maternal vital organs leading to poor placental perfusion, possibly reducing the fetal nutrient and oxygen supply.
- PIH is classified according to one of four levels depending on the woman's symptoms (rarely occurring before 20 weeks of pregnancy): gestational hypertension, mild preeclampsia, severe preeclampsia, and eclampsia.
- Eclampsia is the most severe classification with maternal mortality as high as 15%.

- Eclampsia can result in death of the woman from cerebral hemorrhage, circulatory collapse, or renal failure.
- Fetal prognosis is poor because of hypoxia and *fetal acidosis;* if the fetus must be delivered before term, all the risks of the immature infant will be faced.
- In preeclampsia, fetal mortality is approximately 10%; if eclampsia develops, fetal mortality increases to as high as 25%.
- PIH also may occur 10 to 14 days after birth, although most postpartal hypertension occurs in the first 48 hours after birth.

### ASSESSMENT FINDINGS

#### For gestational hypertension
- Blood pressure 140/90 mm Hg or systolic blood pressure elevated 30 mm Hg or diastolic pressure elevated 15 mm Hg above prepregnancy level
- No proteinuria

#### For mild preeclampsia
- Blood pressure 140/90 mm Hg or systolic blood pressure elevated 30 mm Hg or diastolic pressure elevated 15 mm Hg above prepregnancy level
- Proteinuria of 1+ to 2+ on a random sample
- Weight gain more than 2 lb/week in second trimester and 1 lb/week in third trimester
- Mild edema in upper extremities or face

#### For severe preeclampsia
- Blood pressure of 160/110 mm Hg (noted on two readings taken 6 hours apart while the client is on bed rest)
- Proteinuria 3+ to 4+ on a random sample and 5 g on a 24-hour urine sample
- Oliguria (500 ml or less in 24 hours)
- Cerebral or visual disturbances, such as headache, blurred vision
- Pulmonary edema with shortness of breath
- Extensive peripheral edema
- Hepatic dysfunction
- Thrombocytopenia
- Epigastric pain, nausea and vomiting
- Marked hyperreflexia

### For eclampsia
- Blood pressure greater than 160/110 mm Hg
- Tonic-clonic seizure

## Nursing Implications
- Obtain a thorough *antepartal history and physical examination* on the initial visit to establish a baseline and ongoing to detect changes.
- Assess the client's blood pressure for changes at each antepartal visit, comparing each reading with prepregnancy or early pregnancy levels.
- Monitor the client's weight gain for changes; keep in mind that a weight gain of more than 2 lb/week in the second trimester or 1 lb/week in the third trimester usually indicates abnormal tissue fluid retention.
- Assess the client's deep tendon reflexes frequently for changes and report any hyperactive reflexes immediately.
- Instruct the client to eat a high-protein, moderate-sodium diet to replace the protein lost in the urine.
- Be aware that at one time, stringent sodium restriction was advised to reduce edema, but this is no longer true because stringent sodium restriction may activate the angiotensin system and result in increased blood pressure, further compounding the problem.
- Encourage bed rest in the left lateral recumbent position to avoid uterine pressure on the vena cava and prevent supine hypotension syndrome; keep in mind that bed rest aids in increasing the excretion of sodium, encouraging diuresis.
- Provide emotional support to the client and family; assist with arrangements for work, child care, and other difficulties that may arise from the need for bed rest.
- Explain to the client and family about all aspects of the disorder, including need for compliance and close follow-up, treatments, procedures, and possible effects on the client and the fetus.

### For mild preeclampsia
- Instruct the client regarding need for follow-up visits every 2 weeks; inform the client to notify the physician immediately if symptoms worsen.

### For severe preeclampsia
- Anticipate the need for the client to be hospitalized.

- Prepare for *amniocentesis* to determine fetal maturity or *induction of labor* if the pregnancy is 36 weeks or more.
- Place the client in a private room away from the sounds of women in labor or crying newborns so that she can rest without any possible stimuli that may trigger a seizure.
- Darken the room but avoid using bright lights, which may trigger a seizure.
- Monitor the client's blood pressure at least every 4 hours for changes; monitor blood pressure every hour if it is fluctuating.
- Obtain blood studies, as prescribed, such as complete blood count, platelet count, liver function, blood urea nitrogen, creatinine, and fibrin degradation products to assess for renal and liver function and development of *disseminated intravascular coagulation (DIC),* which often accompanies severe vasospasm; obtain daily hematocrit levels, as prescribed, to monitor blood concentration.
- Anticipate obtaining a type and crossmatch because the client is at risk for premature separation of placenta and resulting hemorrhage.
- Prepare the client for daily examination of optic fundus to detect signs of arterial spasm, edema, or hemorrhage.
- Insert an indwelling urinary catheter to allow for accurate recording of output; report any output less than 600 ml per 24 hours or 30 ml/hour.
- Obtain urine specimens for urinary proteins and specific gravity; collect a 24-hour urine specimen, as prescribed, for protein and creatinine clearance to evaluate renal function.
- Monitor daily weights, using the same scale, at the same time each day for changes.
- Assess fetal status using a continuous *external electronic fetal monitor* or Doppler auscultation every 4 hours.
- Prepare the client for nonstress test or biophysical profile to assess uterine sufficiency.
- Administer oxygen as prescribed to maintain adequate fetal oxygenation and prevent bradycardia.
- Institute safety measures, such as raised siderails, to prevent injury should the client experience a seizure.

- Administer intravenous fluids, as prescribed; monitor the site closely for swelling or irritation, which can trigger a seizure in a severely preeclamptic client.
- Administer hydralazine (Apresoline) or diazoxide (Hyperstat) as prescribed to reduce blood pressure; if used, monitor blood pressure closely, not allowing diastolic blood pressure to go lower than 80 to 90 mm Hg to prevent inadequate placental perfusion.
- Prepare to administer magnesium sulfate (drug of choice) to reduce edema and block peripheral neuromuscular transmission.
- Before administering, check to make sure that urine output is above 25 to 30 ml/hour, respirations are above 12/minute, the client can answer questions, ankle clonus is minimal, and deep tendon reflexes are present; continue these assessments every hour if a continuous infusion is used.
- Administer first intravenously as a loading or bolus dose over 15 to 20 minutes followed by a continuous infusion piggybacked into a main infusion using an electronic pump or controller.
- Monitor serum blood levels and maintain at 4 to 7 mg/100 ml.
- Keep a solution of 10 ml of 10% calcium gluconate at the bedside as the antidote for magnesium toxicity.
- Advise the anesthesiologist, on the day of birth, that the client has been receiving magnesium sulfate; if it is given within 2 hours of delivery, the neonate may be born depressed.
- Carefully assess the fetus for loss of variability in heart rate immediately following magnesium sulfate therapy and for late decelerations with labor contractions.
- Continue magnesium sulfate therapy for 12 to 24 hours following delivery as prescribed to prevent eclampsia; prepare to taper and then discontinue the dose.
- Instruct the client to delay breast-feeding until the medication is discontinued.
- Promote relaxation and provide emotional support, explaining all events and procedures; allow the client to verbalize about her feelings.

*For eclampsia*
- Monitor the client for signs of impending seizure, including a sudden rise in blood pressure, sharp rise in

temperature, blurred vision, severe headache, hyperactive reflexes, epigastric pain, nausea, premonition that something is happening, and urinary output less than 30 ml/hour.

- During the tonic phase:

    Administer oxygen by face mask to protect the fetus; monitor oxygen saturation by pulse oximetry.

    Turn the client on left side or abdomen to prevent aspiration.

    Attach an *external electronic fetal* monitor to evaluate the fetus.

- During the clonic phase:

    Continue to monitor the client closely for changes indicating maternal or fetal distress.

    Continue oxygen administration.

    Administer magnesium sulfate or diazepam (Valium) intravenously as prescribed as an emergency anticonvulsant.

- During the postictal phase:

    Monitor the client's level of consciousness; keep in mind that the client is semicomatose and cannot be roused except by painful stimuli for at least 1 hour and sometimes up to 4 hours.

    Assess the client for the possibility of premature placental separation and *uterine contractions.*

    Keep in mind that the painful stimuli of contractions may initiate another seizure.

    Continuously monitor *uterine contractions* and *fetal heart rate* for changes.

    Assess for *vaginal bleeding* every 15 minutes.

    Keep the client on her side to promote drainage of mouth secretions.

    Allow nothing by mouth (NPO).

    Be aware that when talking at the client's bedside, she may be able to hear even though she does not respond.

    Prepare for delivery once the client's condition stabilizes if the gestational age of the pregnancy is more than 36 weeks.

    Keep in mind that the preferred method of delivery is vaginal.

    Assess the client for spontaneous labor; if it does not occur, prepare for *rupture of membranes* or *induction of labor* by intravenous oxytocin; if this is ineffective, prepare for *cesarean birth.*

# HYPERTHYROIDISM IN PREGNANCY

### DESCRIPTION
- Hyperthyroidism in pregnancy is more commonly seen in pregnancy than *hypothyroidism.*
- It is a preexisting disorder that places the mother and fetus at high risk for problems.
- If undiagnosed, the woman may develop *heart failure* because her rapid heart rate cannot adjust to the increasing serum volume occurring with pregnancy.
- The woman is more prone to symptoms of *pregnancy-induced hypertension* and *premature labor.*

### ASSESSMENT FINDINGS
- Rapid heart rate
- Exophthalmos
- Heat intolerance
- Nervousness
- Heart palpitations
- Weight loss

### NURSING IMPLICATIONS
- Obtain a thorough history and physical examination to establish a baseline.
- Before pregnancy, obtain results of radioactive uptake of [131]iodine; this is not used during pregnancy because the fetal thyroid will also incorporate this drug, resulting in possible destruction of the fetal thyroid.
- Keep in mind that the drugs used to treat hyperthyroidism are teratogens, crossing the placenta and possibly leading to congenital hypothyroidism and enlarged thyroid gland in the fetus; use the lowest dose possible.
- Advise the client to keep a careful record of doses taken so that she does not forget or accidentally duplicate a dose.
- Be aware that surgical treatment to reduce the functioning of the maternal thyroid may be done (not the treatment of choice, however, because of the need for *general anesthesia*); it might be done as an interpregnancy procedure, if the client desires more children.
- If the client's thyroid function was not regulated during pregnancy, assess the neonate for symptoms

of hyperthyroidism, such as jitteriness, tachypnea, and tachycardia, because of the excess stimulation received in utero.

- Obtain a fetal cord blood sample to reveal the level of thyroxine and thyroid-stimulating hormone and indicate if treatment is necessary.
- Advise the client on antithyroid drugs not to breast-feed because these drugs are excreted in breast milk.

## HYPOTHYROIDISM IN PREGNANCY

### DESCRIPTION

- Hypothyroidism is a rare condition in young adults; those women with symptoms of untreated hypo-thyroidism are often unable to conceive because they are anovulatory.
- Because their thyroid cannot increase function to maintain even normal limits, the woman often has a history of early *spontaneous abortion.*
- Most women with hypothyroidism take thyroxine to supplement what their body cannot produce.

### ASSESSMENT FINDINGS

- Easily fatigued
- Tendency for obesity
- Poor tolerance to cold
- Dry skin
- Extreme nausea and vomiting (during pregnancy)

### NURSING IMPLICATIONS

- Be aware that a woman with hypothyroidism needs to consult with her physicians (obstetrician and internist) when she is planning on becoming pregnant.
- Advise the client to come for early diagnosis and close follow-up as soon as she suspects that she is pregnant (1 week past her missed menstrual period).
- Anticipate the need for increased dosage of thyroxine for the duration of pregnancy to simulate the effect that would normally occur in pregnancy; instruct the client in the importance of this increased dosage.
- Following pregnancy, instruct the client that the dosage of thyroxine is tapered gradually back to the prepregnancy level.
- Be certain that the client does not continue her pregnancy dose, or she will pass the line between normal thyroid function and develop hyperthyroidism.

# INCOMPETENT CERVIX

## DESCRIPTION

- Incompetent cervix refers to premature *cervical dilation,* which means the cervix cannot hold a fetus until term.
- It is associated with increased maternal age and congenital development or endocrine factors.
- Trauma to the cervix, such as might have occurred with a dilatation and curettage or traumatic delivery, is often the cause.
- When *uterine contractions* occur, after a short labor the fetus is born, but unfortunately at approximately week 20 of pregnancy when the fetus is too immature to survive.
- Following the loss of one child as a result of an incompetent cervix, a surgical operation, cervical cerclage, can be performed to prevent this from happening again.
- Still newer techniques allow the purse-string sutures to be set before the woman is pregnant, giving her the added assurance that she will not begin aborting before week 14 of pregnancy.
- Women who are discovered to have *cervical dilation* but with membranes still intact at a prenatal visit may have emergent cerclage (sutures placed in the cervix even at this late point).

## ASSESSMENT FINDINGS

- Painless *cervical dilation*
- Pink-stained vaginal discharge
- *Rupture of membranes* and discharge of amniotic fluid
- *Uterine contractions*

## NURSING IMPLICATIONS

- Obtain a thorough history and physical examination to establish a baseline and identify history of incompetent cervix.
- Anticipate *ultrasonography* at approximately 12 to 14 weeks of pregnancy to confirm the health of the fetus.
- Prepare the client for McDonald or Shirodkar procedure, purse-string sutures placed in the cervix by the vaginal route under *regional anesthesia.*

- Anticipate the removal of these sutures at about weeks 38 to 39 of pregnancy so that the fetus may deliver vaginally; if sutures are left in place, prepare the client for *cesarean birth.*
- Be certain to ask clients who are reporting painless *vaginal bleeding* (the symptoms of *spontaneous abortion*) whether they have had past cervical operations.
- Instruct the client in signs and symptoms to report to the physician.
- Provide emotional support and guidance to the client and her partner to help alleviate fears and anxieties.

# INEFFECTIVE UTERINE FORCE

## DESCRIPTION

- Ineffective uterine force refers to *uterine contractions,* the basic force that moves the fetus through the birth canal, that are abnormal.
- There are three types of abnormal *uterine contractions:* hypotonic, hypertonic, and uncoordinated contractions.
- Hypotonic contraction is usually low or infrequent, not increasing beyond two or three in a 10-minute period; the resting tone remains below 10 mm Hg and strength does not rise about 25 mm Hg.
- Hypotonic contractions are most apt to occur during the active phase of labor, when analgesia has been administered too early (before *cervical dilation* of 3 to 4 cm) or when bowel or bladder distention is present and prevents descent or firm *engagement.* They may occur in a uterus overstretched by a *multiple gestation,* a larger than usual single fetus, or *hydramnios* or in a lax uterus from grand multiparity.
- Hypotonic contractions increase the length of labor because so many of them are necessary to achieve *cervical dilation;* because of the exhaustion from a long labor, the uterus may not contract as effectively, thus increasing the woman's chance for *postpartal hemorrhage;* with the cervix dilated for a long period, both the uterus and the fetus are prone to infection.
- Hypertonic contractions are marked by an increase in resting tone to more than 15 mm Hg, occurring frequently and most commonly seen during the latent phase of labor.

- Hypertonic contractions occur because the muscle fibers of the myometrium do not repolarize following a contraction. They tend to be painful and do not allow for optimal artery filling, which may cause the fetus to begin to suffer anoxia early in the latent phase.
- Uncoordinated contractions involve contractions with more than one pacemaker initiating the contraction, or receptor points in the uterus are acting independently of the pacemaker; they occur so closely together that they do not allow good cotyledon filling, making it difficult for the woman to rest or use breathing exercises between contractions.
- All of these types of *uterine contractions* are ineffective, resulting in an ineffective labor.

### NURSING IMPLICATIONS
- Obtain a thorough history and physical examination to establish a baseline and ongoing for changes.
- Assess the client's complaints of and monitor *uterine contractions,* including frequency, duration, and intensity.

***If the client is experiencing hypotonic contractions***
- Anticipate *ultrasonography* to rule out cephalopelvic disproportion.
- Prepare for infusion of oxytocin for *labor induction and augmentation.*
- Assist with artificial *rupture of membranes* to speed labor.
- After delivery, palpate the uterus every 15 minutes and assess *lochia* carefully to ensure that postpartal contractions are adequate for uterine involution.

***If the client is experiencing hypertonic contractions***
- Assist the client with relaxation as much as possible; be aware that the client may become frustrated or disappointed with her breathing exercises for childbirth because they are ineffective in keeping her pain free.
- Evaluate the client's complaints of pain in relation to the quality of her contractions; apply a uterine and *external electronic fetal monitor* if her complaints seem out of proportion for at least a 15-minute interval to ensure that the resting phase of the contractions is adequate and the fetal pattern is not showing late decelerations.

- Encourage the client to rest, and anticipate administering analgesia and sedation.
- Provide comfort measures, such as dimming the lights and decreasing noise and stimulation.
- Anticipate *cesarean birth* if deceleration in *fetal heart rate,* an abnormally long *first stage of labor,* or lack of progress with pushing occurs.
- Provide support to the client and partner and assist them with understanding that although the contractions are strong, they are ineffective and not achieving *cervical dilation.*

***If the client is experiencing uncoordinated contractions***

- Apply a uterine and *external fetal electronic monitor* to assess the rate, pattern, resting tone, and fetal response to contractions for at least a 15-minute interval.
- Anticipate oxytocin administration to help stimulate a more effective and consistent pattern of contractions with a better lower resting tone.
- Provide education and guidance to the client and partner throughout the labor process to promote a safe delivery.

# INFLAMMATORY BOWEL DISEASE IN PREGNANCY

### DESCRIPTION

- Inflammatory bowel disease in pregnancy is a preexisting condition that places the mother and fetus at high risk for problems.
- Crohn's disease (inflammation of the terminal ileus) and ulcerative colitis (inflammation of the distal colon) occur most often in young adults between ages 12 and 30 years (childbearing years).
- The cause of these diseases is unknown, but an autoimmune process may be responsible.
- In both diseases, the bowel develops shallow ulcers and the woman experiences chronic diarrhea, weight loss, occult blood in stool, nausea, and vomiting.
- If the bowel ulceration is extreme, obstruction and fistula formation with peritonitis can occur.
- Crohn's disease can lead to malabsorption, particularly of vitamin $B_{12}$.
- Both diseases can interfere with fetal growth if malabsorption occurs.

### Nursing Implications
- Obtain a thorough *antepartal history and physical examination* to establish a baseline and identify any preexisting conditions.
- Obtain stool specimens for occult blood.
- Monitor the client's weight and report any loss of weight or inability to gain weight.
- Be prepared to administer total parenteral nutrition, as prescribed, to give the gastrointestinal tract total rest.
- Reassure the client that if she is taking sulfasalazine that she may continue during her pregnancy without fear of fetal injury.
- Advise the client, however, that the dosage of sulfasalazine is reduced close to birth because it may interfere with bilirubin binding sites and cause neonatal jaundice.

## INLET CONTRACTION

### Description
- Inlet contraction is defined as a narrowing of the anteroposterior diameter of the pelvis to less than 11 cm, or a maximum transverse diameter of 12 cm or less.
- Inlet contraction is a problem associated with the passage that can cause dystocia, resulting in a failure to progress in labor.
- Inlet contraction is ordinarily due to rickets early in life or an inherited small pelvis.
- The fetal head normally engages at weeks 36 to 38 of pregnancy and proves that the pelvic inlet is adequate.
- When *engagement* does not occur in a primigravida, either a fetal abnormality (larger-than-usual head) or a pelvic fetal abnormality (smaller-than-usual pelvis) is suspected of causing the lack of *engagement*.

### Nursing Implications
- Obtain a thorough *antepartal history and physical examination* to establish a baseline.
- Assist with obtaining pelvic measurements antepartally.
- Be aware that every primigravida should have pelvic measurements taken and recorded before week 24 of pregnancy so that a birth decision can be made.

- Provide guidance and support to the client and partner to alleviate any fears or anxieties.

# INTRAPARTAL FETAL ASSESSMENT

## DESCRIPTION

- Fetal assessment must be undertaken along with maternal assessment as soon as the woman is admitted to a labor unit.
- Although passive in labor, a fetus is subjected to extreme pressure by *uterine contractions* and passage through the birth canal.
- Compression of the umbilical cord and the placenta by *uterine contractions* may compromise the fetal blood and oxygen supply during these times.
- Assessing and interpreting *fetal heart rate* patterns involve evaluating three parameters: the baseline rate, variables in the baseline rate (long-term and short-term), and periodic changes in the rate (acceleration and deceleration).
- By monitoring fetal blood composition, hypoxia in the fetus may be determined before it is apparent on an electrocardiogram or an *external monitoring system.*

## NURSING IMPLICATIONS

- Monitor *fetal heart rate* as well as *uterine contractions* by *electronic fetal monitoring* to ascertain that the *fetal heart rate* remains within normal limits to ensure that labor is not too strenuous for the fetus.
- Assess *fetal heart rate* every 30 minutes during beginning labor, every 15 minutes during active labor, and every 5 minutes during the *second stage of labor.*
- Assess the baseline rate, variables in the baseline rate as well as periodic changes in the baseline rate.
- Assist with fetal blood sampling to determine fetal blood pH and any fetal hypoxia.
- Assist with fetal scalp stimulation to assess acid-base balance in the fetus.
- Perform acoustic stimulation tests to demonstrate that the fetus is reactive.
- Assure the client that the *electronic fetal monitoring* will help her to see that her fetus is doing well.
- Know that infants who have had fetal blood sampling performed should not be delivered by *vacuum*

*extraction* because this can lead to renewed bleeding at the puncture site.

# INTRAPARTAL HISTORY AND PHYSICAL EXAMINATION

## DESCRIPTION

- If the woman is in active labor, the history taken on arrival may be the only history taken until after the baby is born.
- The history taken at this point should include a review of the woman's pregnancy, both physical and psychological events, and a review of past pregnancies, general health, and family medical information.
- Following history taking, the woman needs a thorough physical examination, including pelvic examination to confirm the presentation and position of the fetus and determine the stage of dilation.

## NURSING IMPLICATIONS

- Be patient when obtaining information from the client, pausing to wait until the *uterine contraction* subsides.
- Obtain a current pregnancy history, including gravidity and para, a description of the pregnancy, pattern and place of prenatal care, any complications, childbirth education, plans for labor, and child care.
- Document prior pregnancies (numbers, dates, types of birth, any complications, and outcomes including sex and birth weight of children) and current health status of previous children.
- Ask the client about her past health history and document any previous surgery, heart disease, *diabetes, anemia, tuberculosis,* kidney disease, hypertension, or *sexually transmitted disease* or if she is at high risk for *human immunodeficiency virus (HIV) infection* (multiple sexual partners, history of intravenous drug use, or a sexual partner who uses intravenous drugs).
- Ask the client if any family member has heart disease, a blood dyscrasia, diabetes, kidney disease, cancer, allergies, seizures, congenital defects, or mental retardation.
- Assess the client's overall appearance and note if she is pale, tired, ill, or frightened; any edema; dehydration; or the presence of any open lesions.

- Palpate for enlargement of lymph nodes to detect the possibility of infection.
- Inspect the mucous membranes of the mouth looking for any lesions (herpes) and the conjunctiva of the eyes for color.
- Auscultate the lungs to be certain they are clear and assess the heart sounds.

- Palpate the client's breasts and assess for any lumps or cysts and note their presence for evaluation later (they may be enlarged milk glands).
- Estimate fetal size by *fundal height.*
- Assess *fetal presentation and position* by performing *Leopold's maneuvers.*
- Palpate and percuss the bladder area to detect a full bladder.
- Assess for abdominal scars as abdominal or pelvic surgery can leave adhesions.
- Assess skin turgor for dehydration.
- Inspect the lower extremities for edema and varicose veins.

# INTRAUTERINE DEVICE (IUD)

## DESCRIPTION

- The IUD, a contraceptive method, is a small, plastic object inserted into the uterus through the vagina where it remains in place.
- It is thought that the presence of a foreign object in the uterus interferes with the ability of an ovum to develop as it travels the fallopian tube.
- Another theory related to the IUD's mechanism is that the endometrium of the uterus forms cytoxins that attack and destroy a growing ovum.
- A third theory suggests that a local sterile inflammatory action may result that prevents implantation.
- Copper added to the device appears to affect sperm mobility, decreasing the possibility of sperm being able to traverse the uterine space.
- The two types of IUDs currently approved for use are the Progestasert, a T-shaped device of permeable plastic with a drug reservoir of progesterone in the stem that must be replaced yearly, and the Copper T380, a T-shaped plastic device wound with copper that may stay in for 4 years.

- IUDs place a woman at higher risk than usual for pelvic inflammatory disease (PID) and *ectopic pregnancy.*
- An IUD is not recommended for women who have not been pregnant; who have multiple sexual partners; who have a history of PID; whose uterus is known to be distorted in shape; who have dysmenorrhea, menorrhagia, or a history of *ectopic pregnancy;* who have valvular heart disease, or who have *anemia.*

### NURSING IMPLICATIONS

- Be aware of personal feelings and values about contraception and sexuality.
- Be sensitive to the client's personal, religious, cultural, and social beliefs about birth control.
- Answer the client's questions honestly and openly.
- Perform a thorough history, including the date of the client's last menstrual period.
- Perform a pelvic examination and obtain a Papanicolaou smear and uterine measurements before IUD insertion.
- Know that the device should be inserted during the menstrual flow or before the client has had coitus following the menstrual flow.
- Know that the device can also be inserted immediately after childbirth or before the cervical os closes again.
- Caution the client that she may feel a sharp cramp as the device is passed through the internal cervical os but will not feel it after it is in place.
- Instruct the client that once in place, the device should not be visible except for the dark string that protrudes from the uterus into the vagina.
- Instruct the client that she should check for the string after her menstrual flow and to report any difficulty in locating the string.
- Caution the client that she may notice some spotting or uterine cramping the first 2 or 3 weeks after insertion.
- Caution the client that if she is experiencing the initial spotting that may occur for a few weeks after insertion she should use additional contraception such as vaginal foam.

- Advise the client that she may have heavier than usual menstrual flow for 2 or 3 months accompanied by dysmenorrhea following insertion.
- Advise the client to take precautions to avoid toxic shock syndrome while she has the device in place.
- Instruct the client to be aware of the most common signs of PID, such as fever, lower abdominal tenderness, and dyspareunia.

# LABOR DANGER SIGNS, FETAL

### DESCRIPTION
- Certain signs, evident during labor, indicate the fetal response to labor and birth.
- When these signs deviate too far from normal responses during labor, they may indicate that the fetus is in danger.
- Changes in *fetal heart rate* and a pattern of variable decelerations noted on *electronic fetal monitoring*, *meconium staining* of the amniotic fluid, changes in fetal activity, and *fetal acidosis* are signs of possible danger to the fetus.

### ASSESSMENT FINDINGS
- *Fetal heart rate* >160 bpm (fetal tachycardia)
- *Fetal heart rate* <120 bpm (fetal bradycardia)
- Late or variable decelerations
- Meconium-stained amniotic fluid
- Fetal hyperactivity
- Fetal scalp blood pH below 7.2 (*fetal acidosis*)

### NURSING IMPLICATIONS
- Perform *electronic fetal monitoring* and assess the monitor strip for any deviations from normal.
- Report any abnormal findings to the physician.
- Assist with fetal scalp pH analysis to assess fetal distress.
- Be prepared to administer oxygen by mask to the mother if there is any question that the fetus may be experiencing distress.
- Provide support and reassurance to the client who is fearful for the well-being of her fetus.
- Provide the client and partner with an ongoing account about the well-being of the fetus.

- Be prepared to institute emergency delivery procedures if the fetus is becoming increasingly compromised.

# LABOR DANGER SIGNS, MATERNAL

### DESCRIPTION
- There is a wide variation among individuals in the pattern of labor contractions and maternal responses to labor and birth.
- Certain signs indicate that the course of events is deviating too far from normal.
- Changes in blood pressure (normally rises slightly during the *second* [pelvic] *stage of labor* owing to pushing efforts); pulse (usually increases slightly during the *second stage of labor* owing to the exertion involved); and *uterine contractions,* which normally become more frequent, intense, and longer as labor progresses, may indicate problems.
- A pattern of relaxation must take place between *uterine contractions* so that the intervillous spaces of the uterus can fill and maintain adequate supply of oxygen and nutrients for the fetus.
- Other signs, such as a *pathologic retraction ring,* a full bladder, or a woman who is becoming increasingly apprehensive despite clear explanations of unfolding events, may be signals of problems.

### ASSESSMENT FINDINGS
- Systolic blood pressure >140 mm Hg and diastolic ≥90 mm Hg
- Increase in systolic blood pressure of >30 mm Hg or diastolic increase >15 mm Hg
- Falling blood pressure
- Pulse >100 bpm
- *Uterine contractions* that have become less frequent, less intense, shorter in duration, or longer than 70 seconds
- *Pathologic retraction ring*
- Full bladder
- Increasing apprehension

### NURSING IMPLICATIONS
- Assess maternal vital signs frequently and report any deviations from normal values.

- Monitor *uterine contractions* by *electronic monitoring* and report any change in contraction frequency, intensity, or duration, especially if the relaxation period becomes shortened by longer contractions.

- Observe the client's abdominal contour while auscultating *fetal heart rate* and note any indentation across the abdomen indicating a possible *pathologic retraction ring.*
- Assess for bladder distention evidenced by a round bulge on the lower anterior abdomen.
- Encourage the client to express her fears and worries to assess better the source of her apprehension.
- Provide ongoing information to the client and her partner about her labor progress and fetal well-being.

# LABOR, DYSFUNCTIONAL

## DESCRIPTION
- Dysfunctional labor is a complication of labor involving a problem with power.
- It can occur at any point in labor but is generally classified as primary (occurring at the onset of labor) or secondary (occurring late in labor).
- *Ineffective uterine force,* such as with hypotonic, hypertonic, or uncoordinated contractions, plays a role in dysfunctional labor.
- Dysfunctional labor during the *first stage of labor* can be seen as a prolonged latent phase, protracted active phase, prolonged deceleration phase, secondary arrest of dilation, or prolonged descent.
- Dysfunctional labor during the *second stage of labor* can be seen as an arrest of descent or failure of descent.

## ASSESSMENT FINDINGS
- Low or infrequent contractions (not increasing beyond two or three in a 10-minute period) with a resting tone below 10 mm Hg and strength not rising above 25 mm Hg (hypotonic contraction)
- Frequent contractions with a resting tone greater than 15 mm Hg (hypertonic contractions)
- Erratic contractions (uncoordinated contractions)
- Latent phase longer than 20 hours in a nullipara and 14 hours in a multipara
- Active phase with *cervical dilation* not occurring at a rate of 1.2 cm/hour or more in a nullipara

or 1.5 cm/hour or more in a multipara or lasting longer than 12 hours in a primipara or 6 hours in a multipara

- Deceleration phase extending beyond 3 hours in a nullipara and 1 hour in a multipara
- No progression of *cervical dilation* for more than 2 hours
- Fetal descent occurring at a rate less than 1.0 cm/hour in a nullipara or less than 2.0 cm/hour in a multipara
- No descent occurring for 2 hours in a nullipara or 1 hour in a multipara
- Expected descent not started (*engagement* or movement beyond 0 station has not occurred)

### NURSING IMPLICATIONS

- Anticipate the use of oxytocin to augment labor for hypotonic contractions, uncoordinated contractions, a prolonged active phase, or arrest of descent (if no contraindications).
- Provide *evaluation of fetal well-being* through *electronic fetal monitoring.*
- Provide rest, analgesia, and comfort measures, decreasing lights and stimulation, if the client is experiencing hypertonic contractions or prolonged descent.
- Promote uterine resting and administer adequate fluids for the client with a prolonged latent phase of labor.
- Prepare for possible *cesarean birth* if the cause of the protracted active phase or arrest of descent is fetal malposition or cephalopelvic disproportion.
- If the client is experiencing prolonged descent, anticipate *rupture of membranes;* encourage use of semi-Fowler's, squatting, or kneeling position to help speed descent.
- Assess the time of the client's last meal to determine the possibility of depleting glucose stores with a prolonged labor; if the client is in early labor, allow the client to have some high-carbohydrate fluid such as orange juice or begin an intravenous infusion of glucose.
- Institute measures to minimize stress offering support and explanations of all events and treatments; for example, praise breathing attempts, breathe with the

client, give backrubs, change sheets, and use cool washcloths.
- Urge the client to lie on her side to increase blood supply to the uterus and prevent hypotension.
- Encourage the client to void every 2 hours to keep the bladder empty and aid labor progress.
- Monitor the client for possible fluid and electrolyte losses from prolonged labor; test all voidings for glucose, protein, ketones, and specific gravity for changes.
- Assess the client's abdomen for *pathologic retraction ring* and report immediately.
- Provide emotional support, guidance, and education to the client and partner about the progress of labor and measures to aid the progress.

## LABOR, FALSE

### DESCRIPTION
- Labor is a series of events by which *uterine contractions* expel the fetus and placenta from the woman's body.
- Regular contractions cause progressive *cervical dilation* and sufficient muscular forces to allow the baby to be pushed to the outside.
- False labor involves *uterine contractions,* but these contractions, although strong, are irregular.
- Other characteristics of *true labor* are not present.

### ASSESSMENT FINDINGS
- Irregular *uterine contractions,* located chiefly in the abdomen, with variable intensity and long intervals
- *Uterine contractions* not affected by or relieved with walking
- Bloody show not present (if present, usually brownish rather than bright red)
- No cervical changes
- Decreased number of *uterine contractions* with sedation

### NURSING IMPLICATIONS
- Obtain a thorough history and physical examination to establish a baseline.
- Assess frequency, duration, and intensity of *uterine contractions.*
- Monitor *fetal heart rate.*
- Assess for *cervical dilation* and signs of *true labor.*

- Provide support to the client who is experiencing *false labor;* it is discouraging for a woman who is having what seems like *uterine contractions* only to be told that she is not in *true labor.*
- Anticipate client discharge to home.
- Reassure the client that misinterpreting labor signals is a natural mistake.
- Remind the client that if false contractions have become strong enough to be mistaken for *true labor,* true labor must not be far away.
- Instruct the client in signs of *true labor* and when to return to the health care institution.

## LABOR, INDUCTION AND AUGMENTATION

### DESCRIPTION

- Induction of labor means that labor is artificially started; augmentation refers to assisting a labor that has started spontaneously to be more effective.
- The primary reasons for inducing labor are the presence of preeclampsia, eclampsia, severe *hypertension* or *diabetes,* Rh sensitization, prolonged *rupture of membranes,* intrauterine growth retardation, and postmaturity, or situations in which it seems risky for the fetus to remain in utero.
- Augmentation of labor or assistance to make *uterine contractions* stronger may be necessary when *uterine contractions* are too weak or infrequent to be effective.
- Before induction of labor is begun, the following conditions must be present:
  - The fetus is in a longitudinal lie and at a point of extrauterine viability.
  - The cervix is ripe or ready for birth.
  - The presenting part is *engaged.*
  - There is no cephalopelvic disproportion (CPD).
- Labor induction is a procedure that should be used cautiously with *multiple gestation, hydramnios,* grand parity, maternal age older than 35 years, and presence of uterine scars because it carries a risk of *uterine rupture,* a decrease in the fetal blood supply from cotyledon filling, and premature separation of the placenta.
- Labor induction or augmentation may be accomplished by the administration of oxytocin or by *amniotomy (rupture of membranes).*

- Cervical ripening implies a change in the cervical consistency from firm to soft and is necessary for dilation and coordination of *uterine contractions.*
- Cervical ripening may be accomplished by "stripping the membranes" or separating the membranes from the lower uterine segment or by placing hygroscopic suppositories (suppositories of seaweed that swell on contact with cervical secretions) or prostaglandin gel to urge dilation gradually and gently.

## ASSESSMENT FINDINGS

- History of a condition that would necessitate labor induction
- Ineffective or weak *uterine contractions*
- Presence of conditions allowing for induction or augmentation of labor

## NURSING IMPLICATIONS

- Obtain a health history, including information about fetal maturity.
- Assist with obtaining *ultrasonography* or a lecithin-sphingomyelin ratio to assess fetal maturity.
- Document the use of dilators and sponges, recording the type used and amount used as well as the time.
- Be aware the oxytocin should be administered intravenously (never intramuscularly) so that its effect can be quickly discontinued to prevent hyperstimulation.
- Know that the half-life of oxytocin is about 3 minutes so that with intravenous administration the functioning level ends this quickly.
- Prepare the intravenous solution by using a dilute intravenous form of oxytocin, such as Pitocin or Syntocinon, as prescribed.
- Piggyback the oxytocin solution with a maintenance intravenous solution so that if the oxytocin needs to be shut off abruptly, the intravenous line will not be lost.
- Use an infusion pump to control the small amount of fluid given and to ensure a uniform infusion rate even when the client changes position.
- Make sure that a physician is nearby during the entire procedure to ensure safety.
- Monitor *fetal heart rate* and *uterine contraction* by *electronic monitoring.*

- Assess and document maternal vital signs every 15 minutes.
- Be prepared to administer a beta$_2$-adrenergic receptor drug such as terbutaline sulfate (Brethine) to decrease myometrial activity, as prescribed.
- Assess the client for signs of water intoxication, such as headache and vomiting, since oxytocin has an antidiuretic effect.
- Record intake and output and test urine specific gravity.
- Assure the client that once contractions start by these methods, they are basically normal *uterine contractions.*

## LABOR, MECHANISMS OF (CARDINAL MOVEMENTS OF LABOR)

### DESCRIPTION

- Mechanisms of labor refer to the position changes necessary for passage of the fetus through the birth canal allowing for the smallest diameter of the fetal head (cephalic presentation) always to present to the smallest diameter of the birth canal.
- The cardinal movements of labor are descent, flexion, internal rotation, extension, external rotation, and expulsion.
- Descent is the downward movement of the *biparietal diameter* of the fetal head to within the pelvic inlet; full descent occurs when the fetal head extrudes beyond the dilated cervix and touches the posterior vaginal floor.
- As descent occurs, pressure from the pelvic floor causes the fetal head to bend forward onto the chest; the smallest anteroposterior diameter (the suboccipitobregmatic diameter) is the one presented to the birth canal in this flexed position.
- During descent, the head enters the pelvis with the fetal anteroposterior head diameter in a diagonal or transverse position; the head flexes as it touches the pelvic floor or just below the symphysis pubis, bringing the shoulders into the optimum position to enter the inlet.
- As the occiput is born, the back of the neck stops beneath the pelvic arch and acts as a pivot for the rest of the head; the head thus extends, and the foremost parts of the head, the face and chin, are born.

- In external rotation, almost immediately after the head is born, the head rotates back to the diagonal or transverse position and the aftercoming shoulders are thus brought into an anteroposterior position, allowing the anterior shoulder to be delivered, probably by the downward flexion of the head.
- Once the shoulders are delivered, the rest of the baby is delivered easily and smoothly because of its smaller size.
- The expulsion stage is the end of the pelvic division of labor.

## LABOR, PRECIPITATE

### DESCRIPTION

- A precipitate labor and birth occurs when *uterine contractions* are so strong that the woman delivers with only a few rapidly occurring contractions.
- It is often defined as a labor that is completed in fewer than 3 hours.
- Such rapid labor is likely to occur with multiparity and may follow *induction of labor* by oxytocin or *amniotomy*.
- Rapid labor poses a risk to the fetus because subdural hemorrhage may result from the sudden release of pressure on the head; the woman may sustain lacerations of the birth canal.
- Forceful contractions may lead to premature separation of the placenta and both maternal and fetal risk.
- A precipitate labor can be predicted from a labor graph during the active phase of dilation using the rate as a guideline.

### ASSESSMENT FINDINGS

- Dilation rate >5 cm/hour (nullipara)
- Dilation rate >10 cm/hour (multipara)

### NURSING IMPLICATIONS

- Monitor *uterine contractions* and *fetal heart rate* using *electronic fetal monitoring*.
- Be prepared to administer a tocolytic to reduce the force of contractions.
- Use a labor graph to chart labor progress, especially during the active phase of dilation, to possibly predict a precipitate delivery.
- Inform the multiparous client at 28 weeks of pregnancy that her labor might be shorter than a previous

one so that she can make plans for rapid transportation to the hospital or alternative birthing center.
- Prepare the birthing room for a rapid delivery for the grand multiparous client or a client who has a history of precipitous delivery.

## LABOR, PRELIMINARY SIGNS

### DESCRIPTION
- Preliminary signs of labor are subtle signs that indicate that labor is beginning.
- These include *lightening,* increased level of activity, *Braxton Hicks contractions,* and ripening of the cervix.
- In primiparas, *lightening,* or settling of the fetal presenting part to the level of the ischial spines, occurs approximately 10 to 14 days before labor begins.
- The pregnant woman may have an increased level of activity or burst of energy which is due to an increase in epinephrine release (preparing her body for the work of labor) that is initiated by a decrease in progesterone produced by the placenta.
- In the last week or two before labor begins, the woman usually notices extremely strong *Braxton Hicks contractions,* which she may interpret as *true labor* contractions.
- Braxton Hicks (*false labor*) contractions begin and remain irregular; are felt first abdominally and remain confined to the abdomen; often disappear with ambulation; do not increase in duration, frequency, or intensity; and do not achieve *cervical dilation.*
- *True labor* contractions begin irregularly but become regular and predictable; are felt in the lower back and sweep around to the abdomen in a wave; continue no matter what the woman's activity; increase in duration, frequency, and intensity; and achieve *cervical dilation.*
- Ripening of the cervix is an internal sign seen only on pelvic examination.
- Throughout pregnancy, the cervix feels softer than normal, with the consistency of an earlobe until, at term, it becomes still softer until it can be described as "butter-soft" and tips forward.

### ASSESSMENT FINDINGS
- Increase in activity level
- *Braxton Hicks contractions*

- "Butter-soft" cervix, tipped forward
- *Lightening*

**NURSING IMPLICATIONS**

- Instruct the client in the preliminary signs of labor throughout the antepartal period.
- Assist with pelvic examination to determine *cervical dilation.*
- Assess *fetal heart rate* and *uterine contractions.*
- Remind the client that if false contractions have become strong enough to be mistaken for *true labor,* true labor must not be far away.
- Explain to the client that misinterpreting labor signals is a natural mistake.
- Explain to the client the difference between *true labor* and *false labor.*
- Teach the client how to recognize signs of preliminary and *true labor.*
- Offer the client sympathetic support if she is told that she is not experiencing *true labor* contractions but *Braxton Hicks contractions.*

## LABOR, PREMATURE (PRETERM)

**DESCRIPTION**

- Preterm labor is labor that occurs before the end of week 37 of gestation, occurring in approximately 9% of all pregnancies.
- A woman is considered to be in preterm labor if she is having *uterine contractions* that cause *cervical effacement and dilation.*
- Preterm labor is always serious because if it results in the infant's birth, the infant will be premature.
- The reason for preterm labor is unclear; however, it is frequently associated with dehydration, urinary tract infection, and chorioamnionitis (infection of the fetal membranes and fluid).
- Currently, medical attempts can be made to stop labor if fetal membranes are intact, fetal heart sounds are good, there is no evidence that bleeding is occurring that will affect maternal or fetal welfare, the *cervical dilation* is not more than 3 to 4 cm, and *cervical effacement* is not more than 50%.
- A drug that is able to halt labor is referred to as a tocolytic agent. The following drugs are tocolytic agents:

Calcium channel blockers such as nifedipine
(Procardia), although use is limited owing to
premature closing of fetal ductus arteriosus

Central nervous system depressants such as
magnesium sulfate

Prostaglandin antagonist such as indomethacin
(Indocin)

Beta-adrenergics such as ritodrine hydrochloride
(Yutopar) and terbutaline (Brethine)

- Preterm labor should be halted if possible until the fetus reaches a level of maturity that will allow it to survive in an outside environment.
- If preterm labor cannot be halted, and if the fetus is
  immature, a *cesarean birth* may be planned to reduce
  pressure on the fetal head.

### ASSESSMENT FINDINGS

- Persistent, dull, low backache
- Vaginal spotting
- Feeling of pelvic pressure or abdominal tightening
- Menstrual-like cramps
- Increase in vaginal discharge
- *Uterine contractions*
- Intestinal cramping

### NURSING IMPLICATIONS

- Instruct the client about signs she should watch
  for that may indicate that she is experiencing preterm
  labor.
- Administer intravenous fluid replacement as prescribed to hydrate the client and possibly minimize
  the release of oxytocin.
- Explain the necessity of complete bed rest whether the
  client is hospitalized or cared for at home.
- Obtain vaginal and cervical cultures as well as a clean-
  catch urine specimen to rule out infection.
- Obtain baseline blood data (hematocrit, serum glucose, potassium, sodium chloride, carbon dioxide).
- Record *fetal heart rate* and *uterine contractions* by *electronic monitoring* and observe and report any tachycardia, late decelerations, or variable decelerations.
- Make sure that the client meets the safe criteria for tocolytic administration—no *vaginal bleeding,* no elevated temperature, and no *cervical dilation* of more
  than 4 cm or *cervical effacement* of more than 50%.

- Administer oral tocolytics as prescribed and explain the regimen and the purpose to the client.
- Administer intravenous tocolytic therapy as prescribed by a piggyback method, connected to a mainline intravenous solution so that it can be stopped immediately if effects such as tachycardia or arrhythmia occur.
- Use a microdrip and an automatic infusion pump to administer tocolytic therapy to ensure a constant infusion.
- Obtain maternal vital signs every 15 minutes during the time the flow rate is being increased and thereafter every 30 minutes until contractions halt.
- Auscultate the lungs to assess for rales possibly indicating pulmonary edema.
- Report a maternal pulse rate of more than 120 bpm, blood pressure below 90/60 mm Hg, chest pain, dyspnea, rales, or cardiac arrhythmias while the client is receiving intravenous tocolytics.
- Instruct the client about using a "Daily Fetal Movement Count" to assess fetal welfare.
- Provide adequate nutrition and instruct the client about maintaining a nutritious diet while on bed rest.
- Administer betamethasone to the client as prescribed to attempt to hasten the production of surfactant in the fetal lungs.
- Explain to the client that she may experience some tachycardia and hypotension with the use of ritodrine hydrochloride (Yutopar) or terbutaline (Brethine).
- Be certain that the client with threatened preterm labor is maintaining bed rest while at home.
- Arrange for a homemaker service to care for children or an aging parent, which will help the client to rest completely.

## LABOR, PHYSIOLOGIC RESPONSES TO

### DESCRIPTION

- Labor is a local process involving the abdomen and reproductive organs; however, its intensity also has systemic effects on the cardiovascular, hematopoietic, urinary, musculoskeletal, gastrointestinal, and neurologic systems.
- Labor also has a physiologic effect on temperature regulation and fluid balance.

### Assessment Findings
- Increased cardiac output
- Blood loss 300 to 500 ml
- Increased blood pressure
- White blood count 25,000/mm³ to 30,000/mm³
- Increased respiratory rate
- Increased temperature (slight)
- Diaphoresis
- Urine specific gravity high normal (1.020 to 1.030)
- Concentrated urine with protein trace to 1+
- Increased back pain or pain at pubis during walking
- Loose bowel movement with contractions
- Pain due to contractions and birth

### Nursing Implications
- Monitor maternal vital signs frequently and assess for any deviations other than normal responses to labor.
- Be aware of normal hemodynamic responses to labor and be aware of their implications for the client who has a cardiac problem at the time of birth.
- Consider placing the client in an upright position during the *second stage of labor* if she experiences hypotension during pushing.
- Be aware that a normal rise in white blood count during labor may not be indicative of infection.
- Encourage appropriate breathing patterns to help avoid severe hyperventilation (which can lead to nausea and vomiting) or lengthy breath-holding.
- Administer supplemental fluid replacement by intravenous therapy, as prescribed.
- Instruct the client that intravenous therapy is a prophylactic measure and that the catheter, if inserted, should not interfere with ambulation or turning.
- Ask the client to void every 2 hours during labor to avoid bladder overfilling, which may lead to lessened bladder tone in the postpartal period.
- Explain to the client why she should not eat or why she should limit her intake during labor.

## LABOR, PSYCHOLOGICAL RESPONSE TO

### Description
- Labor can lead to emotional distress because it represents the beginning of a major life change for the woman and her partner.

- Even for the most organized woman, pain reduces her ability to cope and may make her quick-tempered and quick to criticize things around her.
- Increased fatigue, fear, and cultural influences affect a woman's psychological response to labor.

- As birth approaches, a woman is generally tired from carrying extra pounds of weight with her and not being able to sleep well because of an active baby; this results in sleep hunger making it difficult for the woman to perceive situations clearly or to adjust rapidly to new situations.
- Labor moving faster or slower than expected can be a frightening experience and may promote worry and anxiety that her infant may die or be born with an abnormality or that she may not meet her own behavioral expectations.
- Cultural factors influence a woman's experience of labor.

#### Nursing Implications

- Be aware of cultural variations when caring for the client in labor.
- Arrange for an interpreter if the woman does not speak English, which may help lessen her fears.
- Admit the client quickly to a birthing room in an environment free from outside interference, which may help her to focus, control her breathing patterns, and reduce the pain of early contractions as well as help her to organize coping strategies.
- Instruct the client about the labor process early in labor because it serves as a reminder that childbirth is not strange.
- Provide continuing reinforcement and information that the client's labor is progressing as expected.
- Provide ongoing information about the well-being of the fetus during labor to help to allay fears.
- Provide the client with information about procedures to give her knowledge about what is happening and help her feel more in control.

## LABOR, FIRST STAGES OF

#### Description

- The first stage of labor is traditionally called the stage of *cervical dilation*.

- It is divided into three phases: the latent, active, and transition phases.
- The latent phase begins at the onset of regularly perceived *uterine contractions* and ends when rapid *cervical dilation* begins; it lasts approximately 6 hours in a nullipara and 4.5 hours in a multipara.

  > *Uterine contractions* are mild and short (20 to 30 seconds in length).
  > *Cervical effacement* occurs.
  > Cervix dilates to 3 to 4 cm.

- The active phase begins with rapid *cervical dilation* accompanied by stronger *uterine contractions;* it lasts approximately 3 hours in a nullipara and 2 hours in a multipara.

  > *Cervical dilation* goes from 4 cm to 8 cm.
  > *Uterine contractions* are stronger (45 to 60 seconds long and 3 to 5 minutes apart).
  > Increased vaginal secretions and *spontaneous rupture of membranes* may occur.

- In the transition phase, maximum *cervical dilation* occurs and *cervical contractions* reach their peak of intensity.

  > *Cervical dilation* goes from 8 to 10 cm.
  > *Uterine contractions* reach their peak of intensity (60 to 90 seconds long and 2 to 3 minutes apart).
  > *Rupture of membranes* occurs at full dilation (if they have not already done so).
  > *Cervical effacement* is completed.

- The peak of the transition phase can be identified by a slight slowing in the rate of *cervical dilation* when 9 cm is reached; as the woman reaches the end of this stage, an irresistible urge to push begins to occur.

### Nursing Implications

- Obtain a thorough history and physical examination to establish a baseline.
- Instruct the client about the signs and symptoms of *true labor* and need to notify the physician.
- Throughout the antepartal period, prepare the client physically and psychologically for labor.
- On admission to the labor and delivery unit, obtain necessary laboratory tests, including urinalysis, complete blood count, serologic test for syphilis, and type and crossmatch, if indicated.

- Perform perineal preparation and enema, if indicated.
- Assist as necessary with the physical examination, such as *Leopold's maneuvers,* vaginal examination, and assessment of pelvic adequacy.
- Assess the client for spontaneous *rupture of membranes;* anticipate *amniotomy* if this does not occur.
- Monitor maternal and fetal status frequently, assessing vital signs, *fetal heart rate, uterine contractions,* and progress through labor; interpret any changes in fetus and client.
- Assess degree of *cervical dilation, cervical effacement,* station, and *fetal presentation.*
- Allow the client to feel like she has some control over the situation; encourage breathing techniques with contractions and position changes.
    > If the client is in early labor, allow her to be out of bed, walking, sitting up in a bed or chair, kneeling, squatting, or in whatever position she prefers.
    > If the client's membranes have ruptured, encourage her to lie on her side until a fetal monitor shows good baseline variability and no variable decelerations.
- Encourage the client to void spontaneously, if possible, every 2 to 4 hours; assess for bladder distention and anticipate catheterization if client is unable to void.
- Institute measures to prevent hyperventilation; encourage the client to end all breathing sessions with a long deep cleansing breath to help restore carbon dioxide balance.
- Reduce stress by helping the client to perceive labor clearly and providing the opportunity for her partner to provide support as well as being personally available to provide support to the client and partner.
- Provide comfort measures such as touch and wiping forehead with a cool cloth to provide support.
- Respect and promote the partner's activities, acquainting the client and partner with the unit, supplies, and procedures.
- Assess the client's and partner's preparation for childbirth, including attendance at childbirth education classes; review information as necessary.
- Support the client's pain management efforts; administer analgesics as prescribed.

- Limit oral intake of fluids to prevent aspiration if emergency anesthesia is necessary; apply lotion to lips or allow client to suck on hard candy or iced chips to relieve discomfort of dry mouth.
- If labor is prolonged, administer intravenous glucose infusions if oral intake is contraindicated.
- Prepare the client and partner for procedures and events to follow, such as *amniotomy,* and birth preparation.

# LABOR, SECOND STAGE OF

### DESCRIPTION

- The second stage of labor is the period from full *cervical dilation* and *cervical effacement* to the birth of the infant.
- At first, there may be a short period during which the intensity, duration, and frequency of *uterine contractions* may slow somewhat.
- The urge to bear down also grows stronger at this time as the fetus descends into the lower pelvis.
- With retraction of the cervix over the presenting part, fetal descent and negotiation of the pelvis occur rapidly.
- During this stage of labor, all of the woman's energy is directed toward pushing and delivering her child.

### ASSESSMENT FINDINGS

- Full *cervical dilation* and *cervical effacement*
- Momentary nausea and vomiting
- Uncontrollable urge to push or bear down
- Bulging perineum
- Anus everted
- Stool present at anus (possible)
- Crowning

### NURSING IMPLICATIONS

- Monitor maternal and fetal status frequently, assessing vital signs, *fetal heart rate,* and *uterine contractions;* interpret any changes in *electronic monitoring* of fetus and mother.
- Encourage the client as she attempts to push during this stage of labor by informing her of her progress and fetal well-being.

- Instruct the client about effective pushing by telling her to push with the contractions and rest between them.
- Instruct the client not to hold her breath but to breathe out during her contraction while pushing.
- Instruct the multipara whose second stage is moving too quickly to pant with her contractions rather than pushing.
- Assess degree of *cervical dilation, cervical effacement,* station, and *fetal presentation.*
- Graph labor progress after each cervical examination.
- Assess fetal descent and observe for bulging perineum as infant begins to crown.
- Move the client to the delivery room or prepare the birthing room for the impending birth.
- Position the client in the preferred birthing position, remembering to raise both legs at the same time if in the lithotomy position to reduce strain on the client's back.
- Prepare the perineum by cleaning with an antiseptic solution before birth.
- Note and record the time of the birth as determined by the delivery of the entire body of the infant.
- Encourage maternal infant bonding immediately after birth.

## LABOR, THIRD STAGE OF

### DESCRIPTION

- The third stage of labor, or the placental stage, begins with the birth of the infant and ends with the delivery of the placenta.
- There are two separate phases of the third stage; placental separation and placental expulsion.
- Placental separation occurs automatically as the uterus resumes contractions.
- Lengthening of the umbilical cord, a sudden gush of vaginal bleeding, or a change in the shape of the uterus indicates the placenta has loosened and is ready to deliver.
- If the placenta separates first at its center and last at its edges, it tends to fold on itself like an umbrella allowing the shiny fetal surface to present at the vaginal opening and is called a Schultze's placenta.

- If the placenta separates first at its edges, it slides along the uterine surface and presents at the vagina with the maternal side evident and is called a Duncan's placenta.
- Placental delivery or expulsion occurs by the natural bearing down effort of the mother or by gentle pressure on the contracted fundus by the physician.
- If the placenta does not deliver spontaneously, it can be removed manually.

### Assessment Findings

- Uterus palpable as firm, round mass inferior to level of umbilicus
- Beginning of *uterine contractions* again
- Lengthening of umbilical cord
- Sudden gush of vaginal blood
- Change in shape of uterus to discoid shape

### Nursing Implications

- Determine a baseline maternal blood pressure before administration of oxytocin.
- Administer oxytocin intramuscularly or intravenously as prescribed.
- Note and record the time of delivery of the placenta.
- Be aware that pressure should never be applied to a uterus in an uncontracted state or the uterus may evert and hemorrhage.
- Be aware of the cultural beliefs of the couple and ask them if the placenta is of importance to them before it is destroyed.
- Be aware of the client's feelings after birth about the infant and placenta, especially during *episiotomy* repair if necessary.
- Encourage maternal-infant bonding.
- Keep the client and her partner informed of the well-being of the infant if it should develop any problems.
- Lower the client's legs from the stirrups both at the same time to prevent back injury.
- Assess vital signs and palpate the fundus for size, consistency, and position.
- Cleanse the client's perineum and vulva from back to front of any secretions with warm sterile water and a sterile compress, dry with a sterile towel, and apply a perineal pad to absorb vaginal discharge (*lochia*).

- Reassure the client that the shaking and chills she might be experiencing is a normal response probably due to the sudden release of pressure on pelvic nerves after birth or excess epinephrine production during labor.
- Cover the client with a warm blanket and transfer her to a recovery room if she delivered in a delivery room.

## LABOR, TRIAL

### DESCRIPTION
- Trial labor refers to the process allowed by the physician for the woman in labor to see whether labor can progress normally.
- A trial labor is allowed if a woman has a borderline (just adequate) inlet measurement, and the *fetal lie* and position are good.
- A trial labor is allowed to continue as long as descent of the presenting part and *cervical dilation* are occurring.
- If after a definite period (6 to 12 hours) adequate progress in labor cannot be documented, the woman is scheduled for a *cesarean birth*.

### NURSING IMPLICATIONS
- Monitor fetal heart sounds and *uterine contractions* during the trial labor.
- Assess *fetal heart rate* carefully after *rupture of membranes* because if the fetal head is high, there is increased danger of *prolapsed cord* and anoxia in the fetus.
- Offer support to the client and partner that a *cesarean birth* is not an inferior method of birth but an alternative method if the trial labor is not successful.

## LABOR, TRUE

### DESCRIPTION
- Signs of true labor involve uterine and cervical changes.
- The surest sign that labor has begun is the initiation of effective, productive, involuntary *uterine contractions*.
- As the cervix softens and ripens, the mucus plug that filled the cervical canal during pregnancy is expelled.

- The exposed cervical capillaries seep blood owing to pressure exerted by the fetus resulting in blood mixed with mucus, which takes on a pink tinge and is referred to as "show" or "bloody show."
- Labor may begin with the *rupture of membranes,* which the woman may experience by either a sudden gush or scanty, slow seeping of clear fluid from the vagina.
- Early *rupture of the membranes* can be advantageous if it causes the fetal head to settle snugly into the pelvis and can shorten labor.

### Assessment Findings

- Rhythmic, productive, involuntary *uterine contractions,* beginning irregularly but becoming regular and predictable; continue regardless of level of activity, increasing in duration, frequency, and intensity
- Complaints of pain first in lower back and sweeping around to abdomen in a wave
- *Rupture of membranes*
- Pink-tinged or bloody show
- *Cervical dilation*

### Nursing Implications

- Explain the signs of true labor to the client so that she can better prepare for them.
- Obtain a thorough history and physical examination to establish a baseline.
- Monitor *fetal heart rate* and *uterine contractions* throughout labor to evaluate for changes indicating labor progression or possible problems.
- Assess for *premature rupture of membranes.*
- Encourage the client to use the breathing exercises that she and her partner have learned in childbirth education classes to help her deal with the *uterine contractions.*
- Reassure the client that after *rupture of membranes* she will continue to produce amniotic fluid slowly so that she will not have a "dry birth."
- Be prepared to assist with *labor induction* if spontaneous uterine contractions do not occur by 24 hours after *rupture of membranes.*

# LARGE FOR GESTATIONAL AGE

### DESCRIPTION
- An infant is large for gestational age (also termed macrosomia) if the birth weight is above the 90th percentile on an intrauterine growth chart for that gestational age.
- Infants who are large for gestational age have been subject to an overproduction of growth hormone in utero probably owing to mothers with poorly controlled *diabetes mellitus.*
- Other associated causes include multiparous women.
- Conditions associated with large-for-gestational-age infants include transposition of the great vessels, Beckwith's syndrome, and congenital anomalities such as omphalocele.
- *Cesarean birth* may be necessary because cephalopelvic disproportion or *shoulder dystocia.*

### ASSESSMENT FINDINGS
- Prenatal uterine measurement above normal for gestational age
- Birth weight above the 90th percentile
- Immature development despite mature appearance
- Immature reflexes
- Extensive bruising
- Possible broken clavicle or Erb-Duchenne paralysis
- Prominent *caput succedaneum, cephalhematoma,* or molding.

### NURSING IMPLICATIONS
- Perform a nonstress test antepartally to determine placental function.
- Assist with *amniocentesis* to determine lung maturity.
- Perform a thorough physical assessment to establish a baseline.
- Obtain a thorough prenatal and labor history.
- Give adequate nutrition to provide calories for energy.
- Monitor respiratory rate and character as well as heart rate for changes.
- Promote early maternal-infant bonding.
- Observe for signs of hyperbilirubinemia.
- Monitor for signs of hypoglycemia.
- Monitor and maintain body temperature to prevent cold stress.

## LEOPOLD'S MANEUVERS

### DESCRIPTION

- Leopold's maneuvers are a systematic method of observation and palpation to determine *fetal presentation, fetal position,* presenting part, and attitude of the fetus, all important facts to know to help predict the course of labor.
- In Leopold's maneuvers, performed in four consecutive palpation movements, best results are obtained if the palpation is done systematically.
- It is difficult to palpate fetal contour in an obese woman or one with *hydramnios* (excessive amniotic fluid).

### NURSING IMPLICATIONS

- Explain the procedure to the patient and tell her about the information you hope to attain.
- Warm your hands first by washing them in warm water, if necessary, to avoid abdominal muscle contraction and tightness caused by cold hands.
- Have the client empty her bladder before palpation to make her more comfortable and to avoid obscuring fetal contours by a distended bladder.
- Position the client in a supine position with her knees flexed slightly so that her abdominal muscles are relaxed.
- Observe the client's abdomen to determine the appearance of the longest diameter (fetal length) and if the fetus is active where the movement is most apparent (feet).
- For the first maneuver, palpate the anterior surface of the fundus to determine the consistency, shape, and mobility of the presenting part, to form an opinion of what portion of the fetus lies in this fundal area.
- In the second maneuver, palpate the sides of the uterus to determine which direction the fetal back is facing; keep the left hand stationary on the left side of the uterus while the right hand palpates the opposite side of the uterus from top to bottom; then repeat the maneuver with the opposite hands.
- In the third maneuver, grasp the lower portion of the abdomen just above the symphysis pubis between thumb and index finger and try to press the thumb and finger together to determine fetal *engagement.*

- In the fourth maneuver, assess fetal attitude, assuming the fetus has been found to be in a cephalic position, by placing fingers on both sides of the uterus approximately 2 inches above the inguinal ligaments and pressing inward and downward to gain information about the infant's anteroposterior position.

# LIGHTENING

### DESCRIPTION

- Lightening is a *preliminary sign of labor* and is the settling of the fetal presenting part to the level of the ischial spines.
- Lightening causes changes in the woman's abdominal contour as the uterus becomes lower and more anterior.
- Often it gives the woman relief from diaphragmatic pressure and shortness of breath she has been experiencing and thus "lightens" her load.
- In primiparas, it occurs approximately 10 to 14 days before labor begins, probably because of tight abdominal muscles.
- In multiparas, it is not as noticeable and probably occurs on the day of labor or even after labor begins.

# LOCHIA

### DESCRIPTION

- Lochia refers to the postpartal vaginal discharge that occurs from the sloughing of the uterus.
- It is similar to a menstrual flow and consists of blood, fragments of decidua, white blood cells, mucus, and some bacteria.
- The portion of the uterus where the placenta was not attached is fully cleansed by this sloughing process and will be in a reproductive state in about 3 weeks; the placental implantation site takes approximately 6 weeks to be cleansed and healed.
- For the first 3 days after birth, a lochia discharge consists almost entirely of blood, with only small particles of decidua and mucus; because of its red color, it is termed lochia rubra.
- As the amount of blood involved in the cast-off tissue decreases (about the 4th day), and leukocytes begin to invade the area as they do any healing surface, the flow becomes pink or brownish in color; this is termed lochia serosa.

- On about the 10th day, the amount of flow decreases and becomes colorless or white; this is termed lochia alba.
- Lochia alba is present in most women until the 3rd week following birth, although it is not unusual for a lochia flow to last the entire 6 weeks of the puerperium.

### Nursing Implications

- Assess the client's perineal pad drainage for character, amount, color, and presence of any clots.
- Inspect the lochia once every 15 minutes for the first hour, once every hour for the next 8 hours, and then once every 8 hours.
- Keep in mind that during the 1st hour, lochia rubra should be present, possibly with small clots.
- Make sure to check under the client's buttocks so as not to miss bleeding that may be pooling below her.
- Keep in mind that a constant trickle of vaginal flow or soaking through a pad every 60 minutes indicates that the client is losing more than the average amount of blood; notify the physician.
- Instruct the client in proper perineal care; encourage her to change her perineal pads frequently to prevent infection.
- Make certain that the client understands that she must wash her hands after handling the pads and must use only her own personal care equipment so that she does not contract or spread infection.
- Demonstrate good role modeling with handwashing and equipment use.
- Educate the client about how to evaluate lochial flow, including amount (should approximate a menstrual flow), consistency (should contain no large clots), pattern (should be red, changing to pinkish brown, and then white), odor (should not have an offensive odor), and absence (should never be absent during the first 1 to 3 weeks).
- Instruct the client that lochial flow increases on exertion, especially the first few times that she is out of bed, but decreases again with rest.
- Advise the client to notify the physician if any problems occur, such as passing large clots (indicates poor uterine contraction), saturating a perineal pad in less

than an hour (indicates possible poor uterine contraction and hemorrhage), change in color back to red (indicates *retained placental fragments* and decreasing uterine contraction), an offensive odor (indicates infection), or absence of flow (indicates infection).

- Keep in mind that lochia may be scant in amount following a *cesarean birth,* but it is never altogether absent.
- Instruct the client to avoid using tampons until she returns for her postpartal checkup because she is at high risk for toxic shock syndrome until the uterine lining is healed completely.

# LYME DISEASE

### DESCRIPTION

- Lyme disease is a multisystem disease caused by the spirochete *Borrelia burgdorferi* and spread by the bite of a deer tick.
- Infection in pregnancy results in *spontaneous abortion* or severe congenital anomalies.

### ASSESSMENT FINDINGS

- Migratory rash (large, macular lesions with a clear center)
- Pain in large body joints
- History of recent tick bite
- History of being in wooded area

### NURSING IMPLICATIONS

- Complete a thorough history and physical assessment to establish a baseline.
- Educate the client about the importance of reporting any symptoms.
- Advise the client that if she anticipates becoming pregnant or is pregnant that she should avoid areas where she is apt to be bitten by ticks (woods and tall grass).
- Caution her against using tick repellants containing diethyltoluamide as this ingredient is teratogenic.
- Advise her that after coming home from an outing to inspect her body carefully and immediately remove any ticks she finds.
- Be aware that treatment for Lyme disease for pregnant women must be different than that for nonpregnant women because the drugs used for nonpregnant adults

(tetracycline and doxycycline) cannot be used during pregnancy.

# MATERNAL SERUM ASSAY

### DESCRIPTION

- Maternal serum may be used to determine the levels of various hormones for *evaluation of fetal well-being.*
- Substances that can be assessed include diamine oxidase, oxytocinase, progesterone, alkaline phosphatase, and human placental lactogen.
- These substances rise in the maternal blood stream if the fetus is growing well.
- These substances, however, are rarely assessed because information on the fetus can be derived more directly from a single study such as alpha-fetoprotein or a triple screen (maternal serum for alpha-fetoprotein, estriol, and *HCG*).

### NURSING IMPLICATIONS

- Explain the tests to the client and rationale for doing them.
- Obtain the specimen for laboratory analysis.
- Monitor the results and report any deviations from the normal ranges.

# MECONIUM ASPIRATION SYNDROME

### DESCRIPTION

- Meconium aspiration syndrome occurs when the infant inhales meconium-stained fluid in utero or at birth causing severe *respiratory distress.*
- An infant who has hypoxia in utero has a vagal reflex relaxation of the rectal sphincter, which releases meconium into the amniotic fluid.
- Infants born breech may expel meconium into the amniotic fluid from pressure on the buttocks.
- Meconium aspiration can cause severe *respiratory distress* in three ways: by inflammation of the bronchioles because it is a foreign substance, by blocking small bronchioles by mechanical plugging, and by decreasing surfactant production through lung cell trauma.
- Meconium aspiration syndrome can result in hypoxemia, carbon dioxide retention, and intrapulmonary and extrapulmonary shunting as well as a secondary infection of injured tissue, which may lead to pneumonia.

#### Assessment Findings
- *Meconium staining* (greenish to black)
- Difficulty establishing respirations at birth
- Retractions
- Tachypnea
- Cyanosis
- Low *Apgar* score
- Bilateral coarse infiltrations
- Barrel chest
- Diaphragm pushed downward

#### Nursing Implications
- Suction the infant's nose and throat preferably before the first breath is taken to avoid meconium aspiration.
- Prepare to intubate the infant and suction meconium from the trachea and bronchi immediately after birth.
- Be aware that oxygen should not be administered under pressure (bag and mask) until the infant has been intubated and suctioned.
- Obtain specimens for blood gas analysis.
- Obtain a chest x-ray as prescribed.
- Monitor vital signs closely for changes.
- Monitor and maintain body temperature to prevent cold stress.
- Administer antibiotics to the infant, as prescribed.
- Observe the infant closely for signs of congestive heart failure, such as increased heart rate or *respiratory distress.*
- Be prepared to institute extracorporeal membrane oxygenation, as prescribed.
- Perform postural drainage with clapping and vibration to help encourage removal of flecks of remaining meconium from the lungs.
- Provide support to the infant's parents and explain treatment measures to help alleviate their fears and anxieties.

## MECONIUM STAINING

#### Description
- Meconium staining refers to amniotic fluid that is stained with meconium from the fetus.
- Meconium staining may indicate that the fetus is experiencing hypoxia, which stimulates the vagal reflex and leads to increased bowel motility.

- Loss of sphincter control causes escape of meconium into the amniotic fluid.
- Meconium staining may occur in a breech presentation because pressure on the buttocks causes meconium loss.
- Although meconium staining is not always a sign of fetal distress, its correlation is high and should be taken seriously.
- Meconium staining occurs in approximately 10% of all pregnancies.
- It tends not to occur in extremely-very-low-birth-weight infants because the substance has not passed far enough into the bowel for it to be at the rectum in these infants.

### Assessment Findings
- Green-to-black stained amniotic fluid
- Fetal distress (possible)

### Nursing Implications
- Monitor *fetal heart rate* and assess for possible fetal distress.
- Report any signs of meconium-stained fluid to the physician.
- Anticipate the possibility of *meconium aspiration syndrome* in the infant.
- Have appropriate resuscitation equipment available at the birth.

## MULTIPLE GESTATION (PREGNANCY)

### Description
- Multiple gestation occurs when more than one fetus is growing in the uterus.
- Multiple gestation or multiple pregnancy is a complication of pregnancy because the woman's body must adjust to the effects of more than one fetus.
- Multiple birth occurs in only 1% of pregnancies, and it accounts for 11% of neonatal deaths.
- The rate of twinning in the United States is 1 in 84 births; triplets, 1 in 6400 births.
- Single-ovum (monozygotic, identical) twins usually have one placenta, one chorion, two amnions, and two umbilical cords and are of the same sex.
- Double-ova (dizygotic, nonidentical) twins have two placentas, two chorions, two amnions, and two umbilical cords and may be of the same or different sex.

- Multiple gestations of three, four, five, or six children may be single-ovum conceptions, multiple ova conceptions, or a combination of both.
- Multiple gestations often occur as a result of ovulation stimulation by clomiphene (Clomid); with in vitro fertilization, several fertilized ova are introduced into the uterus, resulting in a high possibility of multiple birth.
- Women with multiple gestations are more susceptible to complications such as *pregnancy-induced hypertension, hydramnios, placenta previa, postpartal hemorrhage* and *anemia.*
- There is also a higher incidence of velamentious cord insertion (the cord inserted into the fetal membrane).
- Monozygotic twins can share the same vascular communication, which can lead to an overgrowth of one fetus and an undergrowth of the second (twin-to-twin transfusion).

### Assessment Findings
- Uterine size greater than expected for dates
- Elevated alpha-fetoprotein levels
- *Ultrasonography* positive for multiple pregnancy
- More than one set of fetal heart sounds

### Nursing Implications
- Obtain a thorough *antepartal history and physical examination* to establish a baseline.
- Ensure adequate nutrition by instructing the client to eat six small meals a day rather than three large ones since the growing uterus will compress her stomach and reduce her appetite.
- Review with the client her need for extra rest periods and "shoes off" times during the day to increase tissue perfusion.
- Advise the client to refrain from coitus during the last 2 to 3 months of pregnancy.
- Advise the client to return to the health care facility every month for ultrasound examinations or weekly nonstress tests to document normal fetal growth beginning with the 28th week of pregnancy.
- Encourage the client to adhere to her prescribed bed rest routine during the last 2 or 3 months of her pregnancy.
- Offer support and reassurance to the client as she may be going through many emotional upsets and role changes.

- Monitor *fetal heart rates* and *fundal height* as well as maternal vital signs per facility's protocol.
- Encourage the client to express her fears about the well-being of her multiple fetuses.
- Prepare the client emotionally and physically for labor and delivery of multiple fetuses.

## NEWBORN CIRCULATION

### DESCRIPTION

- In the newborn, changes in the cardiovascular system are necessary at birth because the blood that was formerly oxygenated by the placenta now must be oxygenated by the lungs.
- When the cord is clamped, a neonate is forced to take in oxygen through the lungs.
- As the lungs are inflated for the first time, pressure is greatly decreased in the chest in general and into the pulmonary artery in particular (the artery leading to the lungs).
- The decrease in pressure in the pulmonary artery plays a role in causing the ductus arteriosis to close.
- As pressure increases in the left side of the heart from increased blood volume, the foramen ovale closes because of the pressure against the lip of the structure (permanent closure does not occur for weeks).
- With the remaining fetal circulatory structures—the umbilical vein, two umbilical arteries, and the ductus venosus—no longer receiving blood, the blood within them clots, and the vessels atrophy over the next few weeks.
- The peripheral circulation of the neonate remains sluggish for at least the first 24 hours.

### ASSESSMENT FINDINGS

- Cyanosis of the hands and feet (acrocyanosis)
- Feet feel cold to touch
- High erythrocyte count (6 million/mm³)
- Hemoglobin 17 to 18 g/100 ml
- Hematocrit between 45% and 50%
- Indirect bilirubin 1 to 4 mg/100 ml
- WBC 15,000 to 45,000 cells/mm³
- Prolonged prothrombin time and coagulation time
- Blood levels of vitamin K lower than normal

### NURSING IMPLICATIONS

- Perform a thorough *newborn physical assessment* to establish a baseline and ongoing for changes.
- Warm the heel of the foot to improve accuracy (inaccuracy caused by sluggish peripheral circulation) before obtaining a heel-stick for hemoglobin analysis.
- Be aware that a neonate's high leukocyte count, which is a result of the trauma of birth, may not be indicative of infection unless other signs of infection are present, such as pallor, respiratory difficulty, or cyanosis.
- Administer vitamin K (Aquamephyton) intramuscularly in the lateral anterior thigh immediately after birth.

## NEWBORN PHYSICAL ASSESSMENT

### DESCRIPTION

- A newborn is given a preliminary physical examination immediately after birth to detect such gross observable conditions as meningocele, cleft lip and palate, hydrocephalus, birthmarks, imperforate anus, tracheoesophageal atresia, and bowel obstruction.
- This health assessment must be done rapidly so that the newborn is not exposed for a long period of time, yet it must not be done so quickly that important findings are overlooked.
- The immediate birth appraisal should include auscultation of the chest for heart and respiratory sounds (perhaps already done as part of the *Apgar scoring*).
- In addition to these procedures, a thorough, generalized inspection and tentative determination of gestational age should be included in the immediate birth appraisal.
- Newborn physical assessment should be performed in the delivery or birthing room.
- A more detailed assessment including *newborn reflex* assessment is performed in the newborn nursery after the newborn's temperature has stabilized.

### NURSING IMPLICATIONS

- Observe quickly the appearance of the newborn, looking for obvious anomalies such as meningocele or cleft lip or palate.
- Auscultate the chest and assess heart and respiratory sounds noting any deviations from normal.

- Weigh the newborn without clothes on and without a blanket in the delivery room or birthing room.
- Observe the color of the newborn's skin for cyanosis, jaundice, pallor, birthmarks, lanugo, or forcep marks.
- Obtain heel-stick hematocrit or hemoglobin determination on admission to the term nursery or after the first hour of undisturbed rest.
- Once admitted to the nursery, obtain a complete physical examination of all body systems.
- Evaluate the appearance of the newborn's skin, including color, birthmarks, vernix caseosa, lanugo, milia, desquamation, and skin turgor.
- Obtain length and weight measurements.
- Assess the head, obtaining head circumference measurements, palpating the fontanelles, and inspecting for possible *caput succedaneum* or *cephalhematoma.*
- Evaluate the newborn's eyes, ears, nose, mouth, neck, chest (including chest circumference), abdomen, anogenital area, back, and extremities.

## NEWBORN REFLEXES

### DESCRIPTION

- Mature newborns demonstrate general neuromuscular function by moving their extremities and attempting to control head movement.
- During the physical assessment, a number of reflexes can be tested with consistency by using simple maneuvers.
- Many of the reflexes that are present at birth last only for several months and then disappear.

### NURSING IMPLICATIONS

- Keep the newborn warm while assessing the reflex responses, and choose a time when the newborn is not hungry or is stressed.
- Shine a strong flashlight or otoscope on the eye and observe for a blinking response to the light to elicit the blink reflex.
- Brush or stroke the cheek near the corner of the mouth and observe if the newborn turns toward the direction of the stroking to demonstrate the rooting reflex.
- Touch the neonate's lips and observe for sucking movements to demonstrate the sucking reflex.

- Observe the neonate as he or she nurses from the breast or takes nourishment to assess the swallowing reflex.
- Place one of your fingers in each of the neonate's palms and assess that the neonate will firmly grasp the fingers eliciting the palmar grasp reflex.
- Hold the newborn securely in a vertical position with the feet touching a hard surface and observe the newborn taking several quick, alternating steps to elicit the step (walk)-in place reflex.
- Hold the newborn securely in the same position as for the step (walk)-in place reflex but place the anterior surface of the legs against the edge of a bassinet or table and observe the newborn making a few lifting motions as if to step up onto the table to assess the placing reflex.
- Assess the tonic neck reflex by turning the head to one side and observe that the arm and the leg on the side to which the head turns extend and the opposite arm and leg extend.
- Initiate a startle or Moro reflex by startling the newborn by a loud noise or by jarring the bassinet and observe that the newborn abducts and extends the arms and legs, the fingers assume a typical "C" position, the arms assume an embrace position, and the newborn pulls his or her legs up against the abdomen.
- Stroke the side of the foot in an inverted "J" curve from the heel upward and observe the newborn fan the toes to assess a positive Babinski reflex.

# NEWBORN TEMPERATURE REGULATION

### DESCRIPTION

- The temperature of newborns is about 37.2°C (99°F) at the moment of birth because they have been confined in an internal body organ.
- This temperature falls almost immediately to below normal because of heat loss and immature temperature-regulating mechanisms with the 21 to 22°C (68 to 72°F) temperature of the delivery room adding to this loss of heat.
- Newborns lose heat by four separate mechanisms: convection, conduction, radiation, and evaporation.
- Newborns not only lose heat easily, but also have difficulty conserving heat under any circumstances

because they have little subcutaneous fat to provide insulation and they rarely shiver, which is a means of increasing metabolism and thereby provides heat.

- Newborns can conserve heat by constricting blood vessels.
- Brown fat, a special tissue found in mature newborns, apparently helps to conserve or produce body heat by increasing metabolism.
- A newborn exposed to cool air kicks and cries to increase the metabolic rate to produce body heat, which also increases the need for oxygen and thus increases the respiratory rate.
- Newborns who cannot increase their respiratory rate (immature newborns with poor lung development) in response to increased needs are unable to deliver sufficient oxygen to their systems resulting in anaerobic catabolism of body cells, leading to life-threatening acidosis.
- The neonate also becomes fatigued, placing additional strain on an already stressed cardiovascular system.

### NURSING IMPLICATIONS

- Protect the newborn from drafts from windows or air conditioners to prevent heat loss in the newborn through convection.
- Place a pad or diaper on the scale before weighing the newborn to make sure that the newborn is not placed on an unprotected cold surface to prevent heat loss in the newborn through conduction.
- Protect the newborn from heat loss by radiation by not placing the newborn next to any cold surface such as a window sill.
- Dry the newborn immediately especially the face and head and place a cap on the head and wrap the newborn in blankets to prevent heat loss through evaporation.
- Perform all care quickly to avoid exposing the newborn unnecessarily.
- Perform any procedure (resuscitation, *circumcision*) under a radiant heat source to prevent damaging heat loss.
- Be aware of a neonate whose temperature does not stabilize shortly after birth; the cause should be investigated and measures taken to correct it.

# ORAL CONTRACEPTIVES

## DESCRIPTION

- Oral contraceptives, commonly known as the pill, are composed of synthetic estrogen combined with a small amount of synthetic progesterone.
- The estrogen acts to suppress follicle-stimulating hormone and leuteinizing hormone, thereby halting ovulation.
- Progesterone action complements that of estrogen by causing a decrease in the permeability of cervical mucus, thereby limiting sperm motility and access to ova.
- Progesterone also interferes with endometrial proliferation to such a degree that implantation becomes unlikely.
- When used correctly, oral contraceptives are nearly 100% effective in preventing contraception.
- Positive long-term effects of oral contraceptives are a reduced rate of endometrial and ovarian cancer.
- The woman takes a pill at the same time every day for 21 days, stopping for 7 days and then beginning another cycle.
- Menstrual flow usually starts 4 days after the cycle is complete.
- Certain brands of oral contraceptives are packaged with 28 pills in a disk, the first 7 pills being placebo tablets to eliminate having to count days between cycles; others contain 21 pills in the disk, with the woman refraining from taking a pill for the other 7 days.
- Side effects include nausea, weight gain, headache, breast tenderness, breakthrough bleeding (spotting outside the menstrual period), monilial vaginal infections, mild hypertension, and perhaps depression.
- Poor candidates for oral contraceptive use include women with a history of thromboembolitic disease or a family history of cerebral or cardiovascular accident; women who smoke; women who are older than age 40 years; women who are obese; and women who have high blood pressure, high serum cholesterol levels, breast or reproductive malignancy, undiagnosed vaginal bleeding, migraine headache, epilepsy, sickle cell disease, or pulmonary disease.

- Oral contraceptives may also be prescribed for dysmenorrhea in adolescents, especially if endometriosis is present.
- Oral contraceptives containing only progesterone (for those who cannot take estrogen) allow ovulation to occur but do not allow implantation because the uterine lining does not develop fully.

### NURSING IMPLICATIONS

- Perform a thorough history and physical examination to establish a baseline.
- Be aware of personal feelings and values about contraception and sexuality.
- Be sensitive to the client's personal, religious, cultural, and social beliefs about birth control.
- Answer the client's questions honestly and openly.
- Provide education for the client and partner about family planning methods.
- Teach the woman how to take the oral contraceptives by taking the first pill on a Sunday (the first Sunday following the beginning of a menstrual flow) and one pill everyday thereafter for 21 days and then stop for 7 days, resuming on the Sunday 1 week after she stopped.
- Advise the client that when first taking the pill it is not effective for the first 7 days and that she should use a second form of contraception during this initial 7 days.
- Advise the client that if she misses one pill, she should take it as soon as she remembers and then continue the following day with her usual cycle.
- Advise the client that if she misses two consecutive pills, she should take two pills on the day she remembers and then two pills the following day and then continue the following day with the usual schedule.
- Caution the client who misses two consecutive pills that she should use added protection such as a *spermicide* for the next 7 days because missing two consecutive pills may be enough to allow ovulation to occur.
- Advise the client on oral contraceptives to return for a follow-up visit in 3 months, 6 months, and 1 year for a breast and pelvic examination.
- Instruct the client that taking the pill at bedtime rather than in the morning may eliminate nausea.

- Advise the client that after discontinuing the pill, she may not become pregnant for 1 or 2 months and probably 6 to 8 months.
- Caution the client taking oral contraceptives that if she suspects she has become pregnant to discontinue taking the pill if she intends to continue the pregnancy.
- Counsel the adolescent who desires to take the pill that she should have well-established menstrual cycles for at least 2 years before beginning oral contraceptives.

## OUTLET CONTRACTION

### DESCRIPTION
- Outlet contraction is defined as the narrowing of the transverse diameter to less than 11 cm.
- The outlet or transverse diameter is the distance between the ischial tuberosities in the maternal pelvis.
- Outlet contraction results in cephalopelvic disproportion.
- Outlet contraction, a problem with the passage, can cause failure to progress in labor and can be easily detected during a prenatal visit.

### NURSING IMPLICATIONS
- Obtain a thorough *antepartal history and physical examination* to establish a baseline.
- Assist with obtaining pelvic measurements antepartally.
- Be aware that every primigravida should have pelvic measurements taken and recorded before week 24 of pregnancy so that a birth decision can be made.
- Provide guidance and support to the client and partner to alleviate any fears or anxieties.

## PATHOLOGIC RETRACTION RING

### DESCRIPTION
- Pathologic retraction refers to a condition that occurs when the normal physiologic retraction ring (the boundary between the upper and lower portions of the uterus) becomes prominent and observable as an abdominal indentation.
- Also referred to as Brandl's ring, it is a danger sign that signifies impending rupture of the lower uterine segment if obstruction to labor is not removed.

- It is formed by excessive retraction of the upper uterine segment; the uterine myometrium is much thicker above than below the ring.
- When it occurs in early labor, it is usually from uncoordinated contractions; in the pelvic division of labor, it usually is caused by obstetric manipulation or the result of the administration of oxytocin.
- The fetus is gripped by the retraction ring and cannot advance beyond that point resulting in possible *uterine rupture* and *fetal death.*
- The undelivered placenta is also held at that point, and massive maternal hemorrhage may result.

### Assessment Findings
- Horizontal indentation across abdomen usually during the *second stage of labor.*
- Difficult labor

### Nursing Implications
- Observe the woman's abdomen during contractions.
- Monitor *fetal heart rate* and *uterine contractions.*
- Report the appearance of a retraction ring immediately.
- Prepare to administer amyl nitrate by inhalation or intravenous morphine sulfate to relieve the retraction ring.
- Be prepared to administer a tocolytic to halt contractions.
- Prepare for emergency *cesarean birth.*
- Provide emotional support to the client and partner in regard to her condition and the well-being of her fetus.

## PERCUTANEOUS UMBILICAL BLOOD SAMPLING (PUBS)

### Description
- PUBS (also called cordocentesis or funicentesis) is aspiration of blood from the umbilical vein for analysis.
- Under *ultrasonography,* the umbilical cord is located and then a thin needle is inserted by *amniocentesis* technique into the uterus; it is guided by *ultrasonography* until it pierces the umbilical vein and a blood sample is obtained.
- Blood studies include a complete blood count, direct Coombs, blood gases, and karotyping.

- Kleihauer-Betke tests verify that the sample is fetal blood and not maternal.
- Blood may be transfused in the same manner if the fetus is found to be anemic.
- PUBS carries little additional risk to the fetus or mother over *amniocentesis* and can yield information not available by any other means, especially about blood dyscrasias.

### Nursing Implications
- Monitor the fetus by performing a nonstress test before and after the procedure to assess for *uterine contractions.*
- Monitor fetal and maternal status throughout the procedure.
- Offer the client and partner support throughout the procedure.
- Prepare for *ultrasonography* to monitor for possible intrauterine bleeding after the procedure.
- Administer RHIG to the Rh-negative client to prevent sensitization.

## PERINEAL INFECTION

### Description
- Perineal infection is a complication of the postpartal period.
- Infections of the perineum generally remain localized or manifest the symptoms of any suture line infection.
- A laceration repair or an *episiotomy* is a ready portal of entry for bacterial invasion.

### Assessment Findings
- Pain, heat, and feeling of pressure around suture line
- Normal or elevated temperature
- Inflamed suture line
- Open suture line or sloughing away of one or two sutures
- Appearance of pus

### Nursing Implications
- Observe the *episiotomy* site per protocol.
- Notify the physician of any suspect findings.
- Monitor vital signs, especially temperature, for changes indicating an infection.

- Obtain a culture of inflamed and tender suture line with a sterile cotton-tipped applicator and send specimen to laboratory.
- Offer analgesia for pain as prescribed.
- Prepare the client for possible perineal suture removal to open the area and allow for drainage.
- Keep in mind that packing may be inserted after opening the sutures to help keep them open and promote drainage.
- Administer antibiotic as prescribed.
- Provide sitz baths or warm compresses as prescribed to hasten drainage and cleanse the area.
- Instruct the client to change perineal pads frequently because they may be contaminated by discharge; if left in place for a long time, they might cause vaginal contamination.
- Teach the client to wash her hands after handling perineal pads to prevent transmission of infection.
- Instruct the client to wipe from front to back after a bowel movement to prevent bringing feces forward onto the healing area.

## PERINEAL LACERATIONS

### DESCRIPTION

- Perineal lacerations are a main cause of *postpartal hemorrhage.*
- They usually occur when the woman is delivered from a lithotomy position because this position increases tension on the perineum.
- Perineal lacerations are classified in four categories, depending on the extent and depth of the tissue involved.
- First-degree lacerations involve the vaginal mucous membrane and the skin of the perineum to the forchette.
- Second-degree lacerations involve the vagina, perianal skin, fascia, levator ani muscle, and perineal body.
- Third-degree lacerations involve the entire perineum and reach the external sphincter of the rectum.
- Fourth-degree lacerations involve the entire perineum, rectal sphincter, and some of the mucous membrane of the rectum.

- Unless a secondary infection occurs, even fourth-degree lacerations should heal without long-term dyspareunia or incontinence.

### Assessment Findings
- *Episiotomy* with possible extension
- Ragged suture lines

### Nursing Implications
- Prepare the client for repair of laceration; keep in mind that perineal lacerations are sutured and treated as an episiotomy repair.
- Know that clients with third-degree or fourth-degree lacerations should not be given enemas or rectal suppositories or have their temperature taken rectally to prevent tearing of the sutures.
- Caution ancillary help not to administer enemas or rectal suppositories or use rectal thermometers on the client with third-degree or fourth-degree lacerations to prevent tearing of the sutures.
- Make certain that the degree of laceration is marked on the client's plan of care.
- Provide a diet that is high in fluid to prevent straining during bowel movement, thereby preventing rupture of the sutures.
- Administer stool softeners, as prescribed, to prevent pressure on the suture line during defecation.
- Provide client education regarding perineal care and need for follow-up after discharge.

## PLACENTA, ANOMALIES OF

### Description
- Anomalies of the placenta can lead to delivery complications.
- These anomalies include placenta succenturiata (one or more accessory lobes connected to the main *placenta* by blood vessels); placenta circumvallata (fetal side of the placenta covered to some extent by chorion); battledore placenta (cord inserted marginally rather than centrally); velamentous insertion of the cord (cord separated into small vessels reaching the placenta by spreading across a fold of amnion); vasa previa (umbilical vessels of velamentous cord

insertion crossing cervical os and delivered before the fetus); placenta accreta (unusually deep attachment of *placenta* to the uterine myometrium).

### NURSING IMPLICATIONS

- Always examine the placenta at birth for anomalies.
- Keep in mind that the normal placenta weighs approximately 500 g, is 15 to 20 cm in diameter, and is 1.5 to 3.0 cm thick, and its weight is approximately one-sixth that of the fetus.
- Remember that a placenta may be unusually enlarged in women with *diabetes mellitus* and in certain diseases, such as syphilis and erythroblastosis; it may be so large that it weighs one-half as much as the fetus.

## PLACENTA PREVIA

### DESCRIPTION

- Placenta previa is low implantation of the placenta.
- It occurs in four degrees: implantation in the lower rather than the upper portion of the uterus (low-lying placenta), marginal implantation (the placental edge approaches that of the cervical os), implantation that occludes a portion of the cervical os (partial placenta previa), and implantation that totally obstructs the cervical os (total placenta previa).
- The degree to which the placenta covers the internal cervical os is generally estimated in percentages: 100%, 75%, 30%, and so forth.
- Associated with placenta previa is increased parity, the number of past *cesarean births,* the number of past uterine curettages, smoking, residence at high altitudes, a male fetus, and multiple gestation.
- It is thought to occur whenever the placenta is forced to spread to find an adequate exchange surface.
- The incidence is approximately 3 to 6 per 1000 pregnancies.
- An increase in congenital anomalies in the fetus may occur if the low implantation does not allow for optimal fetal nutrition or oxygenation.

### ASSESSMENT FINDINGS

- Low-lying placenta on *ultrasonography*
- Abrupt, painless bright red *vaginal bleeding* stopping as abruptly as it began

**NURSING IMPLICATIONS**

- Perform a thorough history and physical examination to establish a baseline.
- Caution the client to avoid coitus, to get adequate rest preferably in a side-lying position, and to notify the physician of any sign of *vaginal bleeding*.
- Ask the client the time the bleeding began, her estimation of the amount of bleeding (in terms of cupfuls or tablespoonfuls), whether there was accompanying pain, the color of the blood, what she has done to control the bleeding, whether there were prior episodes of bleeding during the pregnancy, and if she has had prior cervical surgery for an incompetent cervix.
- Observe the perineum for bleeding.
- Obtain vital signs as well as monitor *fetal heart rate* and *uterine contractions*.
- Obtain laboratory specimens for hemaglobin, hematocrit, prothrombin, partial thromboplastin, fibrinogen, platelet count, and type and crossmatch of blood.
- Obtain urine specimen for routine urinalysis.
- Prepare the client for *ultrasonography*.
- Offer support and encouragement to the client and partner.
- Answer the client's questions as best as you can about the well-being of the fetus.
- Administer intravenous fluid replacement as prescribed.
- Be prepared to administer betamethasone to encourage fetal lung maturity as prescribed.

# PLACENTAL FRAGMENTS, RETAINED

**DESCRIPTION**

- Retained placental fragments occurs when the placenta does not deliver in its entirety but separates and leaves fragments behind.
- This results in uterine bleeding because the portion retained keeps the uterus from contracting fully; it is a common cause of *postpartal hemorrhage*.
- It occurs with *placental anomalies*, most likely with a succenturiate placenta, a placenta with an accessory lobe, but it can happen in any instance.

- A placenta accreta, a placenta that fuses with the myometrium (owing to an abnormal decidua basalis layer) that remains after birth, may need to be surgically removed or treated with methotrexate.

### ASSESSMENT FINDINGS
- Excessive postpartal bleeding
- Uterus not fully contracted
- Elevated serum chorionic gonadotropin
- Placental fragments visible on *ultrasonography*

### NURSING IMPLICATIONS
- Thoroughly examine the placenta after birth to make sure it is intact.
- Keep in mind that if the undetected retained fragment is large, the bleeding is apparent in the immediate postpartal period; if the fragment is small, bleeding may not be detected until the 6th or 10th postpartal day.
- Perform fundal checks after birth and assess for height, consistency, and uterine bleeding.
- Assist with dilatation and curettage to remove the retained placental fragments.
- Instruct the client to observe her *lochia* discharge at home and report any tendency for the discharge to change from *lochia* alba to rubra, or a sudden discharge of a large amount of blood.

## PNEUMONIA

### DESCRIPTION
- Pneumonia is the bacterial or viral invasion of lung tissue.
- Following the invasion, an acute inflammatory response occurs with exudate of red blood cells, fibrin, and polymorphonuclear leukocytes into the alveoli.
- Pneumonia poses a serious complication for pregnancy because fluid collecting in alveolar spaces causes limited oxygen–carbon dioxide exchange in the lungs and limited oxygen available to the fetus if the fluid collection is extreme placing the woman and fetus at high risk for problems.
- *Premature labor* may begin if pneumonia develops late in the pregnancy.

### ASSESSMENT FINDINGS
- *Dyspnea*
- Rhonchi or crackles
- Productive cough
- Chills, fever, malaise
- Tachycardia and tachypnea

### NURSING IMPLICATIONS
- Perform a thorough history and physical assessment to establish a baseline.
- Obtain vital signs and assess lung sounds per facility's protocol.
- Obtain sputum cultures for laboratory analysis.
- Be prepared to administer oxygen as needed, especially during labor to ensure adequate fetal oxygenation.
- Monitor *fetal heart rate* and assess for maternal *uterine contractions.*
- Administer antibiotic therapy as prescribed.
- Provide adequate nutrition to ensure adequate fetal growth.
- Provide support and reassurance to the client about her condition and the well-being of her fetus.

## POSITIVE SIGNS OF PREGNANCY

### DESCRIPTION
- Positive signs of pregnancy refer to objective findings indicative of pregnancy.
- They provide diagnostic evidence that a pregnancy exists.

### ASSESSMENT FINDINGS
- Positive *ultrasonography* for fetal outline
- Audible fetal heart sounds
- Palpable fetal movements by the examiner

### NURSING IMPLICATIONS
- Obtain a thorough history and physical examination to establish a baseline.
- Assess the client for *presumptive* and *probable signs of pregnancy.*
- Obtain a serum *HCG* level to confirm pregnancy.
- Develop a teaching plan addressing the essential components of antepartal care, including client counseling

and instructions regarding childbirth education; self-care measures, such as exercise, pain management, breathing techniques, birthing methods, hygiene, *breast care,* physical and sexual activity, sleep, *dental care in pregnancy,* immunizations; and prevention of fetal exposure to teratogens, and management of common discomforts of pregnancy, such as heartburn, *constipation,* nausea and vomiting, breast tenderness, palmar erythema, fatigue, hemorrhoids, varicosities, urinary frequency, palpitations, leukorrhea, backache, headache, *dyspnea, ankle edema,* leg cramps, and *Braxton-Hicks contractions.*

- Offer support and guidance to the client and family; allow time for questions and answers.

## POSTPARTAL DEPRESSION

### Description
- Postpartal depression is a feeling of sadness (postpartal "blues") after childbirth.
- Postpartal depression probably occurs as a response to the anticlimactic feeling following birth and is possibly related to hormonal shifts as estrogen and progesterone levels in the body decline.
- In a few women, this postpartal depression continues beyond the 1 or 2 days after the immediate postpartal period.
- In addition to an overall feeling of sadness, the woman may notice extreme fatigue, an inability to stop crying, increased anxiety about her own or her infant's health, insecurity (unwilling to be left alone or unable to make decisions), and psychosomatic symptoms (nausea and vomiting, diarrhea).
- Depression that continues beyond a few days may reflect a more serious problem.
- Associated with continued depression, the woman often has a multitude of related concerns, such as history of depression, a troubled childhood, stress in the home or work, lack of self-esteem, or lack of effective support people.

### Assessment Findings
- Overall feeling of sadness
- Inability to stop crying
- Increased anxiety about self and infant's health

- Insecurity
- Extreme fatigue
- Psychosomatic symptoms (nausea and vomiting, diarrhea)

### Nursing Implications

- Obtain a health history during the antepartal period to identify potential risk factors for postpartal depression.
- Arrange for counseling during the antepartal period in those clients at risk.
- Help the client arrange good support mechanisms during the antepartal period if she is determined to be at risk for postpartal depression.
- Perform a thorough postpartal health history including demographic information about support and help at home.
- Assess the maternal-infant bonding process.
- Offer support and encouragement and help the client to understand that her initial feeling of depression is normal for a few days after birth.
- Caution the client that if her depression continues beyond a few days she should seek counseling.
- Arrange for follow-up counseling for the client who shows signs of continued depression.

## POSTPARTAL HISTORY AND PHYSICAL EXAMINATION

### Description

- Postpartal history and physical examination is a major component of postpartal care.
- Because a woman is given a fairly complete physical examination during early labor, during the immediate postpartal period it is not necessary to repeat all of this procedure.
- Postpartal history includes information about family profile, pregnancy history, labor and birth history, infant data, and postpartal course.
- Postpartal physical examination includes assessment about nutrition and fluid status, energy level, presence or absence of pain, *fundal height* and consistency, *lochia* amount and character, and circulatory adequacy as well as information gathered from laboratory data.

- Technical aspects of pregnancy, labor, and birth can be learned from the woman's pregnancy and labor and birth chart as well as from the woman herself.
- Assessing this information from the woman herself helps gain insight into the woman's emotions and impressions.

### Assessment Findings

- Assessment findings vary with each client; any deviation from normal should be reported.

### Nursing Implications

- Obtain a health history, including family profile, pregnancy history, labor and birth history, infant data, and postpartal course.
- Obtain laboratory specimens, including hemoglobin, hematocrit, and clean-catch urine for routine urinalysis.
- Perform a physical assessment, including vital signs and areas of physical appearance such as hair, face, eyes, and breast.
- Palpate the uterine fundus and assess the height and consistency.
- Observe the client's *lochia* and assess the color, amount, and odor.
- Assess the perineum and observe for any ecchymosis, hematoma, erythema, edema, intactness, and presence of any drainage or bleeding from any *episiotomy* stitches.
- Assess the rectal area for the presence of hemorrhoids, counting the number, noting appearance, and measuring size in centimeters.
- Offer support and teaching about physiologic changes occurring postpartally.
- Begin reinforcing previous teaching about self-care, newborn feeding, and newborn care measures.

## POSTPARTAL PSYCHOSIS

### Description

- Postpartal psychosis is a mental illness that is characterized by an actual separation from reality.
- As many as 1 woman in 500 presents enough symptoms in the year after birth of a child to be considered psychiatrically ill (this statement represents the current rate of overall mental illness).

- In about two-thirds of these women, the illness develops during the first 6 weeks after birth.
- Because the illness coincides with the postpartal period, it is termed postpartal psychosis.
- Rather than being a response to the physical aspects of childbearing, however, it is probably a response to the crisis of childbearing.
- Nearly one-third of these women have had symptoms of mental illness before pregnancy, and if the pregnancy had not precipitated the illness, a death in the family, the loss of a husband's job, a divorce, or some other major life crisis would probably have precipitated it.
- The woman with a psychosis may deny she has had a child and when the child is brought to her insist that she never was pregnant.

### ASSESSMENT FINDINGS
- Prior history of mental illness
- History of recent major life crisis
- Emotionally sad
- Denial of birth of baby or pregnancy
- Not functioning in reality
- Anger
- Threatening behavior

### NURSING IMPLICATIONS
- Perform a thorough history and include any recent major life crisis.
- Know that with the client who is not functioning in reality, you cannot improve her concept of reality by a simple measure such as explaining what a correct perception is.
- Notify a skilled professional if you observe possible psychotic behavior in the client.
- Do not leave a psychotic client alone and do not leave her alone with her infant while you wait for a skilled professional to arrive.
- Administer antipsychotic medications, as prescribed.
- Arrange for psychiatric counseling for the client.
- Be aware that for some childbearing can trigger mental illness.
- Offer support and encouragement to the family as well as help to arrange for infant care and home support.

# POSTPARTAL REPRODUCTIVE CHANGES

## DESCRIPTION

- During the postpartal period, the reproductive system goes through changes until it returns to its nonpregnant state; this is referred to as involution.
- These postpartal changes involve the uterus, lochia, cervix, vagina, and perineum.
- The uterus will never return to its prepregnant state, but its reduction in size is dramatic, weighing 1000 g after birth, 500 g at the end of the first week, and approximately 50 g in about 6 weeks.
- The woman is in danger of *postpartal hemorrhage* from the uterus until involution is complete.
- *Breast-feeding* women reach involution much quicker because of the release of oxytocin with *breast-feeding* and resulting *uterine contraction.*
- Uterine involution may be retarded by a condition such as *multiple pregnancy, hydramnios,* exhaustion from prolonged labor or a difficult birth, grand multiparity, or physiologic effects of excessive analgesia.
- Uterine involution may be difficult in the presence of *retained placental fragments* or membranes or a full bladder.
- As the placenta and membranes separate from the uterine wall, a uterine flow (*lochia*) consisting of blood, fragments of decidua, white blood cells, and some bacteria begins.
- The portion of the uterus where the placenta was not attached is fully cleansed by sloughing and will be in a reproductive state in about 3 weeks (implantation site in about 6 weeks).
- Contraction of the cervix begins immediately after childbirth. The cervix will not return exactly to its original state but will, on pelvic examination, appear slitlike or stellate (star-shaped) where it was round before.
- Following a vaginal birth, the vagina is soft with rugae present and a diameter that is considerably greater than normal and takes the entire postpartum period to involute.
- After birth, the perineum responds to the stretching of birth with edema, ecchymosis, and tenderness with

the labia majora and minora remaining atrophic and softened and never returns to the prepregnant state.

### ASSESSMENT FINDINGS

- Palpable uterine fundus at the level of the umbilicus within 1 hour following birth and 1 fingerbreadth below umbilicus progressively each postpartum day
- Well-contracted, firm uterus
- Afterpains
- *Lochia* rubra (first 3 days)
- *Lochia* serosa (4th day)
- *Lochia* alba (10th day)
- Ecchymotic, edematous, tender perineum
- *Episiotomy* incision with repair

### NURSING IMPLICATIONS

- Obtain a thorough labor history to establish a baseline.
- Instruct the client about the changes to expect in the postpartum period
- Observe the client's abdomen for contour to detect distention and the appearance of striae or a diastasis.
- Palpate the fundus and assess for position, height, and consistency, per protocol.
- Assess for *lochia* by removing the client's perineal pad and observing the drainage, noting color, amount, and odor.
- Inspect the client's *lochia* every 15 minutes for the first hour, once every hour for the next 8 hours, then once every 8 hours while she is in a health care facility.
- Be certain that when you turn the client to inspect her perineum to check under her buttocks so as not to miss any bleeding that may be pooling beneath her.
- Teach the client when she leaves the health care facility how to assess her *lochia* and to report any unusual findings.
- Observe the client's perineum for ecchymosis, *hematoma,* erythema, edema, intactness, and presence of any drainage or bleeding from any *episiotomy* stitches.
- Instruct the client how to check her perineum at home.
- Provide pain relief for afterpains.

- Provide *episiotomy* care, including the use of cold and hot therapy, sitz baths, medications, and perineal care.
- Instruct the client how and when to perform perineal care at home.

# POSTPARTAL SYSTEMIC CHANGES, CARDIOVASCULAR

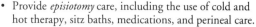

## DESCRIPTION

- After delivery, the cardiovascular system undergoes changes as the body returns to its prepregnant state.
- Diuresis occurring between the 2nd and 5th postpartum days coupled with the blood lost at birth reduces the blood volume in the woman.
- These changes are retrogressive changes whose overall effects are exhaustion and weight loss.

## ASSESSMENT FINDINGS

- Decreased hematocrit
- Decreased hemoglobin
- Elevated plasma fibrinogen level (as in pregnancy)
- Increased white blood cell count
- Slightly lower pulse rate
- Blood pressure readings comparative to prebirth readings (may be slightly decreased with diuresis)

## NURSING IMPLICATIONS

- Perform a thorough *postpartal history and physical examination.*
- Obtain a thorough labor and delivery history.
- Monitor vital signs according to institutional protocol.
- Obtain and monitor laboratory studies and results for possible problems.
- Obtain a blood pressure reading before administering any oxytocin.
- Be aware of possible orthostatic hypotension or dizziness associated with blood loss.
- Advise the client to sit up slowly and "dangle" her legs on the side of the bed before attempting to walk.
- Caution the client not to attempt to walk with her newborn in her arms even if she is only slightly dizzy until her cardiovascular status adjusts better to her blood loss.

# POSTPARTAL SYSTEMIC CHANGES, ENDOCRINE

### DESCRIPTION

- After delivery, the endocrine system undergoes changes as the body returns to its prepregnant state.
- Pregnancy hormones begin to decrease as soon as the placenta is no longer present.
- Fall of estrogen and progesterone causes an increase in prolactin and stimulates milk production.
- Physiologic changes that occur in the woman after childbirth involve progressive changes or the building of new tissue.

### ASSESSMENT FINDINGS

- Negligible level of *HCG* in urine by 24 hours
- Prepregnancy levels of progestin, estradiol, and estrone by week 1
- Elevated estrol for an additional week before reaching prepregnant level
- Increased follicle-stimulating hormone
- Secretion of colostrum
- Increased prolactin allowing breast milk formation (3rd day)
- Gradual return of menstrual flow as follicle-stimulating hormone level is increased

### NURSING IMPLICATIONS

- Perform a *postpartal history and physical examination* to establish a baseline.
- Obtain a thorough labor and delivery history.
- Explain to the client about the expected endocrine changes that are occurring.
- Instruct the client that she will continue to secrete colostrum until breast milk forms on about the 3rd postpartum day.
- Instruct the client that on about the 3rd day, she will notice breast distention and a feeling of heat or throbbing with the production of breast milk.
- Advise her that milk production will continue and will depend on the infant sucking at the breast and the ability of the milk to come forward in the breasts (let-down reflex).

- Caution the client from starting any strict dieting for the first 6 weeks following childbirth because this is a time of new tissue building in her body.
- Advise the client that she should expect her menstrual flow to return within 6 to 10 weeks after childbirth.
- Advise the client that if she is *breast-feeding,* menstrual flow may not return for 3 or 4 months or, in some women, for the entire lactation period.
- Caution the client that the absence of the menstrual flow does not guarantee that she will not conceive during this time; therefore, advise her to take contraceptive precautions.

## POSTPARTAL SYSTEMIC CHANGES, GASTROINTESTINAL

### Description
- After delivery, the gastrointestinal system undergoes changes as the body returns to its prepregnant state.
- These changes are retrogressive changes whose overall effects are exhaustion and weight loss.
- Digestion and absorption begin to be active again in the gastrointestinal system soon after birth.

### Assessment Findings
- Hunger
- Visible hemorrhoids
- Active bowel sounds
- Slow, difficult, and possible painful bowel evacuation

### Nursing Implications
- Perform a thorough *postpartal history and physical examination.*
- Obtain a thorough labor and delivery history.
- Offer the client fluids and something to eat unless she has aftereffects from *general anesthesia.*
- Offer sitz baths, anesthetic sprays, witch hazel or astringent preparations, or preparations such as hydrocortisone acetate as prescribed for hemorrhoid relief.
- Advise the client to assume the Sims' position several times a day to aid in good venous return to the rectal area and also to reduce discomfort.
- Advise the client to increase fluid intake, and administer a stool softener as prescribed to prevent irritation of hemorrhoids by hard stool.

# POSTPARTAL SYSTEMIC CHANGES, INTEGUMENTARY

### DESCRIPTION
- After delivery, the integumentary system undergoes changes as the body returns to its prepregnant state.
- These changes are retrogressive changes.

### ASSESSMENT FINDINGS
- Reddened and prominent stretch marks on the abdomen (striae gravidarum)
- Excessive pigment on the face and neck (chloasma) and on the abdomen (linea nigra)

### NURSING IMPLICATIONS
- Perform a thorough *postpartal history and physical examination.*
- Obtain a thorough labor and delivery history.
- Assure the client that the stretch marks on her abdomen will fade to a pale white (slightly darker pigment in an African-American woman) over the next 3 to 6 months.
- Assure the client that chloasma and linea nigra will be barely detectable in 6 weeks.
- Be aware that if overstretching of the abdominal wall muscles has occurred, this will always be present as a slightly indented, blue-tinged area in the abdominal midline.
- Instruct the client in postpartal exercises, such as head raising or sit-ups, to help return the abdominal wall and ligaments that supported the uterus and were stretched during pregnancy to their former state; otherwise the muscle will remain protuberant and soft.

# POSTPARTAL SYSTEMIC CHANGES, MUSCULOSKELETAL

### DESCRIPTION
- After delivery, the musculoskeletal system undergoes changes as the body returns to its prepregnant state.
- These changes are retrogressive changes whose overall effects are exhaustion and weight loss.

### ASSESSMENT FINDINGS
- Muscle soreness
- Muscle weakness

#### Nursing Implications

- Perform a thorough *postpartal history and physical examination.*
- Obtain a thorough labor and delivery history.
- Offer analgesia as prescribed to relieve muscle aches and soreness.
- Perform a soothing backrub to relieve aching shoulders or back.
- Assess the client who states she has pain on standing by evoking Homan's sign to determine possible *thrombophlebitis.*

## POSTPARTAL SYSTEMIC CHANGES, URINARY

#### Description

- After delivery, the urinary system undergoes changes as the body returns to its prepregnant state.
- These changes are retrogressive changes whose overall effects are exhaustion and weight loss.
- Almost immediately following birth, extensive diuresis occurs to rid the body of the excess fluid accumulated by the body during pregnancy.

#### Assessment Findings

- Transient loss of bladder tone
- Lack of sensation to void
- Displaced uterus with bladder distention
- Increased urine production
- Increased diaphoresis

#### Nursing Implications

- Perform a thorough *postpartal history and physical examination.*
- Obtain a thorough labor and delivery history.
- Assess for bladder distention by palpating or percussing over the abdomen above the symphysis pubis.
- Palpate the fundus of the uterus; a soft boggy fundus may indicate bladder distention.
- Encourage the client to walk to the bathroom and void at the end of the 1st hour postpartum.
- Stay with or close by the client during her first voiding in the event that she becomes dizzy.
- Run water in the sink, offer the client a glass of water, or run warm water over her vulva to assist with voiding.
- Catheterize the client if her bladder is distended and she is unable to void on her own at the end of the 1st hour.

- Monitor intake and output closely to prevent fluid imbalances.

# POST-TERM PREGNANCY

## DESCRIPTION

- Post-term pregnancy is any pregnancy that exceeds a term pregnancy of 38 to 42 weeks' gestation.
- It also is referred to as a prolonged, postmature, or postdate pregnancy. The infant is considered post-gestational, postmature, or dysmature.
- Post-term pregnancy occurs in approximately 10% of all pregnancies.
- Post-term pregnancies include some pregnancies that appear to extend beyond the due date set for them because of a faulty due date, such as women with long menstrual cycles (40 to 45 days) when their child will be "late" 12 to 17 days.
- Prolonged pregnancy can occur in a woman on a high dose of salicylates (for severe sinus headaches or rheumatoid arthritis) because salicylate interferes with the synthesis of prostaglandins, which are thought to be responsible for the initiation of labor.
- Post-term pregnancy is also associated with myome-trial quiescence or a uterus that does not respond to normal labor stimulation.
- Macrosomia may result because the fetus continues to grow, creating a delivery problem; however, the usual effect that occurs is lack of growth.
- The placenta has a growth potential for only 40 to 42 weeks, and after that time it acquires calcium deposits and is unable to function, resulting in a fetus that may suffer from a lack of oxygen, fluid, and nutrients owing to decreased blood perfusion.

## ASSESSMENT FINDINGS

- 40 to 42 weeks' gestation by dates
- *Meconium staining*
- Ogliohydramnios
- Variable decelerations of *fetal heart rate* patterns

## NURSING IMPLICATIONS

- Perform a thorough history, including the date of the client's last menstrual period as well as her menstrual history.
- Perform a nonstress test or a biophysical profile on the client who is 41 weeks' gestation, as prescribed.

- Prepare the client for *ultrasonography.*
- Explain to the client why her due date is being recalculated if the nonstress test, biophysical profile, physical examination, and *ultrasonography* study indicate an infant smaller than a normal-term infant.
- Assist with administration of prostaglandin gel to initiate cervical ripening and labor.
- Monitor *fetal heart rate* and *uterine contractions* and assess for decelerations that would indicate fetal distress and placental insufficiency.
- Assist with amnioinfusion, if prescribed.
- Offer support and encouragement to the client and partner.
- Provide reassurance to the client regarding the well-being of her fetus.
- Prepare for *cesarean birth* if oxytocin is ineffective or if biophysical profile or nonstress test results are not normal or if *ultrasonography* and physical examination indicate a larger than term infant.

## PRESUMPTIVE SIGNS OF PREGNANCY

### DESCRIPTION

- Presumptive signs of pregnancy refer to the subjective findings experienced by the woman but cannot be detected by the examiner.
- These signs are least indicative of pregnancy; taken as single entities, they could easily indicate other conditions.

### ASSESSMENT FINDINGS

- Amenorrhea
- Nausea and vomiting
- Urinary frequency
- Breast tenderness
- Excessive fatigue
- Quickening
- Uterine enlargement
- Linea nigra
- Melasma
- Striae gravidarum

### NURSING IMPLICATIONS

- Obtain a thorough history and physical examination to establish a baseline.
- Obtain a serum pregnancy test to confirm pregnancy.

- Develop a teaching plan addressing the essential components of antepartal care, including client counseling and instructions regarding childbirth education; self-care measures, such as exercise, pain management, breathing techniques, birthing methods, hygiene, *breast care,* physical and sexual activity, sleep, *dental care in pregnancy,* immunizations, prevention of fetal exposure to teratogens; and management of common discomforts of pregnancy, such as heartburn, *constipation,* nausea and vomiting, breast tenderness, palmar erythema, fatigue, hemorrhoids, varicosities, urinary frequency, palpitations, leukorrhea, backache, headache, *dyspnea, ankle edema,* leg cramps, and *Braxton-Hicks contractions.*
- Offer support and guidance to the client and family; allow time for questions and answers.

## PRETERM INFANT

### DESCRIPTION

- A preterm infant is usually defined as a live-born infant born before the end of week 37 of gestation.
- Another criterion used to define a preterm infant is a birth weight of less than 2500 g (5 lb, 8 oz) at birth.
- Infants who are born before week 20 to 24 gestation are generally categorized as products of abortion, not preterm children, because their chances of survival are slight.
- Infants born after the 37th week are considered to be term infants.
- Infants who are born between 30 and 36 weeks' gestation (weighing 1500 to 2000 g) are low-birth weight infants; those born between 26 and 30 weeks' gestation (weighing 1000 to 1500 g) are very-low-birth-weight infants; those born between 24 and 26 weeks' gestation (500 to 1000 g) are extremely-very-low-birth-weight infants.
- All such infants need level III (neonatal intensive care) care from the moment of birth to give them their best chance of survival.
- A lack of lung surfactant makes them extremely vulnerable to *respiratory distress syndrome.*
- Preterm infants of every weight need to be differentiated at birth from *small-for-gestational-age* infants (who also may have a low birth weight) because the

two conditions result from different situations and therefore have different problems of adjustment to extrauterine life.

- A preterm infant is immature and small but well.
- The exact cause of early birth is not known, but there is a high correlation between low socioeconomic level and early termination of pregnancy with lack of nutrition before and after pregnancy being a significant factor.
- Potential problems associated with preterm infants are anemia of prematurity, kernicterus, persistent patent ductus arteriosus, periventricular/intraventricular hemorrhage, *respiratory distress syndrome,* apnea, *retinopathy of prematurity,* and necrotizing enterocolitis.

### Assessment Findings
- Normal prenatal history
- Small and underdeveloped appearance
- Head 3 cm or more larger than chest size
- Ruddy skin
- Acrocyanosis
- Scant vernix caseosa
- Extensive lanugo
- Small anterior and posterior fontanelles
- Few or no sole creases
- Immature ear cartilage
- Absent or diminished sucking reflex (below 33 weeks)
- Markedly diminished reflexes such as the Achilles tendon reflex
- Weak and high-pitched cry

### Nursing Implications
- Provide oxygen to the mother during labor to provide the infant with optimal oxygen saturation at birth.
- Keep maternal analgesia to a minimum if possible to give the infant the best chance of initiating effective respirations.
- Monitor *fetal heart rate* and *uterine contractions.*
- Observe amniotic fluid for presence of meconium and take appropriate measures during birth to avoid *meconium aspiration.*
- Be prepared to resuscitate the infant within 2 minutes after birth to establish respirations and prevent irreversible acidosis.

- Continue to provide oxygen to the preterm infant even after resuscitation.
- Monitor and maintain body temperature to prevent cold stress.
- Monitor vital signs for changes.
- Provide intravenous fluid administration within hours after birth to provide fluid replacement and prevent hypoglycemia.
- Monitor weight, specific gravity, and amount of urine and serum electrolytes to ensure that fluid intake is adequate.
- Measure and monitor urine output by weighing diapers and test urine for ketones and glucose in addition to amount and specific gravity.
- Provide nutrition by gavage or bottle as soon as the infant is stable enough to tolerate them to prevent deterioration of intestinal villi.
- Observe the preterm infant closely after gavage and oral feedings to make sure the full stomach does not cause respiratory distress.
- Encourage maternal infant bonding as soon as possible.
- Provide special time to stroke, hold, rock, and provide nurturing stimulation and comfort to the preterm infant.
- Instruct the parents about any procedures that they will need to be able to do at home.
- Provide support and encouragement to the parents and help them verbalize their feelings and anxiety about having a preterm infant.

## PROBABLE SIGNS OF PREGNANCY

### DESCRIPTION

- Probable signs of pregnancy refer to findings that can be documented by the examiner.
- They are more reliable than *presumptive signs of pregnancy;* however, they still are not true diagnostic findings.

### ASSESSMENT FINDINGS

- Positive serum *HCG* level
- Chadwick's sign (vaginal color change from pink to violet)
- Goodell's sign (cervical softening)

- Hegar's sign (lower uterine segment softening)
- Ballottement (fetal rise against abdominal wall when lower uterine segment tapped)
- Palpable fetal outline
- *Braxton-Hicks contractions*
- Ladin's sign (soft spot anteriorly in middle of uterus)
- McDonald's sign (uterine flexibility against cervix)
- Braun von Fernwald's sign (irregular, soft, enlarged area at implantation site)
- Piskacek's sign (uterine enlargement and softening)
- Uterine souffle (soft blowing sound at rate of maternal pulse)
- Positive *ultrasonography* for gestational sac

### Nursing Implications

- Obtain a thorough history and physical examination to establish a baseline.
- Prepare the client for and assist with pelvic examination.
- Assess the client for *presumptive signs of pregnancy.*
- Obtain a serum *HCG* level to confirm pregnancy.
- Develop a teaching plan addressing the essential components of antepartal care, including client counseling and instructions regarding childbirth education; self-care measures, such as exercise, pain management, breathing techniques, birthing methods, hygiene, *breast care,* physical and sexual activity, sleep, *dental care in pregnancy,* immunizations, prevention of fetal exposure to teratogens; and management of common discomforts of pregnancy, such as heartburn, *constipation,* nausea and vomiting, breast tenderness, palmar erythema, fatigue, hemorrhoids, varicosities, urinary frequency, palpitations, leukorrhea, backache, headache, *dyspnea, ankle edema,* leg cramps, and *Braxton-Hicks contractions.*
- Offer support and guidance to the client and family; allow time for questions and answers.

## PROLAPSED CORD

### Description

- In umbilical cord prolapse, a loop of the umbilical cord slips down in front of the presenting part.
- Prolapse may occur at any time after the membranes rupture and if the presenting part is not fitted firmly into the cervix.

- Prolapsed cord tends to occur with *premature rupture of the membranes,* fetal position other than cephalic presentations, *placenta previa,* intrauterine tumors or cephalopelvic disproportion that prevents firm *engagement* of the fetus, a small fetus, polyhydramnios, and *multiple gestation.*
- Cord prolapse automatically leads to cord compression because the fetal presenting part presses against the cord at the pelvic brim.
- The incidence of prolapsed cord is 1 in 200 pregnancies.
- Management is aimed at relieving pressure on the cord and thereby relieving the compression and the resulting fetal anoxia.
- If the cervix is fully dilated at the time of prolapse, the physician may choose to deliver the infant rapidly, possibly with *forceps delivery,* to prevent a lengthy period of anoxia.
- If dilation is incomplete, the birth method of choice is upward pressure on the presenting part by a practitioner's hand in the woman's vagina until *cesarean birth* is complete.

### ASSESSMENT FINDINGS

- Cord felt as presenting part (rare)
- Presence of cord in vagina after *rupture of membranes*
- Deceleration pattern on fetal monitor

### NURSING IMPLICATIONS

- Monitor *fetal heart rate* and observe for deceleration pattern.
- Monitor and record *fetal heart rate* immediately following *rupture of membranes.*
- Place the client in Trendelenberg or knee-chest position, which causes the fetal head to fall back from the cord if cord prolapse is discovered.
- Prepare the client for relief of cord compression; a hand is placed in the vagina and the fetal head is manually elevated off the cord.
- Administer oxygen at 10 L/min by face mask to prevent fetal anoxia.
- Be prepared to administer a tocolytic to reduce uterine activity.
- Cover any exposed portion of the cord with a sterile saline compress to prevent drying.

- Do not attempt to push any exposed cord back into the vagina because it may cause additional compression by kinking or knotting.

## PSYCHOSOCIAL CHANGES OF PREGNANCY

### DESCRIPTION

- Psychosocial changes of pregnancy occur in response to the physiologic alterations that are occurring and to the increased responsibility associated with welcoming a new and completely dependent person to the family.
- A woman's attitude toward a pregnancy depends a great deal on the environment in which she was raised, the messages about pregnancy her family communicated to her as a child, and the society and culture in which she lives as an adult.
- During the 9 months of pregnancy, a woman runs the gamut of emotions, from surprise at finding herself pregnant (or wishing she were not) to pleasure and acceptance of the fact as she feels the child stir, to fear for her self and the child, to boredom with the process and wishing to get it all over with so that she can get on with the next step of childbearing near the end of pregnancy.
- Once the child is born, she may feel surprised again that it really happened and she has really given birth.
- The 9-month period allows for the woman and her family to prepare emotionally for the birth of the child.
- Emotional responses to pregnancy involve the client, partner, and any siblings.
- Pregnancy is an intrusive process.
- Much of a woman's reaction to pregnancy is one of ambivalence; she wants to be pregnant and yet she is not enjoying it. (It does not mean that the positive feelings counteract the negative feelings so that the woman is left feeling almost nothing toward her pregnancy; the feelings are interwoven.)
- For the partner, accepting the pregnancy means accepting the certainty of the pregnancy and the reality of the child to come and accepting the woman in her changed state; in some cases, a man may develop physical symptoms (couvade syndrome), identifying with the changes in his partner's pregnancy.
- Common responses to pregnancy include grief (before taking on the role of mothering, she has to give up her

present roles), narcissism, introversion, changes in body image and boundary, decreased decision making, emotional lability, and changes in sexual desire.

- During pregnancy, three psychological tasks must be achieved: accepting the pregnancy, accepting the baby, and preparing for parenthood.
- Accepting the pregnancy is the psychological task of the first trimester of pregnancy.
- A diagnosis of pregnancy is a rite of passage.
- Until it is verified by a home test or a health care visit, the uncertainty of symptoms make the pregnancy a vague theoretical possibility and leave room for denial.
- Some women who are surprised to find themselves pregnant immediately experience something less than pleasure and closer to disappointment or anxiety at the news; most women are able to change their attitude toward pregnancy by the time they feel quickening.
- Accepting the baby is the psychological task of the second trimester of pregnancy and usually is related to quickening, which allows the pregnant woman to give the child an identity; she begins to imagine how she will feel at birth and how she will be as a mother.
- This anticipatory role playing helps her to realize that not only is she pregnant, but also there is a child inside her.
- Most women can pinpoint a moment during each pregnancy when they definitely know that they wanted the child.
- For others, acceptance might not occur until labor has begun, after several hours of labor, or when the woman hears the baby's cry or first touches or feeds the neonate; it could take several weeks after the baby is born to accept the new reality.
- Preparing for parenthood is the psychological task of the third trimester when the woman usually begins "nest-building" activities, such as planning the infant's room, buying clothes, choosing names, and "ensuring safe passage" by learning about birth.

### Nursing Implications

- Obtain a thorough history and physical examination to establish a baseline.
- Establish trust early in pregnancy to allow for expression of feelings and problem solving.

- Assess the client's and partner's feelings about the pregnancy.
- Allow them to verbalize their feelings about the pregnancy and how it is affecting their lives and their relationship.
- Explain about the possible responses that each might feel and offer support and guidance in dealing with them.
- Assist the partner with coping with the client's emotional lability to promote acceptance of the mood swings as a part of pregnancy.
- Explain about the possible changes in sexual desire and help the client and partner adjust to the changes, interpreting them as a difference, not as a loss of interest in the sexual partner.
- Encourage the couple to share their feelings with each other and offer support to each other.
- Assist the client and partner with suggestions for preparing siblings.
- Provide anticipatory guidance about pregnancy, labor, and delivery.
- Be aware that a woman's level of acceptance is reflected by how well she follows prenatal instructions.

## PYROSIS

### DESCRIPTION

- Pyrosis (heartburn) is a burning sensation along the esophagus caused by regurgitation of gastric contents.
- Pyrosis is a common discomfort of pregnancy and a common problem interfering with nutrition during pregnancy.
- In pregnancy, it may accompany nausea, but it may persist beyond the resolution of nausea and even increase in severity as pregnancy advances.
- Pyrosis is probably caused by decreased gastric motility.

### NURSING IMPLICATIONS

- Obtain a thorough history and physical examination to establish a baseline.
- Evaluate the client's complaints and any association with dietary intake; perform a dietary recall.
- Advise the client to eat small, frequent meals.

- Encourage the client not to lie down immediately after eating to help prevent reflux.
- Inform the client that aluminum hydroxide or a combination of aluminum and magnesium hydroxide may be prescribed for relief.
- Be certain that the client understands that this "chest pain" is from her gastrointestinal tract and that, although it is called heartburn, it has nothing to do with her heart.

# RENAL DISEASE, CHRONIC

## DESCRIPTION

- Chronic renal disease is a preexisting condition that places the client at high risk during pregnancy.
- In the past, children with chronic renal disease did not reach childbearing age or were advised not to have children because of the high risk for them during pregnancy.
- Today, women with chronic renal disease are having children because pregnancy does not appear to cause progressive deterioration of kidney function; children even have been born to women who have had renal transplants.
- Infants of women with chronic renal disease tend to have intrauterine growth retardation because of lessened placental perfusion.

## ASSESSMENT FINDINGS

- Glycosuria
- Proteinuria
- Elevated blood pressure
- Elevated serum creatinine level
- Edema

## NURSING IMPLICATIONS

- Obtain a thorough history and physical examination at the initial visit to establish a baseline and ongoing to identify changes.
- Obtain a medication history, including use of maintenance corticosteroids; monitor continuation of corticosteroids throughout pregnancy.
- Be aware that the infant may be hyperglycemic at birth because of the suppression of insulin activity by corticosteroids.

- Monitor laboratory tests, including complete blood count for signs of anemia; women may develop severe anemia because of lack of erythropoietin by their diseased kidneys; administer synthetic erythropoietin if indicated.
- Monitor kidney function and blood pressure throughout pregnancy for changes indicating problems; compare pregnancy results with prepregnancy values.
- Be aware that women with an elevated serum creatinine level above 2.0 mg/dL probably should not undertake a pregnancy or the increased strain on already damaged kidneys might lead to renal failure.
- Assess the posttransplant client individually, considering the client's general health, time since the transplant, proteinuria, hypertension, medications used to prevent graft rejection, any signs of graft rejection, and serum creatinine level.
- Keep in mind that women with severe chronic renal disease may require dialysis to aid kidney function, increasing the risk of *premature labor;* if the client requires dialysis, anticipate using progesterone, intramuscularly, before dialysis.
- If hemodialysis is used, schedule it frequently and for short durations to avoid acute fluid shifts.
- Be aware that peritoneal dialysis is preferred because it normally causes less drastic fluid shifts and can be accomplished on an ambulatory basis throughout pregnancy.
- Provide emotional support during pregnancy to alleviate fears and anxieties.
- Allow extra time at birth for bonding because the client may have been too concerned during pregnancy about her health status to begin bonding.
- As necessary, provide extra support to the client that the newborn is well.

## RESPIRATORY DISTRESS SYNDROME (RDS)

### DESCRIPTION
- RDS occurs when a hyalinelike membrane lines the terminal bronchioles, alveolar ducts, and alveoli preventing exchange of oxygen and carbon dioxide.
- RDS of the newborn, formerly termed hyaline membrane disease, most often occurs in *preterm infants,* infants of diabetic mothers, infants born by *cesarean*

*birth,* or infants who for any reason have decreased blood perfusion of the lungs.

- The cause of RDS is a low level or absence of surfactant, the phospholipid that lines the alveoli and resists surface tension on expiration to keep the alveoli from collapsing on expiration.
- Most infants who later develop RDS have difficulty initiating respirations at birth, but after resuscitation they appear to have a period of hours or a day when they are free of symptoms because of an initial release of surfactant.

## ASSESSMENT FINDINGS

- Low body temperature
- Nasal flaring
- Sternal and subcostal retractions
- Tachypnea (more than 60 respirations per minute)
- Expiratory grunting
- Cyanosis
- Fine rales and diminished breath sounds
- Seesaw respirations
- "Ground-glass" appearance on chest x-ray
- Respiratory acidosis

## NURSING IMPLICATIONS

- Perform a thorough physical assessment to establish a baseline and ongoing to detect changes.
- Obtain a prenatal and labor history to identify any possible factors associated with RDS.
- Be prepared for administration of surfactant through endotracheal tube.
- Monitor respirations, breath sounds, and heart rate closely for changes.
- Monitor and maintain ventilatory care, including the administration of oxygen by continuous positive airway pressure or positive end-expiratory pressure.
- Have atropine and prostigmine available if the infant is receiving pancuronium therapy.
- Obtain blood gases as prescribed to evaluate oxygen saturation.
- Monitor and maintain body temperature to identify changes and minimize metabolic demands.
- Administer nutrition intravenously or by gavage feeding to minimize energy expenditure.

## RETINOPATHY OF PREMATURITY

### DESCRIPTION

- Retinopathy of prematurity is an acquired ocular disease that leads to partial or total blindness in children as a result of vasoconstriction of immature retinal blood vessels.
- The causative agent is a high concentration of oxygen, which causes vasoconstriction of immature retinal blood vessels and a secondary proliferation of endothelial cells in the layer of nerve fibers in the periphery of the retina, resulting in detachment and blindness.
- Those infants who are immature and ill and consequently receive oxygen the most are the most susceptible to the condition.

### NURSING IMPLICATIONS

- Obtain $PO_2$ levels by oximetry or trancutaneous monitoring or blood gas monitoring as per order.
- Know that the danger of the disease is greater with $PO_2$ levels of more than 100 mm Hg.
- Administer vitamin E as prescribed. (It reduces the incidence of retinopathy of prematurity by modifying the tissue's response to the effect of oxygen.)
- Prepare for eye examination before discharge from the nursery.
- Anticipate possibility of cryosurgery to delay retinopathy of prematurity.

## Rh INCOMPATIBILITY

### DESCRIPTION

- Rh incompatibility or isoimmunization during pregnancy occurs when an Rh-negative mother is carrying a fetus with an Rh-positive blood type.
- When the Rh-positive fetus begins to grow inside an Rh-negative mother, it is as though her body is being invaded by a foreign agent, or antigen, and her body begins to form antibodies against the invading substance.
- The invading maternal antibodies formed cross the placenta and cause red blood cell destruction (hemolysis) of fetal red blood cells.
- $Rh_o$ (D) immune globulin (RHIG) is a commercial preparation of passive antibodies against the Rh factor

that can be administered to the mother at 28 weeks of pregnancy.
- RHIG can be administered again within 72 hours following delivery of an Rh-positive infant to attain passive antibody protection for future pregnancies.

**NURSING IMPLICATIONS**
- Instruct the client about Rh incompatibility.
- Offer support to the client until she reaches the end of her pregnancy.
- Arrange for antibody titers at the first prenatal visit.
- Monitor titers every 2 weeks during the remainder of the pregnancy if maternal anti-D antibody is elevated.
- Assist with *amniocentesis* at least every 2 weeks to monitor fetal well-being.
- Prepare to administer RHIG to the client at 28 weeks.
- Obtain cord blood samples after delivery.

# RUBELLA

**DESCRIPTION**
- Rubella (German measles) infection in pregnancy usually causes only mild systemic illness in the mother but severe fetal damage when exposure occurs in early pregnancy.
- Maternal rubella infection is a fetal teratogen with the greatest risk to the embryo during the organogenesis period in early pregnancy.
- Fetal damage includes deafness, mental and motor retardation, cataracts, cardiac defects (patent ductus arteriosus and pulmonary stenosis being the most common), retarded intrauterine growth (*small for gestational age*), thrombocytopenia purpura, and dental and facial clefts such as cleft lip and palate.

**NURSING IMPLICATIONS**
- Obtain a thorough history and physical examination to establish a baseline and identify any possible exposure to the virus.
- Caution the client that once she becomes pregnant, she cannot be immunized against rubella.
- Caution the client that following a rubella immunization she should not become pregnant for 3 months.
- Obtain rubella titers in the postpartal period.
- Be aware that clients with low rubella titers should be immunized immediately following a pregnancy.

- Advise pregnant clients to avoid contact with children with rashes since some women, despite demonstrating antibodies against rubella, may become reinfected during pregnancy.
- Isolate an infant born to a mother who had rubella during her pregnancy because the infant is capable of transmitting the disease for up to 8 months after birth.

# RUPTURE OF MEMBRANES, PREMATURE

### DESCRIPTION

- Preterm premature rupture of membranes is rupture of fetal membranes with loss of amniotic fluid before labor begins either at term or earlier in pregnancy.
- Although the cause is unknown, it is associated with infection of the membranes (chorioamnionitis) before rupture.
- Preterm premature rupture of membranes poses a threat to the fetus, especially if this occurs early in the pregnancy, because, following rupture, the seal to the fetus is lost, and uterine and fetal infection can occur.
- *Premature labor* may follow rupture, posing the additional risk of immature birth to the fetus.
- Additional complications include increased pressure on the umbilical cord or *prolapsed cord* (extension of the cord out of the uterine cavity into the vagina), particularly if rupture happens when the fetal head is too small to fit the cervix firmly.
- The fetus may develop a Potter-like syndrome of distorted facial features and pulmonary hypoplasia.

### ASSESSMENT FINDINGS

- Sudden gush of clear fluid from the vagina, with continued minimal leakage
- Vaginal pooling of fluid on speculum examination
- Alkaline reaction with Nitrazine paper test (rupture of membranes turns paper blue; urine leaves the paper yellow, indicating an acidic reaction)
- Positive ferning test (indicates amniotic fluid owing to high content of estrogen in amniotic fluid)

### NURSING IMPLICATIONS

- Perform a thorough history and physical examination to establish a baseline.

- Be prepared to assist with a vaginal speculum examination.
- Perform a nitrazine test to distinguish amniotic fluid from urine.
- Be prepared to obtain a slide test of vaginal fluid to assess for ferning.
- Prepare the client for *ultrasonography* to assess amniotic fluid index.
- Provide support during the examination and explain the procedure to the client and partner if present.
- Reassure the client and partner about the status of her fetus.
- Reassure the client that the amniotic fluid is constantly being formed and that she will not have a "dry labor."
- Monitor *fetal heart rate* and assess for possible fetal distress from cord compression or *prolapsed cord.*
- Encourage the client to adhere to bed rest instructions.
- Advise the client to refrain from tub bathing, coitus, and douching.
- Instruct the client to take her temperature twice a day and to report a fever (a temperature greater than 100.4°F), uterine tenderness, or odorous vaginal discharge.
- Obtain daily white blood cell counts and report any white blood cell counts more than 18,000 to 20,000/mm³, suggesting an infection.
- Be prepared to assist with intrauterine amnioinfusion to supply additional uterine fluid.

# RUPTURE OF MEMBRANES, SPONTANEOUS

## DESCRIPTION

- The spontaneous rupture of membranes occurs when the fetal membranes surrounding the fetus rupture spontaneously, allowing amniotic fluid to escape from the uterus into the vagina.
- In as many as 25% of labors, labor begins with spontaneous rupture of the fetal membranes.

## ASSESSMENT FINDINGS

- Sudden gush or slow loss of clear fluid from vagina
- Nitrazine paper positive for alkalinity (turns blue)
- Positive ferning

### Nursing Implications

- Ask the client to describe the color of the amniotic fluid.
- Be aware that the fluid should be clear; yellow-stained fluid may indicate a blood incompatibility, and green-colored fluid may indicate *meconium staining.*
- Assist with a vaginal examination to determine the presence of amniotic fluid by nitrazine paper or ferning.
- Know that a false nitrazine reading may occur in women with intact membranes who have a heavy, bloody show because blood is also alkaline.
- Obtain *fetal heart rate* and observe for any decelerations.

## SEXUALLY TRANSMITTED DISEASES (STDs)

### Description

- STDs are those which are spread by coitus.
- STDs include candidiasis, trichomoniasis, bacterial vaginosis (*Gardnerella* infection), *Chlamydia trachomatis,* syphilis, *herpes simplex virus type 2,* human papilloma, gonorrhea, group B streptococcal infection, and *human immunodeficiency virus (HIV).*
- Almost all STDs have some effect on the fetus.
- Little disease immunity is developed against a STD once it has been contracted, so it is possible to become reinfected if prevention measures are not taken.

### Assessment Findings

- Positive laboratory findings, such as culture and sensitivity for specific organism
- Positive identification of disease-specific lesions
- Positive symptoms for specific disease

### Nursing Implications

- Perform a thorough history and physical examination to establish a baseline.
- Assist with a vaginal or pelvic examination.
- Advise the client that STDs can be prevented by using "safer sex practices."
- Instruct the client in medication regimen including dosage, frequency, signs and symptoms of adverse effects, and need for compliance.
- Encourage the client to finish her treatment regimen as prescribed.

- Instruct the client and partner about the use of contraceptives.

## SHOULDER DYSTOCIA

### DESCRIPTION

- Shoulder dystocia is a delivery problem that occurs during the *second stage of labor* when the fetal head is born but the shoulders are too broad to enter and be delivered through the pelvic outlet.
- It is hazardous to the mother because it can result in cervical and vaginal tears; it also is hazardous to the fetus because the cord is compressed between the fetal body and the bony pelvis.
- Shoulder dystocia is most likely to occur in women with *diabetes mellitus,* in multiparas, and in postdate pregnancies.

### ASSESSMENT FINDINGS (suspect shoulder dystocia if any of the following occur)

- Prolonged second stage
- Arrest of descent
- Retraction of fetal head during crowning with each *uterine contraction* (instead of protruding with each contraction)

### NURSING IMPLICATIONS

- Offer support and encouragement to the client and her support person during a difficult birth.
- Ask the client to flex her thighs sharply on her abdomen, which widens the pelvic outlet and may allow the anterior shoulder to deliver.
- Be prepared to apply suprapubic pressure to help the shoulder escape from beneath the symphysis pubis.
- Be prepared to provide resuscitation for a potentially compromised neonate.
- Assess the newborn for possible fractured clavicle.

## SMALL FOR GESTATIONAL AGE

### DESCRIPTION

- An infant is small for gestational age if the birth weight is below the 10th percentile on an intrauterine growth curve for that age.
- The infant may be born *preterm* (before week 38 of gestation), may be term (week 38 to 42), or *post-term* (past 42 weeks).

**S**

- Infants who are small for gestational age are distinctly different from infants whose weight is low but who are normal for their gestational age.
- The most common cause is a placental anomaly; either the placenta is unable to obtain sufficient nutrients from the placental arteries, or it is insufficient in transporting nutrients to the fetus.
- In other instances, the placental supply of nutrients is adequate, but the infant is unable to use them, such as in the case with infants with intrauterine infections or chromosomal abnormalities.
- A lack of adequate maternal nutrition may be also be a cause.

### ASSESSMENT FINDINGS

- Prenatal *fundal height* below normal for gestational age
- Poor placental function during a nonstress test
- Decreased fetal size for dates on *ultrasonography*
- Below average weight, length, and head circumference
- Poor skin turgor
- Widely separated skull sutures
- Dull and lusterless hair
- Sunken abdomen
- Dry, yellow-stained umbilical cord
- Increased hematocrit
- Increased red blood cells
- Hypoglycemia

### NURSING IMPLICATIONS

- Perform a thorough physical assessment to establish a baseline.
- Obtain a thorough prenatal history from the client.
- Closely observe respiratory rate and character for changes indicating respiratory distress.
- Monitor and maintain body temperature to prevent cold stress.
- Obtain laboratory specimens as prescribed to evaluate for changes.
- Be prepared to administer intravenous glucose to sustain blood glucose if newborns are unable to suck vigorously enough to take sufficient oral feedings.
- Promote early maternal-infant bonding.

# SPERMICIDES

### DESCRIPTION

- Spermicides are a barrier method of contraception.
- Spermicidal jellies or creams when inserted into the vagina cause the death of spermatozoa before they can enter the cervix.
- These jellies also change the vaginal pH to a strong acid level, which is not conducive to sperm survival.
- The preferred ingredient, nonoxynol 9, apparently also helps prevent *sexually transmitted disease.*
- Another form of spermicide includes a film of glycerin impregnated with nonoxynol 9 that is folded and inserted vaginally. Contact with vaginal or precoital penile emissions dissolves the film and activates a carbon dioxide foam.
- There is also a foam-impregnated sponge available that is moistened with water and then inserted vaginally.
- Other vaginal products are cocoa butter and glycerin-based vaginal suppositories filled with spermicide that when inserted vaginally dissolve and free the spermicidal ingredients.
- Spermicides are contraindicated in women with acute cervicitis because they might further infect the cervix.
- Because the failure rate is about 20%, they are generally inappropriate for women who must prevent conception.

### NURSING IMPLICATIONS

- Be aware of personal feelings and values about contraception and sexuality.
- Perform a thorough history and physical examination to establish a baseline.
- Be sensitive to the client's personal, religious, cultural, and social beliefs about birth control.
- Answer the client's questions honestly and openly.
- Provide education for the client and partner about family planning methods.
- Instruct the client that she should insert the spermicide not more than 1 hour before coitus for the most effective results.
- Advise the client not to douche for 6 hours following coitus to ensure that the cream or jelly has completed its spermicidal action.

- Emphasize to the client that although she may feel safe with her method of barrier contraception, her partner should still wear a *condom* to protect her from *sexually transmitted diseases* if the relationship is not a monogamous one.
- Assure the client that there is no reason to think that the fetus will be affected by the spermicide should she become pregnant.
- Caution the client that products labeled "feminine hygiene" products are for vaginal cleanliness and are not spermicidal: They are not birth control products.
- Caution the client with acute cervicitis to choose another type of contraception as the spermicide will further irritate the cervix.

## STERILIZATION

### DESCRIPTION
- Sterilization is a permanent contraceptive method for reproductive life planning.
- It includes a *tubal ligation* for the woman and a *vasectomy* for the man.
- Sterilization is the most frequently used method of contraception in the United States.

### NURSING IMPLICATIONS
- Perform a thorough history and physical examination to establish a baseline.
- Caution the client that although procedures for the reversal of both male and female sterilization do exist, such techniques are more complicated than the sterilization itself, and the success rates vary greatly.
- Suggest to the client that they consider the possibility of death, divorce, or remarriage when choosing this option.
- Inform the client that these procedures have no effect on sexuality.
- Refer the client and partner to counseling, especially if they are under the age of 25.

## SUBCUTANEOUS IMPLANTS

### DESCRIPTION
- Subcutaneous implants are a form of contraception in which a hormone is implanted subdermally into the

subcutaneous tissue suppressing ovulation and stimulating thick cervical mucus.

- Norplant received Food and Drug Administration approval in 1991 and involves implanting 6 Silastic implants (about the width of a pencil lead) filled with
levonorgestrel just under the skin on the inside of the
upper arm.
- Norplant may remain implanted for a 5-year period.
- Implants are inserted during the menses or no later
than the 7th day of the menstrual cycle to be certain that the woman is not pregnant at the time of
insertion.
- Implants can be inserted immediately after an abortion or 6 weeks after delivery of a baby.
- They can be used during *breast-feeding* with no effect
on milk production.
- The implants are expensive ($150.00), and side effects
include weight gain, headaches, irregular periods, and
an increased incidence of ovarian cysts and possible
depression.

### NURSING IMPLICATIONS

- Be aware of personal feelings and values about contraception and sexuality.
- Perform a thorough history and physical examination
to establish a baseline.
- Be sensitive to the client's personal, religious, cultural,
and social beliefs about birth control.
- Answer the client's questions honestly and openly.
- Provide education for the client and partner about
family planning methods.
- Advise the client that should she desire pregnancy,
fertility returns in about 3 months after the implants
are removed.
- Caution the client about possible side effects and to
report any to her physician.
- Reassure the client that once imbedded, the implants
appear only as lines on the skin, simulating small
veins.

## SUBCUTANEOUS INJECTIONS

### DESCRIPTION

- Subcutaneous injections of a hormone medroxy-
progesterone acetate (DMPA or Depo-Provera) to

suppress ovulation have been approved for contraceptive use.
- Side effects are similar to subcutaneous implants and include menstrual spotting, headache, and weight gain.
- Depo-Provera may impair glucose tolerance in women at risk for diabetes.
- There may be an increased risk for breast cancer and osteoporosis.
- A single injection is given every 3 months.

#### NURSING IMPLICATIONS
- Be aware of personal feelings and values about contraception and sexuality.
- Perform a thorough history and physical examination to establish a baseline.
- Be sensitive to the client's personal, religious, cultural, and social beliefs about birth control.
- Answer the client's questions honestly and openly.
- Provide education for the client and partner about family planning methods.
- Teach the client to do regular breast self-examinations.
- Advise the client to ingest a high amount of calcium and exercise daily to minimize the risk of osteoporosis.
- Advise the client that she must return to a health care provider for a new injection every 3 months for the method to remain reliable.
- Advise the client that she still should insist that her partner use a *condom* to protect her from a *sexually transmitted disease* if her relationship is not a monogamous one.

## SUBINVOLUTION

### DESCRIPTION
- Subinvolution is incomplete return of the uterus to its prepregnant size and shape.
- With subinvolution, at a 4- or 6-week postpartal visit, the uterus is still enlarged and soft, and the woman still has a *lochia* discharge.
- Subinvolution may result from a small *retained placental fragment,* a mild endometritis, or an accompanying problem such as a myoma that is interfering with complete contraction.

- A chronic loss of blood from subinvolution results in anemia and lack of energy, conditions that could lead to interference with maternal-infant bonding because of daily exhaustion.

**ASSESSMENT FINDINGS**
- Uterus still enlarged at 4 to 6 weeks' postpartum
- Uterus soft
- *Lochia* discharge
- Uterus tender on palpation
- *Anemia*

**NURSING IMPLICATIONS**
- Instruct the client before discharge about the normal process of involution and *lochia* discharge.
- Assess the client's *fundal height,* noting size, consistency, and presence of any tenderness.
- Assess any *lochia* discharge, noting color, amount, and odor.
- Instruct the client how to take her medication, such as oral methylergonovine or antibiotics, including any adverse reactions, and to report any problems, especially continuation of *lochia* discharge.
- Obtain necessary laboratory specimens to detect possible *anemia* as a result of excessive bleeding.

# SUDDEN INFANT DEATH SYNDROME (SIDS)

**DESCRIPTION**
- SIDS occurs when a well-nourished infant has been put to bed for a nap and is found dead a few hours later.
- SIDS occurs in about 4 out of 1000 live births.
- SIDS tends to occur at a higher rate in infants of adolescent mothers, infants of closely spaced pregnancies, and underweight male infants.
- Also prone to SIDS are infants with bronchopulmonary dysplasia as well as *preterm infants,* twins, siblings of another child with SIDS, and infants of narcotic-dependent mothers.
- Although the cause is unknown, a number of theories have been advanced, including research that shows a prevalence in infants that sleep prone rather than on the side or back, a viral respiratory or botulinism infection, prolonged and unexplained *apnea,* familial

distorted breathing patterns, and a lack of surfactant in the alveoli.
- Peak ages of incidence are between 2 weeks and 1 year of age.

### Nursing Implications

- Offer to arrange for counseling for the parents by a nurse or someone trained in counseling.
- Offer support and encouragement to the parents; allow parents to express their grief.
- Provide explanations about SIDS; allow parents to ask questions.
- Help the parents to understand that the feelings they are experiencing are not unique.
- Give the parents the number of the local chapter of the SIDS Alliance.
- Offer reassurance to any siblings that they were not at fault for the infant's death even if they wished it dead.
- If another child is born, support the parents through the first few months at least until they are past the point at which the first child died.

## SYSTEMIC LUPUS ERYTHEMATOSUS (SLE)

### Description

- SLE is a multisystem chronic disease of connective tissue that can occur in women of childbearing age: Its highest incidence is in women aged 20 to 40 years.
- With onset of the illness, widespread degeneration of connective tissue, especially of the heart, kidneys, blood vessels, spleen, skin, and retroperitoneal tissue, occurs.
- The most marked skin change is a characteristic erythematous "butterfly-shaped" rash on the face.
- Most serious of the kidney changes are fibrin deposits that plug and block the glomeruli, leading to necrosis and scarring.
- Thickening of the collagen tissue in blood vessels causes vessel obstruction, which could be life-threatening to the woman if the blood flow to the vital organs becomes compromised and to the fetus if blood flow to the placenta is obstructed.
- A number of women with SLE have antiphospholipid antibodies, which increase the tendency to thrombi formation.

- For some women, the chief complaint of the disorder may occur for the first time during pregnancy.
- Infants of women with SLE tend to be small for gestational age owing to decreased blood flow to the placenta.
- The incidence of *spontaneous abortion* and *preterm infant* rises with SLE.

### ASSESSMENT FINDINGS

- Hypertension (occurs with nephritis)
- Hematuria (differentiates SLE from *pregnancy-induced hypertension*)
- Decreased urine output
- Proteinuria
- Edema
- Increased serum creatinine levels over 1.5 mg/dl
- Decreased creatinine clearance level

### NURSING IMPLICATIONS

- Monitor serum creatinine levels to assess kidney function.
- Advise the client to decrease salicylate intake close to birth to reduce the possibility of bleeding in the neonate.
- Be prepared to administer intravenous hydrocortisone during labor to help with stress.
- Assess the neonate for a lupuslike rash, *anemia,* and thrombocytopenia.
- Assure the client that her infant's rash will only last about 6 months and then will fade.
- Be aware that congenital heart block may occur in the neonate; anticipate the possibility that a pacemaker may be necessary.
- Offer support and encouragement to the client and partner, especially if there are problems with the infant.
- Be aware that during the postpartum period, the client may experience an exacerbation of symptoms as corticosteroid levels again fall to normal.

## THROMBOPHLEBITIS

### DESCRIPTION

- Thrombophlebitis is inflammation of the lining of a blood vessel with the formation of clots.

- When thrombophlebitis occurs in the postpartal period, it is usually an extension of an endometrial infection.
- Thrombophlebitis is prone to occur in the postpartal period when blood-clotting ability is high because of increased fibrinogen; dilation of lower extremity veins owing to pressure of fetal head during pregnancy and birth; and the relative inactivity of the period that leads to pooling, stasis, and clotting of blood in the lower extremities.
- Women most prone to thrombophlebitis are those with varicose veins, those who are obese, those who have had a previous thrombophlebitis, women over 30 years old with increased parity who were in a stirrups position for a long time during birth, and those who have a high incidence of thrombophlebitis in their family.
- With femoral thrombophlebitis, the femoral, saphenous, or popliteal veins are involved, often occurring around the 10th postpartum day.
- Although the inflammation site in thrombophlebitis is in a vein, an accompanying arterial spasm often diminishes arterial circulation to the leg as well.
- Pelvic thrombophlebitis involves the ovarian, uterine, or hypogastric veins and occurs later than femoral thrombophlebitis, often around the 14th or 15th day of the puerperium.
- With pelvic thrombophlebitis, an abscess may form (necessitating incision by laparotomy), which may cause tubal scarring and interfere with future pregnancies.

### Assessment Findings

#### Femoral thrombophlebitis

- Elevated temperature
- Chills
- Pain, stiffness, and redness of affected leg
- Leg edema with shiny skin
- Positive Homans' sign

#### Pelvic thrombophlebitis

- Feeling of sudden, extreme illness
- High fever
- Chills
- General malaise
- Pelvic abscess

### NURSING IMPLICATIONS

- Provide prevention of *endometritis* and thrombophlebitis by using good aseptic technique.
- Encourage early ambulation to increase circulation in the lower extremities and decrease the possibility of clot formation.
- Be certain that client does not remain in a lithotomy and stirrups position for more than an hour, and be certain to pad the stirrups to prevent any sharp pressure against the calf of the legs in this position.
- Provide support stockings to the postpartum client who has varicose veins to increase venous circulation and help prevent stasis.
- Instruct the client to put the support stockings on before she rises in the morning and to remove them twice a day to assess the skin underneath.
- Encourage bed rest with the affected leg elevated for the client with a femoral thrombophlebitis.
- Obtain daily blood coagulation levels before administering any anticoagulants.
- Administer anticoagulants, analgesics, and antibiotics, as prescribed.
- Apply heat applications such as a heat lamp or moist, warm compresses as prescribed, making certain that the weight of a hot pack or pad does not rest on the leg, obstructing the flow of blood by its weight.
- Obtain a bed cradle to keep pressure of the bed clothes off the affected leg.
- Measure the diameter of the leg at the thigh and calf level and then compare the measurements in the next few days to note any increase or decrease in size.
- Obtain a record of *lochia* and weigh perineal pads to assess bleeding if the client is on anticoagulant therapy.
- Assess for other possible bleeding signs, such as bleeding gums, ecchymotic spots on the skin, or oozing from an *episiotomy* suture line.
- Reassure the client receiving heparin that she may continue to *breast-feed* her infant as this medication will not be present in breast milk.
- Be prepared to administer protamine sulfate as an antagonist for heparin.
- Instruct the client about heparin administration should she be discharged on subcutaneous therapy.

- Instruct the client that with future pregnancies she should make her physician aware of her difficulty to ensure proper precautions are taken to prevent thrombophlebitis.
- Prepare the client with pelvic thrombophlebitis for surgery.

## TOBACCO USE

### DESCRIPTION
- Tobacco use (cigarette smoking) by a pregnant woman has been shown to have teratogenic effects on the fetus, especially growth retardation.
- Low birth weight in infants of smoking mothers results from vasoconstriction of the uterine vessels, limiting the blood supply to the fetus.
- Part of the influence of cigarette smoking may be related to inhaled carbon monoxide.

### NURSING IMPLICATIONS
- Obtain a thorough history and physical examination to establish a baseline.
- Educate the client about the risks to herself and her fetus at the first prenatal visit and ongoing throughout the pregnancy if the client continues to smoke.
- Encourage the woman to stop smoking during her pregnancy.
- Encourage the woman to reduce the number of cigarettes a day that she smokes to diminish any adverse effects on her fetus.
- Offer support and guidance about smoking cessation; refer to a smoking cessation group, if appropriate.
- Advise the client not to join a smoking cessation group that uses drug therapy because the substitute drug may be as harmful to the fetus as the original smoking.

## TRANSIENT TACHYPNEA OF THE NEWBORN (TTN)

### DESCRIPTION
- TTN occurs when the newborn's respiratory rate remains at a high level between 80 and 120 breaths per minute.
- TTN appears to result from slow absorption of lung fluid.

- It occurs more often in infants who are born by *cesarean birth,* in infants whose mothers received extensive fluid administration during labor, and in *preterm infants.*

- TTN may reflect a slight decrease in production of phosphatidyl glycerol or mature surfactant.
- TTN peaks in intensity at approximately 36 hours of life and then begins to fade until by 72 hours of life, it spontaneously fades as the lung fluid is absorbed and respiratory activity becomes effective.

### Assessment Findings

- Respiratory rate between 80 and 120 breaths per minute
- Mild retractions but no marked cyanosis
- Mild hypoxia and hypercapnia
- Some fluid in the central lung with adequate aeration on chest x-ray

### Nursing Implications

- Perform a thorough labor and delivery history to establish a baseline.
- Assess the newborn's respirations closely, noting rate, depth, and character for changes.
- Observe the newborn closely to see that the increased respiratory effort is not tiring him or her.
- Watch for obvious signs of respiratory obstruction, such as retractions and cyanosis.
- Administer oxygen as prescribed.

## TUBAL LIGATION

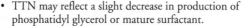

### Description

- Tubal ligation is a procedure that results in *sterilization* for the female client by occluding the fallopian tubes by cautery, crushing, clamping, or blocking the tube, thereby preventing the passage of the sperm into the tube to meet the ova.
- Some other techniques involve instilling silicon gel into the tube as a blocking agent, which can be removed at a later date to attempt to reverse the procedure.
- Tubal ligation can be performed by laparoscopic technique by making a small incision just under the umbilicus and then passing a lighted laparoscope through the incision. Carbon dioxide is pumped into

the incision to lift the abdominal wall. Electrical current is passed through the instrument to coagulate the tissue of the fallopian tube and seal it.

- A minilaparotomy (performed post childbirth or post *abortion*) involves making a small incision transversely across the pubic hair, and then metal or plastic clips or rubber rings seal the fallopian tubes.
- Tubal ligation can be done as soon as day 1 after delivery of a child, although the abdominal distention at this time may make locating the tubes difficult.
- Contraindications to tubal ligation are an umbilical hernia and severe obesity.
- Complications associated with tubal ligation include bowel perforation, hemorrhage, and the risks of using *general anesthesia* with the procedure.
- Tubal ligation should be regarded as a permanent, irreversible procedure.

### Nursing Implications

- Obtain a thorough history and physical examination before the procedure to establish a baseline.
- Provide preoperative teaching regarding deep breathing exercises and coughing.
- Inform the client that she will remain in the hospital a few hours or may be kept overnight after the procedure.
- Advise the client that she should not have unprotected coitus before the procedure since sperm trapped in the tube could fertilize an ovum causing an ectopic pregnancy.
- Inform the client that she may experience abdominal bloating for the first 24 hours after a laparoscopic tubal ligation until the carbon dioxide that was infused during the procedure is absorbed.
- Instruct the client that the procedure will not affect her menstrual cycle.
- Inform the client that she may return to coitus as soon as 2 to 3 days after the procedure.

## TUBERCULOSIS

### Description

- In tuberculosis, lung tissue is invaded by the *mycobacterium tuberculosis,* an acid-fast bacillus.

- Fibrosis, calcification, and a final ring of collagenous scar tissue develop, effectively sealing off the organism from the body and other further invasion or spread.
- Antibodies developed thereafter cause a positive tine or purified protein derivative (PPD) test in the individual.
- Tuberculosis in the pregnant client places her at high risk for problems.
- Recent inactive tuberculosis may become active in the postpartal period, as the lung suddenly returns to its more vertical prepregnant condition and breaks open calcium deposits.

## ASSESSMENT FINDINGS
- Positive chest x-ray
- Chronic cough
- Weight loss
- Hemoptysis
- Night sweats
- Low-grade fever
- Chronic fatigue

## NURSING IMPLICATIONS
- Advise the client that if she has had tuberculosis, it is advisable to wait at least 2 years before attempting to conceive.
- Perform a tine or PPD test for the client in high-risk areas at the first prenatal visit.
- Encourage the client to maintain an adequate level of calcium during pregnancy to ensure that tuberculosis pockets form or are not broken down.
- If the client is receiving isoniazid (INH), encourage her to take her supplemental pyridoxine to prevent peripheral neuritis.
- Do a monthly Snellen test for the client who is receiving ethambutol to detect optic nerve involvement.
- Obtain sputum cultures before allowing the client to hold or care for her baby.
- Caution the breast-feeding mother receiving INH that if her baby is receiving INH she should not breastfeed because this increases the dose to the baby and might be toxic.

## ULTRASONOGRAPHY

### DESCRIPTION

- Ultrasonography, a diagnostic technique, uses intermittent sound waves of high frequency (above the audible range) projected toward the uterus by a transducer that is placed on the abdomen and moved both horizontally and vertically. The sound frequencies that bounce back can be displayed on an oscilloscope screen as a visual image; the frequencies returning from tissues of various thicknesses and properties present distinct appearances.
- It also may be performed using an intravaginal technique.
- It is most likely used for *evaluation of fetal well-being* at least once during a normal pregnancy.
- It can be used to diagnose pregnancy as early as 6 weeks' gestation and later to confirm the presence, size, and location of the placenta and to establish that the fetus is increasing in size and has no gross defects such as hydrocephalus; anencephaly; or spinal cord, heart, kidney, and bladder defects.
- It may be used at term to establish the *fetal presentation and position,* to predict maturity by measurements of the *biparietal diameter,* and during early *stages of labor* to determine the presence of any abnormality such as *placenta previa.*
- It also is used to discover complications of pregnancy, such as the presence of an *intrauterine device, hydramnios* or olgiohydramnios, *ectopic pregnancy,* missed abortion, abdominal pregnancy, *placental previa,* premature separation of the placenta, coexisting uterine tumors, or *multiple gestation.*
- *Fetal death* can be revealed by a lack of heartbeat and respiratory movement.
- Following birth, it can detect *retained placental fragments* or poor uterine involution.

### NURSING IMPLICATIONS

- Explain the procedure to the client and her support person.
- Assure the client that the process does not involve x-ray and that the father of the child or support person may remain in the room during the procedure.
- Encourage the client to drink a full glass of water every 15 minutes beginning an hour and a half before

the procedure to make sure that she has a full bladder during the procedure; caution the client not to void before the procedure.

- Assure the client that the ultrasonography involves no discomfort for the fetus; explain that the only discomfort for her is that she might interpret the contact lubricant touching her abdomen as messy and that she may experience a strong desire to void before the procedure is completed.
- Place a towel under her right buttocks to tip her body slightly so the uterus will roll away from the vena cava to prevent supine hypotension syndrome.
- Be certain the contact gel applied to the client's abdomen has been warmed to room temperature or slightly warmer to prevent uterine cramping.
- Suggest to the client that she ask for a polaroid picture of the sonogram, if one is taken, to enhance the bonding process.
- Assist the client to the bathroom after the procedure and offer her a washcloth or towel to clean the lubricant from her abdomen.

## URINARY TRACT INFECTION

### DESCRIPTION

- A urinary tract infection in a pregnant woman occurs as a result of urinary stasis in ureters that are dilated from the effect of progesterone.
- Glycosuria that occurs with pregnancy can contribute to the growth of organisms.
- The organism most commonly responsible for urinary tract infections is *Escherichia coli.*
- A urinary tract infection can also occur as a descending infection or begin in the kidneys from the filtration of organisms present from other body infections.
- Women with known vesicoureteral reflux develop a urinary tract infection or pyelonephritis more often than others.
- An increased incidence of *preterm labor, premature rupture of membranes,* and fetal loss may be associated with pyelonephritis.

### ASSESSMENT FINDINGS

- Pain in the lumbar region, usually right-sided (because the uterus is pushed to that side by the large

bulk of the intestine on the left side creating stasis), radiating downward
- Tender area where the client experiences pain on palpation
- Complaints of nausea and vomiting, malaise, pain, and frequency of urination
- Slight rise in temperature or extremely elevated (as high as 103 to 104°F [39 to 40°C])
- Urine culture positive for over 100,000 organisms per milliliter of urine.

### NURSING IMPLICATIONS

- Obtain a clean-catch urine specimen for culture and sensitivity.
- Instruct the client about ways to prevent urinary tract infections, such as voiding frequently, wiping front to back after bowel movements, wearing cotton not synthetic fiber underwear, and voiding after intercourse.
- Encourage the client who has a urinary tract infection to increase her intake of fluids by giving her a specific amount to drink every day, up to 3 to 4 L per 24 hours.
- Teach the client how to promote urine drainage by assuming a knee-chest position for 15 minutes morning and evening to shift the weight of the uterus forward, freeing the ureter for drainage.
- Know that sulfonamides are used early in pregnancy to treat urinary tract infections but should not be used near term because they interfere with protein binding of bilirubin, which could lead to hyperbilirubinemia in the neonate.
- Remember also that tetracyclines are contraindicated in pregnancy because they cause retardation of bone growth and staining of fetal teeth.
- Instruct the client in medication regimen and question client if she is adhering to her antibiotic regimen to evaluate compliance.
- Schedule a postdelivery pyelogram, as prescribed for the client who has had frequent urinary tract infections to determine any urinary tract abnormality that might be present to help prevent future infections.

# UTERINE ATONY

## DESCRIPTION

- Uterine atony, or lack of tone, is the most frequent cause of *postpartal hemorrhage.*
- The uterus must remain in a contracted state after birth to allow the open vessels at the placental site to seal.
- Factors that predispose to poor uterine tone and inability to maintain a contracted state include *multiple gestation, hydramnios,* large baby (over 9 lb), presence of uterine myomas, operative delivery, rapid delivery, placenta accreta, *placenta previa,* premature separation of the placenta, deep *anesthesia* or analgesia, *labor induction or augmentation* or assisted with an oxytocin agent, maternal age over 30, prolonged and difficult labor, secondary maternal illness such as *anemia, endometritis, fetal death,* and *disseminated intravascular coagulation.*
- The first step in controlling *postpartal hemorrhage* in the event of uterine atony is to attempt uterine massage to encourage contraction.
- If the uterus cannot remain contracted, the physician invariably orders an intramuscular injection of methylergonovine (Methergine) or a dilute intravenous infusion of oxytocin to help the uterus maintain tone.
- If uterine massage and administration of methylergonovine or oxytocin are not effective, the physician may attempt bimanual compression (one hand inserted into the vagina and the other pushing against the fundus through the abdominal wall).
- It may be necessary to explore the uterine cavity for *retained placental fragments.*
- Uterine packing may be placed to help halt bleeding.
- Prostaglandin $F_{2a}$ may be injected intramuscularly or intramyometrially to initiate *uterine contractions.*
- If all other therapeutic measures fail in achieving uterine atony, ligation of the uterine arteries or hysterectomy, although rare, may be performed.

## ASSESSMENT FINDINGS

- Sudden uterine relaxation
- *Vaginal bleeding (abrupt or seeping)*

- Symptoms of shock and blood loss
  Decreased blood pressure
  Rapid, thready, and weak pulse
  Increased and shallow respirations
  Pale, clammy skin
  Increasing anxiety

## NURSING IMPLICATIONS

- Be cautious and on guard for signs of uterine bleeding in immediate observation of a client in whom any of the predisposing factors are present.
- Palpate the fundus at frequent intervals to ascertain that the uterus is remaining in a state of contraction.
- Assess vital signs and *lochia* per protocol and observe for signs of blood loss and shock.
- Ask the client to turn on her side when inspecting for bleeding to be certain that blood is not pooling underneath her.
- Perform gentle but firm uterine massage while supporting the base of the uterus to encourage uterine involution.
- Remain with the patient following uterine massage to be certain that the uterus is not relaxing again.
- Assess for bladder distention, which interferes with uterine involution.
- Perform a perineal pad count in given lengths of time (half-hour intervals, for instance) to assess better blood loss.
- Weigh perineal pads before and after use (then subtract the difference) to measure vaginal discharge more accurately.
- Be prepared to administer an intramuscular injection of methylergonovine or a dilute intravenous infusion of oxytocin to help the uterus maintain tone.
- Assess the client's blood pressure before administering oxytocin or methylergonovine because these medications can cause hypertension and therefore should not be administered if the client's blood pressure is over 140/90 mm Hg.
- Obtain appropriate laboratory specimens such as crossmatching if it is determined that the client's blood loss requires her to receive blood replacement.
- Observe for side effects of prostaglandin $F_{2a}$ administration, such as nausea, diarrhea, tachycardia, and hypertension.

- Support the client and partner if all efforts fail to produce uterine tone and an emergency hysterectomy must be performed.

# UTERINE RUPTURE

## DESCRIPTION

- Uterine rupture occurs when the uterus undergoes more strain than it is capable of sustaining.
- Although rupture of the uterus is rare, occurring in about 1 in 1500 births, it is always a possibility.
- Rupture occurs most commonly when a vertical scar from a previous *cesarean birth,* hysterotomy, or plastic repair of the uterus tears.
- Rupture can be complete, going through endometrium, myometrium, and peritoneum, or incomplete, leaving the peritoneum intact.
- Contributing factors include prolonged labor, faulty *fetal presentation, multiple gestation,* unwise use of oxytocin, obstructed labor, and traumatic maneuvers using *forceps delivery* or traction.

## ASSESSMENT FINDINGS

- *Pathologic retraction ring* apparent by an indentation across the abdomen over the uterus (impending rupture)
- Sudden, severe pain during a strong *uterine contraction*
- Complaints of a "tearing" sensation
- Stoppage of *uterine contractions*
- Failing *fetal heart rate*
- Change in abdominal contour with two visibly distinct swellings
- Rapid, weak pulse; falling blood pressure; cold, clammy skin; and dilation of the nostrils from air hunger (signs of shock)
- Localized tenderness and a persistent aching pain over the lower segment (incomplete rupture)
- Stoppage of contractions (incomplete rupture)
- Fetal and maternal distress

## NURSING IMPLICATIONS

- Perform *electronic fetal monitoring* for *evaluation of fetal well-being* and *uterine contractions.*

- Be prepared to administer emergency fluid replacement as well as intravenous oxytocin to attempt to contract the uterus to minimize bleeding.
- Be prepared for emergency laparotomy.
- Obtain emergency preoperative laboratory studies.
- Offer support to the client or her support person and inform them as soon as possible about fetal outcome, the extent of the surgery, and the woman's safety.
- Allow the woman and her support person time to grieve about possible loss of her child and her fertility.

## VACUUM EXTRACTION

### DESCRIPTION

- Vacuum extraction is a procedure whereby a disk-shaped cup is pressed against the fetal scalp over the posterior fontanel to assist in vaginal delivery of the fetus.
- When vacuum pressure is applied, air beneath the cup is sucked out, and the cup then adheres so tightly that traction on the cord leading to the cup delivers the fetus.
- Advantages of vacuum extraction over *forceps delivery* include
    The use of less *anesthesia,* making the fetus less depressed at birth.
    Fewer *perineal lacerations* of the birth canal.
- Disadvantages include
    A marked *caput succedaneum* that may be noticeable as long as 7 days after birth.
    Tentorial tears from extreme pressure.

### ASSESSMENT FINDINGS

- Fetal head at the perineum
- Fetus not preterm (softness of preterm scalp would not withstand vacuum extraction)

### NURSING IMPLICATIONS

- Assure the client that *caput succedaneum* swelling is harmless to her infant and it decreases rapidly.
- Assist the client and support person with breathing and pushing exercises during delivery.
- Offer support and encouragement throughout the labor and delivery process, informing the client and partner about events that are happening.

- Perform a thorough *newborn physical assessment* after delivery.

# VAGINAL BIRTH AFTER CESAREAN BIRTH

### DESCRIPTION

- Vaginal birth after cesarean birth refers to the client who has had a previous *cesarean birth* but is now having a vaginal birth.
- It is usually only done for women who have had a previous *cesarean birth* that involved a low transverse uterine incision with the fetus estimated to be less than 4000 g (8 lb, 13 oz).
- Also, there is no evidence of cephalopelvic disproportion.

### NURSING IMPLICATIONS

- Be certain that a physician is readily available during a *trial labor.*
- Have emergency surgical facilities ready.
- Be prepared to institute oxytocin *augmentation* to strengthen *uterine contractions.*
- Monitor *fetal heart rate* and *uterine contractions.* Be sure to obtain baseline *fetal heart rates* previous to *labor augmentation.*
- Anticipate the need for *vacuum extraction* and *forceps delivery* to assist in birth.
- Offer support to the client and encourage her to breathe with *uterine contractions,* push effectively, and accept vaginal birth.

# VAGINAL BLEEDING

### DESCRIPTION

- Vaginal bleeding refers to any deviation from the normal that may occur at any time during pregnancy.
- Some of the serious bleeding complications of pregnancy begin with vaginal bleeding.
- Vaginal bleeding may or may not be serious but should always be investigated because if it occurs in sufficient amount or for sufficient cause, it can impair both the outcome of the pregnancy and the woman's life or future health.
- The primary causes of vaginal bleeding are threatened, imminent, missed, or complete *abortion; ectopic pregnancy;* hydatidiform mole (*gestational trophoblastic*

*disease*); *incompetent cervix; placenta previa,* premature separation of the placenta (*abruptio placentae*); and *premature labor.*

- A woman with any degree of vaginal bleeding during pregnancy should be evaluated for hypovolemic shock.

## ASSESSMENT FINDINGS

- Assessment findings vary with the gestation, severity, and circumstance for the vaginal bleeding and may include
- Vaginal spotting
- Slight cramping
- *Cervical dilation*
- Sudden unilateral lower abdominal quadrant pain
- Painless bleeding
- Sharp abdominal pain followed by uterine tenderness
- Pink-stained vaginal discharge
- *Uterine contractions*
- Signs of hypovolemic shock (increased pulse rate, decreased blood pressure, increased respiratory rate, cold and clammy skin, decreased urine output, dizziness or decreased level of consciousness, decreased central venous pressure)

## NURSING IMPLICATIONS

- Confirm the existence of the pregnancy by asking the client how she knows for certain that she is pregnant and the length of the pregnancy.
- Ask the client how she discovered the bleeding, the duration, intensity, description, frequency, associated symptoms, and her activity before she noticed the vaginal bleeding.
- Perform a health history, including the client's blood type.
- Obtain vital signs and assess for signs of hypovolemic shock.
- Monitor *fetal heart rate* and *uterine contractions.*
- Prepare the client for *ultrasonography* to help determine the source of the vaginal bleeding.
- Place the client flat in bed on her side to maintain optimal placental and renal function.
- Administer intravenous fluids as prescribed to replace intravascular fluid volume.

- Administer oxygen as necessary at 6 to 10 L/minute by face mask.
- Keep the client NPO in the event of surgical intervention to stop the vaginal bleeding.
- Assist with placement of central venous pressure or pulmonary artery wedge catheter to provide more accurate measurement of maternal hemodynamic state.
- Obtain necessary laboratory specimens for cross-matching, fibrinogen, and blood-clotting evaluation.
- Measure maternal blood loss by weighing perineal pads and saving any tissue passed.
- Maintain a positive attitude about fetal outcome.
- Support the client's self-esteem by offering support and encouragement because the sight of the blood, no matter how much, will cause her much worry and anxiety.

## VAGINAL SPONGE

### Description
- Vaginal sponges are a barrier method of contraception.
- Vaginal sponges are impregnated with spermicidal foam, moistened with water, and then inserted vaginally.
- The moisture creates an internal foaming action and contraception protection.
- The sponge can be left in place for 24 hours and continues to be effective during this time.
- A disadvantage of the sponge is that water is necessary to activate it, and this may not always be feasible.

### Nursing Implications
- Be aware of personal feelings and values about contraception and sexuality.
- Perform a thorough history and physical examination to establish a baseline.
- Be sensitive to the client's personal, religious, cultural, and social beliefs about birth control.
- Answer the client's questions honestly and openly.
- Provide education for the client and partner about family planning methods.
- Emphasize to the client that although she may feel safe with her method of barrier contraception, her partner should still wear a *condom* to protect her from

*sexually transmitted diseases* if the relationship is not a monogamous one.
- Assure the client that there is no reason to think that the fetus will be affected by the *spermicide* should she become pregnant.
- Caution the woman with acute cervicitis not to choose this type of contraception as the *spermicide* may further irritate the cervix.
- Caution the client that she should not douche for 6 hours following coitus.

## VASECTOMY

### DESCRIPTION
- Vasectomy is a surgical procedure that results in male sterilization.
- The vas deferens is cut and tied or cauterized or plugged, blocking the passage of spermatozoa.
- This procedure is 100% effective and irreversible, although newer techniques of using silicon plugs and microsurgery can make it reversible to a limited extent.

### NURSING IMPLICATIONS
- Instruct the client that although he can resume sexual coitus within 1 week after surgery, an additional birth control method should be used until two negative sperm reports have been examined.
- Advise the patient to take a mild analgesic and to apply ice packs to the site to manage postoperative pain.
- Allow the client to verbalize fears and anxieties; answer the client's questions honestly and openly to alleviate fears.

## VENOUS THROMBOEMBOLIC DISEASE

### DESCRIPTION
- Venous thromboembolic disease is thrombus formation in the lower extremities due to stasis of blood from uterine pressure, vessel damage, and hypercoagulability.
- As more women delay childbearing until after age 30, the likelihood of deep vein thrombosis leading to pulmonary embolism increases.
- Increased estrogen levels cause increased coagulability.
- Increased blood congestion in the pelvis coupled with poor venous return resulting from pressure

of the uterus leads to stasis and possible thrombophlebitis.
- Increased age is another risk factor for thrombosis formation.
- A particular group of women, women with anti-phospholipid antibodies (aPLA), has been identified as being more susceptible to thrombi formation, *spontaneous abortion, fetal death,* and *pregnancy induced hypertension.*
- Deep vein thrombosis is most common in the post-partal period.

## Assessment Findings
- Calf pain
- Reddened, warm areas on the lower extremities
- Pulmonary embolism (an emergency situation):
  Chest pain
  Sudden onset of *dyspnea*
  Cough with hemoptysis
  Tachycardia or missed beats
  Severe dizziness or fainting from lowered blood pressure

## Nursing Implications
- Be prepared to administer cardiopulmonary resuscitation if client displays signs of pulmonary embolism.
- Obtain a thorough history and physical examination to establish a baseline.
- Teach the client about avoiding the use of constrictive knee-high stockings, not sitting with her legs crossed at the knee, and avoiding standing in one position for a long period of time to prevent the possibility of deep vein thrombosis.
- Anticipate the use of heparin to decrease hypercoagulability, and administer heparin as prescribed.
- Monitor heparin dosage by laboratory analysis of partial thromboplastin time.
- Provide instructions regarding maintaining strict bed rest, heat, and elevation of the extremities to prevent the possibility of embolism.
- Be aware that clients taking heparin during pregnancy should not take any additional injections once labor begins to help reduce the possibility of hemorrhage at birth; keep in mind that they are not routine candidates for *episiotomy* or *epidural anesthesia.*

*Section*
**3**

# Overview of Child Health Care

⊠ ⊠ ⊠

# PRINCIPLES OF GROWTH AND DEVELOPMENT

MENTAL STATUS
HEAD CIRCUMFERENCE
CHEST CIRCUMFERENCE
SKIN
HEAD
EYES
EARS
NOSE
MOUTH
NECK
CHEST
BREASTS
HEART
LUNGS
ABDOMEN
GENITORECTAL AREA
EXTREMITIES
BACK
NEUROLOGIC FUNCTION
**Vision Assessment**
EYE CHARTS
COVER TESTING
COLOR VISION DEFICIT TESTING
**Hearing Assessment**
AUDIOMETRIC TESTS
ACOUSTIC IMPEDANCE TESTING
CONDUCTION LOSS TESTING
**Speech Assessment**
**Developmental Assessment**
**Intelligence**
**Temperament**

▨ ▨ ▨

# FAMILY WITH AN INFANT

**Physical Growth**
STEADILY INCREASING HEIGHT, WEIGHT, AND
HEAD AND CHEST CIRCUMFERENCE
INCREASED BY 50% INCREASE OVER BIRTH
LENGTH BY 12 MONTHS
DOUBLING OF BIRTH WEIGHT BY 6 MONTHS
TRIPLING OF BIRTH WEIGHT BY 12 MONTHS

# FAMILY WITH A TODDLER

STEPLIKE HEIGHT AND WEIGHT INCREASES
   PROTRUDING ABDOMEN
BOW-LEGGEDNESS
HALF OF EXPECTED ADULT HEIGHT BY AGE 2
   4 TO 6 LB WEIGHT GAIN PER YEAR
INCREASED HEAD CIRCUMFERENCE
   1 Inch Between 1 and 2 Years
   1/2 Inch Until 5 Years

**Psychomotor Development**
  BOWEL AND BLADDER CONTROL BY 3 YEARS
  WALKING BY 12 TO 15 MONTHS
  RUNNING BY 2 YEARS
  WALKING BACKWARD AND HOPPING ON ONE
    FOOT BY 3 YEARS
  STAIR CLIMBING WITH BOTH FEET AT ONCE
  MASTERY OF FINE MOTOR SKILLS FOR BUILDING,
    DRAWING, AND UNDRESSING
  RITUALISM, NEGATIVISM, AND INDEPENDENCE

**Development**
  AUTONOMY VS. SHAME AND DOUBT
  ANAL STAGE
  SENSORIMOTOR
    Tertiary Circular Reactions
    Preconceptual Phase
  PRECONVENTIONAL STAGE

**Language**
  SHORT SENTENCES
  300-WORD VOCABULARY BY 2 YEARS
  "WHAT" QUESTIONS

  PARALLEL PLAY
  MAJOR SOCIALIZING MEDIUM
  PUSH-PULL TOYS

**HEALTH PROMOTION**
  **Safety**
  **Emotional Development**
  **Daily Activities**
  **Family Functioning**
**PARENTAL CONCERNS**
  **Toilet Training**
  **Ritualistic Behavior**
  **Negativism**
  **Discipline**

▦ ▦ ▦

# FAMILY WITH A PRESCHOOLER

▦ ▦ ▦

# FAMILY WITH SCHOOL-AGE CHILD

▒ ▒ ▒

# FAMILY WITH AN ADOLESCENT

☒ ☒ ☒

# THE HOSPITALIZED CHILD

⌧ ⌧ ⌧

# PHYSICAL DEVELOPMENTAL DISORDERS

⌘ ⌘ ⌘

# RESPIRATORY DISORDERS

⌗ ⌗ ⌗

## CARDIOVASCULAR DISORDERS

⌗ ⌗ ⌗

# IMMUNOLOGIC DISORDERS

⌗ ⌗ ⌗

# INFECTIOUS DISORDERS

## BLOOD DISORDERS

▨ ▨ ▨

# GASTROINTESTINAL DISORDERS

⊠ ⊠ ⊠

# RENAL AND URINARY TRACT DISORDERS

▨ ▨ ▨

## REPRODUCTIVE DISORDERS

⌘ ⌘ ⌘

# ENDOCRINE DISORDERS

⌘ ⌘ ⌘

# NEUROLOGIC DISORDERS

NEUROLOGIC EXAMINATION
  Cerebral Function
  Cranial Nerve Function
  Cerebellar Function
  Motor Function
  Sensory Function
  Reflex Testing
DIAGNOSTIC TESTING
  Lumbar Puncture
  Ventricular Tap
  Cerebral Angiography
  Myelography

⊠ ⊠ ⊠

# EYE AND EAR DISORDERS

✳ ✳ ✳

# MUSCULOSKELETAL DISORDERS

❊ ❊ ❊

## TRAUMATIC INJURIES

⌘ ⌘ ⌘

# CANCER: LONG-TERM OR FATAL ILLNESSES

✖ ✖ ✖

# COGNITIVE OR MENTAL HEALTH DISORDERS

※ ※ ※

# CHILD ABUSE

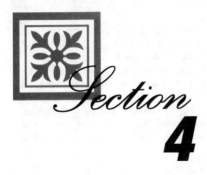

# Child Health
# Care Topics

# ABDOMINAL TRAUMA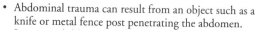

## DESCRIPTION

- Abdominal trauma can result from an object such as a knife or metal fence post penetrating the abdomen.
- In young children, abdominal trauma is generally nonpenetrating and occurs from a direct blow to the abdomen from an object, such as a baseball bat or an automobile dashboard.
- All children who have multiple trauma need observation for abdominal injury.
- Abdominal trauma can include *splenic rupture* or *liver rupture.*

## ASSESSMENT FINDINGS (may or may not be present)

- Abdominal pain
- Respiratory distress from abdominal distention
- Signs of hypovolemia
- Wounds
- Abrasions
- Bruising on the abdomen
- Absent or decreased bowel sounds
- Decreased level of consciousness

## NURSING IMPLICATIONS

- Monitor vital signs, especially pulse and blood pressure, frequently for changes indicating the possibility of hidden abdominal bleeding.
- Insert a nasogastric tube, as prescribed, and check aspirate for frank or occult bleeding; attach to low suction if bleeding is present.
- Insert an indwelling urinary catheter and check for hematuria, indicating possible kidney or bladder trauma.
- Obtain abdominal x-ray film, as prescribed, to rule out fractured pelvis and gastric, *splenic,* or intestinal *rupture.*
- Anticipate the need for abdominal paracentesis.
- Do not administer analgesics so that the location of the pain can help to identify which organs have been injured.
- Explain to the parents and child about treatments, procedures to be performed, and the rationale for them.
- Offer support and guidance to the parents, explaining that an injury need not be obvious at first glance to be serious.

- Anticipate the need for possible surgery and begin parent and child preparation.

# ABUSE, PHYSICAL

## DESCRIPTION

- Physical abuse refers to a type of child abuse in which the action of a caregiver causes injury to a child.
- 10% of all children seen in a hospital emergency department for traumatic injury are victims of child abuse.
- Battered child syndrome, a term used to describe victims of abuse, is one of the leading causes of childhood death and disability.
- Typically, child abuse is associated with physical abuse; however, it can also involve *neglect, psychological abuse, sexual abuse,* and *substance abuse.*
- Theories about child abuse center around a triad of characteristics involving a "special parent," "special child," and "special situation."
- Many parents who abuse their children were abused themselves; these parents typically have less control than other parents, are unfamiliar with normal growth and development of children, have unrealistic expectations of a child, and may be socially isolated with little support. Abuse is strongly associated with parental use of excessive alcohol, which removes inhibitions and self-control.
- Abused children are viewed as "different" by the parents; they may be more or less intelligent or may have been unplanned, or they may have a birth defect or an attention span deficit. Because the child is perceived as different, such as with children born prematurely or having an illness at birth, a good parent-child relationship does not develop.
- Stress, a special situation, may be a response to an event that would not necessarily be stressful to an average parent. It has a greater impact on people who do not have strong internal family support or who have not formed support systems outside the family.
- Child abuse crosses all socioeconomic boundaries because stress occurs at all levels.
- Shame, guilt, and fear of losing the abuser contribute to the child's difficulty in reporting the abuse.
- The abuser may threaten to abandon, injure, or even kill the child if the abuse is reported.

- Nurses are legally obligated to report all suspected cases of child abuse.

**ASSESSMENT FINDINGS** (typically burns or head and hand injuries)

- Curved lacerations such as from a belt buckle
- Circular/linear lesions such as from electrical cord, belt, and clothesline
- Patches of missing hair such as from hair pulling
- Bruises or welts on face, lips, mouth, neck, wrist, ankles, torso, back, buttocks, or thighs
- Bruises or welts clustered over one part of the body
- Injuries to both eyes or both cheeks
- Grab marks on the arms or wrists
- Human bite marks
- Injuries in various stages of healing
- Cigarette burns on buttocks, back, soles of feet, or palms
- Rope burns
- Doughnut-shaped burns on buttocks and perineal area—immersion burns
- Fractured skull, nose, or facial bones
- Dislocated shoulder or hip
- *Subdural hematoma*—head injury from shaken baby syndrome
- Retinal hemorrhages—head injury from shaken baby syndrome
- Low self-esteem, withdrawal, aggression, wariness of parents and other adults, self-injurious behavior, history of running away or *suicide* attempts

**NURSING IMPLICATIONS**

- Suspect physical abuse when the parent cannot explain the child's physical injuries or if the injuries are inconsistent with the parent's explanation or the child's developmental age.
- Use a multidisciplinary approach, including nurses, physicians, social workers, psychologists, and teachers to deal effectively with child abuse and maltreatment.
- Report all confirmed cases of physical abuse to the judiciary system.
- Hospitalize the child with significant physical injury and treat according to the problem.
- Always maintain a nonjudgmental attitude toward the parents.

- Remember that prevention of child abuse is the goal of treatment for the child and the abuser.
- Assess parent-child interactions and listen for feelings of negativity expressed by the parent.
- Provide consistent care and support for the abused child.
- Evaluate the safety of the parent's care.
- Praise abusing parents for the behaviors they do well.
- Talk to the parents away from the child so as to give them the attention they need.
- Advocate courses for parents in parenting and growth and development of children.
- Help children to learn problem-solving techniques so that they are not overwhelmed by mounting problems as adults.
- Foster self-esteem in children to encourage assertive behavior.
- Encourage parents in planned reproduction so children are desired.
- Help parents locate support people in the community.
- Provide role model caring behavior for parents.
- Identify children who may be viewed as special in some way by parents.
- Identify parents who were abused and offer specific help to break the cycle of child abuse.
- Advocate joining Parent's Anonymous for a support to parents who may be potential abusers.
- Advocate counseling for both the adult and child.
- Assess need to remove a child from a home temporarily or permanently.
- Help the child to understand the situation and explain why the child cannot go home with the parents in a nonjudgmental way.
- Carefully follow up on children left in the home and ensure that the pattern of stress and abuse is not recurring.

## ABUSE, PHYSICAL NEGLECT

### DESCRIPTION

- Physical neglect is failure to provide adequate food, clothing, shelter, or education for a child under age 18, resulting in harm or the danger of harm to the child's physical condition.

- It is a more subtle form of child abuse than *physical abuse,* but it can be just as damaging to a child's welfare.
- Neglect may be willful, or it may occur if the parents simply do not realize the normal needs of a child.

### Assessment Findings

- Listless
- Tired
- Unkempt and dirty
- Inappropriate dress for the weather
- Matted hair
- Discolored or stained teeth
- Hungry
- History of stealing or hoarding food
- Chronically absent from school or arriving early and leaving late
- Developmental delays
- Destructive behavior
- Compliant and eager to please

### Nursing Implications

- Assess the suspected child's (or children's) care and compare it to other family members to identify differences.
- Assess parent-child interactions and listen for feelings of indifference expressed by the parent.
- Provide consistent care and support for the child.
- Evaluate the safety of the parent's care; praise parents for the behaviors they do well.
- Talk to parents away from the child so as to give them the attention they need.
- Assess need to remove a child from a home temporarily or permanently.
- Help the child to understand the situation and explain why the child cannot go home with the parents in a nonjudgmental way.
- Carefully follow up on children left in the home and ensure that the pattern of neglect is not recurring.
- Advocate courses for parents in parenting and growth and development of children.
- Teach parents about normal growth and development, including the need for attachment and bonding.

- Assess the child's nutritional status, including height and weight; provide dietary supplements and food intake to ensure adequate nutrition and care of the child.
- Advocate counseling for both the adult and child.
- Report all confirmed cases of neglect to the judiciary system.

## ABUSE, PSYCHOLOGICAL

### DESCRIPTION

- Psychological abuse refers to a type of child abuse that includes constant belittling or threatening, rejecting, isolating, or exploiting the child.
- It can be as damaging to a child as *physical abuse;* it is the most difficult form of abuse to detect because it frequently occurs in the home, and its effects, although severe, may be subtle.
- The child who is psychologically abused will have difficulty becoming an emotionally confident adult.
- Emotional neglect, a type of psychological abuse, is failure to provide adequate nurturing, support, and love to a child under age 18, resulting in harm or the danger of harm to the child's emotional health.
- It may be willful or may result from parents who do not realize the basic normal needs of a child.

### ASSESSMENT FINDINGS

- Parental indifference
- Parental inability to engage in play or social activities with the child
- No signs of warmth or emotional investment made by parent for child
- Parental belittling or degrading of the child
- Frequent parental criticism of child
- Parent stating child is inadequate in some way
- Low self-esteem in child
- No eye contact by child
- Child not seeking adult or parent for comfort
- Developmental delays and *failure to thrive*
- Disruptive behavior (older children)
- Little empathy in play or in social situations (older children)
- Frequent psychosomatic complaints

### Nursing Implications

- Use a multidisciplinary approach, including nurses, physicians, social workers, psychologists, and teachers to deal effectively with child abuse and maltreatment.
- Report all confirmed cases of abuse to the judiciary system.
- Always maintain a nonjudgmental attitude toward the parents.
- Remember that prevention of child abuse is the goal of treatment for the child and the abuser.
- Assess parent-child interactions and listen for feelings of negativity expressed by the parent.
- Provide consistent care and support for the abused child.
- Evaluate the safety of the parent's care; praise parents for the behaviors they do well.
- Talk to the parents away from the child so as to give them the attention they need.
- Help children to learn problem-solving techniques so that they are not overwhelmed by mounting problems as adults.
- Foster self-esteem in children to encourage assertive behavior.
- Help parents locate support people in the community.
- Provide role model caring behavior for parents.
- Advocate joining Parent's Anonymous for a support to parents who may be potential abusers.
- Advocate counseling for both the adult and child.
- Assess need to remove a child from a home temporarily or permanently.
- Help the child to understand the situation and explain why the child cannot go home with the parents in a nonjudgmental way.
- Carefully follow up on children left in the home and ensure that the pattern of abuse is not recurring.
- Advocate courses for parents in parenting and growth and development of children.

## ABUSE, SEXUAL

### Description

- Sexual abuse refers to any sexual contact between the child and an adult.
- It involves the coercion of dependent, developmentally immature children and adolescents in sexual ac-

tivities that they do not fully comprehend, to which they are unable to give informed consent, and that violate the social taboos of family roles.

- It is physically and emotionally destructive, leaving a child unable to trust others and with a sense of ambivalence to intimacy and overall sense of worthlessness.
- It must be investigated for any preschool-age or school-age child with vaginal or rectal bleeding, tenderness, or known sexually transmitted infection.
- Most victims of sexual abuse are extremely reluctant to tell an adult about the abuse.
- Most sexual abusers are family members or close friends.

### Assessment Findings
- Social withdrawal
- Provocative sexual behavior
- Inappropriate knowledge of sexual activities
- Acting out of sexual activities with other children or dolls
- Low self-esteem
- Fearfulness
- History of running away or suicide
- Bruising or bleeding in the external genitalia, vagina, or rectum
- Bruising on the soft or hard palate
- Difficulty walking or sitting
- Genital pain or itching
- Bloody underclothes
- *Sexually transmitted diseases*
- Pain on urination
- Frequent *urinary tract infections*
- Foreign bodies in the vagina or rectum

### Nursing Implications
- Teach children early on that their bodies are their own and they should report anyone who tries to touch their "private parts" to a person whom they trust.
- Help the child to understand that the adult is at fault in sexual abuse cases and that the child is not at all responsible.
- Provide follow-up care by the same person who initially saw the sexually abused child.
- Prevent against *sexually transmitted diseases* and pregnancy with a thorough assessment and evaluation.

- Assist parents (if not the abuser) to obtain counseling regarding their feelings of guilt and anger over their child's sexual abuse.
- Ascertain that help is obtained if other forms of abuse, such as domestic abuse, are occurring in the family.

 ABUSE, SUBSTANCE

### DESCRIPTION
- Substance abuse refers to the use of chemicals to improve the mental state or induce euphoria.
- Drug use occurs in adolescents from a desire to expand consciousness or to feel more confident and mature; it also can occur as a response to peer pressure or may be a form of adolescent rebellion.
- Types of abused substances include cigarettes, alcohol, anabolic steroids, marijuana, amphetamines, cocaine, hallucinogens, and opiates.
- School-age children have available illegal drugs such as cigarettes, alcohol, and cocaine; they also abuse rubber cement and airplane glue, which can cause extensive liver damage or fatal pulmonary edema.

### ASSESSMENT FINDINGS
- Failure to complete assignments
- Poor reasoning ability
- Decreased school attendance
- Frequent mood swings—stupor and lethargy to aggressive behavior
- Violence
- Sleepiness, lack of coordination, drunken appearance
- Deteriorating physical appearance
- Recent change in peer group
- Immaturity
- Negative feelings for parents
- Serum hepatitis or *human immunodeficiency virus (HIV)* positive

### NURSING IMPLICATIONS
- Investigate any symptoms of drug abuse in any age child; perform a thorough history and physical examination to establish a baseline.
- Maintain role modeling behaviors to provide concrete examples of nonchemical productive behavior.

- Teach parents of school-age children the warning signs of drug use: irritability, inattentiveness, and drowsiness.
- Counsel children as young as sixth grade against the use of steroids because it can lead to cardiovascular irregularities, uncontrollable aggressiveness, and possibly cancer later in life.

- Caution children against cigarettes and smokeless tobacco, explaining realistically the physical consequences.
- Help adolescents to reveal any substance abuse patterns.
- Encourage adolescents to find alternate ways of feeling satisfaction in life without substance use.
- Foster growth in adolescents by developing a therapeutic relationship and encouraging verbalization of their feelings.
- Seek out alternate activities with the adolescent that will increase the adolescent's self-esteem.
- Set realistic goals for the adolescent who is chemically dependent.
- Caution adolescents against substance abuse as a preventive measure.
- Counsel that substance abuse is both illegal and harmful.
- Help adolescents to realize that dependence on a chemical to solve problems prevents them from learning to handle life situations and maturing.
- Encourage ownership of the chemical dependency by the adolescent and let the adolescent know only he or she can stop it.
- Teach adolescents that a month of daily alcohol abuse can make them physically addicted.
- Provide continued physical and emotional care for the chemically dependent child to help prevent their return to dependency.

## ACETAMINOPHEN POISONING

### Description

- Acetaminophen is an analgesic, antipyretic agent that does not inhibit platelet aggregation.
- It is now being used as a substitute for aspirin.
- Because parents believe that it is safer than aspirin, they may not be as careful about putting it away; if

the child swallows acetaminophen, they may delay in bringing the child in for help because they think it is a harmless drug.
- Acetaminophen in large doses can cause extreme liver dysfunction.
- Liver toxicity occurs at an acetaminophen load greater than 200 µg/ml by 4 hours and 50 µg/ml by 12 hours.

### ASSESSMENT FINDINGS
- Anorexia
- Nausea and *vomiting*
- *Diarrhea*
- Abdominal pain
- Elevated serum liver enzymes (SGOT and SGPT)

### NURSING IMPLICATIONS
- Immediately administer syrup of ipecac orally to induce vomiting or through a nasogastric tube and perform gastric lavage.
- Follow with administration of acetylcysteine every 4 hours for 72 hours orally.
- Mix acetylcysteine in a carbonated beverage to enhance its taste and aid in swallowing.
- If the child is small, administer the acetylcysteine through a nasogastric tube to avoid problems with swallowing.
- Assess the child for jaundice and tenderness over the liver area.
- Monitor serum liver enzyme levels for changes.

## ACNE

### DESCRIPTION
- Acne is a common adolescent health problem.
- It is a self-limiting inflammatory disease that involves the sebaceous glands that empty into hair shafts, mainly of the face and shoulders.
- It is the most common skin disorder of adolescence, occurring slightly more frequently in boys than in girls.
- The peak age for lesions to occur in girls is 14 to 17 years; for boys, 16 to 19 years.
- Although not proven, genetic factors may influence the development of acne.

- Cigarette smoking may increase the number of inflammatory lesions.
- As androgen levels increase during puberty, sebaceous glands become active; abnormal keratinization of the lining of the ducts occurs, causing obstruction of the ducts.
- The output of sebum (composed of lipids, mainly triglycerides) increases, but because of the narrowing of the ducts, the glands enlarge and sebum becomes trapped forming whiteheads (comedones).
- As the trapped sebum darkens from accumulation of melanin and oxidation of the fatty acid component on exposure to air, blackheads (open comedones) form.
- Bacteria lodge and thrive in the retained secretions, forming papules; leakage of free fatty acid from triglycerides causes a dermal inflammatory reaction.
- If the glands rupture, sebum is extruded into adjacent skin, producing reddened inflammatory cysts.
- Acne is categorized as mild (comedones are present), moderate (papules and pustules are also present), or severe (cysts are present).
- The most common locations of acne lesions are the face, neck, back, upper arms, and chest.
- Flare-ups are associated with emotional stress, menstrual periods, or use of greasy hair creams or makeup that can further plug gland ducts.

### ASSESSMENT FINDINGS

- Whiteheads, blackheads, papules, pustules, or cysts on the face, neck, back, upper arms, and chest
- Complaints of flare-ups

### NURSING IMPLICATIONS

- Obtain a thorough history to determine onset, location, duration, and any relief measures and to identify possible contributing factors.
- Question the client about the effect of the acne on self-image.
- Inspect lesions on physical examination for appearance, location, and distribution.
- Discuss the causes and treatment options for acne.
- Instruct the client to wash the face with mild soap and water twice daily.
- Review any medications prescribed, such as oral tetracycline or retinoic acid cream.

- Instruct the client to check the expiration date on tetracycline and to take on an empty stomach; caution the client to avoid sun exposure while using retinoic acid cream.
- Reinforce the need for no dietary restrictions.
- Assist the client with compliance to prescribed regimen, including return visits for follow-up.
- Assist with measures to promote the client's self-esteem.
- Address any emotional concerns and help with eliminating any factors known to exacerbate the acne (this is individualized).

## ACQUIRED IMMUNODEFICIENCY SYNDROME (AIDS)

### DESCRIPTION

- AIDS is an acquired immunodeficiency spread by contact with the retrovirus *human immunodeficiency virus (HIV)* through blood and body secretions.
- HIV is spread through contact with HIV-infected blood, blood products, body secretions (breast milk or semen), organs, and maternal-fetal blood transfer.
- HIV is not transmitted through casual contact.
- A fetus with a HIV-infected mother has up to a 35% chance of acquiring HIV.
- HIV attacks CD4 (T4 helper/inducer) lymphocytes.
- The destruction of CD4 sites through the virus replication results in loss of ability to initiate a B lymphocyte response.
- The immune response and screening and removing malignant cells from the body are lost.
- HIV infection also destroys or renders other components of the immune system ineffective.
- Severe immunodeficiency results, leaving the child vulnerable to frequent and unusual infections and malignancies.
- Administration of zidovudine (AZT) to HIV-positive women during pregnancy may greatly reduce the rate of placental transmission.
- Increased sexual activity among adolescents has made this group more vulnerable to the growing rate of HIV.
- AIDS is the 9th leading cause of death in children ages 1 to 4 years.

- The incidence of AIDS is higher among African-American and Hispanic children than others.
- HIV may not be clinically evident for years: up to 2 years with neonatally acquired disease and up to 7 years in children infected through other means.

### ASSESSMENT FINDINGS

#### *In the neonate*
- Lymphadenopathy
- Persistent *diarrhea*
- Respiratory tract infections
- *Failure to thrive*
- Thrombocytopenia
- Recurrent bacterial sepsis
- Hepatosplenomegaly
- Encephalopathy
- Loss of developmental milestones
- Disseminated cytomegalovirus
- Herpes simplex viral infection
- Persistent or recurrent candidial infection
- *Chronic otitis media*
- *Pneumonitis carinii infection*
- *Tuberculosis*

#### *In older children and adolescents*
- Fever
- Lymphadenopathy
- Encephalopathy
- Weight loss
- Opportunistic infections
- Thrombocytopenia
- *Nephrotic syndrome*
- Kaposi's sarcoma rarely seen in children with AIDS

### NURSING IMPLICATIONS
- Confirm the diagnosis of AIDS by ELISA or Western blot technique of antibody testing.
- Follow the child's response to therapy by evaluation of CD4 levels.
- Understand and teach the current Centers for Disease Control classification system for HIV in children so that parents will better understand the child's stage.
- Because AIDS is presently incurable and ultimately fatal, support the family and child throughout the diagnosis and disease process.

- Provide time for the family and child to ventilate their fears.
- Allow the emotional needs to be met, such as anticipatory grieving.
- Administer drugs that inhibit the replication of HIV within cells such as AZT, so as to slow the disease progress.
- Teach parents about all aspects of the disease and explain all procedures and their rationales.
- Prevent infection in the immunocompromised child, and administer antibiotics prophylactically if prescribed.
- Teach parents that monthly gamma globulin administration may decrease the overall incidence of bacterial infection.
- Promote as normal a life as possible for the child and provide counseling to maintain self-esteem.
- Administer nutritional supplements as needed.
- Keep in mind that children with HIV need the normal vaccinations of childhood administered; however, the polio vaccine should be inactivated. Be aware that children need pneumonia vaccines at age 2 and influenza vaccinations at age 6 months and then yearly.
- Help the family return to their previous level of functioning so that they can support their child's emotional and physical care needs as well as their own.
- Use universal precautions for all patients to prevent exposure to blood-borne pathogens.
- Remember that pregnant nurses and physicians should follow strict precautions when caring for patients known to be infected with HIV because the possibility of secondary infection (herpes, toxoplasmosis, and cytomegalovirus) being present is great.
- Keep in mind that nursing staff caring for HIV-positive infants abandoned in newborn nurseries and raised by the nursing staff require the same support that a family of an HIV-infected infant requires.

## ADRENAL CORTICAL INSUFFICIENCY, ACUTE

### DESCRIPTION

- Acute adrenal cortical insufficiency is a hypofunction of the adrenal gland.
- In acute adrenal cortical insufficiency, the entire cortical adrenal gland function suddenly becomes insufficient.

- This occurs generally in association with severe overwhelming infections in which there is hemorrhagic destruction of the adrenal glands.
- It is seen most commonly in meningococcemia.
- It also can occur when corticosteroid therapy, which has been maintained at high levels for longs periods of time, is abruptly stopped.
- Acute adrenal cortical insufficiency is a medical emergency.
- Although it is seen less frequently than in the past because of antibiotics that quickly halt the course of infections, it is not an obsolete entity; more conditions now are being treated with corticosteroids, so the chances that acute adrenal cortical insufficiency will occur from sudden withdrawal of steroids are actually increasing.

## ASSESSMENT FINDINGS

- Sudden drop in blood pressure to extremely low levels
- Ashen gray appearance
- Pulselessness
- *Elevated body temperature*
- Marked *dehydration*
- Marked hypoglycemia
- Severely decreased serum sodium levels
- Severely decreased serum chloride levels
- Elevated serum potassium levels
- *Seizures* possible
- Death

## NURSING IMPLICATIONS

- Institute emergency resuscitative measures immediately.
- Monitor the child's hemodynamic status closely for changes.
- Administer intravenous cortisol, such as Solu-Cortef, and deoxycorticosterone acetate (DOCA) and intravenous 5% glucose in normal saline to restore blood pressure, sodium, and blood glucose levels.
- Anticipate administering a vasopressor to elevate blood pressure.
- Administer potassium to replace potassium lost with diuresis to prevent cardiac arrhythmias.
- Monitor serum laboratory results for changes.

# ADRENOGENITAL SYNDROME (CONGENITAL ADRENAL HYPERPLASIA)

### DESCRIPTION

- Adrenogenital syndrome is an inherited autosomal recessive trait.
- The primary defect is an inability to synthesize cortisol from its precursors, occurring at the 21-hydroxylase level.
- When the adrenal gland cannot produce cortisol, the amount of pituitary adrenotropic hormone increases, stimulating the adrenal glands to improve function.
- The adrenal gland then becomes hyperplastic (enlarged), not producing hydrocortisone but overproducing androgen.
- The excessive androgen masculinizes a female child and increases the genital organs in male infants.
- If the child has complete blockage of cortisol formation, aldosterone production also is deficient, and the child cannot retain sodium.

### ASSESSMENT FINDINGS

#### Females

- Enlarged clitoris
- Fused labia
- Normal internal organs
- Sinus between the urethra and vagina (may be present)
- Pubic hair and acne appearing precociously with a deep masculine voice; also absent breast development and menstruation (if undetected at birth)

#### Males

- Sexual precocity appearing by age 6 months
- Enlarged penis, scrotum, and prostate by 3 to 4 years of age
- Presence of pubic hair
- Acne
- Deep male voice
- Testes normal in size (do not enlarge) but appear small in relation to penis
- Increased levels of serum testosterone
- Inability to gain weight (may be sign of salt and water depletion associated with salt-losing form of adrenogenital syndrome)

### Nursing Implications

- Determine the presence of abnormalities in genitalia.
- Administer oral hydrocortisone to replace what is not produced.
- Teach parents about the disease, and explain all treatments and their rationale.
- Teach parents that corticosteroid therapy returns androgen production to normal and needs to continue indefinitely.
- Teach parents about the importance of therapy because the child will be prevented from reaching adult height without it secondary to advanced bone age and long bone closure.
- Identify children with complete blockage of cortisol formation because they are at high risk for irreversible salt depletion and must be identified quickly.
- Administer high amounts of salt and DOCA, a synthetic aldosterone, to children with the salt-losing form of adrenogenital syndrome, to maintain fluid and electrolyte balance.
- Teach parents that a long-acting form of DOCA can be administered once a month intramuscularly.
- Teach the parents that as the child grows older, fluorohydrocortisone may be given orally to aid salt retention.
- Explain to the parents that the child needs periodic analysis of serum cortisol levels and growth measurements to estimate the effectiveness of the therapy.
- If adrenogenital syndrome is identified via chorionic villi sampling early in pregnancy, administer dexamethasone to the mother for the remainder of the pregnancy to prevent masculinization of the female fetus.

## ALLERGIC RHINITIS (HAY FEVER)

### Description

- Allergic rhinitis is an atopic disorder, caused by an immediate hypersensitivity immune response.
- In some children, the tendency for sensitivity to antigens exists, which may be genetic or environmental.
- In these children, higher than normal levels of IgE antibodies are produced, making them more responsive to allergens.

- Children whose parents smoke have twice the incidence of atopic disorders than those with nonsmoking parents.
- The allergens that cause allergic rhinitis are generally pollens or molds.

### ASSESSMENT FINDINGS

- Sneezing
- Nasal engorgement
- Profuse, thin, watery nasal discharge
- Pruritic conjunctivas
- Watery eyes
- "Pebble appearance" of the conjunctiva
- "Allergic salute" from children constantly rubbing their noses
- "Allergic crease"—horizontal crease across the tip of the nose
- "Allergic shiners"—blackened areas under the eyes
- Pale edematous nasal mucous membrane
- Frontal headache
- Eczema and asthma in 50% of the cases
- Recurrent *otitis media*
- Increased eosinophil count of nasal discharge

### NURSING IMPLICATIONS

- Explain to parents the causes of the allergic rhinitis and discuss the options for treatment.
- Administer antihistamines to reverse the action of histamine for children who do not have severe symptoms.
- Teach the child and parent that antihistamines can cause drowsiness and if given for more than 3 days, a rebound effect can occur (nasal mucosa becomes more edematous).
- Explain to parents that skin testing to locate individual allergens is available for children with severe symptoms to the point that they interfere with activities.
- Explain all treatments and rationales to parents and to the child at his or her developmental level.
- Implement hyposensitization therapy once the allergen has been identified.
- Assess the impact of the illness on the child and how it affects his or her interactions with others.
- Offer anticipatory guidance and teaching to maintain as normal a lifestyle as possible.

# ALLERGIES

### DESCRIPTION

- Allergies refer to disorders (hypersensitivity reactions) that occur as a result of an excessive antigen-antibody response when the invading organism is an allergen rather than a simple immunogen.
- There are 4 classifications of hypersensitivity reactions: type I, II, III, and IV.
- A type I response happens immediately; types I, II, and III are mediated by antibodies (humoral response), whereas type IV is mediated by T cells (cell-mediated response).
- Approximately 1 in every 5 children suffers from some form of allergy; the symptoms may be chronic and minor, such as those that occur with *allergic rhinitis,* or acute and severe, as in *anaphylactic shock.*
- Common allergens include dust, mold, and pollen. Other possible causative factors include drugs, foods including milk, and insect stings.
- Regardless of the child's symptoms, there are three goals for therapy: Reduce the child's exposure to the allergen; hyposensitize the child to produce a state of increased clinical tolerance (a state of not responding) to the allergen; and modify the child's response to the allergen with a pharmacologic agent.

### ASSESSMENT FINDINGS (many symptoms are vague)

- Familial history of allergy
- Complaints of "colds all winter," runny nose, or itching eyes
- Rhinitis
- *Urticaria*
- Increased eosinophil count (5% or more on a differential count or eosinophil count of 250 or more cells/mm³)
- Increased IgE antibody levels
- Positive radioallergosorbent test (RAST)
- Weal or flare response on skin testing

**Drug allergies**

- *Urticaria*
- Angioedema
- Allergic *contact dermatitis*
- Pruritus
- Purpura

- Thrombocytopenia
- Hemolytic anemia
- *Anaphylactic shock*
- *Serum sickness*

**Food allergies**
- Fussy eaters
- Hyperactivity (possible)
- Failure to gain weight (milk allergy)
- *Diarrhea* (milk allergy)
- *Vomiting*
- Abdominal pain

**Insect sting allergies**
- Local edema progressing to generalized *urticaria,* pruritus, edema, wheezing, and dyspnea
- *Anaphylactic shock*

### NURSING IMPLICATIONS
- Obtain a thorough history and physical examination to establish a baseline and to help identify any possible allergens; include a family history and exact description of symptoms along with seasonal timing and frequency to establish the underlying causative factors.
- Assist parents and child to keep a chart of when symptoms are worse and better to aid in identification of specific allergen.
- Prepare child and parents for laboratory testing, explaining the purpose and procedure for all tests.
- Anticipate the use of skin testing to identify possible allergens.
- Instruct the child and parents to avoid the use of systemic or aerosol administration of antihistamines or a theophylline derivative for 8 hours before skin testing to prevent inhibition of flare response.
- Be prepared to read the results of skin testing within 20 minutes of the injection; if the child is sensitive to the allergen, a weal or flare response appears at the site of the test.
- Have a syringe filled with 1 mL of epinephrine 1:1000 on hand to counteract an unexpected, but entirely possible, anaphylactic reaction from skin testing.
- Be certain to have the child stay in the health care setting for at least 30 minutes following skin testing, the time a reaction to the injected allergen is apt to occur.

- Educate the parents about environmental control measures, which can make a great deal of difference in their child's symptoms.
- Assist the parents and child with controlling the allergens in the child's environment, such as encasing the child's mattress and pillow in plastic; using only synthetic blankets; removing carpets; using only synthetic, easily washable throw rugs, curtains, and stuffed animals; avoiding the use of scented items, such as perfume and hair spray; not allowing a pet in the child's room; daily wet dusting of child's room; using air-filtration devices and dehumidifiers as appropriate; and suggesting that the child not sit near the blackboard at school.
- Anticipate the need for hyposensitization; instruct parents and child in the procedure and the need for continued follow-up every 3 to 4 weeks to maintain hyposensitization.
- Following hyposensitization, have the child remain in the health care facility for 30 minutes after the injection to monitor for an anaphylactic reaction.
- Instruct the parents that hyposensitization is generally continued for 2 to 3 years; inform them that it does not cure the problem but that it will make the child symptom free or decrease symptoms for a length of time.
- Educate the parents and child about any pharmacologic agents prescribed, such as mast cell stabilizers, antihistamines, epinephrine, or theophylline, including the drug's actions, uses, frequency of dosage, possible side effects, and need for compliance.
- Allow parents and child to verbalize feelings of frustration about the disorder and disruption in the child and family's life and routine functioning.
- Instruct the child to wear a Medic-Alert bracelet identifying the allergy.

### For drug allergies
- Obtain a thorough history to identify any previous drug reactions.
- If drug allergy develops, discontinue the drug immediately and administer antihistamine as prescribed to relieve *urticaria* and *serum sickness.*

- Document on the chart that known drug allergy exists; label the chart and medication record prominently.
- Instruct parents and child to inform all health care persons that a drug allergy exists.

### For food allergies

- Instruct the parents and child to keep a food diary to help identify an offending food, rating each day as either symptom free or a day when symptoms were strongly evident.
- Assist parents with elimination diet, adding one food every 2 to 3 days and evaluating for the development of symptoms.
- Instruct the parents that if symptoms occur, the food must be eliminated from the child's diet permanently.
- If a milk allergy is suspected, place the child on a casein hydrolysate formula; reintroduce milk at a later date; if a true milk allergy exists, be alert to signs recurring when the milk is reintroduced.

### For insect sting allergies

- Begin hyposensitization following the child's first reaction.
- If the child has not been hyposensitized, anticipate using a pressurized inhaler or subcutaneous injection of epinephrine as prescribed.
- Instruct parents and child how to use an emergency insect sting kit and to keep it available at all times, including at school and on trips.
- Educate parents and child about using antihistamine medications, ice to the site, and a tourniquet proximal to the sting to retard absorption should a sting occur.
- Be aware that the initial injection of epinephrine is effective for only 20 minutes; instruct parents and child about the need for emergency transport to the hospital in case additional epinephrine is needed.
- Instruct the child to avoid wearing scented preparations and walking barefoot and to use insecticides when outdoors to minimize insect attraction.

## AMBIGUOUS GENITALIA

### Description

- Ambiguous genitalia refers to external sexual organs in the child that did not follow the normal course of development.

- At birth, the external sexual organs are so incompletely or abnormally formed that it is impossible to determine clearly the child's sex by observation.
- An example of ambiguous genitalia is a male infant with *hypospadias* or a chromosomal female (XX) masculinized in utero by exposure to androgen.
- The most common cause of in vitro virilization of females is congenital cortical hyperplasia syndrome.
- If testosterone is produced in utero but the müllerian duct development was not suppressed, a child may have both ovaries and testes and consequently malformed external genitalia.
- Children with ambiguous genitalia are often termed pseudohermaphrodite.
- Either ovaries or testes are present or neither is present; infants have some external features of both sexes.

### Assessment Findings
- Unidentifiable external genitalia

### Nursing Implications
- Inspect genitalia closely for abnormalities.
- Perform a sex chromatin test to establish the genetic sex of the child.
- Address the concerns and stress that the parents will be experiencing related to ambiguous sex of the child, treatment, and long-term plans.
- Support the parents' decision to have the child with *hypospadias* (urethra opening on the underside of the penis) or *cryptorchidism* (undescended testes) surgically corrected.
- Explore the implications of removal of an enlarged clitoris in a child with the parents and support their decisions for treatment.
- Explain to parents that nonfunctioning organs such as ovaries and testes need to be removed to avoid malignancy later.
- Examine the implications of raising a chromosomally male child as a female if the child does not have an adequate penis, and consider the long-term need for estrogen for secondary sex characteristics to develop.
- Include the cultural and societal ramifications in discussions with parents to identify their attitude concerning this disorder.

- Reassure parents that their child is normal except in this one area.
- Advise additional counseling for the child as he or she grows to adjust to an abnormal appearance or function.

## AMBLYOPIA

### DESCRIPTION

- Amblyopia is "lazy eye" or subnormal vision in one eye.
- This occurs when one eye's vision is significantly different from the other eye, and the child comes to depend on the eye that focuses more readily.
- Children use one eye for vision while resting the other.
- If this "resting" continues for too long, functional vision fades or is lost, and the child becomes functionally blind in one eye.
- Amblyopia can develop from strabismus (crossed eyes).
- With strabismus, a child views two separate images; a child with strabismus suppresses one visual image, causing suppression of central vision in that eye, or amblyopia.

### ASSESSMENT FINDINGS

- 20/50 vision in one eye—normal for preschool
- 20/100 vision in the other eye—lessened vision
- Two dots seen on the Worth 4-dot test on the left eye—nonfunctioning
- Three dots seen on the Worth 4-dot test on the right eye—nonfunctioning

### NURSING IMPLICATIONS

- Screen all preschool-age children for amblyopia by vision testing with an E chart and the Worth 4-dot test.
- Explain to parents and children with amblyopia that it is correctable if treated during the preschool years.
- Explain to parents that after 6 years of age, the prognosis for correction of amblyopia is diminished, and after age 8 years, little improvement can be achieved.
- Inform parents about treatment and how it works by covering the good eye with a patch, thereby forcing the child to develop vision in the poor eye.

- Advise parents and the child that initially it may be difficult adapting to the patch.
- Educate parents and the child that headaches and dizziness may initially be experienced because of the poor vision.
- Stress to parents and children that only with continued use of the patch can the poor eye's vision improve.
- Discuss with parents and the child newer treatments, such as administration of levodopa/carbidopa, in addition to occlusion therapy.
- Answer all questions and support the parents and the child through treatment.

# AMENORRHEA

## DESCRIPTION
- Amenorrhea is the absence of menstrual flow.
- This strongly suggests pregnancy but is not a definitive diagnosis.
- Amenorrhea may result from tension, anxiety, fatigue, chronic illness, extreme dieting, or strenuous exercise.
- With excessive exercise, the ratio of fat to muscle decreases, causing an increase in prolactin production, which results in a decrease in luteinizing hormone–releasing hormone and a decline in follicle-stimulating hormone, follicular development, and estrogen secretion.
- Menstrual cycles return to normal when strenuous exercise is discontinued.
- Amenorrhea also may occur when an adolescent diets excessively secondary to increased prolactin.
- Amenorrhea is primary if an adolescent has never had a menstrual period.
- Amenorrhea is secondary if it occurs after normal menstrual periods.

## ASSESSMENT FINDINGS
- Absence of menses
- Weight loss if excessive dieting the cause
- Low ratio of body fat to body muscle if secondary to excessive exercising

## NURSING IMPLICATIONS
- Establish or rule out a definitive diagnosis of pregnancy.

- Assess the girl's lifestyle, including exercise, stress, diet, anxiety, and sleep habits.
- Evaluate for other possible causes of amenorrhea, including anovulation, blocked endometrial cavity, endocrine changes, medications such as phenothiazines, and metabolic changes.
- Ensure that the girl's dieting habits are healthy.
- Refer any disorders such as *anorexia nervosa* or *bulimia nervosa* to appropriate mental health professionals after a thorough physical examination establishing the girl's physical health.
- Explain to adolescent girls about the occurrence of amenorrhea and teach them about all drugs or procedures necessary for the causative problem.

## ANEMIA, ACUTE BLOOD LOSS

### Description

- Acute blood loss anemia refers to the uncompensated loss of red blood cells as in acute hemorrhage.
- Blood loss sufficient to cause anemia may occur from:
    Trauma such as an automobile accident with internal bleeding.
    Acute nephritis in which blood is lost in the urine.
    In the newborn from disorders such as placenta previa, premature separation of the placenta, maternal fetal or twin-to-twin transfusion or trauma to the cord or placenta as with cesarean birth.
- These patients do not respond to oxygen therapy because they lack red blood cells to transport and use the oxygen.
- This type of blood loss anemia is transitory because a sudden reduction of available oxygen stimulates the bone marrow to regenerate red blood cells.

### Assessment Findings

- Pale skin and mucous membranes
- Shock state
- Tachycardia
- Tachypnea
- Gasping respirations with sternal retractions and cyanosis *(newborns)*

### Nursing Implications

- Institute measures immediately to control the bleeding.
- Address the underlying cause of the bleeding.
- Place the child or infant supine to promote cerebral circulation.
- Maintain body temperature with blankets and an incubator for an infant.
- Administer *blood transfusions* as necessary to replenish erythrocytes.
- If blood is not available, use blood volume expanders, such as plasma and intravenous fluids including normal saline or Ringer's lactate, to maintain blood pressure.
- Limit blood drawing procedures.
- Provide emotional support to parents and child.
- Address teaching needs of parents and child and explain all treatments.

## ANEMIA OF ACUTE INFECTION

### Description

- Acute infection or inflammation, especially in infants, may lead to increased destruction of erythrocytes.
- Impaired production of erythrocytes owing to infection contributes to anemia.
- Common infections associated with anemia are *osteomyelitis, ulcerative colitis*, and advanced renal disease.
- Decreased hemoglobin decreases oxygen carrying capacity.
- Clinical symptoms of low hemoglobin are not apparent until the hemoglobin reaches 7 to 8 g/100 ml.

### Assessment Findings

- Pallor
- Fatigue
- Fever
- Increased white blood cells
- Decreased red blood cells and hemoglobin levels
- Tachycardia
- Tachypnea
- Shortness of breath
- Cyanosis

**NURSING IMPLICATIONS**
- Assess all laboratory values and evaluate the cause of infection.
- Treat the cause of the anemia and provide symptomatic relief with oxygen for hypoxia if anemia is severe.
- Explain all procedures and treatments to parents and child to allay their fears.
- Reveal to parents that once the underlying cause of the anemia is treated, the anemia can be reversed.
- Support the parent and child during the stress of in-hospital care as necessary.

## ANEMIA, APLASTIC

**DESCRIPTION**
- Aplastic anemia results from depression of hematopoietic activity in bone marrow.
- The formation and development of white blood cells, platelets, and red blood cells are all affected.
- Congenital aplastic anemia (Fanconi's syndrome) is inherited as an autosomal recessive trait. The child is usually born with a number of other congenital anomalies and between ages 4 and 12 years begins to manifest symptoms of pancytopenia—reduction of all blood components.
- Acquired aplastic anemia occurs in children who have had excessive exposure to radiation or drugs and chemicals known to cause bone marrow damage.
- Chloramphenicol is the major drug involved in acquired aplastic anemia.
- Other drugs associated with this anemia are sulfonamides, arsenic, hydantoin, benzene, and quinine as well as exposure to insecticides.
- Chemotherapeutic drugs temporarily reduce bone marrow production.
- A serious infection might cause autoimmunologic suppression of bone marrow.
- If children survive past 6 months, their chances for complete recovery are good.

**ASSESSMENT FINDINGS**
> ***Symptoms that reflect low red blood cell count and tissue hypoxia***
- Pallor

- Fatigue
- Anorexia

*Symptoms that reflect reduced platelet formation*
- Bruising and petechiae
- Excessive nosebleeds or gastrointestinal bleeding

*Symptoms that reflect decreased white blood cell count*
- Increase in number of infections
- Poor response to antibiotic therapy

*Signs of heart decompensation*
- Tachycardia
- Tachypnea
- Shortness of breath
- Cyanosis

### NURSING IMPLICATIONS

- Institute measures to decrease tissue oxygenation requirements, such as bed rest and assistance with activities of daily living.
- Allow child and parents to express their frustrations and fears. (This is especially important for the child because anxiety can increase tissue oxygen demands.)
- For an infant, provide a pacifier to calm him or her and encourage parents to stay with the child during the hospitalization.
- Ask about exposure to drugs and investigate the source of the anemia.
- Continue to be conservatively optimistic regarding the course of the disease because some children die.
- For congenital aplastic anemia, administer corticosteroids to decrease erythrocyte destruction and testosterone to increase erythrocyte production in the bone marrow, as prescribed.
- Administer drugs such as antithymocyte globulin or antilymphocyte globulin to suppress abnormal bone marrow activity.
- Supplement blood elements that are being formed in abnormally low numbers.
- Explain to parents of children with acquired aplastic anemia that if the disorder is secondary to a chemical or a drug, the child must not ever be exposed to it again.
- Establish a good rapport with parents to allow them to express their frustrations over the course of the disease, such as with continued abnormal blood results.

# ANEMIA, AUTOIMMUNE ACQUIRED HEMOLYTIC DISORDER

### DESCRIPTION

- Autoimmune acquired hemolytic disorder is a red blood cell disorder in which autoimmune antibodies, abnormal antibodies of the IgG class directed against the child's red cells, attach themselves to red blood cells causing hemolysis.
- This disorder can occur at any age.
- Although normally idiopathic in origin, the disorder can be caused by malignancy, viral infections, or collagen diseases such as *juvenile rheumatoid arthritis* or *systemic lupus erythematosus,* recent upper respiratory infections, measles, (rubella) or *chickenpox* or after administration of certain drugs, such as penicillin.
- In some children, the disorder runs its course without treatment necessary; however, other children require blood transfusions, medications, and possibly a splenectomy.

### ASSESSMENT FINDINGS

- Small round red blood cells
- Increased reticulocyte count
- Positive direct Coombs's test
- Severely decreased hemoglobin levels

#### *Insidious onset*

- Low-grade fever
- Anorexia
- Lethargy
- Pallor
- Icterus from release of indirect bilirubin from the hemolyzed cells
- Dark urine and dark stools

#### *Abrupt onset*

- High fever
- Hemoglobinuria
- Marked jaundice
- Pallor
- Enlarged liver and spleen

### NURSING IMPLICATIONS

- Reduce oxygen tissue requirements of child because hemoglobin levels and oxygen carrying capacity are decreased.

- Assess for signs of respiratory difficulty, and administer oxygen as needed.
- Explain the disorder and all therapeutic interventions to parents and child.
- Support the parent and child through the disorder and encourage them to express their feelings related to the hospitalization.
- Prepare for *blood transfusion* if necessary, ensuring proper crossmatch and assessing for signs of transfusion reactions.
- Administer corticosteroids if prescribed to treat anemia.
- If splenectomy is necessary, prepare the parents and child for the procedure and teach them about the postoperative course.
- Administer immunosuppressive agents, if necessary, to reduce antibody formation.
- Teach parents and child about all drugs administered and their side effects.
- Help parents understand this ambiguous disorder and learn to cope with its unexplainable process.
- Provide parents and child with as much support as needed and reassure them that the child will be well again.

# ANEMIA, HYPOPLASTIC

## DESCRIPTION

- Hypoplastic anemia results from depression of hematopoietic activity in bone marrow.
- It can be congenital or acquired.
- Only red blood cells are affected in hypoplastic anemias.
- Blackfan-Diamond syndrome, a congenital hypoplastic anemia revealed in the first 6 to 8 months of life, affects both sexes and is caused by an inherent defect in red blood cell formation.
- An acquired form of hypoplastic anemia is caused by infection with parvovirus.
- Hypoplastic anemia has an insidious onset, with 25% of children with the congenital form eventually having a spontaneous remission before age 13 years old.
- Acquired hypoplastic anemia causes a reduction of red blood cells transiently, and therefore no therapy is necessary.

- Congenital hypoplastic anemia is treated with corticosteroid therapy, which increases erythropoiesis and packed red blood cells if necessary.

### Assessment Findings
- Muscle weakness, fatigue, and exercise intolerance
- Pale skin, mucous membranes, and conjunctivae
- Headache, dizziness, and irritability
- Normochromic, normocytic red blood cells

### Nursing Implications
- Support the child and family through the diagnosis and explain the pathology as well as associated treatments.
- Administer corticosteroids and explain to the family and child regarding the action and side effects.
- Prevent and assess for complications related to red blood cell transfusions.
- Instruct the family on the need for an iron chelation program because so many transfusions result in hemosiderosis.
- Begin deferoxamine therapy concurrently with transfusions.
- Explain to the child and family that deferoxamine is given 5 to 6 days a week over an 8-hour period.
- Teach the parents how to administer deferoxamine at home and the importance of adequate urination and kidney function (including testing for specific gravity) to excrete iron from the body.
- Encourage parents to find an adequate time period to administer this drug, such as at night but within the designated time frame.
- Assist parents in problem solving.
- Advise the parents on the importance of periodic eye examinations to evaluate for possible cataract formation, which is a drug side effect.
- Promote a positive self-image in the child with a chronic, potentially fatal disease.

## ANEMIA, IRON DEFICIENCY

### Description
- Iron deficiency anemia is the most common anemia of infancy and childhood, most common between 6 months and 2 years of age as well as in adolescent girls who are menstruating.

- Iron deficiency anemia results from inadequate intake of dietary iron.
- Dietary intake of cow's milk contributes to iron deficiency anemia secondary to its poor absorption as well as causing fullness and therefore a low intake of iron-rich foods.
- Children require more daily iron than adults in proportion to their body weight to maintain an adequate iron level.
- A daily intake of 6 to 15 mg is necessary.
- Proper hemoglobin formation does not occur.
- Inadequate iron also leads to red blood cells that are small in size, hypocytic, and pale (hypochromic).
- Infants born with structural defects of the gastrointestinal system, such as chalasia or *pyloric stenosis*, are prone to iron deficiency anemia.
- In children over age 2, the most common cause of iron deficiency anemia is chronic blood loss as a result of gastrointestinal tract lesions.
- Iron deficiency anemia is associated with pica.

### ASSESSMENT FINDINGS

- Pale mucous membranes
- Poor muscle tone, decreased activity
- Irritability from fatigue
- Enlarged heart
- Soft systolic murmur
- Enlarged spleen
- Spoon-shaped or depressed fingernails

### NURSING IMPLICATIONS

- Screen all infants for iron deficiency anemia from 6 months of age.
- Council parents on how to improve their child's diet, such as adding iron-rich foods while decreasing milk intake to maintain the iron levels and prevent recurring anemia.
- Instruct parents to administer a vitamin supplement with iron to toddlers who eat poorly.
- Encourage parents to administer iron elixir with fruit juice because vitamin C enhances iron solubility and absorption.
- Caution parents not to mix iron elixir with milk because milk impedes iron absorption.
- Inform parents that iron elixir darkens stool and may cause constipation.

- Advise parents to increase fluid and fiber in the child's diet to avoid constipation.
- Advise parents to have the child drink water or juice after taking an iron preparation, which can cause temporary tooth staining.
- Instruct parents to supervise the child's environment carefully to keep inedible materials out of the child's reach.

## ANEMIA OF NEOPLASTIC DISEASE

### DESCRIPTION

- Anemia can result from common childhood neoplasms, such as *leukemia* and lymphosarcoma.
- The malignant growths result in normochromic, normocytic anemias because invasion of bone marrow by the malignant cells impairs red blood cell production.
- Accompanying blood loss if platelet formation is decreased also leads to anemia.
- Bone marrow depression from treatment, including chemotherapy and radiation, impairs production of red blood cells, white blood cells, and platelets.

### ASSESSMENT FINDINGS

- Pallor
- Fatigue
- Decreased red blood cells and hemoglobin levels
- Tachycardia
- Tachypnea
- Shortness of breath
- Cyanosis

### NURSING IMPLICATIONS

- Support the child and family through the devastation of diagnosis, treatment, and possible death.
- Provide emotional support and explain all treatments and options.
- Prevent and assess for complications related to cancer and bone marrow depression such as anemia.
- Administer antineoplastic medications cautiously to achieve the goal of remission.
- Depending on the child's condition, anticipate using packed red blood cells to treat anemia.
- Monitor child's blood studies, including complete blood count, for changes.

- Treat any related adverse effects of chemotherapy and radiation.
- Promote adequate hydration and nutrition.

# ANEMIA, PERNICIOUS

## DESCRIPTION
- Pernicious anemia is caused by a deficiency or inability to use vitamin $B_{12}$.
- An intrinsic factor must be present in the gastric mucosa for absorption of vitamin $B_{12}$.
- Lack of intrinsic factor is the most common cause of this anemia.
- If intrinsic factor is deficient, symptoms of this anemia appear by age 2 years.
- Vitamin $B_{12}$ is readily available in food of animal origin.
- Adolescents may be deficient in vitamin $B_{12}$ if they are on a long-term, poorly formulated vegetarian diet.
- A Schilling test measures how much vitamin $B_{12}$ is absorbed in the presence and absence of a dose of intrinsic factor.
- Pernicious anemia is treated with lifelong monthly intramuscular injections of vitamin $B_{12}$.

## ASSESSMENT FINDINGS
- Low serum levels of vitamin $B_{12}$
  ### Children
- Pallor
- Anorexia
- Irritability
- Chronic *diarrhea*
- Papillary atrophy (smooth and beef-red tongue)
- Neuropathologic findings (may be present but are less noticeable) than in adults
  ### Adults
- Ataxia
- Hyporeflexia
- Paresthesia
- Positive Babinski reflex

## NURSING IMPLICATIONS
- Help parents and child understand how pernicious anemia occurs.

- Teach parents and child that when intrinsic factor is absent or deficient, the child needs to have lifelong monthly injections of vitamin $B_{12}$.
- Enlighten the family as to the potential neurologic impairments that can occur without adequate vitamin $B_{12}$.
- Ensure that the family and child has had a chance to have all of their questions answered.
- Continue to facilitate a therapeutic relationship with the family and assist them in conscientiously attending to this deficiency.
- Instruct the family in medication regimen, including administration of vitamin $B_{12}$; monitor for compliance.

## ANEMIA, SICKLE CELL

### Description

- Sickle cell anemia refers to a group of autosomal recessive genetic disorders called hemoglobinopathies and results in abnormally shaped red blood cells.
- The substitution of valine for glutamine within the deoxyribonucleic acid molecule causes this disorder.
- Sickle cell trait and sickle cell disease are the most common hemoglobinopathies in North America, primarily affecting African-Americans.
- Sickle cell anemia is a chronic disorder characterized by moderate anemia.
- The child's red blood cells contain Hgb S and have a shortened life span.
- The child's bone marrow cannot produce sufficient red blood cells to meet the body's needs.
- The erythrocytes become characteristically elongated and crescent-shaped (sickled) under the conditions of acidosis, dehydration, and decreased arterial oxygen tension.
- Sickled red blood cells do not move freely through vessels; blood stasis and further sickling occur.
- The cycle continues, and blood flow halts owing to blocked vessels, and tissue distal to the blockage becomes ischemic.
- The child can compensate for moderate anemia under normal conditions.

- Because young infants with sickle cell anemia have Hgb F, which does not sickle, the disease is not apparent until Hgb S becomes present in sufficient quantities, at about age 6 months.
- Sickle cell anemia can be diagnosed by chorionic villi sampling or from cord blood during an amniocentesis.
- Because of susceptibility to infection, pneumococcal meningitis and *Salmonella*-induced osteomyelitis are frequent illnesses.
- *Cirrhosis* of the liver eventually occurs from infarcts and tissue scarring.
- Kidney function eventually diminishes secondary to scarring.

**ASSESSMENT FINDINGS** (The symptoms of sickle cell disease may be limited to growth retardation and fatigue, with a susceptibility to infection.)
- Fever
- Anemia
- Local disease from stasis of blood in any body part
- Swelling of the hands or feet
- Growth retardation
- Long arms and legs
- Enlarged spleen and liver; protruding abdomen
- Decreased vision from retinal occlusions
- Icteric sclera
- Reduced spleen size secondary to repeated infarction and atrophy
- Priapism or persistent and painful erection

*Sickle cell crisis*
- Sudden, severe, and painful onset
- Fever
- Acute abdominal, back, and extremity pain
- Swollen, painful hands
- *Vomiting* and abdominal tenderness
- Warm, swollen joints
- *Coma, seizures,* and death

**NURSING IMPLICATIONS**
- Ensure that the parents and eventually the child have a strong understanding of sickle cell anemia and the dangers of sickle cell crisis.

- Provide emotional support to families and refer them to appropriate support organizations.
- Provide the family and child with comprehensive information to prevent sickling episodes:

    Make sure the child is properly hydrated.

    Advise on signs and symptoms of dehydration.

    Provide additional fluid in the summer and anticipate ways to provide fluid when it may be limited (field trips).

    Protect the child from infection.

    Maintain routine *immunizations*.

    Ensure that the child gets adequate rest.

    Inform the physician at the first sign of illness.

    Avoid strenuous activity, which increases tissue oxygen requirements.

    Minimize emotional stress, and soothe crying episodes.

    Avoid high altitudes.

    Advise parents to inform all health care personnel of the child's condition even for simple operations such as a tooth extraction.

- Place children from 6 months to 6 years old on prophylactic penicillin to prevent infection.
- Advise all patients with sickle cell anemia to have regular eye examinations to detect for retinal occlusions.
- Reduce metabolic oxygen requirements during a sickling episode by administering oxygen, treating fever with antipyretics, and decreasing pain and agitation with pain medication and application of heat to painful joints.
- Administer fluid and *blood transfusions* if necessary, being alert for signs of reaction.
- Consider exchange transfusions, if crisis is severe, to remove most of sickled cells.
- Help the parent and child adjust to the effects of a chronic disease.

## ANENCEPHALY

### DESCRIPTION

- Anencephaly, the absence of the cerebral hemispheres, occurs when the upper end of the neural tube fails to close in early intrauterine life.
- Anencephaly can be detected at gestational week 16 to 18 by amniocentesis if there is an accompanying open

lesion or by ultrasonography, which reveals an absence of the developing fetal head.
- Childbirth is difficult secondary to the malformed head.
- Anencephaly causes stillbirth because there is no cerebral functioning.
- Because respiratory and cardiac centers are located in the intact medulla, the child may survive for a number of days after birth.
- If anencephaly is found prenatally, parents are given the option of abortion.
- Ethical concerns have been raised regarding the full-term anencephaly child who has transplantable organs.

### Assessment Findings
- Malformed head
- Alpha-fetoprotein present in amniotic fluid
- Absence of cerebral hemispheres

### Nursing Implications
- Provide emotional support to the parents.
- Prepare parents for the appearance of the child.
- Offer anticipatory guidance regarding the grief process.
- Help parents adjust to the child's condition and grieve the loss.
- Ensure the mother's comfort through the labor and delivery process.
- Provide comfort and promote hygiene in the neonate with anencephaly, who may survive for a number of days after birth but who is terminal.
- Encourage parents to visit the child and provide them with privacy.
- Determine whether parents are interested in speaking to an objective member of the health care team concerning transplant of the child's organs.

## ANOREXIA NERVOSA

### Description
- Anorexia is a complex psychological disorder characterized by preoccupation with food and body weight.
- This creates a feeling of revulsion to food to the point of excessive weight loss.
- It begins commonly in early adolescence and affects girls 95% of the time.

- It is more common among sisters and daughters of mothers who have had the disorder.
- Theories related to the disease find that the disorder has both developmental and psychological routes.
- Meades theorizes that the disorder is a phobic-avoidance response to food resulting from the sexual and social tensions generated by the physical changes of puberty.
- Some experts theorize that it reflects a disturbance in the separation-individuation process inherent in adolescence.
- The classic anorexic is a high achiever, a perfectionist, a model child with low self-esteem; the parents are classically overprotective and demanding.
- By excessive dieting, the girl is able to feel a sense of control over her body.
- This disorder can result in severe malnutrition and death from physiologic consequences of malnutrition or suicide.
- The mortality rate is 1% to 15%.
- With counseling, most girls can achieve a full recovery.

### Assessment Findings
- Loss of 20% or more of body weight
- Morbid fear of gaining weight
- History of laxative use, diuretic use, and inducing *vomiting* as well as avoidance of food
- Self-description as fat and unattractive
- Preoccupied with dieting and food, including denial of hunger
- Excessive exercising
- Decreased pulse, blood pressure, and temperature
- Dry, flaky skin and lanugo formation
- Acidosis or alkalosis
- Dependent edema
- *Amenorrhea*
- *Constipation*
- Abdominal pain
- Cold intolerance
- Fatigue and insomnia
- Increasing social withdrawal
- Compulsive mannerisms

### Nursing Implications

- Obtain a thorough history and physical examination to identify the anorexic teenager.
- Refer the patient for psychiatric consultation to avoid grave consequences.
- Assess need for hospitalization for severely malnourished client.
- Assess need for and implement intravenous nutrition or tube feedings, as necessary.
- Provide consistent care from the team approach to avoid confusion.
- Concentrate on the underlying issues but avoid forcing aggressive interpretation of the meaning of symptoms.
- Avoid power struggles around food because the general goal of therapy needs to be establishing and maintaining positive self-image and self-esteem.
- Avoid rapid weight gain because it is too threatening for the client.
- Establish realistic goals for the illness.
- Once the client is stabilized, establish consistent follow-up to ascertain compliance and avoidance of return to previous behaviors.
- Support parents throughout the process and help them to understand the disorder, involving them but not allowing them to control the recovery.
- Establish that counseling will be necessary for 2-3 years to ascertain that self-image is maintained.
- Help the parent and client understand the meaning of the symptoms so as to be aware of any recurrence.

## ANTICIPATORY GRIEF

### Description

- Anticipatory grief refers to a preparatory phase that occurs when parents have some warning of a child's impending death.
- During this phase, parents gradually incorporate the reality of their child's fate into their thoughts.
- Anticipatory grief is necessary for parents to save themselves from the devastation and intolerable grief reaction that comes to parents whose child dies suddenly.

- Anticipatory grief does not shield the parents from experiencing renewed grief once the death occurs.
- A danger of anticipatory grief is when acceptance of the child's death comes too early and the parents stop visiting or have nonuseful visits in which they visit other children.
- This withdrawal process relates to emotional detachment for the parents to shield themselves from the pain of death.

### Nursing Implications
- Encourage all family members to express feelings over impending loss.
- Listen actively to all family members and ensure that the timing of anticipatory loss does not occur so early that the dying child's needs go unmet because of the parental need for self-protection by detachment.
- Help the family to maintain support for the child.
- Assess support systems available to the child and the family.
- Continue to assess the family's level of stress, anticipatory grief, and stage of dying response so as to intervene effectively.

## AORTIC STENOSIS

### Description
- Aortic stenosis is an acyanotic cardiac anomaly that results in obstruction of systemic blood flow (decreased cardiac output).
- Aortic stenosis or stricture of the aortic valve prevents blood from passing freely from the left ventricle into the aorta leading to increased left ventricular pressure and hypertrophy of the left ventricle.
- Eventually, atrial hypertension and pulmonary congestion occur.
- Management of aortic stenosis is balloon stenotomy or surgical repair, dividing the stenotic valve, or dilating an accompanying constrictive aortic ring.
- The initial repair may lead to aortic insufficiency later in life, necessitating further surgery.
- Maternal *rubella* is associated with the development of aortic stenosis.

**ASSESSMENT FINDINGS** (if they exist)
- Rough systolic murmur heard loudest in the second right interspace and transmitted to the right shoulder, clavicle, and up the vessels of the neck
- A thrill present at the suprasternal notch
- Systemic hypoperfusion and *congestive heart failure* (may be present if severe at birth)
- Exercise intolerance (in less severe aortic stenosis)
- Decreased cardiac output
- Chest pain
- Left ventricular hypertrophy
- Sudden death when oxygen supply exceeds oxygen demand

**NURSING IMPLICATIONS**
- Explain disease process, implications, medications, and all procedures to parents.
- Elicit the anxieties and fears the parents have and encourage verbalization.
- Maintain and promote cardiac output and reduce *congestive heart failure.*
- For the infant fatigued from feedings, limit feedings to 20 minutes, ensuring sufficient calories for growth.
- If infant is bottle-fed, use a soft nipple to decrease the energy required to suck.
- Administer diuretics or cardiac glycosides as prescribed.
- Support the parents in their decision-making process regarding surgery.
- Address parents' fear related to the outcome of the cardiac surgery.
- Prepare parents and child for surgery, including expectations for postoperative care.
- Maintain adequate tissue perfusion during the postoperative period.
- Perform routine postoperative assessments.
- Administer antibiotics and assess for signs and symptoms of infection postoperatively.
- Consider need for anticoagulation if aortic valve is replaced with a prosthetic valve.
- Teach parents about any discharge medications, such as warfarin.
- Review steps for follow-up care and emergencies.

# APPENDICITIS

## DESCRIPTION

- Appendicitis is an inflammation of the appendix.
- The appendix, a blind-end pouch attached to the cecum, can become inflamed following an upper respiratory infection or other body infection.
- Overall the cause of appendicitis is obscure.
- Fecal material enters the appendix, hardens, and obstructs the lumen causing inflammation and edema to form, leading to compression of blood vessels, necrosis, and pain.
- Rupture of this necrotic area can result in peritonitis, a potentially fatal condition, if appendicitis is not caught early enough.
- Appendicitis is the most common cause of abdominal surgery in children.

## ASSESSMENT FINDINGS

- Anorexia for 12 to 14 hours
- Nausea and *vomiting*
- Diffuse abdominal pain
- Localized right lower quadrant pain
- Fever and pain (late findings)
- Increased white blood cells
- Acetone in urine
- Right lower quadrant tenderness
- Guarding of the abdomen
- Rebound abdominal tenderness
- Decreased or absent bowel sounds (peritonitis)
- Boardlike rigid abdomen (peritonitis)
- Shallow respirations and fever (peritonitis)

## NURSING IMPLICATIONS

- Document the history and the progression of symptoms.
- Approach the tender area of the abdomen slowly for palpation.
- Assess the parents' state and ability to cope and support them throughout the emergent nature of the admission.
- Encourage the parents and child to verbalize their fears, and although this is usually an emergent situation, take the time to introduce yourself and explain everything that is occurring.

- Explain all procedures to the child honestly even if they will be painful to maintain his or her confidence.
- Prepare the child and parents for surgical removal of the appendix, and explain that it is necessary to avoid rupture.
- Administer fluids and monitor the child's level of hydration to prevent imbalances.

- If ruptured appendix has occurred, position the child in a semi-Fowler's position to drain the infected cecum downward into the pelvis rather than upward to the lungs.
- Perform routine postoperative assessment and care.
- Postoperatively, administer antibiotics and fluid as prescribed, usually for 7 to 10 days.
- Perform dressing changes, as prescribed; examine the wound for signs of healing.
- Note the placement of any drain and report any drain that is expelled because it may need to be replaced to promote drainage of fecal material.
- Teach parents and child which signs and symptoms need to be reported and about any discharge medications.

# ARNOLD-CHIARI DEFORMITY (CHIARI II MALFORMATION)

## DESCRIPTION

- Arnold-Chiari deformity is a neural tube defect that occurs in weeks 16 to 20 of fetal life.
- This specific anomaly is a projection of the cerebellum, medulla oblongata, and the fourth ventricle into the cervical canal.
- The upper cervical spinal cord jackknifes backward, obstructing cerebrospinal fluid flow and causing *hydrocephalus.*
- This deformity is often associated with *meningocele* (lumbosacral *myelomeningocele* is present in approximately 50% of the cases) and spina bifida.
- Prognosis depends on the extent of the deformity and the possibility of surgical intervention.

## ASSESSMENT FINDINGS

- *Meningocele* or spina bifida
- Absent gagging and swallowing reflexes (possible)

#### Nursing Implications

- Assess the child born with this defect and determine what physiologic requirements are needed to sustain life.
- Determine the immediate emotional needs of the parents to promote bonding.
- Encourage parents to touch, hold, and talk to their baby.
- Maintain adequate respirations and institute aspiration precautions.
- Provide adequate nutrition.
- Educate parents regarding pretreatment and posttreatment procedures.
- Assess parents' coping mechanism and self-esteem and provide emotional support.
- Educate parents regarding prevention of infection.
- Encourage parents to seek prenatal screening for any subsequent pregnancies.

## ARTIFICIAL VALVE REPLACEMENT

#### Description

- Artificial valve replacement is used to treat disorders such as congenital heart anomalies (*aortic stenosis*) and diseases such as *Kawasaki syndrome* and *rheumatic fever.*
- Artificial valves can be porcine, bovine, prosthetic, or homograft.
- Prosthetic (synthetic) grafts are the most common because of successful long-term placement.
- The procedure is complicated secondary to the small-sized heart.
- Valve durability is an important consideration.
- The need for long-term anticoagulation must be weighed against the potential for bleeding.
- Following placement of a synthetic valve, a child must be on anticoagulants, most commonly sodium warfarin, or antiplatelet therapy, such as aspirin or dipyridamole, for prevention of thromboembolisms.

#### Assessment Findings

- Audible valvular clicks (with prosthetic valves)

#### Nursing Implications

- Following valve placement, ensure adequate teaching regarding use of anticoagulants and antiplatelet medications.

- Teach the parents and child to assess for signs of bleeding.
- Ensure that the child makes follow-up visits to monitor sodium warfarin blood levels periodically.
- Instruct parents on the importance of prophylactic antibiotics to avoid *endocarditis.*
- Educate adolescent girls on the risk of pregnancy, both because of the increased blood volume and the teratogenic effects of sodium warfarin.
- Discuss appropriate birth control methods with adolescent girls.
- If pregnancy is considered, ensure that the adolescent girl is changed to a heparin regimen.
- Inform parents and child of the potential complication of hemolytic anemia, including how to assess for this in their child.
- Support parents and children, with the goal being that the child lead as normal a life as possible.

## ASPIRATION

### DESCRIPTION
- Aspiration is the inhalation of a foreign object into the airways.
- Prevention is the key to avoiding aspiration, which is common with infants and toddlers.
- Aspiration usually results in choking and a forceful cough causing dislodgement of the object.

### ASSESSMENT FINDINGS
- Universal sign for choking (may be present): hands around throat and coughing
- Increased respiratory difficulty with stridor

### NURSING IMPLICATIONS
- Follow the American Heart Association's recommendations for Heimlich maneuver and resuscitation for infants and children.
- If cough is ineffective and respirations become difficult, use a series of Heimlich subdiaphragmatic abdominal thrusts for children (not infants).
- If child loses consciousness before foreign body is expelled, open the airway and start rescue breathing.
- Keep in mind that Heimlich thrusts are not recommended for infants because of the potential for liver laceration.

- Use a series of back blows and chest thrusts for foreign body obstruction in infants.
- Teach parents of infants and small children to keep small objects out of reach.
- Educate parents to remove all stuffed animals or toys with loose or removable parts.
- Teach parents to avoid feeding children raisins, grapes, seeded foods, hard candy, nuts, or sliced hot dogs.
- Instruct parents to feed an infant in a semireclining position.
- Educate parents not to prop a formula bottle or to cut large holes in nipples.
- Instruct parents not to let infants handle balloons.
- Encourage and teach parents basic pediatric life support and have them invest in this course for anyone caring for their child.

## ASTHMA

### Description

- Asthma is a chronic disorder characterized by hypersensitivity of the trachea and bronchi.
- It is a leading cause of chronic illness in children, affecting children first between ages 2 and 8 and affecting more boys than girls.
- Asthma results in diffuse pulmonary obstructive disease.
- Associated pathophysiologic responses include bronchospasm, mucosal edema, and increased and accumulated thick bronchial secretions.
- These responses reduce the size of the lumen of the airway leading to distress.
- Factors that may trigger severe bronchoconstriction include inhaled irritants, such as cold air, fumes, smoke, inhalation of known allergen, viral upper respiratory infections, and exercise.
- Bronchoconstriction is the result of stimulation of the parasympathetic nervous system, which initiates smooth muscle constriction.
- Drugs used for asthma aim to control or dilate the bronchiole.
- Goals for managing asthma include maintaining airway patency, hydration, and ventilation.

## Assessment Findings

- Chest tightness
- Dyspnea
- Decreased breath sounds
- Wheezing on expiration
- Paroxysmal cough
- Thick, copious, mucoid sputum
- Sputum analysis with white casts
- Increased $PaCO_2$—hypercarbia
- Anxiety and restlessness
- Hyperresonant lungs on percussion
- Expiratory time increased
- Decreased $PaO_2$—hypoxia
- Tachypnea
- Tachycardia
- Difficulty speaking
- Cyanosis
- Respiratory failure
- Shieldlike or barrel-shaped chest
- Clubbing of fingers
- Stunted growth (if steroids have been used)
- Elevated eosinophil count
- Reduced pulmonary function test

## Nursing Implications

- Obtain thorough family history of atopic disease.
- Teach parents about pathology of the disease, normal management, emergency management, medications and their uses and side effects, administration, and how to avoid exposure to allergens.
- Explain all procedures to the child and encourage parents to stay with the child to allay his or her fears.
- Suggest skin testing and hyposensitization to identified allergens.
- Use bronchodilators and corticosteroids to maintain a patent airway.
- Educate parent and child on the dangers of overusing inhalant medication.
- Teach parents and child use of a spacer tube between the inhaler and the mouthpiece for children under 12 years to ensure proper dose administration from metered inhalants.
- Monitor for *dehydration* and teach signs to parents.

- Administer fluids as necessary to hydrate because an asthmatic child can become dehydrated quickly from insensible losses, decreased oral intake, and diuretic effects of some bronchodilators.
- Help parents understand the importance of hydration to help thin bronchiolar secretions.
- Encourage parents and child to verbalize fears related to sudden asthma attacks.
- Support parents and child to help them to understand how to prevent attacks and manage them.

## ATAXIA-TELANGIECTASIA

### DESCRIPTION

- Ataxia-telangiectasia is a primary immunodeficiency disorder resulting in progressive cerebellar degeneration.
- It is a rare genetic disease transmitted as an autosomal recessive trait caused by a defect on the 11th chromosome.
- This disease has both neurologic and immunologic components.
- Endocrine abnormalities may also occur, and there is an increased risk of cancer, particularly *brain neoplasms.*
- Symptoms of this disease vary in severity and onset.
- Increasing cerebellar degeneration and recurrent sinopulmonary infections are hallmarks of the disease.
- Children may develop frequent infections because of the immunologic deficits; there is often evidence of reduced T cell function.
- Death frequently occurs in late adolescence secondary to infection, respiratory failure, or malignant *brain neoplasms.*

### ASSESSMENT FINDINGS

- Telangiectasia (red vascular markings) on the conjunctiva and skin at the flexor creases
- Frequent infections
- Scant tonsillar tissue in the pharynx
- Developmental milestones in infancy not met
- Awkward gait noted when child begins to walk
- Choreoathetosis (rapid, purposeless movements)
- Nystagmus
- Intention tremor
- *Scoliosis*
- Decreased visual field acuity

### NURSING IMPLICATIONS

- Educate parents about what age-appropriate developmental milestones the child should be achieving.
- If a positive diagnosis of ataxia-telangiectasia is made, support the parents and the child, and provide education and time to accept this eventually fatal disease.
- Teach the parents about the importance of prevention of infection and help them to understand the neurologic symptoms.
- Establish a trusting relationship with the family and the child and evaluate their support systems.
- Ensure adequate follow-up and investigate long-term needs.

## ATELECTASIS

### DESCRIPTION

- Atelectasis refers to the collapse of lung alveoli.
- Primary atelectasis occurs in newborns who lack the respiratory strength or the surfactant to expand the alveoli.
- This may occur with immature infants with central nervous system damage or infants with mucous or *meconium plugs* in the trachea.
- With crying, these infants may force air into the alveoli; cyanosis may decrease, differentiating it from cyanotic heart disease at birth.
- Secondary atelectasis results from respiratory tract obstruction, which prevents air from entering part of the alveoli.
- Causes of secondary atelectasis include mucus plugs, aspiration of foreign objects, compression from a *diaphragmatic hernia, scoliosis,* or enlarged lymph nodes.
- Signs of secondary atelectasis depend on the degree of collapse.
- Children with atelectasis are prone to secondary infection that results from stasis of secretions in the lungs.
- Children may need *assisted ventilation* to maintain adequate respiratory function during atelectasis.

### ASSESSMENT FINDINGS

#### *Primary atelectasis*

- Irregular respirations
- Nasal flaring
- Apnea

- Respiratory grunting
- Cyanosis
- Hypotonic and flaccid
- Low Apgar scores

***Secondary atelectasis***

- Asymmetric chest
- Decreased breath sounds on the affected side
- Tachypnea
- Cyanosis
- Collapsed lung on chest x-ray

NURSING IMPLICATIONS

- Establish cause of atelectasis and initiate therapy as prescribed.
- Intervene immediately if the cause of atelectasis is foreign body obstruction.
- Assess child frequently for signs of respiratory distress.
- Maintain loose, nonrestrictive clothing and make sure child's arms are not positioned across the chest where the weight would interfere with deep inspiration.
- Keep the child in a semi-Fowler's position to maximize lung expansion and depress abdominal contents.
- Humidify the child's environment and perform postural drainage to maintain a clear respiratory tract.
- If *assisted ventilation* is necessary, prepare and explain all procedures to the parents and the child to allay their fears as much as possible.

## ATHLETIC INJURIES

DESCRIPTION

- As younger children participate in more sports activities, increasing numbers of injuries are being reported.
- Athletic injuries can include strain, muscle-tendon injury, sprain, and ligament injury.
- A child with a strain or sprain may require crutches for 3 to 4 days to decrease weight-bearing.
- Participation in sports such as football, skiing, or track can lead to knee injuries.
- Knee injuries involve the ligaments surrounding the knee.
- Severe ligament injury takes 8 weeks to heal.
- Arthroscopy has made the repair of ligaments or cartilage a minor procedure and has limited the need for immobilization and casts.

- Severe twisting of the knee causes dislocation of the kneecap.
- Throwing injuries are caused by repeated stress on the upper extremity, which leads to minute tears and fibrous contractures in the muscle.
- Epiphysitis of the medial epicondylar epiphysis (little leaguer's elbow) is caused by stress, which is increased by throwing curve balls and breaking pitches because of the forceful flexion and pronation required; this injury is common in 90% to 95% of pitchers aged 9 to 14.
- Treatment for little leaguer's elbow is rest and immobilization; if not treated adequately, permanent damage can result to the epiphyseal line, and elbow deformity can occur.

## ASSESSMENT FINDINGS
### Knee injuries
- Acute, severe pain
- Localized edema
- Deformed appearance of the knee with dislocation

### Throwing injuries
- Pain
- Tenderness
- Complete loss of elbow extension
- Increased growth, separation, and fragmentation of the medial epicondylar epiphysis on x-ray film
- Limited movement of elbow

### Strains and sprains
- Painful and swollen joints

## NURSING IMPLICATIONS
### Knee injuries
- Ensure that an x-ray film is obtained to rule out fracture.
- Maintain bed rest and ice for 24 hours, followed by heat for mild injuries.
- Consider administration of local anesthetic to minimize pain.
- Teach parents that complete bed rest is necessary for severe injuries in which the knee joint is filled with fluid.
- Prepare the child and parent for aspiration of synovial fluid and need for a compression dressing with ice for 24 hours then heat.

- If complete immobilization is necessary, prepare to assist with cast application.
- Assist with realignment of the kneecap if dislocation has occurred and inform parents of the need to use an immobilizer for 1 week.
- If dislocation is chronic, prepare parents for the potential need for surgery to strengthen the ligaments.
- Monitor and treat severe pain associated with knee injuries.
- Teach the child and parents about cast care, medications, and other treatments as appropriate.

### Throwing injuries

- Teach the child and parents that the arm needs to be rested for 15 to 20 minutes a day with ice pack application to relieve pain.
- Consider systemic phenylbutazone for relief of pain.
- Administer cortisone injections into the elbow musculature if necessary.
- Teach child and parents exercises to strengthen the flexor muscles.
- Inform parents of children with little leaguer's elbow that they need to provide extra protection to the area until the epiphyseal growth centers at the elbow have fused at 14 to 17 years of age.
- Educate parents, who are frequently the coaches, of the need for appropriate warm-up exercises.
- Advise parents that children who are pitchers should be limited to pitching 6 innings per week and that they should not throw curves or break pitches.
- Encourage parents to monitor child's sports activities and provide 3-day rest periods between games.

### Strains and sprains

- Help the parents and child understand that these injuries are truly painful, and because immobilizing devices are not used, strains and sprains can be more painful than fractures.
- Teach parents to use ice on new injuries for 20 minutes.
- Inform parents of proper application of an elastic bandage, which provides firm support.
- Teach child proper use of crutches if they are necessary.

# ATOPIC DERMATITIS

### DESCRIPTION

- Also called infant eczema, atopic dermatitis is a collective term for a group of skin conditions with certain common characteristics.
- Infantile eczema begins between 2 and 6 months and is related to food *allergy*; it also can be caused by pollens, dust, or mold spores.
- With infantile eczema, there is capillary permeability with loss of serous fluid into the tissues.
- Common sites for lesions are scalp, forehead, cheeks, behind the ears, and extensor surfaces of the extremities.
- Infant eczema should clear by the time the child is age 3.
- 50% of infants with atopic dermatitis develop other allergies as they grow older.
- Atopic dermatitis frequently occurs at puberty and ages 16 to 18.
- Atopic dermatitis that occurs at these later ages is prominent on the flexor surfaces of the extremities, the dorsal surfaces of the wrists and ankles, and eyebrows.

### ASSESSMENT FINDINGS

#### *Infantile eczema*

- Irritability
- Poor appetite
- Pruritus
- Erythema
- Papular and vesicular skin eruptions
- Exudate
- Crusting
- Depigmented and shiny skin with healed lesions
- Dry, scaling, and thickening skin
- Linear excoriations
- Secondary infections from open lesions
- Lymph node swelling with secondary infections
- Low-grade fever
- Increased eosinophil count

#### *Atopic dermatitis in older children*

- Depigmentation
- Hyperpigmentation

- Lichenification
- Glossy fingernails
- Pruritus
- Dryness
- Scaling
- Skin thickening

## NURSING IMPLICATIONS

- Ensure that the diagnosis for seborrheic dermatitis is ruled out.
- Suggest screening for *phenylketonuria* because these children frequently have atopic dermatitis.
- Administer skin test to isolate a causative allergen.
- Direct parents to reduce exposure to allergens, such as milk, eggs, citrus juices, and tomatoes, which are most common.
- Institute measures to reduce pruritus and limited secondary infections.
- Teach parents to apply wet dressings to hydrate the skin and remove crusts; however, warn parents to prevent chilling in infants.
- Educate parents on use of emollients to decrease pruritus.
- Administer hydroxyzine hydrochloride (Atarax) for severe pruritus and discomfort.
- Administer topical steroids and teach parents how to apply it properly, reinforcing that the medication will relieve both appearance and discomfort of atopic dermatitis.
- Advise parents to trim the infant's fingernails and cover hands with socks if necessary to prevent scratching.
- If secondary infections occur, administer hydrocortisone mixed with a topical antibiotic.
- Caution parents not to discontinue use of cortisone cream abruptly.
- Teach parents about the side effects of all medications.
- Encourage parents to express their frustrations because these infants are fussy and difficult to soothe.
- Support the family through the course of the disease.
- Listen to parents and reassure them that they are not at fault for the disease.
- Remember that health care workers with herpes simplex should not care for infants with active atopic dermatitis because exposure could cause a generalized reaction in the child.

- Suggest parents humidify the house to reduce skin drying.
- Caution against using harsh laundry detergent and dressing infants in rough-textured, scratchy clothes.
- Advise adolescents on ways to avoid dry skin, such as taking showers instead of baths, using no soap or prescription soap, avoiding swimming in chlorinated pools, and applying skin emollient or moisturizer.
- Caution adolescents on use of *acne* medications because they further dry the skin.
- Help parents and child identify psychological problems that may initiate the scratch-itch cycle.
- Assess the child's adjustment to school and family and the child's self-esteem.

# ATTENTION-DEFICIT HYPERACTIVITY DISORDER (ADHD)

## DESCRIPTION

- ADHD is possibly an umbrella diagnosis for a variety of behavioral-attention problems with a variety of causes.
- ADHD is frequently associated with situational anxiety, *abuse*, and *neglect* and may be one component in the development of some psychiatric disorders.
- Boys are more frequently affected than girls, with an estimated 6% of U.S. schoolchildren having ADHD.
- Children with ADHD are unable to complete tasks because of inattention and impulsivity; they are easily distracted and seem not to listen.
- Impulsivity is paramount in this disorder, acting always before thinking and shifting from one activity to another.
- The child with ADHD exhibits excessive or exaggerated muscular activity, such as excessive climbing or haphazard running.
- Children with ADHD do not have intelligence deficits.
- Both drug and behavior modification treatment methods have been used with success, pointing toward the theory of varying causes.
- ADHD tends to diminish as the child approaches adolescence.
- The child's attention span lengthens, and the ability to filter improves.

- A persistent problem associated with ADHD is lowered self-esteem and reduction in social skills.

## ASSESSMENT FINDINGS

- Unable to sit still in school
- Excessive disorganized activity
- Unable to sit still long enough to eat
- Repetitive activities, such as finger tapping
- Driven or compulsive behavior
- Variability—good moments and bad moments
- Impulsivity
- All-or-none reaction to stimuli (block everything out or unable to filter any stimuli—this is frequently termed short attention span)
- Difficulty with concepts related to sequencing
- Difficulty speaking with prepositions and conjunctions
- Difficulty with reading, math, and spelling because of sequencing
- Abnormal responses to graphesthesia and stereognosis
- Choreiform movements
- Unilateral Babinski reflex or strabismus

## NURSING IMPLICATIONS

- Give the parents time to accept this diagnosis and encourage them to verbalize their feelings.
- Help the parents and the child to understand why the child's behavior has brought them to the attention of the health care system and educate them about ADHD.
- Discuss therapeutic management as it relates to necessary changes in the child's learning environment and support the family with discipline at home.
- Encourage parents to be firm but fair.
- Assure parents of the need for rules to offer stability to the child with ADHD.
- Review normal interactions with families to discover potential areas that could be modified to help the child.
- Remind parents that punishment should follow an offense quickly because a child forgets what he or she did.
- Discuss the important differentiation of being mad at a child's behavior and not at the child.

- Monitor the child's psychosocial well-being, especially as related to anxiety and self-esteem.
- Educate the parent on potential medications helpful in controlling the excessive activity of a child with ADHD, to allow him or her to function in a normal classroom.
- Explain the actions and side effects of all medications prescribed as well as appropriate administration.
- Discuss research related to ADHD and provide family support to reassure the family of their ability to handle the challenges of this disorder.
- Recommend support groups and provide educational material as needed or requested.

## AVOIDANT DISORDER

### DESCRIPTION
- An avoidant disorder is characterized by excessive drawing back from contact with strangers.
- The withdrawal interferes with normal social function or peer relationship development.
- The child typically expresses a desire for affection and acceptance from close family members.
- The child does not have a communication disorder; however, they appear mute with strangers.
- A lack of confidence either develops with or because of the avoidant disorder.
- This disorder occurs from as young as 2 years old, but more often, it manifests in adolescents.

### ASSESSMENT FINDINGS
- Behavior lasting at least 6 months
- Socially withdrawn
- Embarrassed and timid with unfamiliar people
- Increased anxiety with even trivial contact with strangers
- Inarticulate or mute if anxiety is severe
- Unassertive personality
- Lacking confidence

### NURSING IMPLICATIONS
- Suggest to families and clients that this disorder may be treated with family therapy.
- Enlighten families as to the process of family therapy and the insights they will gain into themselves.

- Encourage and support families and clients with this disorder to overcome confidence problems and increase their ability to interact with others.

# BILE DUCT OBSTRUCTION

## DESCRIPTION

- Bile duct obstruction in children commonly occurs from congenital atresia, stenosis, or absence of the duct.
- It also can occur from plugging of biliary secretions, but this is rare.
- When the bile duct is obstructed, bile cannot enter the intestinal tract; it accumulates in the liver.
- Bile pigments (direct bilirubin) then enter the blood stream causing jaundice.
- The jaundice can take up to 2 weeks to develop.
- This delay in development of jaundice differentiates it from physiologic jaundice, which occurs in newborns 24 to 72 hours after birth.
- Because bile salts are not reaching the intestine, absorption of fat and fat-soluble vitamins is poor.
- Absorption of calcium, which depends on vitamin D absorption, also is poor.
- The pressure on the liver leads to cell damage, which, if severe enough, leads to *cirrhosis* of the liver.
- Liver transplantation is necessary, or death from liver failure results.

## ASSESSMENT FINDINGS

- Jaundice
- Increased direct bilirubin
- Elevated alkaline phosphatase levels
- SGOT normal initially, but as the obstruction continues increased back pressure causes liver cell damage and an increased SGOT
- White stools (from lack of bile pigments)

## NURSING IMPLICATIONS

- Differentiate between biliary obstruction versus jaundice secondary to infantile hepatitis because in the latter exploratory surgery under general anesthesia is dangerous.

- Administer magnesium sulfate or dehydrocholic acid to stimulate flow of bile if a mucous plug is suspected.
- Prepare child and parents for surgical intervention; perform preoperative and postoperative teaching if atresia of the bile duct is the cause.

  > Explain to the parents in lay terms that a fistula for bile flow between the liver and the intestine will be created.

  > Support the parents in understanding that a double-barreled colostomy is then created, and the bile flows out of the proximal loop into a collecting bag. Periodically the bile needs to be returned to the distal loop of the intestine.

  > Help the parents to understand that the colostomy is probably temporary and will be closed once biliary flow is established in 6 to 12 weeks.

- Brace the parents for the potential of a permanent colostomy if the atresia is too far back in the liver to be in an operable area.
- Discuss the possibility of the need for a liver transplant if damage is extensive.
- Preoperatively, place the child on a low-fat, high-protein diet and monitor nutritional status.
- Administer water-miscible vitamins and possibly vitamin K if prothrombin levels are high.
- Maintain fluid and electrolytes and administer parenteral fluids for hydration.
- Prepare parents for what the child will look like postoperatively if surgery is necessary (i.e., possible oxygen equipment and restraints).
- Postoperatively, observe for abdominal distention, which could indicate a paralytic ileus.
- Observe for return of bowel sounds before beginning oral intake.
- Monitor for indications of successful surgical repair by evaluating for yellow-brown stools.
- Administer Portagen, a formula with medium-chain fatty acids, if bile flow is inadequate following surgery.
- Provide emotional support throughout hospitalization and explain all therapeutic measures to the parents.
- Encourage parents to stay with their child and participate in care to continue the emotional bond with the infant.

# BITES, MAMMALIAN

## DESCRIPTION

- Dog bites account for 90% of all bites inflicted on humans.
- Cat bites, wild animal bites, and human bites also constitute a threat but occur less commonly in children.
- Bites can potentially cause abrasions, puncture wounds, lacerations, and crushing injuries depending on the size of the animal.
- Infection and long-term scarring with permanent disfigurement are also common concerns associated with bites.
- *Rabies,* from the presence of microorganisms in the mouth of the animal, is also a concern.

## ASSESSMENT FINDINGS

- Puncture marks
- Pain
- Abrasion
- Bleeding
- Laceration
- Crushing injury

## NURSING IMPLICATIONS

- Assess extent of injury.
- Evaluate for any coexisting injury related to crushing injury.
- Assist physician in cleansing the wound.
- Assess need for sutures and assist in procedure.
- Encourage the parents to remain with the child.
- Treat the child's pain and attempt to calm the child.
- Administer pain medication or a sedative depending on the amount of pain and the extent of injury.
- Explain all procedures and need for tetanus prophylaxis if the child's immunization status is unknown.
- Support the parent and the child through the potential for many surgeries, depending on location and extent of injury.
- Help the parents and the child express their fears, anger, and concerns regarding any permanent disfigurement.
- Provide essential consultation information (plastic surgery) and instruct on follow-up visits.

- Include information on signs and symptoms of infection in discharge instructions.

# BITES, SNAKE

## DESCRIPTION
- The copperhead snake and rattlesnake account for most fatal snakebites.
- The snakebite causes a failure of the blood coagulation system.
- Children die of intracranial hemorrhage.
- Venom from coral snakes causes neuromuscular paralysis.
- Snakebites tend to occur during the warmer months.
- Reaction to poisonous snakebite is almost immediate.
- If a child receives appropriate antivenin promptly, the prognosis for a full recovery is good.

## ASSESSMENT FINDINGS
### Local
- White wheal at puncture site
- Puncture marks
- Excruciating pain at site
- Purplish erythema and edema extending rapidly from site
- Sanguineous fluid from bite site
### Systemic
- Dizziness
- *Vomiting*, possibly hemoptysis
- Perspiration
- Weakness
- Epistaxis
- Hematuria
- Subcutaneous or internal hemorrhage
- Dilated pupils
- *Seizures*
- *Coma* and death

## NURSING IMPLICATIONS
- Apply a cold compress at the scene.
- Urge the child to lie quietly.
- Maintain the bitten extremity dependent.
- Suction out venom if suction cup from emergency kit is available.
- Expedite the child's transfer to a health care facility.

- Obtain information on the type of snake that bit the child.
- Perform a skin test of antivenin before administration to avoid an anaphylactic response to the horse serum, which is the base of the antivenin.
- Administer specific antivenin, ensuring that the intramuscular injection is not administered into an edematous body part, which could impede absorption.
- Know that the antivenin can be administered into any limb.
- Institute *tetanus* prophylaxis if immunization status is unknown or if it has been more than 10 years since a *tetanus immunization* was given.
- Attempt to calm the child and the parent and encourage verbalization of their fears.
- Support the child and parents and ensure that no one is to blame for the snakebite.
- Teach the child and parents about safe rules for avoiding snakebites, such as looking for snakes before stepping into underbrush and listening for telltale sounds of a rattlesnake.

## BLOOD TRANSFUSIONS

### DESCRIPTION

- Blood transfusions are used in the treatment of many childhood disorders.
- There are several different components of blood, and therefore the potential to administer the components exists.
- Blood products include whole blood, packed red blood cells, washed red blood cells (the foreign matter is removed to reduce the possibility of blood reaction), plasma, plasma factor such as cryoprecipitate or proplex, platelets, white blood cells, fresh frozen plasma, and albumin.
- The usual amount of blood transfused to a child is 15 ml/kg.
- The rate of administration in a child is 10 ml/kg/hour (unless the child has hypovolemic shock).
- Even if administered slowly, transfusions can cause a strain on a child's cardiovascular system.
- Packed red blood cells are the most common form of transfusion to prevent fluid overload.

- Platelets last only about 10 days, and transfusion of this blood product must be repeated.
- Blood products are used most commonly in children with anemias and primary immunodeficiency disorders.
- Blood product administration has the potential for several side effects and reactions and therefore should be administered carefully and according to hospital protocol.
- Blood products must not be administered with an intravenous glucose or electrolyte solution.
- If blood is administered with a hypertonic solution, fluid is drawn out of the red blood cells, causing them to shrink and rendering them worthless.
- If blood is administered with a hypotonic solution, fluid is drawn into the cells and they burst, rendering them worthless.
- Blood should be administered with an isotonic solution, preferably normal saline, and with a blood filter to filter out impurities.
- Many risks are associated with the administration of a blood product.
- A primary concern is contracting *hepatitis B*, which leads to liver carcinoma and death.
- Blood must be tested for HIV, since this can be transmitted in blood products.

### Nursing Implications

- Assess the need for blood product transfusion.
- Obtain permission from the child's parent or guardian.
- Answer all questions from parents honestly.
- Ensure that the client is identified, unit numbers and the client numbers are correct, and the client's blood type is compatible with that of the product. Also ensure that the product is within its expiration date and that it is administered promptly.
- Have another health care person certified in blood administration review all of the above-listed data, with both of you signing off on the administration.
- Send any obviously contaminated or discolored product back to the blood bank.
- Provide an enjoyable activity for the child during the administration of any blood product so as to avoid problems that may arise when the child gets bored.

- Obtain baseline vital signs before blood product transfusion.
- Obtain vital signs every 15 minutes during the transfusion.
- Observe for any symptoms of blood transfusion reactions, and if they occur, immediately turn the transfusion off and notify the physician.

  Anaphylactic reaction: headache, fever, chills, back pain, dyspnea, hypotension, hemoglobinuria.

  Allergic reaction: pruritus, *urticaria*, wheezing.

  Contaminant in blood: increased fever.

  Circulatory overload: increased pulse, dyspnea.

  Hypocalcemia: muscle cramping, twitching of extremities, *seizures*.

  *Hepatitis*: fever, jaundice, lethargy, tenderness over liver.

  Hemosiderosis: bronzed-colored skin.

- If a reaction has occurred, send samples of blood and urine from the child to the laboratory and send the intact unit of blood back to the blood bank for testing.
- If the reaction is severe, administer oxygen if necessary.
- Administer antihistamine to reduce symptoms of reaction.
- Monitor for signs of circulatory overload during and after administration of blood products.
- Administer calcium gluconate if muscle cramping develops secondary to hypocalcemia related to blood transfusion.
- Support self-esteem and altered body image if hemosiderosis (iron deposits cause bronze-colored skin) occurs.
- If patient is admitted with fever, jaundice, lethargy, and tenderness over liver, obtain a thorough transfusion history because these are signs of *hepatitis*.

## BLOUNT'S DISEASE

### DESCRIPTION

- Blount's disease is retardation of growth of the epiphyseal line on the medial side of the proximal tibia (inside the knee) resulting in bowed legs.
- This is a serious disturbance of bone growth and requires treatment.

- Bracing or osteotomy may be necessary to correct this deformity or prevent it from becoming more severe.

### Assessment Findings

- Medial aspect of the proximal tibia as sharp and beaklike in appearance on x-ray film.
- Bowed legs

### Nursing Implications

- Ensure the definitive diagnosis of Blount's disease by confirming x-rays.
- Explain to parents why their child requires treatment or surgery, whereas another child on the block may have a similar appearance and is expected to outgrow the problem (developmental *genu varum*, which presents as bowing of the legs; however, the condition corrects itself).
- Prepare the child and the parents for any necessary surgical intervention.
- Assess for signs of altered nutrition, impaired physical mobility, altered skin integrity, infection, and pain postoperatively.
- Prepare the child for discharge by informing the child and the parents of any special instructions or medications.

## BODY TEMPERATURE, ELEVATED

### Description

- Elevated body temperature in the infant and child can cause febrile convulsions.
- Because these convulsions arise with sudden fever, they are preventable. The *seizure* associated with fever is tonic-clonic in nature and generally lasts 15 to 20 seconds.
- Elevated body temperature is defined as fever greater than 102°.
- Treatment of children who have had a febrile convulsion is to prevent further episodes of high fever.
- The child with two or more febrile convulsions may be placed on maintenance phenobarbital.
- The child who has had a febrile convulsion needs to have the underlying cause of the fever determined and treated.

- A child does not normally suffer neurologic impairment from a febrile convulsion.

### Nursing Implications

- Educate parents to report fever of greater than 101°F in their infant or child.
- Inform parents of the importance of giving acetaminophen to keep fever below 101°F.
- Inform the parents of other ways of cooling the child, such as by sponging the child with tepid water.
- Educate the parents on the importance of avoiding aspirin, not giving the child a cool bath because the child could slip, not using cool water because it could cause shock in the immature nervous system, not using alcohol because it could be inhaled or absorbed through the skin in toxic amounts, and not administering oral medications when the child is drowsy or postictal.
- Advise parents if all attempts to cool the child fail that they should transport the child to a health care facility.
- Administer treatment depending on the underlying cause of the fever.
- Assist with a lumbar puncture to rule out *meningitis*.
- Administer antipyretic drugs to keep the fever below seizure level.
- Begin antibiotic therapy as prescribed.
- Assure the parents that febrile convulsions do not lead to brain damage.
- Support the parents and the child throughout the hospitalization, ensuring that they are prepared for all procedures and understand all treatments.
- Encourage the parents to stay with the hospitalized child to allay the child's fear.
- Educate the parents on any discharge medication's actions or side effects.

## BONE MARROW TRANSPLANTATION

### Description

- Bone marrow transplantation involves the transfer of bone marrow from a donor (through aspiration) and its intravenous infusion to a recipient.
- Bone marrow transplants are most successful when the patient has not been sensitized by receipt of previous blood transfusions.

- Success also depends on compatibility (HLA) of donated marrow to the child's blood.
- Identical twins are the ideal donors, followed by parent or sibling. Sometimes registered donors at bone marrow banks are a closer match than a parent or a sibling.
- There is no guarantee that a graft will be accepted or that improvement will occur; with a good match, however, it is effective 80% of the time.
- This is a common procedure for children with blood disorders such as acquired *aplastic anemia, leukemia,* and some forms of immune dysfunction.
- Marrow cells begin to migrate from the child's blood stream into the marrow almost immediately after infusion.
- If the transplant is accepted (engraftment occurs), red blood cells can be detected in peripheral blood in about 3 weeks.
- White blood cells and platelet cells may not return to normal for up to 1 year posttransplant.
- After discharge, the child continues to require blood replacement, and therefore isolation at home needs to be continued.
- Follow-up visits are required for 1 year to ascertain that the child is free of infection while white blood cells rise to normal levels.
- Graft versus host disease is a potentially lethal complication of bone marrow transplantation that is an immunologic response of donor T cells against the tissue of the recipient.

### ASSESSMENT FINDINGS

#### *Preoperatively with cyclosporine administration or irradiation*
- Nausea
- *Vomiting*
- *Diarrhea*

#### *Post bone marrow transplantation in recipient*
- Fever
- Chills

### NURSING IMPLICATIONS
- Explain all procedures and answer all questions that the parents and child may have regarding the procedure.

- Prepare parents for the potential complications associated with infection postoperatively and the potential for death.
- Encourage parents or siblings to express feelings of guilt or frustration if they exist regarding incompatibility.
- Ascertain that the child receiving the transplant understands he or she is not responsible for the outcome.
- Elicit any anxiety that the family has.
- Remember that to prevent rejection of the bone marrow by the recipient's T cells, cyclosporine is administered to the recipient preoperatively to suppress immune function.
- Prepare the child for total body irradiation to destroy the child's marrow.
- Inform donors that they will remain in the hospital for 24 to 48 hours to ascertain that the aspiration site is not infected.
- Be aware that circulatory overload and pulmonary emboli from unfiltered particles are potential complications that occur during transfusion of the bone marrow into the recipient.
- Institute protective isolation for the recipients.
- Prepare the child for painfulness of some procedures, and support the child throughout procedures.
- Let the donor know that the although the donation is not painful (done under general anesthesia), the sites will be tender and the donor will be tired for several days.
- Assess the donor's aspiration sites for redness or pain and monitor temperature.
- Before the donor's discharge, teach donor to watch for signs of infection and to report them to the transplant coordinator.
- Administer the donated marrow as prescribed via intravenous infusion, over 60 to 90 minutes. (Do not use a blood filter because this would filter out the marrow tissue.)
- Assess for signs of circulatory overload or pulmonary emboli.
- Treat common reactions of fever and chills with acetaminophen, diazepam, or diphenhydramine hydrochloride as prescribed.

- Monitor white blood cell count daily.
- Prevent graft versus host disease by administering methotrexate or cyclosporine and irradiating blood products before infusion of bone marrow.
- Assess for symptoms of graft versus host disease (rash and general malaise beginning 7 to 14 days post-transplant with latent infections becoming active, high fever, *diarrhea,* and liver and spleen enlargement).
- Assess for alteration in recipient's growth and development secondary to extended isolation at hospital and at home.
- Encourage family to provide schoolwork if appropriate and help them realize that school books and papers can be gas sterilized for use in protective isolation.
- Support the family throughout the hospitalization, and refer them to appropriate support or community groups.
- Prepare the child and parents for discharge, and encourage them to call the transplant coordinator regarding even the simplest questions.
- During follow-up appointments, pursue appropriate activities for the child and discuss avoiding overprotecting the child.

## BREAST HYPERTROPHY

### DESCRIPTION

- Breast hypertrophy is an abnormal enlargement of breast tissue secondary to low progesterone levels during the establishment of regular menstrual cycles.
- Normally breast development halts after puberty when progesterone levels rise to mature strength.
- With breast hypertrophy, breast growth may continue for several years.
- Breast hypertrophy can lead to physical and emotional stress.
- Adolescent girls with breast hypertrophy have many self-image issues related to their new appearance.
- Breast reduction is an option; however, removal of a large amount of glandular tissue could interfere with future breast-feeding.
- A woman with breast hypertrophy must do breast self-examination conscientiously because a cancerous lesion may easily escape detection.

### Assessment Findings
- Pain and fatigue in back of shoulders
- Slouching and poor posture in an attempt to minimize breast size

### Nursing Implications
- Support the adolescent girl in her concerns regarding her self-image.
- Encourage the girl to verbalize her feelings and discuss options such as breast reduction with her and her parents.
- Help the girl to understand that changes in her self-concept must come from within and that surgical reduction only reduces physical discomfort.
- Inform a woman with breast hypertrophy that pregnancy and lactation will make her breasts even larger because they become filled with milk.
- Ensure that the woman with breast hypertrophy understands the importance of and how to perform a breast self-examination.

## BREATH HOLDING

### Description
- Breath holding is a neurologic phenomenon revealing the immaturity of a child's neurologic control.
- Breath holding occurs in young children when they are stressed or angry.
- This is different than children who deliberately hold their breath during temper tantrums or with *seizures*.
- A child breathes in and forgets to breathe out because he or she is upset.
- The child becomes cyanotic, slumps to the floor, and momentarily loses consciousness.
- The loss of consciousness allows the child to begin breathing again.
- The child's color returns, and he or she is revived.

### Assessment Findings
- Stress or anger present
- Child not breathing out
- Child cyanotic and then slumps to the floor '

### Nursing Implications
- Confirm the differential diagnosis between breath holding, temper tantrums, and *seizures* by having the parents describe the actual episodes.

- Explain to parents and child that this breath holding occurs because of the immaturity of the child's neurologic control.
- Reassure the child and parents that although this is frightening, the child will be all right.
- Explain to the family that no treatment is recommended.
- Teach the family how to differentiate between signs of temper tantrums, breath holding, and *seizures*.
- Educate the family on basic pediatric cardiopulmonary resuscitation (CPR) as an important skill, which may also make them feel more reassured.

# BRONCHIAL OBSTRUCTION

## DESCRIPTION

- Bronchial obstruction can occur when an aspirated object not large enough to obstruct the trachea obstructs the right main bronchus.
- The right main bronchus is obstructed because it is straighter and has a larger lumen than the left bronchus in children over 2 years.
- Alveoli distal to the obstruction collapse causing atelectasis.
- If the foreign object allows air in but not out, the right lung can become hyperinflated, leading to a *pneumothorax*.
- Common objects aspirated include bones, nuts, coins, safety pins, and popcorn. Mucous plugs can also obstruct airways.
- Objects coated with oil that swell with moisture, such as popcorn, not only can cause obstruction, but also lipid *pneumonia*, which is difficult to treat.
- Most objects that are aspirated can be removed by laryngoscopy or bronchoscopy.

## ASSESSMENT FINDINGS

- Violent cough
- Dyspnea
- Localized wheezing
- Pain
- Choking and distress
- Chest film positive for radiopaque object
- Hemoptysis
- Fever

- Purulent sputum
- Leukocytosis

### Nursing Implications
- Teach parents which foods are commonly aspirated and advise them not to give them to children under school age.
- Teach parents the signs of an obstruction and have them bring their child to an emergency room if suspected.
- Quickly orient the child to the emergency room, and explain the treatment to the child and parents.
- Allow the parents to accompany the child if possible.
- Attempt to allay the child's and parents' fears, and let the parents know they should not feel guilty about giving the child the aspirated food.
- Prepare the child for bronchoscopy or laryngoscopy.
- Observe the child throughout the procedure for further distress and after the procedure to detect bronchial edema and airway obstruction.
- Keep the child NPO (give nothing by mouth) for 1 hour postprocedure.
- Assess the child's gag and swallowing and monitor first fluids closely to ensure the child does not aspirate.
- Offer the child cool fluids to reduce throat pain.
- Apply external ice packs and administer humidified air to reduce bronchial edema and liquefy bronchial secretions.

## BRONCHIOLITIS

### Description
- Bronchiolitis refers to an inflammation of the fine bronchioles secondary to an acute respiratory viral infection in children under age 2.
- The peak incidence of bronchiolitis is 6 months.
- Bronchiolitis most commonly occurs during winter and spring months and occurs in boys more than girls.
- The respiratory syncytial virus (RSV) is the most common underlying cause of bronchiolitis.
- RSV can be spread by respiratory droplet for up to 9 days.
- The inflamed bronchioles become edematous, and respiratory secretions accumulate, occluding the bronchiolar lumen.

- The narrowed airways compromise expiration and cause air to be trapped in the alveoli.
- Hyperinflation occurs followed by atelectasis.
- The inadequate ventilation leads to hypoxemia and hypercapnia.
- The acute phase of bronchiolitis lasts 2 to 3 days, after which the child's condition improves rapidly.
- Many children with numerous instances of bronchiolitis in early life go on to develop *asthma*.

## ASSESSMENT FINDINGS

- Nasal drainage
- Sneezing
- Coughing
- Poor appetite or inability to suck
- Low-grade infection
- Tachypnea
- Nasal flaring
- Intercostal and subcostal retractions on inspiration
- Inspiratory crackles
- Expiratory wheezing
- Dyspnea
- Tachycardia
- Productive or congested cough
- Cyanosis and hypoxia
- Low oxygen saturation levels
- Laboratory analysis of nasal washings positive for RSV

## NURSING IMPLICATIONS

- Maintain the child with adequate oxygenation, and institute humidified oxygen therapy if necessary to counteract cyanosis and preserve hydration.
- Prevent spread of the infection with respiratory isolation and good hand washing.
- Administer prescribed antibiotic if causative organism is unknown.
- Administer ribavirin by aerosol if causative organism is RSV.
- Caution the parents about the dangers and teratogenic side effects of this drug.
- Explain to parents about their child's condition and about bronchiolitis.
- Help the parents to understand that this child did not have a simple cold and that they should not feel guilty.

- Help the parents to understand that although this can be a life-threatening disorder without treatment, with appropriate treatment, the child will be much better in a few days.
- Institute fluid therapy to maintain hydration and liquefy secretions.
- Maintain the child in a semi-Fowler's position to facilitate breathing.
- Promote airway clearance via chest physiotherapy because bronchodilators are often ineffective in infants because they have inadequate bronchiole muscles to respond to the drug.
- Institute full respiratory assistance, and assist with extracorporeal membrane oxygenation if necessary to maintain adequate oxygenation.
- Maintain adequate nutrition because feeding often increases the work of breathing.
- Administer parenteral or enteral fluids if the child is unable to take oral feedings.
- Provide sufficient rest periods to help conserve the child's energy for breathing.
- Encourage the parents to verbalize their fears over the illness of their small child.
- Recommend that parents assist with the care of their child as much as possible.
- Explain all procedures and equipment to the parents and support them throughout the hospitalization.

## BRONCHITIS

### DESCRIPTION

- Bronchitis is an inflammation of the major bronchi and the trachea.
- This inflammation is usually secondary to an upper respiratory tract viral infection, which spreads to the bronchi.
- It is seen in children under age 2 and more often in the winter.
- Infants with acute bronchitis can develop acute respiratory distress.
- The associated cough is pronounced at night and can wake a child from sleep. The cough may persist for up to 10 days.

- The child's signs and symptoms persist for about a week and then fade.

## ASSESSMENT FINDINGS

- Gradual development of a hoarse, hacking, productive cough
- "Noisy rattling breathing"
- Wheezing
- Rhonchi
- Fine or coarse rales
- Increased percussion sounds secondary to hyperinflated alveoli
- Signs of respiratory distress
- Fever
- Leukocytosis
- Increased erythrocyte sedimentation rate
- Chest film with diffuse alveolar hyperinflation and hilus markings

## NURSING IMPLICATIONS

- Explain to the concerned parents what bronchitis is and that normally the child does not require hospitalization.
- Teach the parents appropriate interventions to relieve the child's symptoms.
- Have the parents maintain the child on bed rest and provide plenty of fluids.
- Instruct the parents to keep air warm and moist and that a bronchodilator may be prescribed to dilate the bronchi.
- Teach the parents how to use a bronchodilator and also about any antibiotics prescribed if the infecting organism is a bacterium.
- Advise the parents to administer an expectorant if the child's mucous is viscous.
- Recommend against cough syrups because the child's cough should not be suppressed but encouraged to expectorate accumulating secretions.
- Keep in mind that cough suppressants may be used at night if the child has trouble sleeping.
- Teach the parents to administer antipyretics, such as acetaminophen, to reduce fever.
- Educate the parents on worsening signs of respiratory dysfunction, and advise them to seek medical atten-

tion for their child if they occur or if the child does not improve after a week.

# BULIMIA NERVOSA

## DESCRIPTION

- Bulimia nervosa is an eating disorder that is characterized by episodes of binge eating followed by self-induced vomiting.
- This is classified in the *Diagnostic and Statistical Manual of Mental Disorders* (DSM-IV).
- It typically occurs in late adolescence and primarily affects girls.
- The adolescent is aware of the eating disorder but is unable to control it.
- Bulimia nervosa can last for months to years with periods of normal eating interspersed.
- The adolescent may vacillate between periods of binging and fasting.
- A girl with bulimia nervosa exhibits great concern about her weight and makes repeated attempts to control it via dieting, *vomiting*, use of cathartics, or diuretics.
- Frequent weight fluctuations occur secondary to the binging and fasting.
- The binging is of high caloric food and is done in secret.
- Following a binging episode, the girl experiences abdominal discomfort and vomits to relieve it and to improve self-concept.
- Bulimia nervosa can lead to serious physical complications related to the frequent vomiting and use of laxatives and diuretics.
- Erosion of teeth, esophageal tears, fluid and electrolyte abnormalities, and *cardiopulmonary arrest* can occur.
- This can be a difficult disorder to assess because bulimic girls may be only slightly underweight as compared with anoretic girls.
- The primary problem is thought to be related to poor self-esteem and a need to control.
- Counseling for the disorder is recommended and aimed at increasing self-esteem and a sense of control.

## ASSESSMENT FINDINGS

- Weight within normal range with frequent fluctuations

- Recurrent episodes of rapid food consumption
- Abdominal pain after binge eating
- Self-induced *vomiting*
- Laxative use
- Preoccupation with body image and weight
- Excessive exercise
- Poor impulse control
- Constant dieting
- Awareness of abnormal eating patterns
- Tooth enamel loss
- Chronic sore throats
- Esophageal irritation or tears
- Electrolyte imbalances, such as hyponatremia, hypokalemia, hypochloremia, and *metabolic acidosis*

### Nursing Implications
- Perform a thorough history to obtain essential information to aid in a definitive diagnosis.
- Assess for the serious physical complications associated with bulimia nervosa.
- Advise the client and her family that counseling is necessary to address the psychological issues of self-esteem and control.
- Explain that the goal is to restore normal eating habits; however, increasing self-esteem and promoting self-control are the issues.
- Assist the client and parents with necessary adjustments; offer positive feedback with successes.

## BURN TRAUMA

### Description
- A burn is injury to body tissue caused by excessive heat.
- Burns are the second cause of accidental injury in children between the ages of 1 and 4 years old.
- Burns are more serious in children because of their small body surface area.
- Scalding water or biting electrical cords are common burn causes in toddlers.
- Thermal burns occur at temperatures greater than 40°C.
- Electrical burns affect a larger area than where the entry occurs because of transmission through the skin and underlying tissues.

- Older children suffer from burns associated with flames.
- Some burns are secondary to child abuse.
- 50% of burns are preventable.
- Depth of burns is described as superficial (first degree), partial thickness (second degree), and full thickness (third degree).
- Partial-thickness burns can be first-degree and second-degree burns.
- Burns are classified as severe (second-degree burn over greater than 20% of body or third-degree burn over greater than 10% of body), moderate (second-degree burn over between 10% and 20% of body or less than 10% of body surface), or minor (first-degree or second-degree burns over less than 10% of body or third-degree burns over less than 2% of body). Location of burn is considered in the classification system.
- Many burns are compound, involving first-degree, second-degree, and third-degree burns.
- Location of burn injury is important to note, especially as related to the consequences of throat or face burns.
- If adhesions form during healing of hand or leg burns, full range of motion can be inhibited.
- Burns of the genitalia and feet can easily become infected if the child is sent home after initial treatment.
- Genitalia burns can cause urinary meatus edema and obstruction.
- A child with a moderate or severe burn requires swift care to ensure survival without disability caused by scarring, infection, or contracture.
- All body systems may be affected by a burn injury and must be evaluated to ensure survival.
- Fluid shifts that occur in the first 24 hours must be addressed to avoid circulatory collapse as well as altered renal function.
- Epinephrine and norepinephrine release in the burn victim leads to compensatory hypertension.
- Aldosterone and antidiuretic hormones increase to conserve water.
- The metabolic rate increases in burn victims, and they must receive adequate nutrition to avoid protein breakdown and acidosis.

- Curling's ulcer and paralytic ileus can occur in burn victims.
- Burn victims have a decreased protection from infection at a time when they are especially prone to infection.
- *Pseudomonas* is commonly found in burn wounds.
- Eschar, a tough leathery scab that forms over moderate or severely burned areas, can put pressure on underlying vessels and nerves and thereby may necessitate an escharotomy.

## ASSESSMENT FINDINGS

### *Superficial burn, such as scalds or severe sunburns*
- Superficial epidermis is involved
- Painful
- Area of burn blanches to pressure

### *Partial-thickness burn*
- Entire epidermis involved with sweat glands and hair follicles intact
- Erythematous
- Blisters
- Moist from exudate
- Very painful

### *Full-thickness burn: flames*
- Epidermis and dermis involved
- Adipose tissue, fascia, muscle, and bone may also be involved
- White or black burned area
- Not painful (the nerves have been burned)

## NURSING IMPLICATIONS

- Teach parents that prevention is the key to most burns, and instruct them in how they can take an active role in that prevention.
- Undress a child completely to remove the heat source, and fully assess the area of burn injury.
- Determine what caused the burn to evaluate better the degree of the burn and institute appropriate treatment.
- Institute measures to maintain the patient's airway because smoke inhalation can be more serious than the burn injury.
- Clarify as to whether any preexisting medical condition is present.

### *Mild or first-degree burns*
- Apply an analgesic and antibiotic ointment and a gauze bandage. Evaluate the need for debridement and assist in any treatment required. Teach the parents to keep the bandage dry and have them return for a follow-up in 2 days.

### *Moderate-to-severe burns*
- Monitor arterial blood gases and evaluate for the need of assisted ventilation.
- Address all needs of the child and the parents, being supportive throughout the painful experience and hospitalization.
- Provide analgesics for pain relief as needed and before dressing changes and debridement.
- Maintain hydration and monitor volume status because a great deal of plasma can be lost through the burn site and into tissue.
- Carefully monitor vital signs and assess for changes in circulatory status as well as signs of infection.
- Ensure that the child is receiving appropriate nutritional requirements to meet increased metabolic needs.
- Assess gastric pH and bowel sounds to avoid complications of Curling's ulcer and a paralytic ileus.
- Assist with appropriate treatments as prescribed: topical application of silver nitrate and bandages, open or closed burn therapy, escharotomy, debridement, and preparation for grafting.
- Address all psychosocial needs of the child and the parent during this long hospitalization from social isolation, family coping, to potential for permanent disfigurement.
- Provide diversional activities for the child, and encourage parents to be with the child as much as possible.
- Promote the child's verbalization of fears, anger, and self-image problems as well as parents' frustration and anger.
- Prepare the child and family for transition to home.

## CANCER, ACUTE LYMPHOCYTIC LEUKEMIA (ALL)

### DESCRIPTION
- ALL is the most frequent type of leukemia in children.
- It accounts for one-third of all instances of leukemia.

- The malignant cell involved is the immature lymphocyte, the lymphoblast.
- With the rapid proliferation of lymphocytes, the production of red blood cells and platelets falls, and invasion of body organs by the rapidly increasing white blood cell elements begins.
- The highest incidence for ALL is in children between 3 and 5 years of age.
- The prognosis for children under 2 years or over 10 years at the time of first occurrence is not as good as in those between 2 and 10 years.
- The incidence of ALL is slightly higher in males than females, and the disease is seen more often in white children than in children of other races.
- Children with Down syndrome or Fanconi's syndrome are more likely to develop leukemia than are other children.
- It occurs more often in identical twins than in other siblings.
- The cause in children is unknown.
- Radiation, exposure to chemicals, or genetic factors may have some influence on the occurrence.

## ASSESSMENT FINDINGS

- Pallor
- Low-grade fever
- Lethargy
- Petechiae and bleeding from oral mucous membranes
- Abdominal pain
- *Vomiting*
- Anorexia
- Bone and joint pain
- Headache
- Unsteady gait
- Generalized lymphadenopathy
- Variable leukocyte count
- Marked leukocytosis of blast cells
- Decreased platelet count
- Decreased hematocrit
- 25% blast cells present on bone marrow aspiration

## NURSING IMPLICATIONS

- Obtain a thorough history and physical examination to establish a baseline.

- Instruct the child and parents in all aspects of the disease and treatments.
- Assist with administration of *chemotherapy* as needed; monitor child for signs and symptoms of effects related to *chemotherapy*.
- Administer allopurinol during *chemotherapy*, as prescribed to reduce the formation of uric acid.
- Monitor fluid status carefully; encourage fluids, if not contraindicated, to prevent *dehydration* and maintain safe uric acid excretion.
- If central nervous system involvement occurs, prepare the child and parents for *radiation therapy* and intrathecal *chemotherapy*.
- Allow the child therapeutic *play* with needles, syringes, or intravenous tubing, so that they can work through their feelings about the intrusive procedures.
- Handle the child gently to minimize pain; use comfort devices and reposition frequently to prevent skin breakdown.
- Assist with preparing the child and family for *bone marrow transplantation* or immunotherapy if standard therapy is ineffective.
- Allow the child and parents to verbalize feelings; offer support, guidance, and instructions as necessary.
- Help the child adjust to changes in body image.
- Encourage adequate nutritional intake; offer suggestions for supplements to provide a high-protein, high-calorie bland diet.
- Refer the child and parents to cancer support groups and community services as appropriate.
- Instruct the child and family in signs and symptoms of infection and bleeding and measures to prevent or control them.

## CANCER, ACUTE MYELOGENOUS LEUKEMIA (AML)

### DESCRIPTION
- AML is overproliferation of granulocytes.
- Granulocytes grow so rapidly that they are often forced into the blood stream in the blast stage.
- This overproduction of granulocytes limits the production of red blood cells and platelets.
- AML accounts for 20% of all childhood leukemia.

- This disorder increases in frequency in late adolescence and is the most common type of leukemia in adulthood.

## ASSESSMENT FINDINGS

- Petechiae and bleeding from oral mucous membranes
- History of upper respiratory infection secondary to increased susceptibility to infection with immature granulocytes
- Fatigue
- Low-grade fever
- Periosteal pain
- Liver enlargement
- Spleen enlargement
- Gingival hypertrophy
- Perirectal necrotic lesions

## NURSING IMPLICATIONS

- Obtain a bone marrow aspiration and biopsy specimen, necessary to confirm diagnosis.
- Inform and teach the parents about the prognosis, disease, and cell classification system of M1–M6.
- Teach the parents and child regarding all aspects of the disease and treatments.
- Administer *chemotherapy* (most commonly used drugs are doxorubicin and cytosine) as prescribed, and teach the parents and child regarding the drugs and their side effects.
- During *chemotherapy* administration, keep in mind that the patient requires allopurinol to decrease the uric acid created by the great number of destroyed cells being evacuated from the blood.
- Monitor fluid and electrolyte status and assess for *dehydration.*
- Assess the need to provide replacement therapies for low leukocytes, erythrocytes, or platelets during *chemotherapy* administration and during remission.
- Promote the child's and family's expression of their fears and anxieties through appropriate interventions, such as *play therapy* for the child; offer support, guidance, and instruction throughout the child's illness.
- Anticipate the changing needs of the child and family through the chemotherapy and remission periods.

- Inform the child and parents of the potential need for *bone marrow transplantation* following initial remission to ensure new growth of normal granulocytes.
- Monitor and teach the child and parents regarding proper nutrition, signs of recurrence, and signs of infection.

## CANCER, BRAIN NEOPLASMS

### DESCRIPTION

- Brain tumor is the second most common form of cancer in children and the most common solid tumor form.
- Brain tumors occur in children between 1 and 10 years old with 5 years old being the peak incidence.
- Childhood brain tumors normally occur at the midline in the brain stem or cerebellum located beneath the tentorial membrane, making them difficult to remove without damaging normal brain tissue.
- Usually 4 to 6 months pass before actual symptom diagnosis of brain tumor.
- Suspected brain tumors require thorough neurologic examination, skull films, bone and brain scans, sonogram or magnetic resonance imaging, cerebral angiography or computed tomography scan, and myelography (may be necessary for tumors suspected of having seeded into the spinal column).
- Nuclear magnetic resonance may detect small tumors earlier than a computed tomography scan.
- A lumbar puncture must be done cautiously, or the release of cerebrospinal fluid may cause the brain stem to herniate.
- Therapy for brain tumors depends on the location and the extent of the tumor and may include a combination of surgery, *radiation therapy,* and *chemotherapy.*
- *Radiation therapy* and *chemotherapy* are important because most tumors cannot be totally removed because of their location.
- Long-term neurologic and pituitary dysfunction and intellectual retardation are not unusual in survivors of pediatric brain tumors, especially when treated with high doses of cranial radiation at a young age.
- One-fourth of all brain tumors in children are **cerebellar tumors, usually cerebellar astrocytomas,** which are benign, slow-growing cystic tumors, and treatment is surgical removal.

- *Medulloblastomas* are fast-growing malignant tumors most often found in the cerebellum in 3- to 5-year-old children, with metastasis occurring via spread through the cerebrospinal fluid and treated with surgery, *chemotherapy*, and *radiation therapy*. Survival rate is 40%.
- *Ependymomas* are tumors of the floor of the fourth ventricle that grow with intermediate speed in 2- to 6-year-olds; they are highly radiosensitive and are treated with *chemotherapy* and *radiation therapy* after surgical removal with a 50% survival rate.
- *Brain stem tumors (gliomas)* are tumors of the support tissue of the brain and occur almost exclusively in children; they are insidious and difficult to remove surgically; however, *radiation therapy* and *chemotherapy* can reduce the tumor size with recurrence expected in 6 months and limited survival rate.
- *Cerebral tumors* are usually astrocytomas and occur in school-age children, with removal difficult. Chances of a full recovery following surgery and *radiation therapy* are encouraging.
- *Tumors of the optic nerve* occur almost exclusively in children and tend to be astrocytomas; they are removed surgically and treated with *radiation therapy*, with vision lost in the operative eye because the optic nerve is removed.
- *Craniopharyngiomas* are tumors located near the upper surface of the pituitary gland in the sella turcica in school-age children; corticosteroids are administered before and after surgical removal to correct deficits in cortisone production with the potential for hormonal therapy and human growth therapy needed.

**ASSESSMENT FINDINGS**
### *Brain neoplasms—general*
- *Increased intracranial pressure* signs
    Intermittent headache worse in the morning
    Vision changes, especially diplopia
    *Vomiting* occurs on rising
    Enlarged head circumference
    Lethargy
    Projectile *vomiting, coma* (late signs)
- Nystagmus
- Cranial nerve paralysis
- Visual field deficits
- Ataxia

- Personality changes: lability and irritability
- *Seizures*

### Cerebellar tumors
- Signs of *increased intracranial pressure*
- Ataxia
- Head tilt
- Nystagmus

### Medulloblastomas
- Signs of *increased intracranial pressure*
- Ataxia
- *Hydrocephalus* with fourth ventricle compression

### Ependymomas
- *Hydrocephalus*
- Head tilt
- Ataxia
- Nystagmus
- *Vomiting* because the vomiting center of the brain is under the fourth ventricle

### Brain stem tumors (gliomas)
- Paralysis of the 5th, 6th, 7th, 9th, and 10th cranial nerves
- Paralysis of conjugate gaze (inability of eyes to work together)
- Ataxia
- Horizontal nystagmus
- Hemiparesis
- Positive Babinski reflex

### Cerebral tumors
- Headache
- *Vomiting*
- Motor weakness
- Spasticity

### Tumors of the optic nerve
- Exophthalmos
- Nystagmus
- Strabismus
- Optic atrophy

### Craniopharyngiomas
- *Increased intracranial pressure* from blocked cerebrospinal fluid flow
- Visual field deficits
- Diminished pituitary activity: growth retardation and sexual immaturity

- Excessive urinary output from decreased anti-diuretic hormone secretion
- Hypothermia or hyperthermia from diminished functioning of the hypothalamus

## NURSING IMPLICATIONS

- Be alert to danger signs whenever a child is brought to a health care facility with any neurologic assessment findings, especially patterned *vomiting* or headaches.
- Observe a child suspected of brain tumor for signs of *increased intracranial pressure.*
- Record vital signs accurately so that subtle changes can be noted.
- Maintain safety precautions and keep bed side rails up.
- Describe completely any *seizure* activity that is witnessed so as to help localize the point of maximum brain pressure.
- Allow the child with suspected brain tumor or parent time to absorb the shock of the diagnosis and support them throughout the hospitalization.
- Help a family understand that brain tumor symptoms are insidious and they need not feel any guilt for not having recognized them.
- Encourage the family to express their fears and anxiety, and encourage parental participation in care as much as possible.
- Refer parents to other people familiar with the care of children with brain tumor, and encourage them to ask specific questions to the neurosurgeon.
- Make parents understand that brain surgery is never minor because of the importance of brain tissue, and prepare them for how their child will look and act after surgery.
- Inform the parents that after brain surgery, the child can be expected to remain comatose for several days owing to brain irritation and edema.
- Allow the child opportunities to express feelings about intrusive procedures through *play* with puppets or hospital equipment.
- Remember that the child may hear you even if he or she is unconscious.
- Before surgery, prepare the child in a positive way for a shaven head and emphasize that hair grows fast.

- Make a preoperative visit to the intensive care unit (ICU) with the child.
- Postoperatively, position the child's head as prescribed, generally on the unoperated side with the head of the bed flat or slightly elevated.
- Apply a neck brace or cast to stabilize the head and neck, especially if surgery was in the low occipital area.
- Assess vital signs and temperature frequently.
- Maintain intravenous fluids and administer mannitol as prescribed to decrease cerebral edema.
- Monitor head dressing, and assess drainage and for signs of infection.
- Help the child gradually increase independence in self-care.
- Orient the child and parents regarding postoperative radiation and chemotherapy.
- Encourage the child to be allowed as much normal activity as possible after discharge.
- Persuade family and school (school nurse) to take an active role helping the child readjust to school.

## CANCER, EWING'S SARCOMA

### DESCRIPTION

- Ewing's sarcoma, a type of tumor derived from connective tissue, such as bone and cartilage, muscle, blood vessels, or lymphoid tissue, is a malignant tumor occurring most often in the bone marrow of the diaphyseal area (midshaft) of the long bones.
- Ewing's sarcoma spreads longitudinally through the bone.
- This sarcoma primarily affects young adolescents and school-age children; bone tumor may arise during adolescence because of the rapid bone growth at this time.
- Metastasis is usually present at the time of diagnosis.
- The lungs and the bones are the most common sites for metastasis, eventually followed by central nervous system and lymph node metastasis.
- 50% of children achieve a 5-year survival rate when treated with surgery, *chemotherapy, radiation therapy* or a combination.
- Older children have a higher survival rate than younger children.

## ASSESSMENT FINDINGS
- Intermittent pain at the site of the tumor eventually becoming constant and severe
- "Onion-skin" appearance around the tumor on x-ray film

## NURSING IMPLICATIONS
- Investigate symptoms of pain in the legs of this age group.
- Obtain an x-ray film, computed tomography scan, and bone scan as prescribed to determine if Ewing's sarcoma is present and if metastasis has occurred.
- Assist with other diagnostic procedures, such as bone marrow aspiration and an intravenous pyelogram.
- Prepare the parents and the child for the need for a tumor biopsy for definitive diagnosis.
- Do not allow the child to bear weight on the affected extremity during testing to avoid pathologic fracture if a large area of the bone is involved in the tumor.
- Instruct the parents and the child on what Ewing's sarcoma is and optional treatment modalities.
- Give the child and parents time to ask questions and support them through the stages of acceptance of this cancer.
- Prepare the child and parent for limb amputation only if the tumor is extensive at diagnosis.
- Familiarize the parents and child with the usual therapy combination of surgery to remove the primary tumor, *radiation therapy,* and *chemotherapy.*
- Support the child and parents through all phases and complications associated with the sarcoma and the treatments.
- Teach the parents and child about the need to avoid all infections if treated with *chemotherapy* or high-dose *radiation therapy* to the leg.
- Allow the child or young adolescent chances to verbalize or express their fears and frustrations.
- Prepare the child for discharge to home, and educate the child and parents on any discharge medications or activity restrictions.

# CANCER, HODGKIN'S DISEASE

## DESCRIPTION
- Hodgkin's disease is malignancy of lymphoid tissue.
- A proliferation of lymphocytes and special Reed-Sternberg cells is found.

- Hodgkin's disease accounts for 4 in every 1 million cancers and is more common in males than in females.
- Peak incidence of Hodgkin's disease is between the ages of 15 and 34; it is rarely seen in children under 5 years of age.
- Hodgkin's disease occurs more frequently in children with *rheumatoid arthritis* or *systemic lupus erythematosus.*
- In some children, there is an abnormal distribution of human leukocyte antigens to suggest that the disease may be inherited.
- Metastasis with Hodgkin's disease is via the lymphatic system, with metastasis to the lung, liver, and bone marrow late in the disease.
- Confirmation of Hodgkin's disease is made by node biopsy in addition to supporting studies, including bone marrow, liver function, chest and abdominal computed tomography, lymphangiogram, and abdominal biopsy to identify the stage of the disease.
- Four subcategories of Hodgkin's disease include lymphocyte predominant, nodular sclerosing, mixed cellularity, and lymphocyte depletion.
- The most frequently occurring subcategories in children are nodular sclerosing and lymphocyte predominant.
- The category with the best prognosis is lymphocyte-predominant type, and the worst for a child is lymphocyte-depletion type.
- The disease is staged according to regional involvement using a staging laparotomy with partial or total splenectomy and liver and bone marrow biopsy.
- Treatment of Hodgkin's disease depends on the clinical stage determined by the staging laparotomy; it may consist of *radiation therapy* and *chemotherapy.*

### ASSESSMENT FINDINGS

- One rubbery-feeling, painless lymph node, usually cervical
- Anorexia
- Weight loss
- Malaise
- Fever
- Elevated sedimentation rate
- Decreased red blood cells

- Elevated serum copper level
- Enlarged mediastinal nodes on chest film
- Enlarged lymph nodes of the abdomen

### NURSING IMPLICATIONS
- Promptly recognize early signs of Hodgkin's disease.
- Explain to the child and the parents the disease process and the need to evaluate fully the stage of Hodgkin's disease the child is in.
- Prepare the child for the staging laparotomy and explain that the recovery is painful with the abdominal incision.
- Support the child and family throughout the course of the illness.
- Institute appropriately prescribed treatment guided by the results of the exploratory laparotomy.
- Prevent complications associated with impaired immune defenses.
- Address the child's and family's fear related to the disease.
- Assist the child in managing other adverse affects of *chemotherapy*, such as hair loss and related body image disturbance.
- Monitor for fluid and electrolyte disturbances, which can occur during treatment with the nausea and *vomiting*.
- Monitor nutritional intake and ensure adequate calories.
- Encourage adolescents to attend regular school during periods of remission, and promote as normal a life as possible.
- Support the child and adolescent throughout the long course of the illness and encourage verbalization of feelings to express concerns of coming out of remission.

## CANCER, NEUROBLASTOMA

### DESCRIPTION
- Neuroblastomas are tumors that arise from the cells of the sympathetic nervous system; cells are undifferentiated and highly invasive and occur most frequently in the abdomen near the adrenal gland or spinal ganglia.
- They are the most common abdominal tumor in childhood.

- Neuroblastoma occurs primarily in infants and preschool children; it is slightly more common in boys than in girls.
- There is an association between the development of neuroblastomas and fetal alcohol syndrome, *Hirschsprung's disease*, and *neurofibromatomosis.*
- Common sites of metastasis include bone marrow, liver, and subcutaneous tissue.
- Neuroblastoma has four stages: Stage I involves a tumor that is encapsulated and can be completely removed by surgery; stage II involves a tumor that cannot be completely removed by surgery, or there is lymph node involvement; stage III tumors extend beyond the midline, and regional lymph nodes may be involved bilaterally; stage IV has distant metastases at diagnosis with involvement of bone, eye, or liver.
- Most children are at stage IV at diagnosis.

### Assessment Findings
- Palpable abdominal mass
- Excessive sweating
- Flushed face
- *Hypertension*
- Abdominal pain
- *Constipation*
- Loss of motor function in lower extremities
- Weight loss and anorexia
- Dyspnea
- Difficulty in swallowing
- Neck and facial edema
- Jaundice
- Blue or purplish colored nodules on arm or legs
- Positive results of computed tomography scan, intravenous pyelogram, arteriogram, gallium bone scan, or bone marrow aspiration.
- Urine analysis positive for catecholamines or vanillylmandelic acid and homovanillic acid.

### Nursing Implications
- Obtain a thorough history and physical examination to establish a baseline.
- Obtain urine sample for analysis.
- Prepare the child for a computed tomography scan, gallium scan, bone marrow aspiration, intravenous pyelogram, or ateriogram as prescribed for diagnosis.

- Prepare the child and parents for surgery to remove the tumor.
- Prepare the child and parents for *chemotherapy* and *radiation therapy* if the child has stage III involvement.
- Offer emotional support and guidance to the child and parents during this disease; allow the child and parents to verbalize their feelings.

## CANCER, NON-HODGKIN'S LYMPHOMA

### DESCRIPTION

- Non-Hodgkin's lymphoma refers to a malignant disorder of the lymphocytes.
- The malignancy involves the stem cells and lymphocytes in varying degrees of differentiation.
- In the pediatric population, diffuse lymphoblastic, undifferentiated, and large cell lymphomas are commonly seen.
- Spread of non-Hodgkin's lymphomas is through the blood stream rather than directly by lymph, so it is unpredictable; metastatic spread to the central nervous system tends to occur early.
- The most common age of occurrence for non-Hodgkin's lymphoma is between 5 and 15 years old.
- A slightly higher incidence exists in males than in females.
- The cause of non-Hodgkin's lymphoma may be an oncogenic virus.
- These disorders are more commonly found in children with altered immune states, such as in agammaglobulinemia, *acquired immuno deficiency syndrome (AIDS)*, and those receiving long-term immunotherapy.
- The lymphomas can be divided into diffuse lymphoblastic lymphomas and diffuse undifferentiated lymphomas.
- Cells can be classified as T cell, B cell, or non-T or non-B type.
- The prognosis for recovery is best if cells are non-T or non-B; it is worse if cells are B cell type.
- Diagnosis is confirmed by biopsy of the affected lymph nodes and bone marrow analysis.
- Chest film, lymphangiogram, gallium scan, liver scan, spleen scan, and computed tomography scan define areas of metastasis.

- Burkett's lymphoma, a rare non-Hodgkin's lymphoma, is a rapidly growing tumor initially requiring surgical removal of the primary tumor followed by *chemotherapy.*
- Other non-Hodgkin's lymphomas are treated by *radiation therapy* to the lymph notes and by systemic *chemotherapy.*
- Intrathecal *chemotherapy* may be included in the therapy because non-Hodgkin's lymphoma tends to metastasize to the central nervous system.
- Autologous *bone marrow transplantation* with bone marrow that was removed before invasion of the lymphoma to the central nervous system allows more aggressive *chemotherapy* to be used.
- 80% to 90% of children with non-Hodgkin's lymphoma with minimal symptoms achieve remission.
- In a small percentage of children, the disorder may transform to *acute lymphocytic leukemia.*

### ASSESSMENT FINDINGS

#### Diffuse lymphoblastic type
- Lymp node enlargement, especially the neck and chest
- Cough or chest cold with mediastinal lymph swelling
- Edema of the face if mediastinal nodes press on the veins returning blood from the head

#### Diffuse undifferentiated types
- Abdominal mass (if abdominal nodes are involved)
- Abdominal pain
- *Diarrhea*
- *Constipation*

#### Burkitt's lymphoma
- Detectable painless mass
- Enlarged submaxillary or abdominal lymph nodes

### NURSING IMPLICATIONS

- Evaluate any complaints related to lymph node enlargement in this age group carefully.
- Refer  any child seen at a health care visit and found to have an abdominal mass or other lymph node enlargement to a physician for further evaluation.
- Explain the diagnosis of non-Hodgkin's lymphoma to the child and family.

- Discuss the available options, and support the family during the initial shock of knowing their child has a metastatic disease.
- Encourage families and inform them of the 80% to 90% survival rate.
- Relate to the child and family the different stages of *chemotherapy.*
- Explain all hospital diagnostic and therapeutic procedures to the family and to the child in language appropriate for the particular developmental stage of the child.
- Prepare the child with Burkitt's lymphoma for surgical removal of the primary tumor.
- Caution parents and children of the side effects of chemotherapeutic agents.
- Support the child and allow him or her to express feelings through appropriate therapeutic intervention.
- Support the parents in helping the child through all phases of therapy.
- Carefully evaluate for electrolyte imbalances, renal functioning, and adequate hydration in the child receiving *chemotherapy.*
- Provide information to the parents and child requiring autologous *bone marrow transplantation* about the procedure and post-operative care.
- Monitor for side effects of intrathecal *chemotherapy.*
- Institute infection control measures to prevent complications of immunosuppression and bone marrow depression.
- Evaluate nutritional status of the child and provide adequate calories and nutrients.
- Encourage the parents to bring in healthy foods that the child likes, and have the child work with a nutritionist.
- Monitor for *constipation* related to administration of chemotherapeutic agents, and provide stool softeners if necessary.
- Promote a positive self-image for the child.
- Promote the child's and family's expression of their fears and anxieties through appropriate interventions, such as *play therapy* for the child, and offer support, guidance, and instruction throughout the child's illness.
- Anticipate the changing needs of the child and family through the cycles of *chemotherapy* and remissions.

# CANCER, OSTEOGENIC SARCOMA

## DESCRIPTION

- Osteogenic sarcoma is a malignant, rapidly growing tumor of the osteoid tissue, most commonly the metaphyses of long bones.
- Osteogenic sarcomas most commonly occur in the distal femur, proximal tibia, and proximal humerus.
- This malignancy may be secondary to radiation therapy for other malignancies.
- These tumors occur more often in boys than in girls.
- Children with *retinoblastoma* have a higher incidence of osteogenic sarcoma, implying a probable hereditary influence.
- These cancers may also be caused by viruses in other animals.
- A biopsy specimen of the area confirms the diagnosis.
- The prognosis for osteogenic sarcoma has improved; 50% to 60% of adolescents diagnosed early and treated aggressively can be cured.

## ASSESSMENT FINDINGS

- Height taller than average (indicating rapid bone growth)
- Pain and swelling at the tumor site
- Warmth at the site (secondary to the increased vascularity of the area of the tumor)
- Pathologic fracture of the bone
- Increased serum alkaline phosphatase (secondary to rapidly growing bone cells)

## NURSING IMPLICATIONS

- Evaluate any reports of pain or swelling near the knee for the possibility of a malignant process.
- Prepare the child and parents for a biopsy of the site to confirm the diagnosis of osteosarcoma.
- Discuss the treatment options for each individual case with the parents and child, and inform them of the improved prognosis in recent years.
- Ensure that the parents and child understand that trauma to the area did not cause the malignant process.
- Obtain laboratory tests, such as a complete blood count, urinalysis, chest film, chest scan, and bone scan to assess if metastasis has occured.

- Do not allow weight bearing on the weakened bone because it may cause pathologic fracture.
- Discuss with the family the potential need to use *chemotherapy* to shrink the size of the tumor before surgical removal.
- Alleviate the parents' fears about postponing surgery by explaining that this is a normal intervention before surgery.
- Provide the child and family with information on the *chemotherapy*, and support them through the administration and potential side effects.
- Prepare the parents and the child for surgical removal of the tumor if the tumor is small and the child has reached adult height.
- Tell the parents and child that the single bone can be removed and replaced with an internally placed bone or metal prosthesis to preserve the child's leg.
- Inform the child with extensive tumor involvement and parents that the leg may be amputated at the joint above the tumor.
- Allow the child and family time to grieve and encourage them in verbalization of their feelings.
- Prepare the family for the need for a total hip amputation if necessary.
- Prepare the child with metastasis to the lungs from the sarcoma and family for a thoracotomy.
- Continue to support the child and family through all phases of the hospitalization.
- Educate the family and child on discharge instructions and potential need for rehabilitation and follow-up *chemotherapy*.
- Encourage the child in the knowledge that he or she can receive full remission and fulfill life potentials with a prosthesis.

## CANCER, RETINOBLASTOMA

### DESCRIPTION
- Retinoblastoma is a malignant tumor of the retina of the eye.
- This rare tumor accounts for only 1% to 3% of childhood malignancies.
- A small amount of cases of retinoblastoma (about 10%) develop because of an inherited autosomal

dominant pattern; it most often occurs as a spontaneous development.

- Children with the inherited type tend to develop bilateral disease; those with the spontaneous type may or may not have the tumor in both eyes.
- Retinoblastoma occurs early in life, from about 6 weeks of age through the preschool period.
- It occurs equally in boys and girls, and there is no preference for the right or left eye.
- One tumor or many individual tumors may be present and may be located on the retina or in the vitreous fluid or extend backward into the choroid, the optic nerve, and the subarachnoid space.
- The tumor metastasizes readily along the optic nerve to the subarachnoid space and brain, quickly involving the second eye.
- Metastasis to distant body sites, such as the bone marrow and liver, occurs because of the rich blood supply to the brain.
- Treatment depends on the size of the tumor: If the tumor is small at the time of diagnosis, it may be treated with cryosurgery; if the tumor is large, eye enucleation can be done; if metastasis is present, *radiation therapy* and *chemotherapy* are used.
- The long-term survival rate for children with retinoblastoma is as high as 90%.

### Assessment Findings

- Pupil appears white or described as "cat's eye" on examination
- Red reflex absent
- Strabismus (as eye becomes nonfunctional)
- Family history (possible with inherited type)
- Intraocular calcification or tumor on computed tomography or ultrasonography
- Metastasis positive on lumbar puncture, liver and skeletal survey, and bone marrow biopsy

### Nursing Implications

- Obtain a thorough history and physical examination to establish a baseline.
- Encourage the parents of children with a family history to have the child examined at least three times yearly until they reach 5 years of age.
- Prepare the child for examination under general anesthesia if a tumor is suspected.

- Prepare the child and parents for diagnostic tests used to establish the diagnosis and determine metastasis; provide necessary follow-up care.
- Prepare the child and parents physically and psychologically for surgery; include preoperative and postoperative teaching about all aspects of surgery.
- Be aware that following eye enucleation surgery, three-dimensional vision is distorted; if both eyes are involved, bilateral resection results in blindness.
- Following enucleation:
    Observe the pressure dressing site for bleeding.
    Monitor vital signs frequently for changes.
    Anticipate restraining the child if someone cannot be with the child constantly to keep him or her from tugging at the dressing and removing it.
    Assist with removing the eye dressing as prescribed after 48 hours and applying a small eye patch.
    Irrigate the empty socket with normal saline or apply antibiotic ointment as prescribed.
    Provide teaching to the parents regarding follow-up and use of eye prosthesis.
    Instruct the parents that the eye prosthesis need not be removed and cleaned daily; in children this age, leaving the prosthesis in place prevents the child from playing with it.
- With *radiation therapy*, monitor the child's white blood cell count closely for changes.
- Assist with administering *chemotherapy*, as indicated.
- Explain to and instruct the child and parents about all treatment plans, including the type, frequency, and duration of the therapy.
- Assess the child for possible side effects of *radiation therapy* and *chemotherapy*.
- Provide emotional support and guidance to the child and parents to help them cope with this disease; allow the child and parents to verbalize feelings and fears regarding the treatments and prognosis.
- Provide time for discussion to help them work through their decision.

## CANCER, RHABDOMYOSARCOMA

### Description

- Rabdomyosarcoma is a tumor of striated muscle that arises from the embryonic mesenchyme tissue that forms muscle, connective, and vascular tissue.

- The peak age of incidence is 2 to 6 years; a second peak occurrence is during puberty.
- Six different subtypes of tumors can be identified.
- Common sites of occurrence are the eye orbit, paranasal sinuses, uterus, prostate, bladder, retroperitoneum, arms, and legs.
- Central nervous system invasion occurs from direct tumor extension; distant metastasis most commonly occurs in lungs, bone, or the bone marrow.
- The primary treatment is surgical removal of the tumor followed by *radiation therapy* and *chemotherapy.*
- Prognosis depends on the size of the tumor and whether metastasis was present at the time of initial diagnosis, ranging from 80% (if all the tumor can be removed and no lymph node metastasis has occurred) to 20% (if metastasis to lung or bone was present at the time of the initial diagnosis).
- In children who do survive, long-term complications, such as cataract formation, bone neoplasm, gastrointestinal stricture, and hemorrhagic cystitis may occur from the extensive radiation used in the primary therapy.

ASSESSMENT FINDINGS (relate to site of tumor)
### Orbit
- Proptosis
- Visible and palpable conjunctival or eyelid mass
### Neck
- Hoarseness
- Dysphagia
- Visible and palpable mass in neck
### Nasopharynx
- Airway obstruction
- *Epistaxis*
- Dysphagia
- Visible mass in nasal or nasopharyngeal passages
### Paranasal sinuses
- Swelling
- Pain
- Nasal discharge
- *Epistaxis*
### Middle ear
- Pain
- *Chronic otitis media*
- Hearing loss

- Facial nerve palsy
- Mass protruding into external ear canal

***Bladder and prostate***

- Dysuria
- Urinary retention
- Hematuria
- *Constipation*
- Palpable lower abdominal mass

***Vagina***

- Mass protruding from uterus or cervix into vagina
- Abnormal vaginal bleeding

***Trunk, extremities***

- Visible and palpable soft tissue mass

***Testicles***

- Visible and palpable soft tissue mass

### NURSING IMPLICATIONS

- Prepare the child and parents physically and psychologically for surgery.
- With *radiation therapy,* monitor the child's white blood cell count closely for changes.
- Assist with administering *chemotherapy,* as indicated.
- Explain to and instruct the child and parents about all treatment plans, including the type, frequency, and duration of the therapy.
- Assess the child for possible side effects of *radiation therapy* and *chemotherapy.*
- Provide emotional support and guidance to the child and parents to help them cope with this disease; allow the child and parents to verbalize feelings and fears regarding the treatments and prognosis.

## CANCER, TESTICULAR CANCER

### DESCRIPTION

- Testicular cancer is rare today (only 1% of all malignancies).
- It usually occurs between ages 15 and 35 years and often in association with cryptorchidism.
- If discovered early, testicular cancer is one of the most curable cancers.
- Metastasis occurs rapidly.

### ASSESSMENT FINDINGS

- Painless testicular enlargement
- Complaints of heavy feeling in the scrotum
- Abdominal and back pain (if metastasis)

- Weight loss and general weakness (if metastasis)
- Gynecomastia (possible)
- Human chorionic gonadotropin and alpha-fetoprotein detected in blood serum (tumor markers)

### Nursing Implications

- Teach self-testicular examination to boys to permit early detection.
- Provide appropriate care for patients undergoing orchiectomy and subsequent *radiation therapy* or *chemotherapy.*
- Explain the option of using gel-filled prosthesis following orchiectomy to provide a symmetric appearance.
- Inform the patient about "sperm banking" options before *radiation therapy* because this treatment results in infertility in the opposite testis.

## CANCER, WILMS' TUMOR

### Description

- Wilms' tumor (nephroblastoma) is a malignant tumor that rises from the metanephric mesoderm cells of the upper pole of the kidney.
- It accounts for 20% of solid tumors in childhood with no increased incidence for sex or race.
- Discovery usually occurs between 6 months and 5 years of age (peak at 3 to 4 years).
- Wilms' tumor occurs in association with congenital anomalies, such as aniridia (lack of color of the iris), *cryptorchidism, hypospadias,* pseudohermaphroditism, cystic kidneys, hemangioma, and *talipes deformity.*
- Prognosis is best if cells are mostly differentiated epithelial cells; it is worst if cells are undifferentiated stromal cells.
- Metastasis is most often to the lungs, regional lymph nodes, liver, bone and eventually brain.

### Assessment Findings

- Firm, nontender, abdominal mass
- Hematuria (may be present)
- Low-grade fever (may be present)
- *Hypertension* (may be present)
- Anemia (may be present)
- Mass displacing normal kidney structure on intravenous pyelogram

- Points of metastasis detected by sonogram or computed tomography

#### NURSING IMPLICATIONS

- Place a sign reading "No abdominal palpation" over the child's bed because handling appears to aid metastasis.
- Prepare the child and parents for staging procedures to predict therapy and prognosis.
- Support the family emotionally during staging and throughout the course of therapy.
- Anticipate the need for surgery (usually nephrectomy), *radiation therapy*, and *chemotherapy*, and begin parent and child preparation.
- Explain the need for follow-up to monitor for tumor recurrence and complications of therapy, which may include small bowel obstruction, liver damage, nephritis, interstitial *pneumonia*, *scoliosis*, hypoplasia of the ileum and lower rib cage, different growth rates in the two femurs, sterility in girls, and development of a secondary tumor.
- Inform parents that in most protocols, if there is no recurrence in 2 years, the child is considered cured.

## CANDIDIASIS

#### DESCRIPTION

- Candidiasis is a fungal infection caused by *Candida albicans.*
- Newborns born vaginally of mothers with candidal vaginitis may develop thrush (oral *Candida* infection).
- *Candida albicans* also can cause one form of diaper dermatitis.
- *Candida albicans* does not improve with normal diaper rash measures, such as talcum, ointment, or exposure to air.
- Adolescent girls can develop candidal vaginitis.
- Girls with frequent candidal infections should have diabetes mellitius ruled out.
- Nystatin, an antifungal drug, is effective against all forms of candidiasis.
- Candidiasis can become a generalized systemic infection, especially in newborns, which is a serious disease.

#### ASSESSMENT FINDINGS
##### *Thrush*

- Painful, erythematous buccal membranes

- White plaques on the buccal membranes
- Poor appetite because of inflammation and pain

**Candida albicans** *diaper dermatitis*
- Bright red shiny rash
- Sharply defined edges
- Satellite papules or pustules

*Candidal vaginitis*
- Vulvar reddening
- Vaginal burning and itching
- White patches on the vaginal wall
- Thick cream cheese–like vaginal discharge

### Nursing Implications
- Teach parents the importance of good handwashing before and after diaper changes.
- Inform parents of the signs of candidiasis in their child.
- Instruct parents to apply nystatin ointment 3 times daily to affected diaper rash area and avoid all other ointments or powders until the area is clear.
- Instruct parents to keep the area as dry as possible with frequent diaper changes.
- Teach parents to administer nystatin slurry orally 4 times a day for oral thrush, by dropping into the child's mouth after feedings to remain in contact with the lesions.
- Educate the adolescent girl with candidal vaginitis to use nystatin vaginal suppositories at bedtime once daily for 7 days.
- Inform the girl that vaginal discharge is expected and she should use a sanitary napkin.
- Urge the girl to refrain from coitus or to have her partner use a condom during treatment to prevent reinfection.
- Instruct the girl not to interrupt the treatment even during menstruation.

## CARDIAC CATHETERIZATION

### Description
- A cardiac catheterization is performed to obtain information about structural heart defects, blood flow and pressures within the systemic and pulmonary circulations, and oxygen content in the various chambers of the heart.

- After administration of local anesthesia to numb the insertion site, a radiopaque catheter is passed through a vein in the arm, leg, or neck into the heart.
- Left-sided heart catheterization is performed through a venous or arterial approach. Venous approach is via a right femoral vein; the catheter is advanced to the right atrium, punctures the intra-atrial septum, and enters the left atrium. Femoral approach is via a femoral or brachial artery.
- Right-sided heart catheterization is done via a venous approach using the right femoral vein or a vein in the antecubital fossa.
- The vessel chosen for catheterization must not be infected or obscured by a hematoma at the time of the catheterization.
- Dye may be injected for angiography to visualize the heart chambers and vessels.
- Cardiac catheterization has a mortality rate of 0.5%.
- Most fatalities occur in infants under 7 months secondary to cardiac perforation or arrhythmia.
- Bleeding at the insertion site is a potential complication because heparin is introduced into the catheter to reduce clot formation and thrombophlebitis from catheter irritation.
- Arrhythmias may occur during passage of the catheter through the heart chambers or during injection of a contrast medium; however, they usually are transient and stop with catheter withdrawal.

### Nursing Implications

- Prepare the parent and child for the procedure, using developmentally appropriate materials.
- Inform the child that the room will have a lot of equipment and the lights will be low for the procedure.
- Explain the purpose of the procedure to the parents and ensure that all their questions have been answered.
- Maintain the child NPO (nothing by mouth) 4 hours preprocedure to reduce the danger of vomiting and aspiration.
- Ensure that the child has had a recent chest film, electrocardiogram (ECG), blood for crossmatch, and a patent intravenous line preprocedure.
- Monitor child's ECG, vital signs, and pain or anxiety during the procedure and treat appropriately.

- Postprocedure, assess vital signs every 15 minutes for the first hour and then every hour until discharge.
- Evaluate for bleeding: Assess catheter insertion site, distal pulses, color, and temperature of affected extremity.
- Keep the child flat for 3 to 4 hours to reduce oozing and postural hypotension.
- Administer fluids as prescribed to prevent *dehydration* while monitoring urine output and for signs of *congestive heart failure.*
- Assess for signs of infection at the insertion site, and evaluate temperature (which can be elevated with *dehydration* or low with hypothermia following the procedure).
- Watch for signs of all potential complications, including reaction to dye, and notify the physician immediately to examine the child.
- Teach the parents in preparation for discharge that the child can resume regular activity and to report a fever over 101.3°F, redness, swelling, or drainage at the catheter insertion site.
- Instruct the parents to change the groin dressing if it becomes soiled.
- Begin preparation for surgical intervention, if the results of the catheterization indicate surgery is necessary.

## CARDIAC SURGERY

### DESCRIPTION
- Cardiac surgery is available because of pulmonary bypass, in which the venous blood is diverted to the heart-lung machine, oxygenated, and returned to the arterial system.
- During cardiac surgery, hypothermia is used to reduce the child's metabolic needs and to stop the heart from beating.
- The heart, which remains bloodless, is opened and operated on, and although it is not pumping, it receives adequate oxygen supply from the bypass procedure.
- Associated complications from cardiac surgery include hemorrhage, cardiac tamponade, shock, heart block or arrhythmias, *congestive heart failure*, post–cardiac surgery syndrome, postperfusion syndrome, and death.

NURSING IMPLICATIONS

- Obtain preoperative cardiac parameters and vital signs for a baseline comparison of postoperative measures.
- Obtain height and weight measurements for blood volume estimates on the heart-lung machine and for calculation of appropriate medication dosages.
- Prepare the child and family for surgery and the postoperative environment, correcting any misconceptions they may have.
- Encourage the child and family to visit the intensive care unit (ICU) preoperatively to alleviate anxiety over who will be caring for the child.
- Explain all procedures to both the child and the parent in a clear, calm, and competent manner.
- Encourage the child and family to express their fears.
- Invite parents to reinforce your teaching and be involved in their child's care as much as possible.
- Teach the child the importance of pulmonary toilet postoperatively, and orient them to different oxygen equipment and chest tube apparatus.
- Keep in mind that postoperatively the child will have full cardiac and hemodynamic monitoring as well as ventilatory assistance.
- Monitor the child for adequate tissue perfusion postoperatively.
- Evaluate ventilatory status, hemodynamic parameters, electrocardiogram (ECG), and urine output; report any parameters outside of normal limits.
- Rewarm the hypothermic child with blankets and a hyperthermia unit.
- Assess the child's ventilatory status, mode of ventilation, arterial blood gases, and readiness for weaning from the mechanical ventilator.
- Monitor chest tube drainage and hemoglobin for signs of bleeding or cardiac tamponade.
- Maintain the child on a ventricular demand pacemaker at a low rate to ensure that the child has a heart rate should a sudden arrhythmia develop.
- Monitor pleural tubes for patency, and ensure that they are securely taped to avoid accidental dislodgment and pneumothorax.
- Administer cardiac support medication and intravenous fluids as prescribed, with intravenous fluid being administered judiciously by an intravenous pump to prevent overload on the heart.

- Assess fluid and electrolyte studies for abnormalities, and administer replacements as prescribed.
- Use measures to prevent pooling of secretions in the lung postextubation, such as incentive spirometry and turning, coughing, and deep breathing (TCDB).
- Ascertain that the child's pain is addressed and not impeding pulmonary efforts.
- Prepare the child for removal of chest tubes and pleural tubes, and provide emotional support during the procedure.
- Observe the child for signs of infection and administer prophylactic broad-spectrum antibiotics as prescribed.
- Evaluate the child's incision for drainage, erythema, and stability.
- Begin the child on oral fluids gradually, 24 hours postoperatively, if bowel sounds are present and the child is able to eat.
- Monitor nutritional intake and evaluate the need for supplemental nutrition.
- Increase the child's mobility as soon as possible and encourage parents' involvement with the child during the postoperative period.
- Encourage the parents to verbalize their anxieties, and provide support and teaching for them.
- Prepare the parents and child for the transition to the step-down cardiac unit.
- Explain to parents before discharge what activities the child may participate in, about the need for a follow-up appointment, and about any medications the child will be taking.
- Make a referral to a community health nurse to support the child and family during the child's initial week at home.

## CARDIAC TRANSPLANT

### DESCRIPTION

- Cardiac transplant, a surgical procedure, replaces the child's original heart (except for the right atrium, which contains the sinoatrial node) with a donor heart.
- This may be necessary for children with hypoplastic left ventricle or extensive cardiomyopathy from any cause.
- The transplanted heart is kept chilled for 2 to 3 hours before transplant via pulmonary bypass technique.

- The new heart is transplanted, and before surgical closure, hemodynamic monitoring lines and pacing wires are implanted.
- Postimplantation, the new heart can respond normally except for autonomic nervous system control.
- Remnant P waves from the residual original heart appear on the electrocardiogram (ECG) tracing because the SA node is intact.
- The child will require immunosuppressant therapy, such as cyclosporine A, prednisone, and azathioprine, for life.
- Rejection of the transplant, the number one cause of death in cardiac transplant patients, is assessed by cardiac catheterization with cardiac biopsy manifested as tissue necrosis.
- Most children adjust well to cardiac transplant and are able to grow and develop normally.

**NURSING IMPLICATIONS**
- Prepare the child and family for the surgical experience.
- Ensure that the transplant coordinator has answered all of their questions.
- Be aware that postoperatively the heart rate varies secondary to the amount of blood arriving rather than by nervous system control.
- Reposition the child slowly because of the inability of the heart to respond autonomically to hemodynamic fluid changes (it will not be able to increase its rate because of low blood pressure).
- Monitor the child for alterations in cardiac output, impaired gas exchange, infection, and altered nutrition.
- Evaluate for arrhythmias because injury to the donor SA node can occur during transport or transplant.
- Administer immunosuppressant agents as prescribed, and begin family teaching about the drugs as soon as possible.
- Assess for signs of rejection of the transplant: Hyperacute rejection is manifested by coronary thrombosis and can occur immediately; acute rejection is manifested by low-grade fever, tachycardia, and ECG changes and occurs 7 to 10 days postoperatively; long-term rejection may begin a year postoperatively.
- Keep in mind that the child needs to return to the transplant center for yearly cardiac catheterization and evaluation of his or her progress.

- Instruct the family in signs and symptoms to report to the physician.
- Ensure that the child and family have received all discharge instructions and have a follow-up appointment arranged.

## CARDIOPULMONARY ARREST

### DESCRIPTION

- Cardiopulmonary arrest refers to the absence of heart and respiratory function.
- This occurs in children with heart disease, airway obstruction secondary to a foreign body or obstruction from the tongue and epiglottis, accident trauma, anaphylactic allergic reactions, central nervous system depression, drowning, and electrocution.
- Respiratory failure is the most common cause of cardiac arrest.
- Cardiac arrest occurs secondary to an anoxic heart muscle.
- Clearing the airway, ventilating the lungs, and circulating the blood by cardiac compression can provide adequate oxygenation to major body organs for several minutes until additional personnel arrive to initiate advanced cardiopulmonary resuscitation (CPR).
- The outcome of the secondary measures depends on how well and how promptly initial measures are performed.

### ASSESSMENT FINDINGS

- Unresponsiveness
- Absent respirations and breath sounds
- Absent pulses
- Absent heart sounds
- Cyanosis

### NURSING IMPLICATIONS

- Call the child's name while shaking him or her; if no response, call for help and turn the child on his or her back and begin CPR according to the American Heart Association's guidelines.
- Remember ABCs of resuscitation: airway assessment, breathing, and circulation.
- Use a one-way mask for mouth-to-mouth resuscitation for protection from body secretions, if available.

- Open the airway using the head tilt-chin lift method or jaw thrust maneuver.
- If not breathing, administer two slow breaths (seal the mouth and nose for an infant under age 1; seal the mouth and pinch the nose tightly for a child age 1 to 8).
- After two ventilations, feel the brachial pulse in a child less than 1 year or the carotid pulse in a child older than 1 year; if no pulse, begin cardiac massage by chest compression.
- Observe the child's chest with each breath delivered to ensure it rises; if not, the child has an obstructed airway.

   In the newborn, generate chest compressions by using two fingers or a thumb pressed on the midsternum about a finger breadth below the nipple line at a rate of 100 beats per minute, depressing the sternum ½ to 1 inch.

   In a child age 1 to 8, apply the heel of one palm for compressions, over the sternum, measuring two fingerbreadths up from the sternal-costal notch at a rate of 80 to 100 beats per minute, depressing the sternum 1 to 1½ inches.

   Use a 1:5 breath to compression ratio.

   Remember not to inflate lungs and compress at the same time.

   Ensure that the hands come off the chest between compressions to allow the heart to fill more readily.

- Respond to the airway obstruction, of any cause, according to the American Heart Association's guidelines because it is the highest priority.
- Consider tracheal intubation if unable to clear the obstruction.
- Continue CPR until equipment for intubation is available.
- Establish vascular access.
- Administer emergency drugs once available, including oxygen, epinephrine, atropine, calcium chloride, dextrose, isoproterenol, and lidocaine, as prescribed.
- Monitor electrocardiogram (ECG) and administer defibrillation as prescribed for ventricular fibrillation and sustained unstable ventricular tachycardia.
- Reassure the child that is revived that everyone is there helping to relieve the child's fear.

- Comfort the child and parent, and provide reassurance that everything is all right.
- Allow the parents to see the child as soon as possible.
- Explain to parents and the child the need to perform follow-up procedures, such as ECG monitoring and arterial blood gas analysis to prevent another emergency and to establish the cause of the arrest.
- Manage the child who remains intubated or in a *coma* in the intensive care unit, monitoring respirations, vital signs, and organ function and supporting the parents.
- Involve the parents in all decisions regarding the child, and help them to understand the child's condition.
- Support the parents through all difficult ethical decisions that may be required.

## CATARACT

### Description

- Cataract is a marked opacity of the lens, which may be present at birth or become apparent in early childhood.
- It can result from trauma to the eye if the lens is injured.
- Opacity on the anterior surface of the lens is secondary to birth injury or contact between the lens and the cornea during intrauterine life.
- Opacity at the edge of the lens is secondary to nutritional deficiency during intrauterine life (rickets or *hypocalcemia*).
- Central cataracts are secondary to *rubella* infection during pregnancy or may be familial.
- Other conditions may simulate the appearance of cataract and must be ruled out.
- If surgical removal of the lens is delayed past 6 months, amblyopia may result.

### Assessment Findings

- Leukocoria
- Normal red reflex appears white
- Lack of response to a smile and inability to grasp an object, nystagmus (infants)
- Blurred vision (older children)

### Nursing Implications

- Teach the parents about the condition and about the operative and postoperative course.
- Inform the parents that the child will have some discomfort but not acute pain.

- Explain to the parents that the child will be fitted with contact lenses after surgery.
- Cover the eye with a patch if necessary postoperatively.
- Administer a sedative to the child postoperatively to keep child still for 24 hours.
- Avoid anything that may increase intraocular pressure and injure the suture line, such as nausea or *vomiting* or crying.
- Introduce fluids cautiously to avoid nausea and *vomiting*.
- Encourage the parents to stay with and comfort the child.
- Notify the physician of signs of increased intraocular pressure, such as unusual restlessness, fussiness or crying, and manifestations of pain, which could be caused by hemorrhage or occlusion of the canal of Schlemm, indicating a developing glaucoma.
- Administer a mydriatic to dilate the pupil and steroids to prevent adhesions.
- Support parents to carry out procedures necessary for long-term management.

## CAT-SCRATCH DISEASE

### DESCRIPTION

- Cat-scratch disease is caused by cat-scratch disease virus, most commonly occurring in preschool children who receive scratches from infected cats.
- Incubation period is 3 to 10 days; mode of transmission is by a bite or a scratch from a cat or kitten.
- Children with human immunodeficiency virus (HIV) are extremely susceptible to the virus.
- Cat-scratch disease virus is similar to herpes simplex.
- One episode of the disease provides lifetime immunity.
- No passive artificial immunity exists.
- Positive diagnosis occurs with a positive skin test of cat-scratch disease antigen, along with history of a scratch and aspiration of sterile pus from enlarged lymph nodes.
- Treatment is aimed at relief of symptoms.

### ASSESSMENT FINDINGS

- Single skin papule or pustule lasting 1 to 3 weeks
- Severe local lymphadenopathy, usually head, neck, and axillary nodes, 2 weeks after the scratch

- Nodal enlargement for 3 months
- Node suppuration of sterile pus (in some children)
- Low-grade fever
- Malaise
- Encephalitis or meningitis (may occur)

**NURSING IMPLICATIONS**
- Confirm positive diagnosis and discuss the disease and its treatment with the parents.
- Instruct parents to administer analgesics for painful adenopathy.
- Prepare parents and child for node aspiration if necessary to relieve pain.
- Teach parents about antibiotics, including administration and side effects, if they are prescribed to shorten the course of the disease.
- Advise parents that the cat does not need to be destroyed because fewer than 10% of children scratched by an infected cat contract the disease, and the child with the disease has immunity.

## CELIAC DISEASE (MALABSORPTION SYNDROME: GLUTEN-INDUCED ENTEROPATHY)

**DESCRIPTION**
- Celiac disease, a rare inherited disorder, is a sensitivity or immunologic response to protein, particularly the gluten factor of protein in grains.
- It occurs in children of a northern European background and is associated with Down syndrome and *diabetes mellitus.*
- On ingestion of gluten factor by affected children, changes occur in the intestinal mucosa preventing absorption into blood.
- Most notable is an inability to absorb fats.
- Deficiencies in fat-soluble vitamins occur.
- Rickets can occur because of deficiency of vitamin D.
- Hypoprothrombinemia can occur from deficiency of vitamin K.
- Children affected may develop anemia and hypoalbuminemia.
- Symptoms appear at 6 to 18 months of age.
- Children gradually fall back in normal growth and height.

- Once placed on a gluten-free diet, children improve and gain weight.
- Children with celiac disease who develop any type of infection are prone to celiac crisis, which involves severe *vomiting*, *diarrhea*, and need for fluid and electrolyte replacement.

### ASSESSMENT FINDINGS
- Steatorrhea
- Malnutrition, anorexia, and irritability
- Distended abdomen
- Plump face with spindly extremities

### NURSING IMPLICATIONS
- Focus the care of the child on nutritional counseling, which the child should continue for life.
- Teach parents which foods contain gluten and must be avoided.
- Help parents recognize foods that have fillers that contain gluten; teach parents to be careful shoppers and to read labels.
- Encourage small frequent feedings initially because the child is anorectic.
- Examine creative ways to help the child eat new foods.
- Monitor a child's stool for consistency and appearance and number.
- Explain to parents that disappearance of steatorrhea is a good indicator of the child's ability to absorb nutrients.
- Administer iron and folate to correct anemias.
- Advise parents that these children require water-miscible forms of vitamins A and D.
- Prepare parents for the child's anger over not being able to eat some of old favorites (e.g., hot dogs).
- Ready the parents for problems of finding food in a school cafeteria and for difficulties during the holidays.
- Encourage parents to teach children how to recognize appropriate foods.

## CELLULITIS

### DESCRIPTION
- Cellulitis is an inflammation of the deepest layers of the skin.

- It occurs on the extremities, the face, or surrounding wounds.
- Abscess and tissue destruction occur if untreated with antibiotics.
- Damaged skin, poor circulation, and diabetes mellitus favor the development of cellulitus.

### Assessment Findings
- Local heat
- Edematous, reddened area
- Pain
- Fever
- Malaise
- Chills
- Headache

### Nursing Implications
- Inspect extremities of patients prone to cellulitis.
- Administer antibiotics as prescribed.
- Apply warm soaks to affected area to relieve pain and inflammation.
- Avoid pressure to affected area.
- Teach clients who are susceptible to cellulitis to inspect their extremities everyday.

## CELLULITIS, PERIORBITAL

### Description
- Periorbital cellulitis is an inflammation around the orbit of the eye.
- Periorbital cellulitis occurs in children as an extension of a superficial infection after an open break in the skin.
- A mosquito bite or scratch near the eye can develop into cellulitis.
- Periorbital cellulitis is always serious because the eye globe fulls snugly into the orbit in children.
- Permanent damage to the optic nerve or the eye globe from compression results from the swelling if it is not treated.
- The extent of inflammation can be detected by sonogram.

### Assessment Findings
- Swelling
- Inflammation

##### Nursing Implications
- Advise the family of the child with periorbital cellulitis on the importance of therapy.
- Admit the child into the hospital.
- Administer intravenous antibiotics as prescribed.
- Answer all questions that the family has, and encourage them to stay with the child to alleviate any fears the child may have.

## CEREBRAL PALSY

#### Description
- Cerebral palsy is a nonprogressive disorder of upper motor neuron impairment that results in motor dysfunction and in some cases impaired cognitive function.
- It is the most common permanent disability in children.
- Cerebral palsy is most often caused by brain anoxia, which leads to cell destruction, before, during, or shortly after birth.
- Other causes of cerebral palsy include neurologic injury secondary to metabolic disturbances, congenital infections, and central nervous system infections.
- The premature neonate is most susceptible to cerebral palsy.
- Kernicterus from neonatal hyperbilirubinemia can cause this disorder, usually of the athetoid type.
- Associated defects with this disorder include deafness, mental retardation, ocular difficulties, and hyperactivity.
- Cerebral palsy is classified according to the degree and type of motor dysfunction.
- Spastic type, occurring in 50% of the cases, is excessive tone in the voluntary muscles; it is characterized by hypertonic muscles, abnormal clonus, exaggeration of deep tendon reflexes, positive Babinski sign, and continuation of neonatal reflexes.
- Athetoid or dyskinetic cerebral palsy, occurring in 20% of the cases, involves abnormal involuntary movement and may involve all of the extremities as well as the face and the neck; movements increase under stress and anxiety.
- Ataxic type, occurring in 5% of the cases, has an awkward wide-based gait; it may involve the cerebellar

rather than the cerebral functions, and although coordination problems exist, they improve with age.

- Mixed cerebral palsy, occurring in 25% of the cases, is characterized by symptoms of both spasticity and athetoid movements; it results in a severe degree of impairment.
- Children with cerebral palsy may have sensory disturbances, such as strabismus, refractive disorders, visual perception problems, and visual field defects, as well as speech disorders, such as abnormal rhythm or articulation. They may have *attention-deficit hyperactivity disorder* also.
- Cerebral palsy is diagnosed from neurologic findings and patient history.
- Goals of medical management include promoting locomotion, communication, and self-care skills.
- Braces may reduce or prevent deformity.
- Surgery may be necessary to improve muscle function.
- Physical therapy, speech therapy, and devices that aid in communication are used.
- Medication to reduce spasticity has little effect.
- Anticonvulsants are used to control seizures.

### Assessment Findings

#### Spastic cerebral palsy
- Asymmetric crawling
- Unilateral hand preference by age 3
- Quadriplegia, monoplegia, hemiplegia, or diplegia
- Astereognosis
- Impaired speech and *mental retardation* (may accompany quadriplegia)
- Drooling

#### Athetoid cerebral palsy
- Writhing movements of tongue and extremities while awake
- Drooling
- Dysarthria

#### Ataxic cerebral palsy
- Unable to perform finger-nose test
- Unable to perform rapid repetitive movements

#### Mixed
- Severe delays in both motor and speech development
- Ataxia and athetoid movements present together

**NURSING IMPLICATIONS**
- Help the parents cope with the diagnosis of this disease and explain that it is nonprogressive.
- Support the parents in their grief and disappointment.
- Establish realistic short-term goals involving the parents and dealing with the individuality of their child's disease.
- Assist the parents and child with braces, and help them to understand the importance of preventing contractures.
- Teach the parents how to do passive and active range of motion exercises with the child.
- Encourage self-care activities and promote the child's independence.
- Role model for the parents, praising the child when independent actions are made.
- Assist the parents with modifying the environment to ensure safety.
- Encourage rest in children with cerebral palsy because the disorder expends tremendous amounts of energy.
- Provide adequate nutrition, and help the parents to find a feeding program that works.
- Teach the parents to provide stimulating activities for the child because the child cannot pursue them.
- Encourage exposure to the outside world to promote growth and development.
- Advocate that a child is placed in a school setting consistent with his or her intellectual abilities.
- Promote alternative forms of communication, and ensure that the child receives appropriate physical and speech therapy.
- Promote a positive self-image in the child, and encourage the parents to help the child reach his or her full potential.
- Encourage the parents to join the Cerebral Palsy Foundation and to look at all options of support.

# CHEMOTHERAPY

## DESCRIPTION
- Chemotherapy refers to the administration of antineoplastic drugs.
- In many cases, a combination of chemotherapeutic agents is used to interfere with cellular growth, division, and reproduction.

- Chemotherapy is scheduled over a period of time so that all cells can eventually be destroyed.
- Chemotherapy may be the primary cancer treatment or used in conjunction with other treatments.
- To avoid multiple venipunctures, venous access devices such as Hickman catheters or implanted ports are used; however, these devices may also cause soft-tissue injury resulting from accidental administration through an infiltrated or leaking intravenous line.
- Chemotherapeutic agents affect all cells, especially those that proliferate rapidly, such as bone marrow, hair, skin, and epithelial lining of the gastrointestinal tract, thereby accounting for many of the adverse reactions to chemotherapy.
- Several categories of antineoplastic drugs exist:
    Antimetabolites, such as methotrexate, closely resemble natural products; however, the cell cannot function with them in its structure and dies.
    Plant alkaloids, such as vinblastine (Velban), interfere with cell mitosis.
    Antibiotics, such as doxorubicin (Adriamycin), impair DNA synthesis and thereby destroy the malignant cell.
    Enzymes, such as L-asparaginase, interfere with enzymatic activity.
    Steroids, such as prednisone, bind to DNA and inhibit mitosis as well as RNA synthesis, thereby preventing the formation of new cells.
    Immunotherapy causes the stimulation of the body's immune system to destroy foreign or malignant cells.
- All chemotherapeutic agents have both side effects and toxic effects.

### Nursing Implications

- Provide support to the child and family throughout all phases of cancer treatment and refer them to appropriate support groups.
- Monitor for the wide range of adverse effects that accompany chemotherapy.
- Evaluate the degree of nausea and *vomiting* and watch for associated fluid and electrolyte imbalances.
- Provide the child with an antiemetic, as prescribed, before, during, and after chemotherapy.

- Limit food intake during chemotherapy to minimize nausea and vomiting.
- Encourage the child to consume clear liquids in small-to-moderate amounts.
- Use relaxation techniques to help reduce nausea, as appropriate.
- Maintain adequate nutrition, suggesting different foods or methods of preparation.
- Stay with the child during mealtimes and encourage the parents to also.
- Allow the child to make choices about food when possible.
- Implement oral hygiene measures to prevent and minimize ulcer development, which may interfere with food intake.
- Apply a topical anesthetic and administer topical antibiotics as prescribed if ulcers develop.
- Provide a bland diet and avoid citrus products.
- Keep the child's perianal area meticulously clean to prevent rectal ulcers, which increase the risk of sepsis.
- Leave ulcerated skin exposed to air.
- Administer stool softeners and maintain adequate fluid intake to prevent constipation.
- Reassure the child with hair loss (alopecia) that it is temporary and hair will grow back once treatment ends.
- Suggest ways to minimize the effects of hair loss before it occurs, such as with a baseball cap or hats.
- Teach the child to apply sunscreen and cover the head before environmental exposure to prevent injury from sun or cold.
- Assure children with cushingoid appearance that they will return to normal after therapy.
- Promote a positive self-image for the child.
- Invent diversional games that a child can be involved in despite accompanying neuropathy secondary to chemotherapy.
- Attempt to keep the child free of infection.
- Monitor for subtle signs of infection.
- Administer appropriate antibiotics or antifungals as prescribed.
- Assess laboratory values and provide protective isolation if *neutropenia* exists.
- Treat any related tumor pain.

## CHICKENPOX (VARICELLA VIRUS)

### DESCRIPTION

- Chickenpox is a highly contagious virus spread by direct or indirect contact with saliva or a vesicle.
- It is common in children 2 to 8 years old, occurring primarily from January to May.
- Potential complications include secondary bacterial infections, such as *cellulitis* and abscesses, *pneumonia,* and *encephalitis.*
- Chickenpox is extremely serious if it occurs in immunocompromised children.
- Incubation period is 10 to 21 days with communicability 1 day before rash and 5 to 6 days after its appearance when vesicles have crusted.
- After contracting the virus, a person has lifetime immunity to chickenpox.
- Because the same virus causes herpes zoster, it may be reactivated at a later time as herpes zoster.
- A chickenpox lesion begins as a macule and in 6 to 8 hours progresses to a papule, then a vesicle, and then it crusts.
- If the scab from crusting is allowed to fall off naturally and lesions do not become secondarily infected, scarring does not occur.
- Scabs removed prematurely may leave a white, round, slightly indented scar at the site.

### ASSESSMENT FINDINGS

- Extremely pruritic rash

  ***Prodromal phase***
- Slight fever
- Malaise
- Anorexia
- Headache

  ***Acute phase***
- Small red macules on trunk, followed by eruption of 3 to 4 macules daily on trunk, face, scalp, extremities, and mucous membranes

### NURSING IMPLICATIONS

- Advise parents about administering antihistamines to control pruritus and the importance of preventing scratching.
- Teach parents that antihistamines may cause drowsiness or hyperactivity and insomnia.

- Encourage use of other methods to relieve the pruritus, such as cool compresses, calamine lotion, baking soda, or oatmeal baths.
- Have the parents cut the child's fingernails short, and inform them that applying pressure to the lesions may lessen the itching.
- Advise the parents to administer antipyretics for fever.
- Caution parents not to administer aspirin to control fever because of the risk of *Reye's syndrome.*
- Teach parents of children over age 2 to give oral acyclovir suspension to reduce the number of lesions and shorten the course of the illness.
- Teach parents about the adverse effects of acyclovir, such as diarrhea.
- Direct parents to keep the child isolated until lesions have crusted and dried.

## CHILDHOOD PSYCHOSIS (PERVASIVE DEVELOPMENTAL DISORDERS: *INFANTILE AUTISM*)

### DESCRIPTION

- Childhood psychosis is marked by serious distortions in psychological functioning.
- Deficits in language, perceptual, and motor development may exist.
- Defective reality testing and an inability to function in social settings are also associated with these disorders.
- Lack of responsiveness to others, gross impairment in communications skills, and bizarre responses to the environment all develop within the first 30 months of age.
- *Infantile autism* is a rare disorder occurring 3 times more often in boys than in girls; although the cause is unknown, it is linked to cerebellar and limbic system anomalies that probably occurred in utero associated with maternal *rubella, phenylketonuria, meningitis,* and *encephalitis.*
- 75% of children with *infantile autism* are mentally retarded.
- Some children may eventually lead independent lives, although social ineptness and awkwardness are apt to remain.

### ASSESSMENT FINDINGS

- Social isolation
- Stereotyped behaviors

- Resistance to change in routine
- Insensitivity to pain
- Inappropriate emotional expressions
- Disturbances of movement
- Poor speech development
- Specific, limited intellectual problems

#### NURSING IMPLICATIONS

- Assist parents in understanding this complex disorder.
- Provide ongoing support and available resources to parents.
- Help parents to accept the child and the disorder.
- Suggest behavior modification therapy for controlling some of the bizarre mannerisms.
- Encourage parents to understand that as the child grows he or she will develop an awareness and attachment to parents and other familiar adults.
- Advise the parents to look at reputable day care programs, to promote the child's social awareness.

## CHOANAL ATRESIA

#### DESCRIPTION

- Choanal atresia refers to an obstruction, either unilateral or bilateral, of the posterior nares.
- Choanal atresia prevents newborns (who up to age 3 months are natural nose breathers) from drawing air through the nose and down into the nasopharynx.
- The condition may be congenital or may be caused by an obstructing membrane or bony growth.
- Treatment for bilateral atresia involves piercing of the membrane or surgical removal of the bony growth.

#### ASSESSMENT FINDINGS

- Respiratory distress at birth or immediately after the infant quiets and tries to breathe through the nose
- Air hunger when mouth is closed
- Air hunger and cyanosis at feedings

#### NURSING IMPLICATIONS

- Assess for choanal atresia, by gently compressing first one nostril and then the second; if present, struggling secondary to air hunger occurs.
- Pass a soft no. 8 or 10 F catheter through the posterior nares to the stomach in the delivery room. If the

catheter does not pass bilaterally, the diagnosis of choanal atresia is confirmed.

- Ensure adequate hydration and glucose levels by administering intravenous fluids for infants with difficulty feeding.
- Help the parents to understand the anatomic problem and how surgical intervention may be required.
- Insert an oral airway, if necessary.
- Provide the parents with emotional support and information.
- Allow the parents to see their child as soon as the procedure is over.
- Prepare the parents and the infant for discharge and answer any questions the parents may have.

# CIRRHOSIS

### DESCRIPTION
- Cirrhosis is fibrotic scarring of the liver.
- Although rare in children, it may occur as a result of congenital biliary atresia or as a complication of chronic illnesses.
- Chronic illnesses associated with cirrhosis include protracted hepatitis, *sickle cell anemia,* and *cystic fibrosis.*
- Liver function becomes impaired when fibrotic infiltrates replace normal liver cells.
- The liver's ability to detoxify toxic substances, synthesize protein, produce prothrombin, and produce bile become impaired.
- Decreased hepatic blood flow also results in portal hypertension, ascites, esophageal varices, hypersplenism, and compromised heart function.
- There is no known cure for cirrhosis of the liver once infiltration begins.

### ASSESSMENT FINDINGS
- Fatty stools
- Avitaminosis of fat-soluble vitamins
- Symptoms of hemorrhage
- Anemia
- Jaundice
- Hypoglycemia

### NURSING IMPLICATIONS
- Explain all procedures to the child with this chronic disease and the parents.

- Focus care on allowing the child to be as comfortable as possible.
- Provide appropriate nutrition and instruct the parents on the need for a high-protein, high-carbohydrate, and medium-chain-triglyceride diet.
- Prepare parents for the need of a liver transplantation.
- Explain to parents how a liver transplantation will prolong the child's life; however, it is associated with a lifelong commitment towards medical treatment.
- Administer cholestyramine to stimulate bile flow and reduce reabsorption of bile into the circulation to minimize jaundice.
- Monitor for any bleeding episodes, and teach the parents to test for blood in stools.
- Treat associated complications, such as ruptured esophageal varices, emergently because a child loses large quantities of blood quickly.
- Provide emotional support for the family and the child, and encourage verbalization of feelings, especially as related to the potential for liver transplantation.

## CLEFT LIP AND PALATE

### DESCRIPTION

- Cleft lip and palate is the fusion of the maxillary and median nasal processes, occurring during weeks 5 and 8 of intrauterine life.
- Cleft lip is more prevalent among males than females, occurring in 1 in 1000 live births.
- Cleft lip may occur from transmission of multiple genes or by teratogenic factors, such as avitaminosis or viral infection during the 5th and 8th weeks of gestation.
- Cleft palate is a opening of the palate on the midline and may involve just the anterior hard palate or the posterior soft palate or both.
- Cleft palate may be a separate anomaly but most often occurs in conjunction with a cleft lip.
- Alone cleft palate occurs more frequently in females than in males and may be the result of polygenic inheritance or environmental influences.
- With cleft lip, the incidence is 1 in 1000 live births; as a single entity, cleft palate occurs in 1 in 2500 live births.

## Assessment Findings
### Cleft lip
- Small notch in the upper lip to a total separation of the lip and facial structure up into the floor of the nose.
- Upper teeth and gingiva may be absent.
- Flattened nose (because the incomplete fusion of the upper lip has allowed it to expand in a horizontal direction)
- Unilateral or bilateral deviation

### Cleft palate
- Opening on the anterior hard palate, soft palate, or both
- Other congenital anomalies (because cleft palate is a component of many syndromes)

## Nursing Implications
- Monitor the client for altered nutrition preoperatively.
- Teach the parents how to support the child in an upright position and feed the child gently by using a commercial cleft lip nipple.
- Teach the parents the importance of slow gentle feeding to avoid aspiration.
- Be aware that the infant may be able to suck on nipple or breast-feed before surgery depending on the extent of the clefts.
- If surgical repair is going to be done immediately, encourage the mother to breast-feed because it can occur as early as 7 to 10 days postoperatively.
- Keep in mind that infants with cleft lip need to be bubbled well after feeding owing to tendencies to swallow air.
- Offer small sips of fluid between feedings to keep the mucous membrane moist and prevent cracks and fissures that could lead to infection.
- If surgery is delayed past introduction of solid foods (approximately 6 months), teach the parents to offer soft foods because coarse food could invade the nasopharynx and cause aspiration.
- Postoperatively, keep the infant NPO (nothing by mouth) at least 4 hours.
- Assess for respiratory distress related to local edema.
- Suction as needed to remove excess mucus.
- Avoid anything that puts tension on the suture line.

- Clean and maintain the suture line to avoid infection.
- Do not allow milk as a first fluid because milk curds tend to adhere to the suture line.
- Use a Breck feeder during the immediate postoperative period, not breast-feeding or bottle-feeding because they would place too much tension on the suture line.
- Following palate surgery, offer liquids for 3 to 4 days postoperatively.
- Offer fluid that the parent tells you the child likes.
- Provide a soft diet until healing is complete.
- Do not allow a child to use a spoon because it will put pressure on the soft palate.
- Assess psychosocial impact of potential scar on the child and parents.
- Prepare the parents for high risk of ear infection related to altered slope of eustachian tube with cleft palate surgery.
- Prepare the parents for potential for altered communication related to cleft palate, the goal being effective communication by age 2.

## COLIC

### DESCRIPTION

- Colic is paroxysmal abdominal pain that generally occurs in infants under 3 months of age.
- It may occur as a result of overfeeding, swallowing too much air while feeding, or a formula too high in carbohydrate.
- Formula-fed infants are more likely to have colic than breast-fed infants.
- Infants with colic still thrive; however, the condition is distressing and frightening to the whole family.
- Colic interferes with parental sleeping and may interfere with the formation of the parent-child relationship.
- Mothers of colicky infants have reported psychological distress.
- Colic usually disappears at 3 months when digestion becomes easier, and the child can maintain a more upright position, allowing less gas to form.

### ASSESSMENT FINDINGS

- Abrupt discomfort with difficulty soothing the crying

- Legs pulled up onto a tense abdomen
- Red, flushed face
- Clenched fists
- Vigorous sucking from bottle, then stopping when another wave of intestinal pain occurs
- Crying and pain lasting for 3 hours a day for 3 months

### Nursing Implications

- Treat colic as a family problem.
- Obtain a thorough history to rule out similar symptom diagnosis, such as intestinal obstruction or infection.
- Determine the infant's feeding pattern and recommend a change in formula or increased burping.
- Recommend a change in maternal eating habits if infant is breast-fed, such as eliminating gassy foods.
- Advise parents to use a bottle with a disposable bag and to feed the infant in a quiet, nonstimulating atmosphere.
- Recommend the use of a pacifier to soothe the infant.
- Have the parents place the infant in the infant seat for ½ hour after feeding then lay the infant on the stomach with a folded towel under the abdomen.
- Teach the parents other ways to attempt to sooth the colicky infant, such as taking the infant for a ride; rubbing his or her back; or inserting a rectal thermometer into the rectum the length of the bulb, which helps relieve intestinal gas.
- Recommend measures that may increase peristalsis and move gas through the intestines to relieve pain, such as offering a bottle of warm glucose water.
- Support the parents in all the efforts they make, and let them know it is all right to let the infant cry for short intervals (5 to 15 minutes).

## COMA

### Description

- Coma refers to an unconsciousness from which a child cannot be roused.
- Coma is a symptom of an underlying disorder.
- *Head trauma* is the most likely underlying cause of coma.
- Other potential causes include *seizure*, metabolic disturbances such as *diabetes mellitus, dehydration*, severe hemorrhage, or drug ingestion.

- A child's response to coma depends on the initial cause.
- A modified version of the Glasgow Coma Scale is used to classify comas accurately in children.

    A Glasgow score of 3–8 indicates severe trauma, with under 5 carrying a severe prognosis.

    A Glasgow score of 9–12 indicates moderate trauma.

    A Glasgow score of 12–15 indicates a slight trauma.

**ASSESSMENT FINDINGS** (vary with the underlying cause)

- Decreased pulse rate, decreased respiratory rate, and increased blood pressure (increased intracranial pressure)
- Increased respirations *(diabetes)*
- Increased pulse rate and a decreased blood pressure (hemorrhage)
- Increase or decrease in vital sign measurements (drug ingestion)
- Irregular breathing (medullary pressure from brain injury)
- Ineffective or absent swallowing reflex (brain stem compression)
- Fixed and dilated pupils bilaterally (irreversible brain stem damage; may also occur with atropine-like drug poisoning)
- Unilateral dilated pupil (cranial nerve damage)
- Eyes deviated downward and laterally (tentorial tear and herniation of the temporal lobe into the torn membrane)
- Papilledema (increased intracranial pressure for greater than 24 hours)
- Lack of doll's eye reflex (compression of the oculomotor nerves or brain stem involvement)
- Posturing (cerebral compression and dysfunction)

**NURSING IMPLICATIONS**

- Admit any child unconscious for more than a transient period of time to a hospital.
- Place the child on the side to avoid tracheal aspiration.
- Assist with endotracheal intubation if signs of respiratory difficulty are present.
- Establish an intravenous route.
- Obtain a history to determine the circumstances immediately before the time the child became comatose.

- Perform a thorough neurologic examination every 30 minutes, including Glasgow score testing, assessment for doll's eye reflex, and observing for posturing.
- Count respirations and pulse to obtain baseline values.
- Obtain appropriate laboratory studies to determine the cause of coma, such as blood glucose, blood electrolytes, blood urea nitrogen, liver function tests, blood gas studies, lumbar puncture, and toxicology tests.
- Observe for pupillary response and signs of increased intracranial pressure. It is important to relieve any increases in intracranial pressure before permanent brain damage occurs.
- Prepare a client with a tentorial tear for emergency surgery to alleviate temporal compression.
- Examine the retina of the eye for papilledema.
- Maintain the child's body function in an optimum state until the child reawakens.
- Monitor skin integrity, and change the child's position every 2 hours.
- Perform passive range of motion exercises to all extremities to help maintain muscle tone and prevent contractures 3 times a day.
- Provide appropriate nutrition as prescribed via intravenous, nasogastric, or gastrostomy route.
- Ensure appropriate maintenance of route administration, and evaluate for associated complications.
- Give mouth care at least twice a day, and instill artificial tears to keep eyes from drying.
- Support the family throughout this difficult period.
- Assist the child with understanding the events once he or she has awakened.
- Answer all of the child's questions honestly and evaluate for any permanent damage.
- Provide follow-up care and discuss the potential need for rehabilitation if the child was in a comatose state for a prolonged period of time.

## CONCUSSION

### DESCRIPTION
- A concussion is a head injury that results from a hard, jarring shock.
- A coup injury occurs when a concussion is on the side of the skull that was struck.

- A contrecoup injury occurs when a concussion is on the opposite side of the brain from the site of injury.
- As the brain recoils from the head injury, it strikes the posterior surface of the skull and a second injury occurs.
- Children have at least a transient loss of consciousness at the time of the injury.
- The treatment for a child recovering from a concussion consists principally of observation for signs of intracranial bleeding or edema.

### Assessment Findings
- Loss of consciousness
- Vomiting
- Irritability on regaining of consciousness
- Convulsion within minutes of the injury
- Amnesia of the events leading up to the injury or the injury
- Headache

### Nursing Implications
- Obtain a skull radiograph to rule out skull fracture, and observe the child for 24 hours to rule out severe brain trauma, edema, or bleeding.
- Avoid asking many questions about the accident because some children with amnesia of the event are frightened by the amnesia.
- Instruct parents who will be observing their child at home to rouse the child every 1 to 2 hours, and instruct them on how to check level of consciousness.
- Have the parent ask the child to name a favorite toy.
- Advise parents to rouse the child once during the night and to assess that the pulse is greater than 60 beats per minute.
- Give the parents the telephone number to call if they have any questions about their child's care.
- Encourage parents to notify the physician if any suspicious change of behavior occurs.

## CONDUCT DISORDERS

### Description
- Conduct disorders represent the most common psychiatric diagnosis of children and adolescents.
- They are seen more frequently in males than in females, particularly when property or violent crimes are

involved; however, the prevalence of conduct disorders in girls is increasing, which means that male predominance may be reduced over time.
- Etiologic factors include genetic predisposition, neurologic deficits, and sociologic factors related to poverty and cultural disadvantages.
- In addition, the home environment is frequently characterized by rejection, frustration, and harsh, inconsistent discipline; parents may have an unstable marital relationship; and children may have had a series of stepparents or foster parents.

### Assessment Findings
- Aggressive behavior, including purse snatching, mugging, or robbery with confrontation
- Persistent truancy, lying, or vandalism
- Inability to demonstrate a normal degree of affection, empathy, or ability to bond with others
- Few meaningful peer relationships
- Strong egocentrism
- Guilt or remorse lacking
- Manipulation of others without effort to return favors

### Nursing Implications
- Obtain a thorough history and physical examination to establish a baseline.
- Administer medications, such as neuroleptics or lithium carbonate, as prescribed.
- Assist parents with measures to modify the home environment so that it is more consistent and less rejecting.
- Anticipate the possibility of having to remove the child from the home to a structured day care environment; explain to the child that this is not rejection.
- Instruct parents in behavior therapy and limit setting.
- Provide information to parents about support groups, such as Tough Love International.

## CONGENITAL HEART DEFECTS, ATRIAL SEPTAL DEFECT (ASD)

### Description
- ASD, an acyanotic congenital heart defect, is an abnormal opening between the two atria resulting in blood flow from the left atrium through the

opening into the right atrium (oxygenated to unoxygenated) because of the higher pressures in the left side of the heart.

- Increased right atrial blood volume is ejected into the right ventricle, and eventually right ventricular hypertrophy occurs.
- Small ASDs are generally well tolerated.
- Surgical intervention is the recommended treatment with suturing and closure of the defect.
- Maternal rubella is associated ASDs.
- ASDs occur more commonly in girls than in boys.
- Females are prone to emboli during pregnancy if surgery is not done.
- The prognosis is good with uncomplicated heart surgery.
- Before and after any congenital heart defect repair, children may require prophylactic administration of antibiotics to prevent infectious *endocarditis.*

## ASSESSMENT FINDINGS

- Crescendo-decrescendo systolic ejection murmur over second or third intercostal space (pulmonic area)
- Wide, fixed splitting of second heart sound (S2)
- Enlarged right side of the heart
- Separation of the atrial septum
- Dyspnea, cough, tachypnea, chest retractions, orthopnea, wheezing, crackles, and rhonchi (indicate *congestive heart failure*/pulmonary edema)

## NURSING IMPLICATIONS

- Assess and evaluate heart sounds, including murmurs, in all children.
- Address parents' knowledge deficit and teach them about the normal physiology of the heart and the pathophysiology of the congenital heart defect with resultant complications.
- Explain all procedures and rationales for treatment to the child and parents.
- Invite verbalization of fears and discussion of concerns from the family.
- Support the child and parents throughout the hospitalization.
- Promote cardiac output for the child with ASD.
- Prepare the child and parents for potential surgical procedure to correct the anomaly.

- Support the parents, and answer all questions they may have regarding specific procedures.
- Prepare the child and parents for the surgical experience and postoperative management.
- Observe for jaundice postoperatively resulting from red blood cell destruction if a newly constructed valve is placed.
- Assess, evaluate, and treat arrhythmias common postoperatively secondary to edema.
- Monitor carefully for signs of infection and administer antibiotics as necessary.
- Provide essential postoperative instruction to avoid pulmonary complications.
- Instruct the parents and child for discharge planning on potential limitations, awareness of unusual symptoms, medications prescribed, and their side effects.

# CONGENITAL HEART DEFECTS, COARCTATION OF AORTA

### DESCRIPTION
- Coarctation of the aorta, an acyanotic congenital heart defect, is a narrowing of the lumen of the aorta owing to a constricting band.
- Because it is difficult for blood to pass through the stricture, pressure is high proximal to the coarctation and low distal to it.
- Cardiac output is reduced with this anomaly.
- Severe aortic coarctation manifests at infancy, causing evidence of congestive heart failure and severe systemic hypoperfusion.
- Before and after any congenital heart defect repair, children may require prophylactic administration of antibiotics to prevent infectious *endocarditis*.

### ASSESSMENT FINDINGS
- Absent femoral pulses
- Absent brachial pulses if obstruction is proximal to the left subclavian
- Cool pale extremities
- Hypertension of the upper extremities, which may lead to headaches and *epistaxis*

### NURSING IMPLICATIONS
- Check femoral pulses in all newborns.
- Monitor oxygenation and pulmonary status in all children with coarctation of the aorta.

- Address parents' knowledge deficit and teach them about the normal physiology of the heart and the pathophysiology of the congenital heart defect with resultant complications.
- Explain all procedures and rationales for treatment to the child and parents.
- Invite verbalization of fears and discussion of concerns from the family.
- Support the child and parents throughout the hospitalization.
- Promote cardiac output for the child with coarctation of the aorta.
- Monitor for and reduce respiratory distress and pulmonary congestion.
- Promote fluid loss for the child with right-sided heart failure.
- Evaluate the most appropriate time for surgical intervention for the child with coarctation of the aorta (usually between 2 and 4 years of age); however, self-esteem of the child must be considered.
- Advise that girls must have this defect corrected before child-bearing age secondary to the heart's inability to handle the extra blood volume.
- Prepare the child and parents for potential surgical procedure to correct the anomaly.
- Support the parents, and answer all questions they may have regarding specific procedures.
- Prepare the child and parents for the surgical experience and postoperative management.
- Assess, evaluate, and treat arrhythmias common postoperatively secondary to edema.
- Monitor carefully for signs of infection and administer antibiotics as necessary.
- Provide essential postoperative instruction to avoid pulmonary complications.
- Remind the child and the family before discharge that the surgical procedure resulted in increased blood flow to the abdomen, which may cause pain and abdominal discomfort as a short-term problem.
- Instruct the parents and child for discharge planning on potential limitations, awareness of unusual symptoms, medications prescribed, and their side effects.

# CONGENITAL HEART DEFECTS, DUPLICATION OF AORTIC ARCH

## DESCRIPTION
- Duplication of the aortic arch is an acyanotic heart defect that causes decreased pulmonary blood flow.
- Duplication of the aortic arch occurs because of the persistence of embryonic vascular precursors of the aorta and stem branches of the aorta.
- Children with this defect experience symptoms of respiratory difficulty in the first year of life.
- Surgical repair involves removal of duplicated tissue, and the prognosis is excellent if uncomplicated.
- Before and after any congenital heart defect repair, children may require prophylactic administration of antibiotics to prevent infectious *endocarditis.*

## ASSESSMENT FINDINGS
- Respiratory difficulty secondary to compression of the trachea or esophagus or both
- Dysphagia

## NURSING IMPLICATIONS
- Assess and evaluate lung sounds and oxygenation status of the child with duplication of the aortic arch.
- Address parents' knowledge deficit and teach them about the normal physiology of the heart and the pathophysiology of the congenital heart defect with resultant complications.
- Explain all procedures and rationales for treatment to the child and parents.
- Invite verbalization of fears and discussion of concerns from the family.
- Support the parents and child throughout the hospitalization.
- Monitor for and reduce respiratory distress and pulmonary congestion for the child with duplication of the aortic arch.
- Promote fluid loss for the child with right-sided heart failure.
- Prepare the child and parents for potential surgical procedure to correct the anomaly.
- Support the parents and answer all questions they may have regarding specific procedures.

- Prepare the parents and child for the surgical experience and postoperative management.
- Assess, evaluate, and treat arrhythmias common postoperatively secondary to edema.
- Monitor carefully for signs of infection, and administer antibiotics as necessary.
- Provide essential postoperative instruction to avoid pulmonary complications.
- Instruct the parents and child for discharge planning on potential limitations, awareness of unusual symptoms, medications prescribed, and their side effects.

# CONGENITAL HEART DEFECTS, ENDOCARDIAL CUSHION DEFECT

### DESCRIPTION

- Endocardial cushion defect, an acyanotic heart defect, is a common congenital anomaly associated with Down syndrome.
- Defective endocardial cushion development causes openings in the lower atrial septal wall and upper ventricular septal wall as well as atrioventricular valve defects.
- Blood flows from the left atrium and ventricle through the openings into the right atrium and ventricle, increasing pulmonary blood volume.
- *Cardiac catheterization* and x-ray films confirm the diagnosis.
- Surgical intervention is necessary and may involve a valve repair to avoid future valvular insufficiency.
- Before and after any congenital heart defect repair, children may require prophylactic administration of antibiotics to prevent infectious *endocarditis.*
- Children who require a prosthetic valve replacement require anticoagulant or antiplatelet therapy.

### ASSESSMENT FINDINGS

- *Cardiac catheterization* and x-ray positive for defect.
- Systolic murmur

### NURSING IMPLICATIONS

- Assess and evaluate heart sounds, including murmurs, in all children.
- Address parents' knowledge deficit and teach them about the normal physiology of the heart and the pathophysiology of the congenital heart defect with resultant complications.

- Explain all procedures and rationales for treatment to the child and parents.
- Invite verbalization of fears and discussion of concerns from the family.
- Support the child and parents throughout the hospitalization.
- Monitor for and reduce respiratory distress and pulmonary congestion.
- Prepare the child and parents for surgical procedure to correct the anomaly.
- Explain to the parents that the procedure may involve a septal repair and a valve repair to avoid valvular insufficiency later.
- Support the parents, and answer all questions they may have regarding specific procedures.
- Prepare the parents and child for the surgical experiences and postoperative management.
- Assess, evaluate, and treat arrhythmias common postoperatively secondary to edema.
- Monitor carefully for signs of infection, and administer antibiotics as necessary.
- Provide essential postoperative instruction to avoid pulmonary complications.
- Instruct the parents and child for discharge planning on potential limitations, awareness of unusual symptoms, medications prescribed, and their side effects.

# CONGENITAL HEART DEFECTS, HYPOPLASTIC LEFT HEART SYNDROME

### DESCRIPTION

- In hypoplastic left heart syndrome, a cyanotic congenital heart defect, the left ventricle of the heart is nonfunctional.
- There may be mitral or aortic valve atresia with hypoplastic left heart syndrome.
- As the right ventricle attempts to maintain the entire heart action, right ventricular hypertrophy occurs.
- Cyanosis is mild to moderate as unoxygenated blood is shunted across the foramen ovale.
- Children with this defect seldom live longer than 1 month.
- Medical and surgical intervention are of limited success.
- *Cardiac transplant* is an option when available.

### ASSESSMENT FINDINGS

- Cyanosis as desaturated blood from the pulmonary artery enters the aorta
- Tachypnea
- *Congestive heart failure*
- Systemic hypoperfusion

### NURSING IMPLICATIONS

- Assess and evaluate heart sounds, respiratory rate, and lung sounds.
- Promote support of cardiac output and attempt to decrease all excess oxygen demands.
- Address parents' knowledge deficit and teach them about the normal physiology of the heart and the pathophysiology of the congenital heart defect with resultant complications.
- Explain all procedures and rationales for treatment to the child and parents.
- Invite verbalization of fears and discussion of concerns from the family.
- Support the child and parents throughout the hospitalization.
- Administer prostaglandin therapy to maintain a patent ductus.
- Schedule smaller, more frequent feedings to provide sufficient calories for growth to the infant with a cyanotic anomaly.
- Investigate current research into newer improved surgical techniques and advocate for the child and family the best medical and surgical treatment.
- Help the parents begin to cope with the potential for a needed *cardiac transplant* or death if a donor heart is not available.
- Prepare the child and family for *cardiac transplantation*, and ensure they fully understand this lifesaving procedure, which will have an impact on all of their lives.

## CONGENITAL HEART DEFECTS, PATENT DUCTUS ARTERIOSUS (PDA)

### DESCRIPTION

- PDA, an acyanotic congenital heart defect, is an accessory fetal vessel that connects the pulmonary artery to the aorta.

- Normal closure occurs between birth and 3 months.
- If it fails to close, blood is shunted from the aorta, because of increased aortic pressure, through the ductus to the pulmonary artery.
- With PDA, shunted blood returns to the left atrium, to the left ventricle, out the aorta, and back to the pulmonary artery.
- This ineffective flow of blood causes left ventricular hypertrophy and may increase pressure in the pulmonary circulation.
- Maternal rubella is associated with defects such as PDA.
- Before and after any congenital heart defect repair, children may require prophylactic administration of antibiotics to prevent infectious *endocarditis.*

### Assessment Findings

- Wide pulse pressure
- Continuous (systolic, diastolic), machinery murmur auscultated at the upper left sternal border or under the left clavicle in older children
- Left ventricular enlargement on electrocardiogram

### Nursing Implications

- Assess and evaluate heart sounds, including murmurs, in all children.
- Address parents' knowledge deficit and teach them about the normal physiology of the heart and the pathophysiology of the congenital heart defect with resultant complications.
- Explain all procedures and rationales for treatment to the child and parent.
- Invite verbalization of fears and discussion of concerns from the family.
- Support the parents and child throughout the hospitalization.
- Promote cardiac output for the child with a PDA.
- Monitor for and reduce respiratory distress and pulmonary congestion for the child with a PDA.
- Administer oral or intravenous indomethacin, a prostaglandin inhibitor.
- Monitor for side effects of this drug.
- Prepare the parents for the need for surgical intervention to close the ductus arteriosus if medical management fails.

- Support the parents, and answer all questions they may have regarding specific procedures.
- Prepare the parents and child for the surgical experience and postoperative management.
- Assess, evaluate, and treat arrhythmias common postoperatively secondary to edema.
- Monitor carefully for signs of infection, and administer antibiotics as necessary.
- Provide essential postoperative instruction to avoid pulmonary complications.
- Instruct the parents and the child for discharge planning on potential limitations, awareness of unusual symptoms, medications prescribed, and their side effects.

## CONGENITAL HEART DEFECTS, TETRALOGY OF FALLOT

### DESCRIPTION

- In tetralogy of Fallot, the most common cyanotic congenital heart defect, decreased pulmonary blood flow exists.
- Four anomalies are present with tetralogy of Fallot: pulmonary artery stenosis, intraventricular septal defect, dextroposition of the aorta, and hypertrophy of the right ventricle.
- Before and after any congenital heart defect repair, children may require prophylactic administration of antibiotics to prevent infectious *endocarditis.*

### ASSESSMENT FINDINGS

- Mild cyanosis with mild pulmonary artery obstruction
- Severe cyanosis with severe pulmonary artery obstruction

### NURSING IMPLICATIONS

- Assess and evaluate heart and lung sounds in all infants suspected of tetralogy of Fallot.
- Address parents' knowledge deficit and teach them about the normal physiology of the heart and the pathophysiology of the congenital heart defect with resultant complications.
- Explain all procedures and rationales for treatment to the child and parent.
- Invite verbalization of fears and discussion of concerns from the family.

- Help the parents to understand the importance of not allowing the infant to overexert himself or herself and increase oxygen needs.
- Place the infant in a knee-chest position if a hypoxic episode occurs.
- Administer propranolol (Inderal) for heart spasm.
- Prepare the parents for the temporary surgical procedure, which creates a shunt between the aorta and the pulmonary artery.

- Help the parents to understand a full repair will be necessary at a later date.
- Support the parents and child throughout the hospitalization.
- Promote cardiac output and decrease oxygen demands while increasing oxygen supply.
- Monitor for and reduce respiratory distress, and administer oxygen as prescribed.
- Schedule smaller, more frequent feedings to provide sufficient calories for growth to the infant with a cyanotic anomaly.
- Assess, evaluate, and treat arrhythmias common postoperatively secondary to edema.
- Monitor carefully for signs of infection, and administer antibiotics as necessary.
- Provide essential postoperative instruction to avoid pulmonary complications.
- Instruct the parents and child for discharge planning on potential limitations, awareness of unusual symptoms, medications prescribed, and their side effects.

## CONGENITAL HEART DEFECTS, TOTAL ANOMALOUS PULMONARY VENOUS RETURN ▓

### DESCRIPTION

- Total anomalous pulmonary venous return, a cyanotic heart defect, is a disorder in which the pulmonary veins return to the right atrium or the superior vena cava instead of to the left atrium.
- For blood to reach the left side of the heart, it must be shunted through a patent foramen ovale or *patent ductus arteriosis.*
- Until the heart is repaired, children with cyanotic heart defects are prone to *congestive heart failure* and anoxic episodes.

- Before and after any congenital heart defect repair, children may require prophylactic administration of antibiotics to prevent infectious *endocarditis.*

### Assessment Findings
- Pulmonary congestion
- Respiratory infection
- Mild to severe cyanosis depending on degree of pulmonary venous obstruction
- Decreased cardiac output and systemic hypoxia (possible)
- Fatigue
- Absent spleen

### Nursing Implications
- Assess and evaluate heart and lung sounds and evaluate oxygenation status in children with total anomalous pulmonary venous return.
- Monitor for signs of pulmonary infection.
- Address parents' knowledge deficit and teach them about the normal physiology of the heart and the pathophysiology of the congenital heart defect with resultant complications.
- Explain all procedures and rationales for treatment to the child and parent.
- Invite verbalization of fears and discussion of concerns from the family.
- Support the child and parents throughout the hospitalization.
- Monitor for and reduce respiratory distress and pulmonary congestion.
- Maintain and promote adequate cardiac output, and administer vasoactive medications if necessary to support cardiac output and oxygenation.
- Schedule smaller, more frequent feedings to provide sufficient calories for growth to the infant with a cyanotic anomaly.
- Support the parents, and answer all questions they may have regarding specific procedures.
- Prepare the child and parents for the surgical experience and postoperative management.
- Instruct the parents as to how the surgical therapy for total anomalous pumonary venous return involves reimplanting the pulmonary veins into the left atrium.

- Administer prostaglandin E₁ until the surgery occurs to maintain a patent ductus arteriosus.
- Assess, evaluate, and treat arrhythmias common postoperatively secondary to edema.
- Monitor carefully for signs of infection, and administer antibiotics as necessary.
- Provide essential postoperative instruction to avoid pulmonary complications.
- Instruct the parents and child for discharge planning on potential limitations, awareness of unusual symptoms, medications prescribed, and their side effects.

# CONGENITAL HEART DEFECTS, TRANSPOSITION OF THE GREAT VESSELS

## DESCRIPTION

- Transposition of the great vessels, a cyanotic congenital heart defect, is a disorder in which the aorta arises from the right ventricle instead of the left.
- The pulmonary artery arises from the left ventricle instead of the right.
- The creation of two separate circulatory systems occurs.
- For survival to occur, a communication between the left and right sides of the heart must occur (such as with a *patent ductus arteriosus*).
- Until the heart is repaired, children with cyanotic heart defects are prone to *congestive heart failure* and anoxic episodes.
- Before and after any congenital heart defect repair, children may require prophylactic administration of antibiotics to prevent infectious *endocarditis*.

## ASSESSMENT FINDINGS

- Cyanosis from birth
- No murmur to various murmurs (depending on the shunting of blood through atrial or ventricular defects or through the ductus arteriosus)
- Enlarged heart

## NURSING IMPLICATIONS

- Assess and evaluate heart sounds, including murmurs, in all children.
- Maintain adequate oxygenation and decrease oxygen demand when applicable.

- Address parents' knowledge deficit and teach them about the normal physiology of the heart and the pathophysiology of the congenital heart defect with resultant complications.
- Explain all procedures and rationales for treatment to the child and parent.
- Invite verbalization of fears and discussion of concerns from the family.
- Support the parents and child throughout the hospitalization.
- Promote cardiac output and administer prescribed medications.
- Monitor for and reduce respiratory distress and pulmonary congestion.
- Schedule smaller, more frequent feedings to provide sufficient calories for growth to the infant with a cyanotic anomaly.
- Prepare the child and parents for potential surgical procedure to correct the anomaly.
- Support the parents, and answer all questions they may have regarding specific procedures.
- Advise parents of children with transposition of the great vessels without an associated septal defect that a pull-through operation may be done in the first few days of an infant's life to enlarge the opening of the foramen ovale and create an artificial septal defect.
- Administer prostaglandin $E_1$ to keep the ductus arteriosus open.
- Inform parents that a Mustard procedure or the Arterial switch procedure to restructure the heart is necessary for the child's survival.
- Prepare the parents and child for the surgical experience and postoperative management.
- Assess, evaluate, and treat arrhythmias common postoperatively secondary to edema.
- Monitor carefully for signs of infection, and administer antibiotics as necessary.
- Provide essential postoperative instruction to avoid pulmonary complications.
- Instruct the parents and child for discharge planning on potential limitations, awareness of unusual symptoms, medications prescribed, and their side effects.

# CONGENITAL HEART DEFECTS, TRICUSPID ATRESIA

### DESCRIPTION

- In tricuspid atresia, a cyanotic congenital heart defect, the tricuspid valve is completely closed causing obstruction of blood flow from the right atrium to the right ventricle.
- Blood crosses the foramen ovale into the left atrium.
- A *patent ductus arteriosis* permits pulmonary blood flow.
- As long as the fetal shunts remain open, the child can obtain adequate oxygenation of blood.
- Surgery consists of construction of a subclavian-to-pulmonary artery shunt.
- Before and after any congenital heart defect repair, the child may require prophylactic administration of antibiotics to prevent infectious *endocarditis.*

### ASSESSMENT FINDINGS

- Cyanosis at birth (mild to severe depending on the size of the ductus arteriosus)
- Tachypnea
- Dyspnea

### NURSING IMPLICATIONS

- Assess and evaluate heart and lung sounds in all children.
- Monitor a child with tricuspid atresia for alteration in pulmonary function, and evaluate level of cyanosis.
- Address parents' knowledge deficit and teach them about the normal physiology of the heart and the pathophysiology of the congenital heart defect with resultant complications.
- Explain all procedures and rationales for treatment to the child and parent.
- Invite verbalization of fears and discussion of concerns from the family.
- Support the child and parents throughout the hospitalization.
- Promote fluid loss for the child with right-sided heart failure.
- Prepare the child and parents for potential surgical procedure to correct the anomaly.
- Support the parents, and answer all questions they may have regarding specific procedures.

- Administer prostaglandin E₁ before surgery.
- Teach the family that subclavian-to-pulmonary artery shunts deflect more blood to the lungs.
- Inform families about the option of a Fontan procedure, which restructures the right side of the heart.
- Prepare the parents and child for the surgical experience and postoperative management.
- Assess, evaluate, and treat arrhythmias common postoperatively secondary to edema.
- Monitor carefully for signs of infection, and administer antibiotics as necessary.
- Provide essential postoperative instruction to avoid pulmonary complications.
- Instruct the parents and child for discharge planning on potential limitations, awareness of unusual symptoms, medications prescribed, and their side effects.

# CONGENITAL HEART DEFECTS, TRUNCUS ARTERIOSUS

## DESCRIPTION

- In truncus arteriosus, a cyanotic congenital heart defect, one major artery or trunk arises from the left and right ventricles in place of a separate aorta and pulmonary artery.
- There is usually an accompanying *ventricular septal defect.*
- It is surgically restructured by creating separate vessels from the "common" trunk.
- Until the heart is repaired, children with cyanotic heart defects are prone to *congestive heart failure* and anoxic episodes.
- Before and after any congenital heart defect repair, children may require prophylactic administration of antibiotics to prevent infectious *endocarditis.*

## ASSESSMENT FINDINGS

- Pulmonary congestion
- Cyanosis (may not be present because of the excessive pulmonary blood flow)

## NURSING IMPLICATIONS

- Assess and evaluate heart and lung sounds in all children with truncus arteriosus.
- Monitor for any associated murmurs in this population.

- Address parents' knowledge deficit and teach them about the normal physiology of the heart and the pathophysiology of the congenital heart defect with resultant complications.
- Explain all procedures and rationales for treatment to the child and parent.
- Invite verbalization of fears and discussion of concerns from the family.
- Support the parents and child throughout the hospitalization.
- Promote cardiac output, and administer medications as prescribed.
- Monitor for and reduce respiratory distress and pulmonary congestion and any associated *ventricular septal defect.*
- Schedule smaller, more frequent feedings to provide sufficient calories for growth to the infant with a cyanotic anomaly.
- Prepare the child and parents for potential surgical procedure to correct the anomaly.
- Inform parents that a repair involves restructuring of the common trunk to create separate vessels.
- Support the parents, and answer all questions they may have regarding specific procedures.
- Prepare the parents and child for the surgical experience and postoperative management.
- Assess, evaluate, and treat arrhythmias common postoperatively secondary to edema.
- Monitor carefully for signs of infection, and administer antibiotics as necessary.
- Provide essential postoperative instruction to avoid pulmonary complications.
- Instruct the parents and child in preparation for discharge about any potential limitations, awareness of unusual symptoms, medications prescribed, and their side effects.

## CONGENITAL HEART DEFECTS, VENTRICULAR SEPTAL DEFECT (VSD)

### DESCRIPTION

- VSD, an acyanotic congenital heart defect, is the most common of all congenital cardiac defects.
- An opening is present in the septum between the two ventricles.

- Pressure in the left ventricle is greater than in the right ventricle, and blood therefore shunts from left to right across the septum.
- Decreased cardiac output and right ventricular hypertrophy occur.
- Before and after any congenital heart defect repair, the child may require prophylactic administration of antibiotics to prevent infectious *endocarditis.*

### ASSESSMENT FINDINGS
- Loud, harsh pansystolic murmur
- Palpable thrill

### NURSING IMPLICATIONS
- Assess and evaluate heart sounds, including murmurs, in all children.
- Address parents' knowledge deficit and teach them about the normal physiology of the heart and the pathophysiology of the congenital heart defect with resultant complications.
- Explain all procedures and rationales for treatment to the child and parent.
- Invite verbalization of fears and discussion of concerns from the family.
- Support the parents and child throughout the hospitalization.
- Promote cardiac output for the child with a ventricular septal defect.
- Monitor for and reduce respiratory distress and pulmonary congestion for the child with VSD.
- Explain to parents that 60% of all VSDs close spontaneously.
- Prepare the parents and child for the surgical experience and postoperative management.
- Support the parents through surgery, which requires extracorporeal circulation for a quiet heart.
- Assess for arrhythmia postoperatively because edema in the septum may interfere with conduction.
- Monitor carefully for signs of infection, and administer antibiotics as necessary.
- Provide essential postoperative instruction to avoid pulmonary complications.
- Instruct the parents and child for discharge planning on potential limitations, awareness of unusual symptoms, medications prescribed, and their side effects.

# CONGESTIVE HEART FAILURE

### Description

- CHF occurs secondary to other diseases, such as *rheumatic fever, Kawasaki disease, congenital heart defect,* or infectious *endocarditis.*
- This results in the myocardium of the heart being unable to pump adequate blood and nutrients to the systemic circulation to meet the body's metabolic needs.
- Blood pools in the heart (increased preload) or in the pulmonary or venous circulation.
- Compensatory mechanisms assist the failing myocardium to maintain cardiac output.
- Compensatory mechanisms include ventricular hypertrophy, stimulated sympathetic nervous system response to increase heart rate that increases the heart's force of contraction and causes peripheral vasoconstriction, and increased aldosterone and antidiuretic hormone release in response to decreased drop in renal blood flow causing sodium and water retention.
- A child with CHF who maintains cardiac output via compensatory mechanisms may be asymptomatic under normal conditions.
- Children have limited heart capacity for compensating, and symptoms appear when the heart can no longer maintain adequate cardiac output.
- Right-sided heart failure occures when the right ventricle cannot pump blood into the pulmonary circulation, and blood accumulates in the right ventricle leading to venous congestion.
- Left-sided heart failure occurs when the left ventricle cannot pump blood into the aorta, and blood accumulates in the left ventricle, left atrium, and pulmonary vein leading to pulmonary hypertension and pulmonary congestion.
- Right-sided CHF and left-sided CHF rarely exist separately because each side of the heart eventually affects the other.

### Assessment Findings

- Tachycardia
- Tachypnea
- Sweating
- Fatigue
- Restlessness

- Anorexia
- Galloping rhythm (secondary to ventricular dilatation)

*Right-sided heart failure*
- Hepatomegaly
- Abdominal pain
- Edema

*Left-sided heart failure*
- Dyspnea
- Rales
- Bloody sputum
- Cyanosis
- Decreased blood pressure and peripheral pulses

### Nursing Implications

- Support heart function, and help the parents deal with the present crisis.
- Improve tissue oxygenation by elevating the head of the bed, putting the bed in a semi-Fowler's position, or placing the infant in an infant seat.
- Administer humidified oxygen as prescribed for the child with dyspnea or cyanosis.
- Discuss the oxygen equipment with the child, and explain how it will make the child feel better.
- Encourage turning, coughing, and deep breathing (TCDB) for the older child.
- Monitor skin color, respiratory rate, breath sounds, quality and quantity of respiratory secretions, and blood oxygen saturation or arterial blood gases.
- Enhance cardiac output and administer cardiac glycosides, such as digoxin, as prescribed.
- Consider sedating the child to encourage bed rest and decrease oxygen demands.
- Reduce cardiac demands by eliminating unnecessary nursing care and clustering necessary care to allow for rest.
- Involve the parents in the plan of care, and ensure that they understand the importance of adequate rest periods.
- Involve the parents in medication instruction from the start to begin to prepare them for home administration.
- Maintain fluid restrictions, and monitor weight to prevent fluid overload.
- Promote fluid loss to reduce preload by administering diuretics and angiotensin converting enzyme inhibitors as prescribed.

- Evaluate fluid balance and electrolyte levels.
- Promote physical growth by providing sufficient calories.
- Provide high-calorie, low-sodium diet.

- Examine alternate routes of nourishment, such as gastrostomy, if the child is too tired to consume adequate nutrients.
- Provide reassurance to parents and point out subtle signs of improvement.
- Encourage the child to engage in quiet activities, such as reading or playing cards.
- Offer reassurance to the child that the medication and the oxygen he or she may need will make his or her heart stronger.
- Explain all discharge medications' actions, side effects, and dosages with the parents and ensure proper understanding.
- Ensure proper follow-up, expecially concerning appropriate understanding of medications and what the parents should be assessing for as side effects.
- Review *cardiopulmonary resuscitation* (CPR) techniques with parents to prepare them in case of an emergency.

## CONJUNCTIVITIS

### DESCRIPTION
- Conjunctivitis is inflammation of the conjunctiva.
- A number of causes of conjunctivitis exist with the most serious being opthalmia neonatorum, which occurs in newborns exposed to gonococcus bacillus.
- Inclusion blennorrhea occurs approximately 10 days after birth from contact with chlamydial organisms; in older children, it is referred to as "swimming pool conjunctivitis" because it is contracted there.
- Acute catarrhal conjunctivitis (pinkeye) is caused by *haemophilus influenzae* and *Streptococcus pneumoniae;* it may also occur secondary to a virus, an irritation, or from a foreign body.
- Herpetic conjunctivitis occurs from the herpes simplex virus and may accompany facial herpes lesions; it can spread easily and become a corneal infection with resultant opacity and permanent scarring.
- Allergic conjunctivitis occurs in children with hypersensitivity reactions to specific allergens and causes conjunctival changes; it is seasonal and is most often secondary to pollen.

### ASSESSMENT FINDINGS
- Watery eyes
- Reddened conjunctiva (fiery red with acute catarrhal conjunctivitis)
- Light sensitivity
- Pustular drainage
- Pain
- Pinpoint vesicles on the conjunctiva (with herpetic conjunctivitis)
- Edema of the eyelids and conjunctiva with severe itching (with allergic conjunctivitis)

### NURSING IMPLICATIONS
- Evaluate any eye problems referred by a parent.
- Establish a definitive diagnosis, especially as related to a specific organism.
- Ensure that a foreign body is not the cause of the conjunctivitis; if so, treat appropriately as prescribed (e.g., eye washes).
- Teach parents of children diagnosed with inclusion blennorrhea that systemic erythromycin is necessary.
- Advise parents of children with acute catarrhal conjunctivitis that they must administer the antibiotic ointment or the eyedrops for a full 7 days.
- Refer all children with a confirmed diagnosis of herpetic conjunctivitis to an opthalmologist for care.
- Ensure that a child with herpetic conjunctivitis is not receiving steroids because this could spread the infection to the cornea.
- Administer idoxuridine or trifluorothymidine, which are specific drugs used in treating the herpesvirus.
- Advise parents of children with hypersensitivity reactions who are prone to allergic conjunctivitis to reduce exposure to specific allergen if possible.
- Suggest over-the-counter antihistamines to reduce the allergic reaction.
- Reassure the child with allergic conjunctivitis that the problem should dissipate once the season has passed.
- Instruct the parents how to administer eye drops or ointments properly.

## CONSTIPATION

### DESCRIPTION
- Constipation refers to the difficulty passing hardened stools and may occur in children of any age.
- Constipation is painful and can cause anal fissures.

- A cycle begins in which the distressed child may suppress the urge to defecate; eventually the rectum becomes distended from the presence of stool.
- When the child passes a stool, it is large and firm and more painful than if the child had not suppressed the urge to defecate.
- Severe constipation, coupled with *diarrhea* and encopresis (involuntary release of stool) occurs when the rectum can hold no more.
- Some children may begin holding stool for emotional reasons; however, it quickly becomes a physical ailment.
- Treatment must include counseling to correct the initial emotional problem as well as treatment for the physical symptoms.
- Treatment is initially aimed at softening the stool to allow easy passage and to help the child form normal bowel habits.

### ASSESSMENT FINDINGS
- Hard painful passing of stool
- Hard stool in rectum
- Anal fissures
- Abdominal pain

### NURSING IMPLICATIONS
- Assess a child's bowel habits at each routine physical examination.
- Ascertain that the child is having constipation versus defecation of normal stool over longer periods of time.
- Prepare the child for initial treatment of an enema if necessary.
- Teach parents about the need for a prescribed stool softener, such as docusate sodium (Colace).
- Discuss with the child and family about the need for a high-fiber and high-in-fluid diet.
- Review with the child and family the importance of establishing a normal elimination pattern.
- Suggest to the child and parents that the child attempt to evacuate his or her bowels at the same time every day to form a habit.
- Recommend to parents the need to avoid power struggles over toileting issues with the child.
- Refer the child and family to an appropriate counselor to address any emotional issues that may have contributed to the problem.

- Follow up with the family and child in 2 weeks to ensure that the child is able to follow a recommended diet and is having a soft bowel movement without pain at least every other day.

## CONTUSION

### DESCRIPTION

- A contusion, also called a bruise, in an injury that does not break the skin; it may be caused by a blow to the body.
- The application of cold may limit the development of a contusion.
- Contusions can occur anywhere in the body.
- Brain contusions are a tearing or laceration of brain tissue.
- Symptoms of brain contusions depend on the lacerated brain area.
- If bleeding exists with the brain contusion, surgery may be indicated.
- Prognosis for brain contusion depends on the extent of injury and complications, such as increased intracranial pressure.
- Ocular contusions can be caused by blunt trauma, affecting the eyelid and surrounding tissue.
- Ocular contusions may be simple, such as a black eye, or more complicated, such as an orbital fracture, which inhibits eye globe movement and requires surgical intervention.

### ASSESSMENT FINDINGS

- Swelling
- Discoloration
- Pain

*Brain contusion*
- Focal *seizure*
- Eye deviation
- Loss of speech

*Ocular contusion*
- Vision disturbances
- Ocular motion disturbances
- Dilated, fixed, or cloudy pupil
- Loss of vision
- Visible blood in the anterior chamber

### Nursing Implications

- Assess the extent of contusion injury.
- Instruct the parents to apply ice or cold packs for simple contusions.
- Explain to the parents and the child that reabsorption of blood in the tissue takes 1 to 3 weeks.
- Evaluate for signs and symptoms that would indicate a need or a referral to an ophthalmologist or admission into the hospital for further evaluation and potentially surgery.
- Inform the parents that tissue hemorrhage may extend across the nose and surround the other eye the day after the ocular injury.
- Monitor changes in level of consciousness in children with a brain contusion.
- Provide adequate preparation and teaching for the family and the child who may need surgical intervention with ocular or brain contusions.

## COXSACKIEVIRUS

### Description

- The coxsackievirus is any of 30 serologically different enteroviruses.
- Coxsackievirus A has 24 subdivisions.
- Coxsackievirus B has 6 subdivisions.
- These viruses primarily affect children during warm weather.
- The coxsackievirus resembles the virus responsible for poliomyelitis.
- The most common disease caused by coxsackievirus A is herpangina.
- Other diseases associated with coxsackievirus infections are hand-foot-and mouth disease, epidemic pleurodynia, myocarditis, pericarditis, aseptic meningitis, and several exanthems.
- There is no known preventive measure against these viruses.
- Isolation of infected persons and treatment of related symptoms are the goals of treatment.
- The infections are usually benign and self-limiting.

### Assessment Findings
#### *Herpangina*
- Abrupt increase in temperature to 104–105° F
- Fever for 1 to 4 days

- Anorexia
- Sore throat with difficulty swallowing
- *Vomiting*
- Graying vesicles in the mouth, which change to shallow ulcers

### NURSING IMPLICATIONS
- Teach prevention of the spread of all viruses with good hand-washing techniques.
- Conduct community teaching for day care workers on the prevention of disease.
- Isolate children diagnosed with any coxsackievirus until lesions are dry and healing.
- Provide supportive care and instruct the parents to:
  - Administer antipyretics for the fever.
  - Maintain the child on soft or liquid diet while the mouth and throat are sore.
  - Apply a local anesthetic to ulcers in mouth (viscous lidocaine [Xylocaine]) to combat pain; however, do not let the child swallow the local anesthetic because it could lead to aspiration from decreased gag reflex.
- Inform the parents that there are generally no complications from these viruses.

## CRANIOSYNOSTOSIS

### DESCRIPTION
- Craniosynostosis is premature closure of the sutures of the skull occuring at birth or in utero.
- Closure in utero may be idiopathic, secondary to rickets, or caused by irregularities of calcium or phosphate metabolism.
- Craniosynostosis is associated with other skeletal defects.
- Cardiac anomalies, *choanal atresia,* or defects of elbows and knee joints also are associated with craniosynostosis.
- Premature closure of the suture line compromises brain growth.
- Premature coronal suture line closure causes facial deformity; the orbits of the eyes become misshapen, and increased intracranial pressure occurs, leading to exophthalmos, nystagmus, papilledema, strabismus, and atrophy of the optic nerve with loss of vision.

- Premature closure of the coronal suture line is associated with syndactyly (a congenital anomaly characterized by fusion of the fingers or toes).
- Premature coronal suture line closure must be surgically corrected to prevent eye and brain damage from inhibited brain growth.
- Premature closure of the sagittal suture line causes the child's head to grow anteriorly and posteriorly.
- Premature sagittal suture closure may require frequent monitoring and observation.

### ASSESSMENT FINDINGS

- Abnormal head circumference or growth
- Facial deformity
- X-ray confirmation of fused suture line
- Exophthalmos
- Nystagmus
- Papilledema
- Strabismus
- Atrophy of the optic nerve
- Loss of vision

### NURSING IMPLICATIONS

- Measure head circumference on all children under 2 years of age at every health maintenance visit.
- Compare infant's head circumference with past measurements and with standard measurements.
- Evaluate for any changes, and refer to physician for detection of craniosynostosis and prevention of brain compression.
- Observe all children with premature closure of the fontanelles for craniosynostosis.
- Monitor head circumference in all children with syndactyly.
- Evaluate for associated abnormalities, such as cardiac anomalies, *choanal atresia,* or defects of elbow and knee joints.
- Educate the parents on the dangers of inhibited brain growth, and prepare them for surgical intervention if necessary.
- Allow parents time to understand the implication of the diagnosis, and support the family throughout any potential hospitalization.
- Monitor postoperatively for signs of *increased intracranial pressure* secondary to swelling at the surgical site.

- Teach parents about any medications required at discharge, and ensure proper support and medical attention to associated anomalies.

# CROHN'S DISEASE

### DESCRIPTION

- Crohn's disease is an inflammation of segments of the intestine, usually affecting the terminal portions of the ileum.
- This is one of two diseases classified as inflammatory bowel disease.
- All layers of the intestinal mucosa develop ulcerations.
- The wall of the colon becomes thickened, and the surface is inflamed, leading to a cobblestone appearance of mucosa.
- Malabsorption and associated increased risk of bowel cancer exist with Crohn's disease.
- The cause of Crohn's disease is unknown; however, it tends to be familial.
- Crohn's may represent an alteration in immune system response or an autoimmune process because an increased number of immunoglobulins are present on the intestinal mucosa.
- Psychological factors, such as emotional stress, seem to exacerbate signs and symptoms.
- Surgery is avoided with Crohn's disease because recurrence in another part of the bowel may occur and it does not decrease the risk of colon cancer.
- Dietary management with replacement of nutrients and vitamins is necessary.

### ASSESSMENT FINDINGS

- Mild-to-moderate *diarrhea*
- Steatorrhea
- Abdominal pain
- Bloody stools
- Malnutrition
- Anorexia and weight loss
- *Dehydration* and electrolyte abnormalities
- Recurring fever
- Severe growth delays
- Delayed sexual maturation
- Rectal fistula

### NURSING IMPLICATIONS

- Know that the diagnosis of Crohn's disease is confirmed with a biopsy after ulcerations are seen via sigmoidoscopy.
- Inform the parents about the disease and its management.
- Rest the bowel by maintaining the child NPO (nothing by mouth) and administering corticosteroids as prescribed.
- Advise the parents that parenteral nutrition is necessary during the acute exacerbations to allow the bowel to rest.
- Keep in mind that ensuring adequate rest and nutrition for these children is a lifetime goal.
- Evaluate electrolytes and fluid status, and replete deficiencies as necessary.
- Monitor glucose and assess for signs of hyperglycemia or hypoglycemia for a child on total parenteral nutrition (TPN) or enteral feedings.
- Attempt to ensure a steady administration rate of supplemental nutrition to avoid fluctuations in glucose.
- Promote return to home during this period with adequate referral to home care nursing agencies.
- Teach parents to monitor for signs of infection related to intravenous line sepsis with TPN administration.
- Provide education of a high-protein, high-carbohydrate, high-vitamin diet to the family and the child when food in reintroduced after the rest period.
- Assess intake and output when reintroducing food to ensure adequate nutrients and calories without *diarrhea.*
- Stress the importance of maintaining the dietary regimen and drug therapy even in remission to avoid exacerbations of Crohn's disease.
- Provide emotional support to the family and the child, and help them to adjust to this chronic problem.

## CROUP

### DESCRIPTION

- Croup is an inflammation of the larynx, trachea, and major bronchi, commonly occuring between 6 months and 3 years of age.
- Croup is usually caused by a viral infection, such as parainfluenza virus or *Haemophilus influenzae.*

- Croup is one of the most frightening diseases in early childhood because symptoms of respiratory distress appear so suddenly.
- The danger of croup is the potential for glottal obstruction from the laryngeal inflammation.
- Severe symptoms typically may last several hours and subside in the morning, possible recurring the next night.

## Assessment Findings

- Upper respiratory infection at bedtime
- Barking (distinctive harsh brassy) cough during the night
- Inspiratory stridor
- Marked respiratory retractions
- Extreme respiratory distress
- Cyanosis (may be present)

## Nursing Implications

- Instruct the parents in the home management of symptoms, including filling a room with steam, such as with running a hot shower and bringing the child into the bathroom.
- Inform the parents to transport the child to the emergency department if at-home measures (hot shower) do not abate the child's symptoms.
- Apply cool, moist air via an air tent once the child arrives in the emergency room.
- Advise the parents to remain constantly with the child for observation and to reduce anxiety.
- Administer dextramethasone to reduce airway edema.
- Administer racemic epinephrine via nebulizer for bronchodilation.
- Begin intravenous therapy to maintain the child's hydration status.
- Offer sips of liquid, if able to take, to maintain hydration and moist secretions.
- Measure intake and output and urine specific gravity to evaluate hydration.
- Keep the child calm, and do not elicit a gag reflex because this can cause laryngospasm with total occlusion of the airway.
- Monitor for restlessness, tachycardia, tachypnea, stridor, and cyanosis because they indicate increased respiratory distress.

- Maintain a continuous record of vital signs and activity to assess for increasing respiratory rate and restlessness.
- Continuously monitor pulse oximetry and transcutaneous $PO_2$ to document if hypoxia is occuring.
- Obtain arterial blood gases to determine adequate oxygenation if pulse oximetry is not available.
- Prepare for and assist with *tracheotomy* or *endotracheal intubation* if necessary.
- Monitor for associated complications of a tracheotomy, such as infection, *atelectasis*, tracheal tube occlusion, tracheal bleeding, granulation or stenosis, and delayed stoma healing.
- Explain the condition of croup to the parents and discuss appropriate care after discharge, which may include continued use of humidity and assurance of adequate hydration.
- Inform parents that croup runs its course in 3 to 7 days; allow them to verbalize any concerns they may have on returning home.

## CRYPTORCHIDISM

### DESCRIPTION

- Cryptorchidism, a reproductive disorder in males, is failure of one or both testes to descend from the abdominal cavity to the scrotum.
- The testes normally descend into the scrotal sac during intrauterine life but may descend up to 6 weeks after birth.
- Testes descend secondary to stimulation of testosterone.
- Cryptorchidism may be secondary to fibrous bands at the inguinal ring, inadequate length of spermatic vessels, or lower than normal levels of testosterone production.
- Premature infants are often born with undescended testes.
- The right testis remains undescended more often than the left.
- Poor examining technique may cause the testes to retract and cause a misdiagnosis of undescended testes.
- Laparoscopy is effective in identifying undescended testes.

- The warmth of the abdominal cavity may inhibit development of testes and affect spermatogenesis; therefore, early detection is important.
- After puberty, sperm production deteriorates in undescended testes, possibly undergoing a malignant change.
- Anchoring the testes to the scrotal sac may not prevent malignancy but does allow the boy to perform testicular self-examinations for early prevention.
- Because testes arise from the same germ tissue as kidneys, kidney function should be evaluated in this population.

### Assessment Findings

- Testes at the inguinal ring (true undescended testes)
- Testes still in the abdomen (ectopic testes)

### Nursing Implications

- After confirmation of cryptorchidism, explain the condition to the parents and possible treatment options.
- Advise the parents to wait 1 year for treatment because sometimes the testes descend spontaneously during the first year of life.
- Teach the parents about the administration of chorionic gonadotropin hormone to stimulate testicular descent in the preschool child.
- Advise the parents on necessary surgical intervention if pharmacologic intervention fails.
- Focus on parent and child teaching of preoperative procedures and postoperative care if an orchiopexy is needed.
- Ensure that boys who are old enough to understand are adequately prepared for this surgery.
- Assure the boy that his penis will not be cut off and use anatomically correct pictures to describe the procedure.
- Assume the preschool child fears mutilation, and encourage verbalization of these fears through picture drawing.
- Prepare the parents of the potential need for an internal support structure and what it will look like postoperatively.
- Inform the parents that although this may be a day-surgical procedure, the child will have activity

limitations until the second day after surgery, when the tension suture is released.

- Ascertain that the child's suture line is healing well postoperatively without signs of infection.
- Address the boy's feeling about the surgery and his body.
- Teach testicular self-examination to the boy when he reaches puberty.

## CUSHING'S SYNDROME

### DESCRIPTION

- Cushing's syndrome is caused by overproduction of the adrenal hormone cortisol.
- This may result from benign increased ACTH production but is more often associated with a malignant tumor of the adrenal cortex.
- Signs and symptoms of Cushing's syndrome reflect excessive amounts of circulating cortisol.
- Children on high doses of synthethic corticosteroids for a long period of time develop the same symptoms of Cushing's syndrome.
- Cushing's syndrome is often suspected as the cause of childhood obesity.
- A dexamethasone suppression test confirms the diagnosis of Cushing's syndrome.

### ASSESSMENT FINDINGS

- Polyuria, fat collection in the child's face, neck, and trunk, and obesity and hypertension (from increased glucose production)
- Protein loss and muscle wasting
- Osteoporosis
- Decreased humoral immunity
- Hyperpigmentation (from melanin-stimulation properties of ACTH)
- Signs of abnormal masculinization or feminization (from overproduction of androgen or estrogen)
- Purple striae on the child's hips, abdomen, and thighs (from collagen deficit)
- Growth cessation
- Elevated plasma cortisol levels
- Elevated urinary free cortisol levels
- Elevated fasting glucose
- Hypokalemia

- Alkalosis
- Enlarged adrenal gland on computed tomography scan or ultrasonography
- Poor wound healing
- Peptic ulcer secondary to increased gastric acid production
- Mental or emotional disturbances

### NURSING IMPLICATIONS

- Confirm the diagnosis of Cushing's syndrome with appropriate laboratory data and test results.
- Explain to parents and children the cause of Cushing's syndrome and the appropriate medical and surgical interventions.
- Prepare the child and parents for the surgical experience if the causative factor is an adrenal tumor.
- Instruct the family and child on the need for replacement cortisol therapy indefinitely, and educate them regarding the implications and the therapy.
- Discuss the prognosis depending on if the tumor is benign or malignant.
- Honestly answer questions on the rapidity of metastasis with this type of malignant tumor.
- Encourage the child required to take corticosteroids that then develops Cushing's syndrome to discuss concerns about weight gain and appearance.
- Advise children to wear loose-fitting clothing to disguise fat around the waist and upper back.

## CYSTIC FIBROSIS

### DESCRIPTION

- Cystic fibrosis is a hereditary disorder causing widespread dysfunction of the exocrine glands; it is caused by an autosomal recessive trait that occurs predominantly in whites and affects both sexes equally.
- Mucous secretions of the body, especially the pancreas and lungs, are abnormally thick and have difficulty flowing through gland ducts.
- There is a marked electrolyte change in the secretions of the sweat glands.
- The pathophysiology of cystic fibrosis is the inability to transport small molecules across cell membranes, leading to *dehydration* of epithelial cells in the airway and pancreas.

- Cystic fibrosis shortens life expectancy; however, with the available option of lung transplantation, life expectancy is increasing.
- This disorder can be found by chorionic villi sampling or amniocentesis early in pregnancy.
- Boys with cystic fibrosis may not be able to reproduce because they may have tenacious plugging of the vas deferens.
- Girls may have thick cervical secretions making it difficult for sperm to penetrate.
- The pancreas of children with cystic fibrosis eventually atrophies from plugged ducts, which causes an increase in back pressure; the pancreatic enzymes are not produced.
- Children are unable to digest fat, protein, and some sugars.
- Initial misdiagnosis in infants of a milk *allergy* occurs often.
- Infants with cystic fibrosis are not breast-fed because there is not sufficient protein in breast milk for them.
- The lungs of children with this disorder plug with thick mucous in the bronchioles causing bronchial obstruction, ventilatory problems, and bacterial infection.
- The most frequent lung infections are caused by *Stapyhlococcus aureus, Pseudomonas aeruginosa,* and *Haemophilus influenzae.*
- Cystic fibrosis eventually leads to secondary emphysema with overinflated alveoli accompanied by chronic hypoxia and hypercapnia.
- *Atelectasis*, bronchiectasis, and *pneumonia* occur.

### Assessment Findings

- Chloride: sodium concentration of sweat 2 to 5 times above normal
- Steatorrhea
- Foul-smelling stool
- Protuberant abdomen
- Malnutrition with emaciated extremities
- Loose flabby folds of skin on the buttocks
- Fat-soluble vitamin deficiencies
- Meconium ileus (first obvious sign in infants)
- Nausea
- Colicky abdominal pain
- Decreased breath sounds

- Hypoxia
- Hypercapnia
- Fever
- Productive cough
- Tachypnea
- Wheezing
- Rhonchi
- Barrel chest
- Clubbed fingers
- Failure to gain back initial weight lost as a newborn by 4 to 6 weeks

### NURSING IMPLICATIONS

- Carefully evaluate for passage of stool and meconium in a newborn.
- Monitor the infant's weight and note if the child regains initial loss of weight by 4 to 6 weeks.
- Note any child seen at a health visit with complaints from the mother that the child has a feeding problem because the child always appears hungry. (These children absorb only about 50% of their intake and then eat so ravenously that they swallow air, which is then manifested as colic.)
- Assess type and frequency of stool and whether there is a foul odor with it.
- Note any child seen frequently in the health care setting between 4 and 6 months because of frequent respiratory infections, a chronic cough, and failure to gain weight.
- Support the parents and child through initial tests for duodenal analysis of pancreatic enzymes, sweat testing, chest film, and pulmonary function tests.
- Explain all procedures and answer any questions that the parents may have.
- After confirmation of cystic fibrosis occurs, spend time with the parents to help them understand this multifaceted disease.
- Promote airway clearance, and control respiratory infections and teach the parents the importance of maintaining adequate hydration in this population.
- Provide supplemental high humidity oxygen if prescribed.
- Encourage a child on bed rest to make frequent position changes every 2 to 4 hours so that all lobes of the lungs drain by being in a superior position.

- Observe the hospitalized child frequently to assess for rapid deterioration in pulmonary status.
- Provide respiratory hygiene and mouth care to aid with the disagreeable taste and odor of secretions.
- Maintain adequate rest and comfort to avoid exhaustion, and ensure that the child is adequately rested before eating.
- Educate the parents on the use of bronchodilators if prescribed to combat airway narrowing and to help the child expel mucus.
- Teach the parents how to perform chest physiotherapy and breathing exercises, and support them as they begin to realize the lifelong commitment to maintenance of a clear airway.
- Prepare the parents for the expectation of acute pulmonary infections, which will need to be treated with intravenous and inhaled antibiotic therapy.
- Instruct the parents on how to promote digestive function in their child.
- Place the infant on Probana, a high-protein formula.
- Place the child on a high-calorie, high-protein, moderate-fat diet.
- Supplement the diet with water-miscible forms of vitamins A, D, and E.
- Inform the parents of the need to add extra salt to food, expecially in hot months, because of the excess salt lost in perspiration.
- Instruct parents that medium-chain triglycerides are used with the diet because they are more readily digested than other oils.
- Educate the parents and child that before each meal and snack they need to take a synthetic pancreatic enzyme to replace the enzyme they cannot produce.
- Instruct the parents on different methods of administering these large capsules.
- Educate the parents on how to assess for dietary absorption by monitoring their child's stool and weight.
- Monitor skin integrity in this population as related to acid stools and frequent periods of prolonged bed rest from pulmonary complications.
- Assess for rectal prolapse after stools.
- Observe family dynamics and assess for ineffective or compromised coping.

- Provide assistance and support to the parents regarding home care of these children.
- Promote a normal childhood and have the child attend regular school if possible.
- Allow the child to participate in physical fitness activities as tolerated.
- Ensure that the child has routine health assessments and maintains adequate *immunizations*.
- Encourage parents to verbalize their frustrations and put them in contact with support agencies such as the Cystic Fibrosis Foundation.

# DACRYOCYSTITIS

### DESCRIPTION
- Dacryocystitis is the inflammation of the nasolacrimal duct.
- This affects the school-age and adolescent child with sinusitis.
- Dacryocystitis is secondary to dacryostenosis, which causes stasis of fluid.
- Nasal mucosa is swollen, and infected mucus is forced back into the nasolacrimal duct causing increased pressure on the duct, resulting in extrusion of purulent drainage into the inner canthus of the eye.

### ASSESSMENT FINDINGS
- Acute pain at the inner canthus of the eye (referred to eye pain or back of the eye pain)

### NURSING IMPLICATIONS
- Confirm diagnosis of dacryocystitis, and explain the process to the child and parents.
- Administer systemic antibiotics if prescribed.
- Educate the parents on administration of systemic or local antibiotics.
- Assure the parents and the child that vision will not be affected.
- Explain to the child and parents that a procedure involving probing of the duct to remove accumulated debris may be necessary.
- Advise children prone to dacryocystitis (chronic allergic children and children with frequent sinusitis) that antihistamines can keep the nasal mucosa from becoming edematous.

## DEHYDRATION, HYPERTONIC

### DESCRIPTION

- Hypertonic dehydration occurs when there is decreased fluid intake and or increased fluid loss.
- Conditions that may precipitate hypertonic dehydration include fever, nausea (which prevents fluid intake), profuse *diarrhea,* and conditions that cause polyuria.
- With hypertonic dehydration, electrolytes concentrate in the blood.
- Fluid is shifted from the interstitial and intercellular spaces to the blood stream because of the increased osmotic pressure of the blood.
- Dehydration of interstitial and intracellular compartments then occurs.
- Because fluid shifts to the extracellular space, hypovolemic shock is less likely than with other forms of dehydration.

### ASSESSMENT FINDINGS

- Thirst
- Fever
- Dry, flushed skin
- Decreased saliva and tears
- Hemoconcentration as reflected by elevated red blood cell count and increased hemoglobin
- Elevated sodium, chloride, and bicarbonate levels
- Decreased blood pressure
- Decreased urine output
- Elevated urine specific gravity
- Stupor
- Irritability

### NURSING IMPLICATIONS

- Assess the child's hydration status, monitor fluid intake and output (including amount of *diarrhea*), and check urine specific gravity.
- Weigh the child daily and establish the degree of fluid loss and *dehydration.*
- Monitor skin turgor and assess mucous membranes.
- Cleanse the perineal area to prevent perineal irritation with *diarrhea.*
- Check infants for bulging fontanelles.
- Carefully monitor laboratory values, such as serum sodium and blood urea nitrogen.

- Monitor for decreased perfusion by assessing hemodynamic status, skin temperature and color, capillary refill time, and peripheral pulses.
- Provide replacement fluid and maintenance fluid as needed.
- Administer intravenous fluids as prescribed.
- Administer fluid and electrolyte solutions by mouth if the child is alert and able to ingest oral fluids.
- Educate parents on solutions such as Pedialyte, which are available without a prescription for children who are mildly dehydrated.
- Inform the parents on how to monitor fluid loss and to notify the physician if more severe signs of dehydration occur.
- Teach the parents what signs of dehydration to be aware of.
- Conserve the child's energy and provide rest.

## DEHYDRATION, HYPOTONIC

### Description
- A high loss of electrolytes relative to fluid loss occurs with hypotonic dehydration.
- Conditions that precipitate hypotonic dehydration include excessive gastrointestinal *vomiting*, low intake of salt with extreme therapeutic diuresis, and conditions that cause extreme loss of electrolytes such as *adrenocortical insufficiency* or diabetic acidosis.
- Serum sodium and chloride are low and water then shifts into the intracellular spaces even further reducing extracellular volume.
- The kidneys also excrete more fluid in an attempt to excrete the excess water and bring the proportion of electrolytes to fluid back into balance.
- This leads to secondary extracellular dehydration.
- Hypovolemic shock is a serious complication of hypotonic dehydration.

### Assessment Findings
- Decreased blood pressure
- Cardiovascular collapse
- Oliguria
- Anuria
- Poor skin turgor
- Cool, clammy skin

- Rapid respirations
- Rapid thready pulse
- Sunken fontanelles
- Weight loss
- Hemoconcentration as reflected by elevated red blood cell count and increased hemoglobin
- Stupor
- Irritability

### NURSING IMPLICATIONS
- Assess the child's hydration status, monitor fluid intake and output, and check urine specific gravity.
- Weigh the child daily and establish the degree of fluid loss and dehydration.
- Check infants for sunken fontanelles.
- Carefully monitor electrolytes, renal function tests, and hemodynamic parameters.
- Monitor for decreased perfusion by assessing hemodynamic status, skin temperature and color, capillary refill time, and peripheral pulses.
- Obtain data concerning the underlying condition and treat that as prescribed (i.e., diabetic acidosis).
- Provide replacement fluid and maintenance fluid as needed.
- Administer intravenous fluids as prescribed.
- Administer fluid and electrolyte solutions by mouth if child is alert and able to ingest oral fluids.
- Educate parents on solutions such as Pedialyte, which are available without a prescription for children who are mildly dehydrated.
- Inform the parents on how to monitor fluid loss and to notify the physician if more severe signs of dehydration occur.
- Teach the parents what signs of dehydration to be aware of.
- Conserve the child's energy and provide rest.

## DEHYDRATION, ISOTONIC

### DESCRIPTION
- Isotonic dehydration occurs when the body loses more water than it absorbs or absorbs less fluid than it excretes.
- This results first in a decrease in the volume of blood plasma.

- The body compensates for this condition by shifting interstitial fluid into the blood vessels.
- Fluids and electrolytes are lost in equal proportions, and the patient maintains a normal serum sodium level.
- When compensatory mechanisms are used up, the volume of the plasma falls rapidly, and cardiovascular collapse occurs.
- Conditions that may precipitate isotonic dehydration include *diarrhea* and nausea and *vomiting*.

### ASSESSMENT FINDINGS

- Thirst
- Weight loss
- Dry skin
- Poor skin turgor
- Sunken eyeballs
- Anterior fontanelle depression
- Gray or ashen appearance secondary to inadequate peripheral circulation
- Rapid and weak pulse
- Decreased blood pressure
- Oliguria
- Stupor
- Irritability

### NURSING IMPLICATIONS

- Assess the child's hydration status, monitor fluid intake and output (including the amount of *diarrhea*), and urine specific gravity.
- Weigh the child daily and establish the degree of fluid loss and dehydration.
- Monitor skin turgor and assess mucous membranes.
- Prevent perineal irritation with *diarrhea*.
- Check infants for depressed anterior fontanelle.
- Carefully monitor laboratory values.
- Monitor for decreased perfusion by assessing hemodynamic status, skin temperature and color, capillary refill time, and peripheral pulses.
- Treat the underlying cause of the isotonic dehydration (if *vomiting* is secondary to *chemotherapy,* administer antiemetic).
- Provide replacement fluid and maintenance fluid as needed.
- Administer intravenous fluids as prescribed.

- Administer fluid and electrolyte solutions by mouth if able.
- Educate parents on solutions such as Pedialyte, which are available without a prescription for children who are mildly dehydrated.
- Inform the parents on how to monitor fluid loss and to notify the physician if more severe signs of dehydration occur.
- Teach the parents what signs of dehydration to be aware of.
- Conserve the child's energy and provide rest.

## DELAYED PUBERTY

### Description
- Delayed puberty refers to a late development of maturation; it can be anxiety producing for both females and males.
- There may be a family history of late maturation.
- Girls who have not begun to menstruate by 17 years of age are started on estrogen after pathology has been ruled out.
- Boys, distressed over their lack of development, may be started on testosterone supplements to stimulate hair and genital growth.

### Nursing Implications
- Complete a thorough physical examination to reveal whether some secondary sex characteristics are present or if endocrine stimulation is beginning.
- Assure the adolescent that development is simply delayed and it can occur on its own.
- Administer estrogen to girls and testosterone to boys if necessary.
- Educate the adolescent on use of the medication supplements as well as dosage and side effects.

## DEPRESSION, CHILDHOOD

### Description
- Childhood depression results from a combination of genetic factors, biochemical abnormalities, and stress.
- The incidence of childhood depression ranges from 0.3% for preschoolers to 14% for adolescents.
- Manifestations of childhood depression vary with the developmental level.

- Depression in children is of growing concern as the suicide rate for children and adolescents increases.
- Depression is diagnosed when 5 or more of the listed assessment findings exist for more than 2 weeks.
- Psychotherapeutic counseling is necessary to discuss the problems.
- Family and individual counseling may be necessary to help the child regain self-esteem and the family to understand the level of depression that has occurred.
- Antidepressant medication may be used in treatment.

### Assessment Findings

- Loss of interest or pleasure
- Significant weight loss or gain
- Depressed mood
- Insomnia
- Psychomotor agitation
- Feelings of worthlessness or excessive inappropriate guilt
- Diminished concentration
- Recurrent thoughts of death
- Suicidal ideation

### Nursing Implications

- Obtain a thorough history from the child and parents; perform a physical examination and diagnostic workup to rule out physiologic causes.
- Differentiate between depression and normal sadness, when a child cannot remember the last time they felt happy or had a good time.
- Recognize signs and symptoms of depression, and provide necessary referrals for treatment for any suspected childhood depression to avoid depression worsening to the point of school failure or suicide.
- Teach the child and parents about antidepressant medication, such as tricyclic antidepressants or monoamine oxidase inhibitors.
- Provide psychosocial interventions, such as modeling, role-playing, and positive reinforcement, to enhance social behavior and decrease the incidence of depression.

# DERMATITIS, CONTACT

### DESCRIPTION

- Contact dermatitis is an inflammation of the skin after exposure to a specific allergen.
- This is an example of delayed, or type IV, hypersensitivity response.
- A patch test may be used to identify contact dermatitis allergens.

### ASSESSMENT FINDINGS

- Erythema
- Papules
- Vesicles
- Pruritus (may be intense)

### NURSING IMPLICATIONS

- Evaluate for contact dermatitis and investigate as to the child's body part that is affected.
- Determine if the diaper detergent is causing a dermatitis around the diaper area.
- Determine if the onset of puberty and use of cosmetics is causing facial contact dermatitis.
- Determine if *allergy* is to nickel with oozing at the site of newly pierced ears.
- Assess hands and feet of children to determine if the culprit is poison ivy.
- Remove the identified allergen.
- Administer sedatives if necessary to relieve discomfort during intense periods of pruritus.
- Treat present contact dermatitis with dressings wet with water, saline, or Burrow's solution to relieve itching.
- Educate parents on the use of calamine lotion and baths with oatmeal for itching.
- Teach parents how to apply corticosteroid creams to reduce itching and promote healing.

# DERMATITIS, DIAPER

### DESCRIPTION

- Diaper dermatitis is frequently referred to as diaper rash and is the result of prolonged skin contact with urine or feces.
- Diaper dermatitis can be avoided and its recurrence abolished by frequent diaper changes and with the

use of certain protective creams depending on the severity of the diaper rash.

- If diaper dermatitis is secondary to fungal infection, as represented by a shiny, red, beefy-looking rash with sharply defined edges and satellite papules, treatment should be with an antifungal medication, such as clotrimazole (Lotrimin) or nystatin.
- Good hand washing is essential to prevent the spread of *Candida* organisms because they are spread via direct contact.

### Assessment Findings
- Reddened skin and erythema
- Skin scaling
- Skin papules, vesicles, and ulcerations

### Nursing Implications
- Obtain a careful history from the parents to ascertain that the dermatitis is not from a new brand of detergent or disposable diaper.
- Instruct parents of children with mild diaper dermatitis to change the diaper after each voiding and bowel movement; gently clean the area with warm water and mild soap; and apply a water barrier ointment, such as petroleum jelly or zinc oxide.
- Instruct parents of children with moderate diaper dermatitis to keep the diaper area clean and dry with measures used for mild diaper dermatitis, apply hydrocortisone cream 3 times a day, and expose the diaper area to air for 30-minute periods.
- Instruct parents of children with severe diaper dermatitis to use the above-listed measures and also apply Neosporin G cream to the diaper area 3 times a day.
- Inform parents not to use disposable diapers or rubber pants with cloth diapers until the rash disappears.
- Instruct parents to prevent recurrence of diaper dermatitus by avoiding commercial diaper wipes, keeping diaper area clean and dry with frequent changes, and applying a water barrier ointment with each change.
- Treat diaper dermatitis secondary to *Candida* infection with antifungal cream.
- Instruct parents and day care workers on the importance of excellent hand washing technique after each diaper change to prevent spread of infection.

# DERMATOMYOSITIS

### DESCRIPTION

- Dermatomyositis is a disease of the connective tissue involving characteristic pruritic or eczematous inflammation of the skin.
- Dermatomyositis involves degeneration of skeletal muscle fibers.
- The cause of this disorder is not known.
- In 15% of the cases, the condition develops with an internal malignancy.
- Viral infection and antibacterial medication are associated with an increased incidence of dermatomyositis.
- The symptoms begin insidiously, and the child can no longer perform tasks that they could previously manage, such as competing in gym class.
- A muscle biopsy is done to confirm lack of electrical activity in muscle fibers.
- Treatment is aimed at increasing muscle strength, and corticosteroids may be used.
- Children who survive past 1 year have a good prognosis for prolonged remissions.

### ASSESSMENT FINDINGS

- Muscle weakness
- Swollen upper eyelids, confluent rash on cheeks
- Pruritus
- Subcutaneous calcifications (skin feels firm)
- Creatinine in urine (from muscle breakdown)

### NURSING IMPLICATIONS

- Assess the child for any changes in muscular performances.
- Explain to the child and parents about the disease process once diagnosis has been confirmed.
- Improve muscle strength with administration of corticosteroids and immunoglobulins.
- Explain all procedures and educate the child and parent about all medications administered.
- Honestly answer the child's and parents' questions regarding prognosis, with the aim being to maintain the child in remission.
- Support the child and parents throughout all phases of the disease process.

# DIABETES INSIPIDUS

**D**

## DESCRIPTION

- Diabetes insipidus refers to a disorder related to a decreased release of antidiuretic hormone (ADH) by the posterior pituitary gland.
- Less water is reabsorbed at the distal tubules of the kidneys, resulting in a great deal of fluid being lost from the body.
- Diabetes insipidus may be caused by genetic transmission; be the result of a lesion, tumor, or injury to the posterior pituitary; or be idiopathic.
- A rare form of diabetes insipidus results from adequate release of ADH; however, the kidney nephrons are not sensitive to the ADH.
- Diabetes insipidus usually presents gradually with a diagnosis made by a urine concentration test or a vasopressin administration test.

## ASSESSMENT FINDINGS

- Polydipsia
- Polyuria
- Urine specific gravity 1.001 to 1.005
- Bed wetting
- Weight loss
- *Dehydration*
- Computed tomography or x-ray film positive for lesion or tumor (possible)

## NURSING IMPLICATIONS

- Be alert to parental complaints of bed wetting in a previously toilet-trained child.
- Evaluate for any complaints of polyuria, polydipsia, or weight loss.
- Monitor for signs of dehydration that result from loss of large amounts of fluid.
- Educate the child and parents about the disorder of diabetes insipidus once diagnosis is confirmed.
- Follow up with appropriate diagnostic studies and client education about the cause.
- Prepare the child and parents for potential surgical removal of a causative tumor.
- Teach the child and parents about pharmacologic control of diabetes insipidus with intramuscular or intranasal administration of desmopressin (DDAVP).

- Assure that the parents and child understand proper route of administration, the action of the medication, and any potential side effects.
- Inform the parents that intranasal DDAVP is not effective if the child has an upper respiratory infection.
- Assess child and parental level of understanding in how to evaluate the effectiveness of treatment.
- With kidney resistance to ADH, inform the child and parents that excessive thirst can be relieved by lowering the child's take of sodium and protein and administering diuretics.

# DIABETES MELLITUS, INSULIN DEPENDENT (IDDM)

- IDDM is caused by an absolute or relative insulin deficiency or resistance.
- It is the most common endocrine disorder in children.
- The cause is multifactorial, including genetics and autoimmune and environmental factors.
- An autoimmune destruction of the islet cells of the pancreas occurs in predisposed persons.
- The lack of insulin causes glucose to remain in the blood stream leading to hyperglycemia.
- Compensatory mechanisms, such as the kidneys excreting excess urine, attempt to lower the serum glucose.
- The body breaks down fat for energy because it is unable to use the glucose as a source of energy.
- Untreated children are acidotic secondary to the buildup of ketone bodies in their blood from fat metabolism, dehydrated secondary to the polyuria, and electrolyte imbalanced secondary to the loss of electrolytes in urine.
- Disturbances in carbohydrate, protein, and fat metabolism occur.
- With the lack of necessary components to grow, the child is short in stature and underweight.
- Treatment of IDDM is aimed at controlling serum glucose with insulin therapy, dietary modifications, and exercise program.

### ASSESSMENT FINDINGS
- Polyuria
- Polydipsia

- Polyphagia
- Fasting blood glucose level above 120 mg/dl; random blood glucose level above 200 mg/dl
- Glucosuria
- Nocturnal enuresis
- Weight loss
- *Constipation*
- Fatigue and malaise
- Nausea, *vomiting*, and abdominal pain if acidotic
- Fruity breath odor if acidotic
- *Coma*

### Nursing Implications

- Explain at length and review frequently what the disease process implies once diagnosis is confirmed.
- Support the parents and child with newly diagnosed IDDM giving them time to understand the disease, and answer all questions they may have.
- Teach the parents and child about diabetes management.
- Keep in mind that restoring the child's blood glucose to normal is one of the initial nursing goals.
- Teach insulin therapy at length with follow-up education to ensure understanding.
- Evaluate parental and child insulin administration and technique.
- Teach the parents and child how to evaluate effectiveness of insulin therapy.
- Education on how to monitor and document blood glucose and urine ketones is necessary.
- Start a dietary management plan in conjunction with the family and a dietitian.
- Stress that the child should not eat concentrated carbohydrates, and suggest alternative sugar-free juices, candy, and jelly.
- Monitor the child's intake, and ensure that the child consumes snacks at prescribed times.
- Review exchange lists for meal planning with the child, allowing the child as much independence as possible.
- Teach the child and parents signs of hypoglycemia and hyperglycemia and appropriate treatments of each.
- Promote an atmosphere in which the parents and child feel free to ask questions.

- Assure that the parents and child understand the dangers and potential complications of IDDM as well as the related signs.
- Teach the child about the importance of exercise and how it relates to IDDM.
- Educate the parents why it is important to monitor blood glucose closely when the child becomes ill.
- Help the child and parents to live with a chronic disease.
- Provide the family with alternate support group information as well as American Diabetes Association information.

## DIARRHEA

### DESCRIPTION

- Diarrhea refers to the frequent passage of watery stools.
- The primary cause of diarrhea is bacterial or viral invasion of the gastrointestinal tract.
- Bacterial infectious diseases that cause diarrhea include *Salmonella,* shigellosis, and staphylococcal food poisoning.
- Diarrhea in infants is serious because they have limited extracellular fluid reserve and can quickly become dehydrated.
- Breast-feeding may actively prevent diarrhea, especially that caused by *Campylobacter Campylobacterjejuni.*
- Mild diarrhea occurs with a loss of 2.5% to 5% of body weight.
- Severe diarrhea in a child can cause a 5% to 15% loss of body weight quickly.
- Any child with a 10% body weight loss is very ill and needs hospitalization.
- Therapeutic management of diarrhea depends on the severity and includes fluid and electrolyte replacement.

### ASSESSMENT FINDINGS

- 2 to 10 loose watery bowel movements per day
- Fever of greater than 101°F
- Anorexia
- Irritability
- Dry mucous membranes
- Rapid pulse

- Warm skin
- Normal urine output

***Severe diarrhea***
- Loose green diarrhea every few minutes
- Explosive bowel movements
- Fever greater than 103°F
- Tachypnea
- Weak rapid pulse
- Cool skin
- Listlessness
- Lethargy
- Depressed fontanelle
- Sunken eyes
- Poor skin turgor
- Scanty urine output
- Concentrated urine specific gravity
- Elevated hemoglobin/hematocrit
- *Metabolic acidosis*

### NURSING IMPLICATIONS
- Evaluate any reports of diarrhea in infants and children reported by parents.
- Assess for signs and symptoms of *dehydration* and assess for weight loss.
- Encourage parents of infants that are breast-fed to continue breast-feeding.
- Recommend to parents that the child may need to rest the gastrointestinal tract for a short time.
- After 1 hour, the parents should begin to offer water or an oral rehydration solution such as Pedialyte in small amounts.
- Inform the parents that it is okay to treat any associated fever.
- Caution parents not to use over-the-counter antidiarrheal medication because it is usually too strong for infants and small children.
- Educate parents on the importance of washing hands after diaper changes to prevent spread of infection.
- Introduce lactose-free formula before the return of breast milk for the infant who develops lactose intolerance following diarrhea.
- Encourage parents of children with a greater than 10% body weight loss to admit the child into the hospital.

- Assess severity of *dehydration,* and replace fluids and electrolytes as prescribed to achieve balance.
- Obtain a stool culture to determine the causative organism.
- Determine a child's renal status before administration of potassium replacement.
- Promote hydration and comfort with intravenous fluids and by applying vaseline to dry lips and offering a pacifier.
- Maintain the child NPO (nothing by mouth) for the first several hours for a gastrointestinal rest.
- Offer clear oral fluids slowly in small amounts.
- Evaluate tolerance to oral intake.
- Gradually increase the diet, adding a soft diet and monitoring tolerance.
- Do not use a rectal thermometer on a child with diarrhea.
- Treat fever with antipyretics.
- Monitor fluid intake and output, and maintain patency of all intravenous lines.
- Assess for skin breakdown related to presence of diarrheal stool on skin.
- Change diapers frequently and wash area with soap and water.
- Cover diaper area with petroleum jelly (Vaseline) or A&D ointment.
- Encourage parental participation in care of the child, and support them and the child throughout the hospitalization.

## DIPHTHERIA

### DESCRIPTION

- Diphtheria is a communicable bacterial infection caused by *Corynebacterium diphtheriae* (bacillus), spread by direct or indirect contact.
- Diphtheria vaccine is included in routine *immunizations* for infants, and therefore this disease has been almost eradicated in the United States.
- When diphtheria is diagnosed, prompt treatment is necessary.
- The incubation period for diphtheria is 2 to 6 days.
- Diphtheria bacilli become infected by a virus and invade and grow in the nasopharynx of children, producing an exotoxin that causes massive cell necrosis and inflammation.

- The bacilli reproduce rapidly in this environment.
- The exotoxin is absorbed from the membrane surface and spread into the systemic circulation.
- Diphtheria can affect the heart, including myocarditis with congestive heart failure and conduction disturbances.
- The nervous system can be affected with severe neuritis and paralysis of the diaphragm and pharyngeal and laryngeal muscles.
- Airway obstruction from inflammation is a potential threat with diphtheria.
- The period of communicability for diphtheria is 2 to 4 weeks if untreated and 1 to 2 days if treated with antibiotics.
- Contracting diphtheria provides lifelong natural immunity.
- Diphtheria toxin, given as part of the DPT vaccine, provides active artificial immunity.
- Diphtheria antitoxin provides passive artificial immunity.
- Diagnosis of diphtheria is made by clinical appearance and on a throat culture.
- Treatment of diphtheria is with intravenous administration of antitoxin in large doses, antibiotics, and supportive care.
- The antitoxin is grown from a horse-serum base, and a skin or conjunctiva test is necessary to rule out allergic reaction before administration of an intravenous dose.

### Assessment Findings

- Gray membrane on the nasopharynx
- Purulent nasal discharge
- Brassy cough

### Nursing Implications

- Maintain accurate *immunization* records for all children.
- Teach parents the importance of updating a child's *immunizations* to avoid communicable diseases and their sequelae.
- Refer parents unable to afford *immunizations* to agencies that fund them.
- Administer DPT *immunizations* according to schedule unless contraindicated.

- Assess and document signs of potential diphtheria infection for prompt recognition and treatment.
- Administer skin or conjunctiva tests to rule out reaction to horse serum from the antitoxin.
- Be prepared to administer epinephrine for a sudden anaphylactic reaction to the horse serum.

- Administer antitoxin and antibiotics as prescribed.
- Maintain the child on bed rest during the acute stage of the illness.
- Observe pulmonary status carefully to prevent airway obstruction.
- Assist with *endotracheal intubation* if necessary.
- Monitor for potential complications related to diphtheria, including cardiac and neurologic complications.
- Advise parents of the importance of early treatment and communicability period.
- Evaluate any children with potential contact with the infected child for recognition and prompt treatment of the disease.

## DISSEMINATED INTRAVASCULAR COAGULATION (DIC)

### DESCRIPTION

- DIC is an acquired disorder of blood clotting.
- It is a paradoxic disorder with increased coagulation and a bleeding defect occurring at the same time.
- DIC may occur with trauma, sepsis, shock, or other underlying stimulus.
- In DIC, an imbalance occurs between clotting activity and fibrinolysis.
- Extreme clotting occurs initially, and clotting factors (platelet and fibrin) are depleted from the general circulation.
- A secondary coagulopathy occurs at the same time with fibrinolysis occurring.
- Fibrin degradation products inhibit the action of fibrin, and therefore decreased clotting occurs.
- Therapeutic management of DIC is to identify the cause; treat with replacement coagulation factors, red blood cells, and heparin; and halt the coagulopathic process.

### ASSESSMENT FINDINGS
- Bleeding from puncture sites
- Ecchymosis
- Petechiae
- Cyanotic or mottled cold extremities
- Neurologic symptoms (possible)
- Renal symptoms (possible)
- Decreased platelet count
- Prolonged prothrombin time and partial thromboplastin time
- Decreased fibrinogen
- Elevated fibrin split products

### NURSING IMPLICATIONS
- Observe all children with serious illness carefully for signs of increased bleeding.
- Educate the parents and child about the clotting disorder and ensure that they comprehend its paradoxic nature.
- Administer heparin for DIC to halt the coagulation process.
- Administer platelet, fresh frozen plasma, fibrinogen, or cryoprecipitate to restore clotting function.
- Evaluate for neurologic or renal system damage from brain or kidney vessel occlusions.
- Support the child's cardiovascular and pulmonary systems during the acute stages of DIC.
- Explain all procedures to the parents and child to allay their fears.
- Monitor the effectiveness of treatment by evaluating coagulation studies.

## DYSMENORRHEA

### DESCRIPTION
- Dysmenorrhea is painful menstruation.
- This pain is related to the release of prostaglandins (primarily $PGF_2$) in response to tissue destruction during the ischemic phase of the menstrual cycle.
- $PGF_2$ causes smooth muscle contraction in the uterus.
- Dysmenorrhea is classified as either primary, if it occurs in the absence of organic disease, or secondary, if it occurs as a result of organic disease.
- Dysmenorrhea can be a symptom of an underlying illness, such as pelvic inflammatory disease, uterine myomas, or endometriosis.

- Up to 80% of adolescents have discomfort with menstruation.
- 10% have discomfort that interferes with daily activities.

### ASSESSMENT FINDINGS

- Bloating and light cramping 24 hours before the onset of menses.
- Colicky sharp pain and cyclic pain, which is superimposed on a dull and nagging pain across the lower abdomen
- Aching or pulling sensation in the vulva and inner thighs
- Mild diarrhea with abdominal cramping
- Breast tenderness
- Nausea and *vomiting*
- Headache
- Facial flushing

### NURSING IMPLICATIONS

- Encourage verbalization of any problems with menstruation in the adolescent.
- Evaluate complaints of abdominal cramping in the adolescent.
- Suggest the oral intake of ibuprofen, which is a strong prostaglandin inhibitor, or aspirin for the relief of pain.
- Advise on alternate comfort measures, including decrease of sodium intake a few days before an expected period, use of abdominal breathing, application of heat to abdomen during menstruation, abdominal massage, or use of low-dose oral contraceptives to prevent ovulation if necessary.

## ENCEPHALITIS

### DESCRIPTION

- Encephalitis is inflammation of the brain tissue and possibly the meninges.
- The cause of encephalitis may be bacterial, viral, protozoan, or fungal.
- Enteroviruses are the most common cause followed by arboviruses.
- Many of the viruses are borne by mosquitoes.
- Encephalitis also can be the result of direct invasion of the cerebrospinal fluid during a lumbar puncture.

- Encephalitis also may occur as a complication of *measles, mumps,* or *chickenpox.*
- Initial complications related to encephalitis involve the cardiac, respiratory, and neurologic systems related to brain stem involvement.
- Encephalitis can cause residual neurologic defects after recovery.
- Complete recovery is possible; however, many children's health and abilities may be changed forever.

**ASSESSMENT FINDINGS** (symptoms may be gradual or sudden onset)

- Headache
- High temperature
- Nuchal rigidity
- Kernig's sign
- Ataxia
- Muscle weakness
- Paralysis
- Diplopia
- Confusion
- Irritability
- Lethargy
- *Coma*
- Cerebrospinal fluid with elevated leukocyte count and elevated protein and glucose levels
- Widespread cerebral involvement on electro-encephalogram (EEG)

**NURSING IMPLICATIONS**

- Educate parents on what encephalitis is, the seriousness of the disease, and the need to treat the cause quickly.
- Evaluate the child with encephalitis symptoms quickly so as to confirm and treat the disease promptly.
- Assist with a lumbar puncture, informing the child of all parts of the procedure and allowing the parent to be with the child as soon as possible.
- Administer antipyretics to control fever.
- Monitor vital signs frequently to assess for cardiac or pulmonary changes, which may be due to brain stem involvement.
- Evaluate for changes in ventilation, which may require *assisted ventilation.*

- Administer antibiotics if the causative organism is viral.
- Administer anticonvulsants to treat or as prophylaxis for *seizures.*
- Evaluate for neurologic changes or behavioral changes.
- Administer steroids to decrease brain edema and decrease intracranial pressure if indicated.
- Administer appropriate pharmacologic agents dependent on the cause of encephalitis.
- Support the parents through acceptance of this serious disease, and prepare them for the potential complications.
- Encourage the family to stay with the child, and prepare the child for all invasive and noninvasive procedures.
- Provide teaching regarding any discharge medications.
- Ensure that the child and family have a follow-up appointment to assess further for any neurologic deficits.
- Suggest follow-up care for the family after the hospitalization to help them deal with grief, shock, and anger, especially if the neurologic deficit is severe (*mental retardation*).
- Educate all parents and community health officials on the importance of monitoring any outbreaks of encephalitis.
- Suggest ways to prevent encephalopathy.
- Suggest mosquito repellents in endemic areas.
- Maintain aseptic technique during any invasive procedures, especially during lumbar punctures.
- Ensure that children receive routine *immunizations.*

## ENCEPHALOCELE

### DESCRIPTION

- An encephalocele is a cranial *meningocele* or *meningomyelocele.*
- This a *neural tube defect* that is characterized by a saclike cyst containing brain tissue, cerebrospinal fluid, and meninges, which protrudes through a congenital defect in the skull and is associated with brain defects.
- This defect may be visible at birth if not found during intrauterine life.
- This defect occurs in the occipital area of the skull or may be a nasal or nasopharyngeal defect.

- Encephalocele is generally covered fully by skin but may be open with the potential for infection.
- Encephalocele may or may not contain portions of the ventricular system.
- Tests are used to verify the actual size of the encephalocele and if it is a solid substance or fluid in the sac.
- Discovery of alpha-fetoprotein in amniotic fluid or maternal serum leads to further tests that can detect encephalocele.

### NURSING IMPLICATIONS

- Familiarize parents preparing to give birth to a child with a known *neural tube defect* as to what to expect.
- Prepare for a cesarean birth to protect the sac and avoid increased pressure and potential injury.
- Help parents who have unexpectedly given birth to a child with a *neural tube defect* to cope with the disorder and understand it.
- Assess the child born with an encephalocele closely and monitor as if high-risk infant until stable.
- Protect the sac from injury with proper positioning and devices.
- Educate the parents on the need for surgical closure of the defect if it is open to reduce the chance of infection.
- Caution the parents that the surgery is a risk in itself and will not change the already existing brain defects.
- Support the parents during the surgical procedure because it normally takes place within 24 hours of birth.
- Help the parents to absorb the realization of having a potentially disabled child.
- Give the parents time to ask questions and allow them to grieve for the loss of "healthy baby."
- Prepare the parents for potential complications of hydrocephalus or infection.
- Ensure adequate nutritional intake postoperatively.
- Evaluate on an ongoing basis the extent of mental and physical functioning in the child.
- Support the parents as they begin to care for their child.
- Refer the parents to associated organizations to maximize support to them.
- Ensure that the parents have a telephone number to call in case of emergency or questions.

# ENCOPRESIS, FUNCTIONAL

## DESCRIPTION

- Functional encopresis is the repeated passage of feces in places not culturally acceptable.
- This incontinence of stool is considered primary if the child was never fully toilet trained.
- This disorder is considered secondary if the problem occurs after toilet training had been effective.
- Functional encopresis is characterized as an emotional problem and may be a manifestation of a poor parent-child relationship.
- Stress is associated with functional encopresis.
- The stress may be a sibling's birth or visiting a strange house and fear of asking to use the bathroom.
- Functional encopresis may be secondary to extreme constipation in some children.
- This disorder leads to lowering of self-esteem and further stress on the parent-child relationship.

## NURSING IMPLICATIONS

- Document the number and type of bowel accidents a child has.
- Investigate any stress factors in a child's life.
- Evaluate the parent-child relationship.
- Perform a physical examination on the child, including a rectal examination to ensure proper anal sphincter control.
- Recommend that parents administer 1 to 6 tablespoons of mineral oil daily for 2 to 3 months if constipation and pain are occurring.
- Teach parents that if long-term mineral oil is necessary, the child will need supplemental water-soluble vitamins because they can be removed from the gastrointestinal tract with mineral oil.
- Encourage children to defecate in the morning before school to decrease the chance of encopresis at school.
- Educate the parents on the importance of not punishing a child for encopresis.
- Teach the parents to pay little attention to the bowel accidents and to give praise for days when encopresis does not occur.
- Refer the family and child to a family therapist for further evaluation if the problem continues so as to avoid low self-esteem in the child and to foster a healthy parent-child relationship.

# ENDOCARDITIS

## DESCRIPTION

- Endocarditis is the inflammation and infection of the endocardium or valves of the heart.
- This may occur with any child; however, it is more common as a complication of congenital heart disease.
- The infection associated with endocarditis is usually streptococcal, staphylococcal, or fungal in origin.
- The streptococcal infection can occur with dental work or *urinary tract infections.*
- Progression of the disease leads to valvular vegetation.
- Eventually the lining of the heart is destroyed, including underlying muscle and valves.
- The onset of endocarditis is typically insidious.
- Treatment is aimed at identification and treatment of the invading organism with antibiotics and supportive measures to reduce *congestive heart failure.*
- Prognosis is good.

## ASSESSMENT FINDINGS

- Pallor
- Anorexia
- Weight loss
- Arthralgia
- Malaise
- Chills
- Heart murmurs
- *Congestive heart failure*
- Petechiae of the conjunctiva or oral mucosa
- Hemorrhages of the fingernails or toenails
- Left upper quadrant pain secondary to spleen infarction
- Splenomegaly
- Proteinuria
- Hematuria
- Leukocytosis
- Increased sedimentation rate
- Positive blood cultures of invading organism
- Echocardiogram revealing vegetative growths on the heart valves

## NURSING IMPLICATIONS

- Evaluate all children with a known *congenital heart defect.*

- Prevent the incidents of endocarditis in this population with prophylactic use of antibiotics before invasive procedures, including dental work.
- Be alert to signs and symptoms of endocarditis in this population.
- Evaluate for any signs and symptoms, and refer to physician for further workup.
- Prepare the parent and child for the hospital experience, and support them in better understanding the disease process.
- Administer intravenous penicillin as prescribed to treat streptococcal infection.
- Discover and appropriately treat the invading organism.
- Monitor for serious *congestive heart failure*, and administer diuretics as prescribed.
- Maintain the child on bed rest during the acute stages to help rest the heart.
- Prepare the child for continued medical and possibly surgical intervention depending on the severity of damage caused by the endocarditis.
- Provide long-term follow-up care to be certain that the invading organism is completely eliminated and the disease is halted.
- Provide continued follow-up care to monitor the functional heart muscle.
- Support the parents and child throughout this difficult disorder and with the potential complications.

## ENDOTRACHEAL INTUBATION

### DESCRIPTION

- Endotracheal intubation is the placement of an endotracheal tube through the mouth or the nose through the larynx into the trachea.
- Endotracheal intubation is used to maintain a patent airway, prevent aspiration, allow tracheal suctioning, and administer positive pressure ventilation.
- Endotracheal intubation requires that the child (except for newborns) be lightly anesthetized.
- No sedation is used in the unconscious child.

### NURSING IMPLICATIONS

- Quickly prepare the child and parents if endotracheal intubation is emergent.

- Answer all questions and support the child and family when endotracheal intubation is planned.
- Assist with placement of the endotracheal tube.
- Auscultate breath and abdominal sounds to confirm placement.
- Continue to auscultate for bilateral breath sounds every 2 hours.
- Ensure that the endotracheal tube is taped in a secure position, and use a bite block for oral intubations if necessary.
- Record position of the endotracheal tube at tooth/lip line every shift to ensure maintenance of proper position.
- Keep in mind that during endotracheal intubation and while the child is intubated, the child is NPO (allowed nothing by mouth) and is unable to speak.
- Use a capnometer to monitor exhaled carbon dioxide.
- Suction the trachea as needed for removal of secretions.
- Monitor that the ventilatory mode, rate, tidal volume, positive end-expiratory pressure, and or pressure support are as prescribed and document.
- Ensure the endotracheal tube's patency and that it is securely taped at all times.
- Monitor vital signs, and evaluate for any changes.
- Turn the patient every 2 hours, and assess for skin integrity.
- Administer parenteral fluids and nutrition as prescribed.
- Record intake and output, and monitor for pulmonary overload.
- Tell the child everything that is being done and why it is being done.
- Provide emotional support to the child and the parents.
- Use restraints if necessary to protect the child from removing the endotracheal tube.
- Allow the child alternate methods of communication, such as writing.
- Encourage the parents to stay with the child and allay his or her fears.
- Tell the parents to bring the child's favorite stuffed animal or blanket to provide comfort.
- Explain the course on intubation with the parents and update them daily.

# ENURESIS

### DESCRIPTION

- Enuresis is the involuntary passage of urine.
- Most children with enuresis experience bed wetting.
- This occurs after the child has attained or is expected to attain bladder control, usually occurring at age 5 to 7 years old.
- Enuresis affects more boys than girls.
- Organic causes for enuresis are difficult to find; however, diagnostic testing may be done to rule out organic disease.
- Conditions that promote enuresis include a small bladder, immature neurologic control of the bladder, and children who are deep sleepers.
- Primary enuresis occurs if bladder training was never achieved.
- Acquired or secondary enuresis occurs if the bladder control was established but lost.
- Enuresis may be classified as functional or nocturnal.
- Functional enuresis is repeated involuntary or intentional urination, occurring during the day or at night.
- This occurs after children have attained or are at the age to attain bladder control.
- Functional enuresis occurs in 8% to 12% of children age 8 and younger.
- This disorder is found in girls more than boys and tends to be familial.
- The primary cause of functional enuresis is unknown; however, stress may play a factor.
- Functional enuresis is characterized as an emotional problem, contributing to a child's feelings of failure and low self-esteem and rejection by parents and peers.
- Nocturnal enuresis is involuntary urination that occurs at night during the deep stage IV of NREM sleep.
- It also occurs with the shift into a REM sleep pattern.
- Children with nocturnal enuresis at home also have it at the hospital.
- Bed wetting is associated with small bladder capacity but may be organic or secondary to family stressors or bladder or urinary tract infections.

- Parents can become frustrated with the constant laundering of bed linens.
- Management strategies vary but may include behavioral therapy, bladder-stretching therapies, drug therapy, and family and child support.

## NURSING IMPLICATIONS

- Investigate on admission to the hospital what the child's bowel and bladder habits are.
- Evaluate any complaints of enuresis in children.
- Document how often and how frequently during the day or night this occurs.
- Identify if the problem is primary or secondary enuresis.
- Obtain a clean-catch urine specimen to rule out bacteriuria.
- Evaluate urine specific gravity to rule out a defect in urine concentration.
- Prepare the parents and child for any diagnostic testing that must be done to rule out organic causes.
- Identify any predisposing stressors, and evaluate the family dynamics to rule out functional enuresis.
- Discuss the situation at length with the parents, and review current treatment recommendations.
- Encourage the parents to limit evening liquid intake and possibly to awaken the child during the night so as to avoid bed wetting.
- Involve the child in frank discussion of the enuresis.
- Caution the family to avoid punishing, embarrassing, shaming, or diapering the child.
- Discuss potential pharmacologic interventions, and educate the parents and child on prescribed medication and route of administration (e.g., intranasal ADH).
- Instruct the parents and child on bladder stretching exercises, which may be helpful in some children.
- If the child is experiencing functional enuresis:

    Obtain information on the parents and if functional enuresis existed in their childhood.
    Assess the level of stress in the family.
    Identify stress factors in a family with the family and the child.
    Offer the child a frank discussion of why these stress factors exist, and attempt to help the child cope better within the dynamics of the family.

Evaluate the effect of functional enuresis on the
whole family, and assess the child's self-esteem.
Recommend that evening liquids be eliminated.
Advise that the family and child see a family
therapist if the problem is ongoing.

# EOSINOPHILIA

## DESCRIPTION

- Eosinophilia refers to an increase in eosinophils,
  which constitute 1% to 3% of the white blood cells in
  the body.
- They increase in number with allergic disorders, such
  as *atopic dermatitis.*
- Eosinophilia also occurs with parasitic infections.

## NURSING IMPLICATIONS

- Determine the underlying cause for eosinophilia.
- Monitor laboratory studies for eosinophilia.
- Assess for worsening allergic reaction and need to as-
  sist medical interventions.
- Use appropriate nursing implications for related dis-
  ease processes.

# EPIDURAL HEMATOMA

## DESCRIPTION

- An epidural hematoma refers to bleeding into the
  space between the dura and the skull.
- This occurs with severe head trauma.
- Epidural hemorrhage is usually an arterial bleed, commonly a rupturing of the middle meningeal artery.
- Because it is arterial in nature, the bleed is intense and
  causes rapid brain compression.
- The child typically loses consciousness momentarily
  after the injury and after regaining consciousness may
  appear well for minutes to hours.
- The closer the symptoms occur to the time of injury,
  the more severe the epidural hematoma.
- Surgical intervention is necessary to reduce cortical
  pressure by removing the accumulated blood and to
  cauterize or ligate the torn artery.

## ASSESSMENT FINDINGS

### *Signs of cortical compression*

- *Vomiting*
- Loss of consciousness

- Headache
- *Seizures*
- Hemiparesis
- Unequal dilatation or constriction of the pupils
- Decorticate posturing
- Impaired respiratory and cardiovascular function

### Nursing Implications

- Be alert for symptoms of epidural hematoma with any *head trauma.*
- Refer changes in neurologic status to the physician immediately to ensure prompt treatment.
- Prepare the parents for the emergency surgical procedure and support them in understanding the need for immediate intervention.
- Monitor the child postoperatively for signs of rebleeding.
- Treat cerebral swelling and monitor for systemic alterations resulting from the cortical depression.
- Carefully monitor intake and output.
- Explain to the child what has occurred, and encourage the child to ask questions.
- Advocate that the parents stay in the hospital with the child to allay his or her fears.
- Treat any other associated traumatic injuries.
- Assess for any residual neurologic damage, and involve physical therapy and rehabilitation services in the child's care if necessary.
- Prepare the parents and the child for discharge and educate them regarding any discharge medications.
- Support the parents of the child with residual deficits or who died, and refer them to the appropriate services.

## EPIGLOTTITIS

### Description

- Epiglottitis is inflammation of the epiglottis most commonly seen in the child age 3 to 6 years.
- Although rare, epiglottitis creates an emergency situation because the swollen epiglottis prevents the airway from opening.
- The cause of epiglottitis is either bacterial or viral; *Haemophilus influenzae* type B is the most common bacterial cause.

- Echovirus and respiratory syncytial virus also cause epiglottitis.
- The child usually has a history of a mild upper respiratory infection.
- Inflammation spreads to the epiglottis, and severe symptoms develop.
- Inspection of the edematous epiglottis with a tongue blade can initiate the gag reflex, which can cause complete obstruction.

## ASSESSMENT FINDINGS

- Inspiratory stridor
- High fever
- Hoarseness
- Sore throat
- Difficulty swallowing with excessive drooling
- Cherry red, swollen epiglottis
- Leukocytosis

## NURSING IMPLICATIONS

- Evaluate all toddlers with epiglottitis symptoms.
- Obtain blood cultures for evaluation of septicemia.
- Maintain a patent airway and prepare for insertion of artificial airway if obstruction occurs.
- Prepare the parents and child if a *tracheotomy* or *endotracheal intubation* is necessary.
- Never initiate the gag reflex with children with symptoms of epiglottitis unless a means of providing an artificial airway is present.
- Keep the child as calm as possible to avoid precipitation of obstruction.
- Obtain lateral neck x-ray films to reveal enlarged epiglottis.
- Explain to the parents and child what epiglottitis is and how serious its manifestations can be.
- Accompany the child on all tests in case obstruction occurs.
- Administer moist air to reduce the epiglottal inflammation.
- Administer oxygen as prescribed if child is cyanotic.
- Prepare the parents and child for all procedures, and orient them to the hospital routine.
- Administer antibiotics intravenously as prescribed, such as cefuroxime or chloramphenicol.

- Administer intravenous fluids for hydration, and monitor intake and output.
- Support families throughout the hospital experience.
- Encourage the parents to stay with the child.
- Prepare the child and the parents for discharge, and educate them regarding any restrictions or medications.
- Recommend that parents receive counseling for the child that was not brought to the hospital soon enough and died from complete obstruction.

## EPISTAXIS

### DESCRIPTION

- Epistaxis, nosebleed, is extremely common in children.
- It can occur from trauma; lack of humidification; respiratory infection; after strenuous exercise; and in association with a number of systemic diseases, such as *rheumatic fever* and *measles*.
- Epistaxis can occur with nasal polyps, sinusitis, and *allergic rhinitis*.
- There is a familial predisposition to epistaxis.

### ASSESSMENT

- Visible bleeding
- Blood in nasopharynx
- Slight choking sensation

### NURSING IMPLICATIONS

- Keep the child with nosebleed in an upright position.
- Slightly tilt head forward to minimize the amount of blood pressure in nasal vessels and to keep blood moving forward not back into the nasopharynx.
- Apply pressure to the sides of the upper nose with your fingers.
- Calm the child because crying increases pressure in the blood vessels of the head and prolongs bleeding.
- If bleeding continues, apply epinephrine 1:1000 to constrict blood vessels and control bleeding as prescribed.
- Assess the need for a nasal pack.
- Investigate potential cause in the child who has chronic nosebleeds.
- Teach parents the importance of keeping the child in an upright position and to apply firm manual pressure for future nosebleeds.

# EXSTROPHY OF THE BLADDER

## DESCRIPTION

- Exstrophy of the bladder, a midline closure defect that occurs during the first 8 weeks of gestation, refers to the bladder lying open and exposed on the abdomen.
- This occurs more frequently in males than females.
- Treatment of exstrophy of the bladder is surgical closure of the bladder and anterior wall if possible.
- A second-stage operation may be necessary to create a urethra.
- Bladder removal may be necessary with continent urinary reservoir constructed if bladder tissue is limited.

## ASSESSMENT FINDINGS

- Absence of anterior bladder wall
- Absence of anterior skin covering on the lower abdomen
- Bright red bladder without ability to contain urine
- Forceful drainage of urine from the open bladder
- Unformed or malformed penis in males
- Pelvic bone defects
- Epispadias
- Excoriated skin around the exposed bladder

## NURSING IMPLICATIONS

- Monitor fetal ultrasonography results, which would reveal exstrophy of the bladder.
- Explain the implications of exstrophy of the bladder and that surgical correction is necessary.
- Help the parents to cope with this difficult diagnosis in their unborn child.
- Review anatomy with the parents so they understand which procedure may need to be done.
- Promote parental and newborn bonding.
- Cover the exposed bladder with sterile petroleum gauze to minimize infection and to protect the bladder surface from injury.
- Assess for skin integrity around the site of the bladder and treat preventively with A&D ointment to avoid breakdown and risk of infection.
- Prevent further separation of the symphysis by bringing the infant's legs together and applying an ace wrap.
- Place the diaper under the infant and do not separate the legs to apply the diaper.

- Promptly change all soiled diapers to avoid bladder contamination with feces.
- Position the infant on his or her side to allow the free flow of urine.
- Do not bathe the child in a tub to avoid risk of infection from water entering the ureters.
- Help parents learn how to care for the child, and support them through the process.
- Prepare the family for discharge home if the bladder repair is not going to be immediate, and provide follow-up care.
- Monitor children with exstrophy of the bladder as they begin to walk to detect a waddling gait, indicating pelvic bone defects.
- Maintain the incision line clean, dry, and free of infection after surgery.
- Administer analgesics and antispasmodics for bladder contractions, which occur the first few days after surgery.
- Assist with fitting the child with an external fixation device to prevent the nonfused pubic bone from separating and putting stress on the suture line.
- Prepare the parents and child to expect stress incontinence from the constructed urethra, after the second stage of the surgical repair.
- Depending on the surgical procedure, be aware that the child may need to learn to catheterize himself or herself.
- Help the child and parents adjust to a continent urinary reservoir.
- Prepare the child for exposure to this condition as he or she reaches school age.
- Assess the child's and adolescent's adjustment to the reservoir and the reservoir's functioning during follow-up appointments.
- Refer the child or parents who are having adjustment problems to a family or child psychologist.

## EXTREMITIES, CONGENITAL ANOMALIES OF

### DESCRIPTION

- Absent or malformed extremities is a physical developmental disorder.

- They are congenital bone defects that may result from drug ingestion during pregnancy, virus invasion during pregnancy, or amniotic band formation in utero, although in most instances, the cause of the anomaly cannot be established.
- Parents often feel devastated at the child's birth and search to discover the cause of the defect.
- Children with a congenital extremity loss do not grieve over the lost extremity as do adults or older children, which means that they are often better prepared to move on to rehabilitation.

## ASSESSMENT FINDINGS

- Missing or deformed extremities or part(s) of an extremity
- Possible positive pregnancy history for complications, such as drug ingestion or virus invasion

## NURSING IMPLICATIONS

- Obtain a thorough maternal history to identify any possible contributing factors.
- Assist parents to deal with the deformity; allow parents to grieve for the loss of the "perfect child."
- Introduce the parents to the rehabilitation team soon after birth to help them move past the helplessness they feel to more positive action.
- Provide information about the deformity, such as the arms that appear as seal flippers will not grow to be normal.
- Assist parents with decision making regarding corrective surgery (if this is an option) or prosthesis.
- Allow the parents and child to visit another child who uses a prosthesis.
- Introduce the prosthesis early to prevent a child from adjusting to a missing extremity, such as writing with the feet or sliding across the floor when walking.
- Help the parents to think of interesting activities to introduce so that the child uses the prosthesis rather than having the child feel like the prosthesis is only a ritual.
- Assist the child in mastering the use of the prosthesis and mastering a positive body image as a whole person.
- Arrange for supportive services, including home health care, community support groups, and agencies.

# FAILURE TO THRIVE (REACTIVE ATTACHMENT DISORDER)

### Description

- Failure to thrive refers to a syndrome in which the infant falls below the 3rd percentile for weight and height on standard growth charts.
- Organic causes of failure to thrive include cardiac disease.
- Nonorganic failure to thrive exists secondary to a disturbance in the parent-child relationship.
- Failure to thrive has both physical and emotional factors.
- Nonorganic and mixed failure to thrive are considered a form of child *neglect*.

  The parent in this situation has little emotional attachment to the child, and an accompanying lack of food may be present.

  Some children are offered the food but are too lethargic from emotional deprivation to take it.

  The child may become increasingly fussy and irritable, thereby further hindering a parental-infant bond.

  In some instances, the practitioner may find the attachment disorder began prenatally with an unwanted pregnancy or crisis during pregnancy.

- Management of the failure-to-thrive child is to ensure weight gain in the infant by placing him or her on a diet appropriate for his or her ideal weight.
- Severe failure to thrive must be treated aggressively to avoid permanent neurologic damage secondary to protein deficits and interference with brain metabolism.

### Assessment Findings

- Weight loss
- Motor and social developmental delays
- Poor muscle tone
- Lethargy
- Delayed or absent speech
- Diminished crying
- Distended abdomen from poor abdominal muscle tone

### Nursing Implications

- Identify mothers at high risk for poor parenting during pregnancy to provide careful follow-up postnatally.
- Seek optional care situations for the mother who needs "respite care" from the child.
- Provide consultation to a therapist to assist the mother with her feelings.
- Assess all infants and children against the standard growth chart at each health maintenance visit.
- Carefully evaluate any weight loss, assessing eating patterns and evaluating the parental-infant bond.
- Obtain a detailed history from the parents on the pregnancy.
- Determine if the cause for failure to thrive is organic or nonorganic with a complete health history and physical examination.
- Give parents support and education regarding the significance of weight loss and information about the disorder.
- Provide an age-appropriate diet with adequate calories for growth.
- Carefully record the child's intake and output, and weigh the child everyday.
- Assess stool pH for acidity, which indicates lack of absorption of carbohydrates.
- Evaluate the infant's ability to suck, and record any signs of gastrointestinal discomfort during or after eating.
- Limit the number of nurses caring for the infant; use one primary "mother" nurse to facilitate a nurturing relationship.
- Encourage a nurturing environment, and role model nurturing behavior.
- Advocate that the parents stay in the hospital with the child or visit frequently.
- Provide age-appropriate stimulation for the child.
- Evaluate if the child should be sent home or to foster care if *neglect* is suspected.
- Involve social services in the care of the family and child from the onset of hospitalization.
- Provide definitive follow-up for the family for several months to evaluate for a change toward a more posi-

tive infant-parent attachment and to maintain the gains made during the hospitalization.

# FIFTH DISEASE (ERYTHEMA INFECTIOSUM)

## DESCRIPTION

- Fifth disease is the fifth childhood exanthem, caused by parvovirus B19.
- The incubation period is 6 to 14 days with the period of communicability uncertain.
- The mode of transmission of this virus is by droplet.
- There is no immunity for fifth disease.
- Children affected are usually between 2 and 12 years old.
- The first symptom is a rash, which erupts in three stages.
- After the rash has faded, it may reappear if exposure to a skin irritant, such as sunlight, hot, or cold, occurs.
- There are no known complications of fifth disease.

## ASSESSMENT FINDINGS

- Intensely red facial rash
- Maculopapular lesions that coalesce on the cheeks to form a "slapped face" appearance, and fading in 1 to 40 days
- Rash on the extensor surfaces of the extremities 1 day after the facial rash appears
- Rash on the flexor surface and the trunk 1 day later
- Hand and trunk lesions lasting 1 or more weeks
- Lacelike rash appearance on fading (fades from the center outward)

## NURSING IMPLICATIONS

- Evaluate the skin rash and explain to the parents and child about fifth disease.
- Ensure that the parents and child understand the course of the disease.
- Reassure the parents and child that the disease does not have any known complications.
- Educate the parents on common comfort measures for rashes, including:
  Light clothing to avoid overheating.
  Adequate fluid intake to maintain hydration.
  Cutting child's fingernails to avoid injury from scratching.

Teaching child to press on area rather than scratch for itching.

Administering analgesics as needed.

Bathing child in lukewarm water with a few teaspoons of baking soda to sooth itching.

# FRACTURES

## DESCRIPTION

- A fracture is a break in the continuity or structure of bone.
- Children commonly have long bone fractures secondary to frequent falls in childhood.
- In fractures in children, bone bends rather than breaks because the bone is more porous.
- Epiphysial lines may cushion a blow so bone does not break.
- Healing occurs more rapidly in children secondary to overall increase in bone growth.
- A hematoma forms at the site of the break after a fracture has occurred; over several days, granulation tissue develops; over the next several weeks, osteoblasts invade the new tissue, and calcium is deposited to form new bone.
- When callus formation is extensive enough to inhibit movement at the fracture site, clinical healing or clinical union has occurred.
- Complete healing does not occur until all the temporary callus is replaced by mature bone cells and the bone has regained normal shape and contour.
- Several types of fractures exist:

  Comminuted—bone is broken into fragments.

  Compound—the bone is broken and piercing the skin.

  Compressed—one bone is forced or pressed against another.

  Displaced—the ends of the broken bone are not in good alignment for healing.

  Greenstick—an incomplete fracture with the periosteum divided only on one side (common in early childhood because of the resilience of immature bone).

  Pathologic—a fracture that occurs because of a bone defect, such as at the site of a bone neoplasm.

Simple—the fracture is straight and in good alignment.
Spiral—a fracture that results from a twisting motion.

- Fractures that occur at the epiphyseal line are always serious because they may affect bone growth.
- Compound fractures are usually the result of trauma and may cause serious injuries because of severed bone potentially lacerating nerves and blood vessels and from infection.
- Falls may cause compound or comminuted fractures.
- A number of complications are associated with traumatic fractures, including fat embolus, compartment syndrome, and interference with growth.
- Open reduction, a surgical technique, is used to stabilize, align, and repair the bone.
- Internal fixation devices may be necessary to stabilize the bone further.
- After open reduction, the area is usually casted to provide support.
- Forearm fractures usually occur from landing on an outstretched arm; in children, most fractured forearms involve the distal third of the arm.
- Volkmann's ischemic contracture is a vascular complication of casts that causes nerve injury or severe impairment of circulation.
- For fracture of the proximal third of the radius, the child should be admitted for observation of circulatory or nerve impairment.
- If compression is present and undetected within 6 hours, permanent damage to the arm results.
- Elbow fractures occur if a child falls and stops the fall with a hand, transmitting the force of the blow to the distal humerus and causing supracondylar fracture of the humerus.
- Clavicle fractures occur from a fall when the child's outstretched hand transmits the force of the blow to the clavicle.
- Clavicle fracture may also occur during birth, especially in infants with broad shoulders.
- Fractures of the femur occur from motor vehicle accidents or falls from considerable heights.
- Child *abuse* should be investigated in fractures of the femur in infants because few normal instances could cause this.

- Fractures of the femur can cause extensive blood loss because of the size of the bone broken.

#### ASSESSMENT FINDINGS
- Pain
- Swelling
- Deformity

#### NURSING IMPLICATIONS
- Splint the extremity of any child seen in the emergency department with symptoms of fracture to avoid further damage and to reduce pain and movement.
- Do not force a deformed extremity into a splint.
- Place sandbags on the sides of the deformed extremity to immobilize it.
- Investigate the cause of injury for any associated injury.
- Explore the family dynamics and establish if injury may be related to child *abuse.*
- Obtain an x-ray film to establish fracture and type.
- Administer antitetanus vaccine if child's skin has been broken.
- Establish an intravenous line for a child with a compound fracture with potential for other injury.
- Monitor for blood loss, and implement replacement therapy if necessary.
- Assess and treat pain with appropriate analgesic.
- Monitor for any signs of fracture complications.
- Treat the following types of fractures and educate the family appropriately:

Comminuted—prepare for open reduction to set the bone.

Compound—monitor for osteomyelitis from outside contamination.

Displaced—prepare the child for a pin or traction to approximate the break and allow healing.

Greenstick—(this fracture will heal quickly) prepare the child and the family for the potential need to break the bone completely before casting for alignment.

Pathologic—support the child through this complication of the major illness.

Simple—inform the family that healing time will be fairly short.

Spiral—prepare the family for the difficulty in bringing this type of fracture into good bone alignment for healing.

- For forearm fractures, anticipate using traction if necessary.
- Prepare to reduce and stabilize fractures of the humerus with an arm cast, a splint, or traction, depending on the position of the fracture.
- Carefully monitor for circulatory stasis so that Volkmann's contracture does not occur.
- Elevate casted extremity on a pillow or suspend the hand by a strip of gauze to reduce edema.
- Immobilize the arm of the newborn with a clavicle fracture against the chest.
- Reassure parents that clavicle splints are adequate therapy for fractured clavicles.
- Initiate traction in the fractured femur so as to ensure proper bone alignment before casting.
- Carefully assess for any signs of bleeding with fractured femurs.
- Use Bryant's traction for a child less than 2 years with a fractured femur.
- Use *skeletal traction* for the child over 2 years with a fractured femur.
- Treat painful muscle spasms with muscle relaxants and analgesics.
- Advise parents of the importance of keeping follow-up appointments, especially with epiphyseal separations so as to detect and treat abnormal bone growth promptly.
- Assist with the application of a cast when alignment is confirmed.
- Educate parents and children on cast care:
  Protect the cast and extremity from further injury.
  Keep the extremity elevated on a pillow for the first day.
  Do not touch the cast with anything but your palm until it is dry.
  Be alert for signs of swelling and circulatory compromise.
  Assess fingers or toes for color and warmth every 4 hours for the first 24 hours.
  Problem solve with the child the affects the cast will have on the child's daily life.
  Stress the importance of never putting anything in the cast.
  Blow cool air into the cast for itching.

Keep the cast dry.
Keep the follow-up appointment.
- Educate the family regarding any discharge instructions and medications.
- Reassure the parents and the child that the bone will heal.

# FRIEDREICH'S ATAXIA

## DESCRIPTION
- Friedreich's ataxia is an abnormal condition that causes progressive cerebellar and spinal cord dysfunction.
- The primary pathologic feature of the disease is pronounced sclerosis of the posterior columns of the spinal cord with possible involvement of the spinocerebellar tracts and the corticospinal tracts.
- This is an autosomal recessive hereditary disorder.
- Typically, symptoms occur in late adolescence.
- The characteristic gait with this disorder is caused by a high-arched foot, hammer toes, and *scoliosis.*
- All of the signs and symptoms are progressive.
- There is no curative treatment for Friedreich's ataxia.
- Treatment is palliative, and death occurs as a result of myocardial failure secondary to cardiac muscle fiber degeneration.

## ASSESSMENT FINDINGS
- Unsteady gait (ataxia) and stance
- Positive Babinski reflex
- Absent deep tendon reflexes
- Slurred speech
- Head tremors
- Tachycardia
- Cardiac failure
- Thoracic scoliosis

## NURSING IMPLICATIONS
- Observe for any associated signs and symptoms of Friedreich's ataxia at health maintenance visits of adolescents.
- Support the parents and child during education of the disorder once diagnosis is confirmed.
- Discuss potential corrective surgical options to maintain the child in an ambulatory state as long as possible.

- Examine the need for spinal fusion possibly to correct spinal scoliosis.
- Prepare the parents and the child for all tests, hospital admissions, and surgical procedures.
- Encourage the family to discuss their fears and concerns.
- Maintain the child as independent as possible, and openly discuss the occurrence of progression of the disease.
- Honestly discuss the course of the disorder, and encourage the family and the child to grieve over the child's loss of functioning and threat of death.

## FROSTBITE

### Description

- Frostbite is tissue injury that is caused by exposure to the freezing cold.
- The cells at the site of injury actually die.
- Cold exposure causes peripheral vasoconstriction; oxygen supply is eventually diminished leading to necrosis and cell death.
- Frostbite in children usually affects fingers and toes, occurring most frequently when skiing or snowmobiling for long periods with inadequate clothing.
- Frostbite of the buccal membrane occurs occasionally during the summer from popsicles and causes no permanent effects.

### Assessment Findings

#### *Extremity*

- White or erythematous area with edema
- Numbness in affected extremity
- Pain
- Necrosis
- Tissue sloughing

#### *Buccal membrane*

- Redness
- Edema
- Pain

### Nursing Implications

- Evaluate any potential exposure cases by careful history taking of actual trauma.
- Assess exposed area and warm it slowly.

- Administer analgesic as the area is rewarmed and extreme pain occurs.
- Apply a dressing to injured area to prevent secondary infection.
- Assess body temperature to evaluate for early signs of infection.
- Help the parents and child cope with the loss of any extremities.
- Assess the family dynamics, and rule out any potential signs of disturbance or potential *neglect.*
- Encourage follow-up appointments, and refer to counseling to adapt to the loss of a body part.
- Teach parents of children with buccal membrane frostbite to offer them soft foods for a day or two.
- Educate parents, children, teachers, and sports coaches on the dangers of environmental trauma and early symptom evaluation and detection.

## FURUNCULOSIS (BOILS)

### DESCRIPTION
- Furunculosis is an acute skin disease caused by staphylococci or streptococci.
- The furuncle is an infection of the hair follicle.
- The infection should run its self-limiting course without rupture of the lesions and further spread of infection.

### ASSESSMENT FINDINGS
- Localized redness
- Pain
- Edema of the surrounding skin
- Yellow pustule forming at the site of the hair follicle

### NURSING IMPLICATIONS
- Urge the child diagnosed with furunculosis not to scratch or pick the lesions so that the infection does not spread or become cellulitis.
- Educate the parents about the need to allow the infection to run its course.
- Teach parents ways to prevent the child from rupturing the lesions, such as cutting the child's nails and providing diversional activities.
- Inform the parents to administer analgesics for pain.

- Monitor for spread of the infection to surrounding area or signs of cellulitis.
- Ask the parents to inform the health care center if the child displays any signs of cellulitis or if the child develops a new-onset fever.
- Urge the parents and child to return to the health care center for follow-up appointment.

## GALACTOSEMIA

### DESCRIPTION

- Galactosemia, an inborn error of metabolism transmitted as an autosomal recessive trait, is a disorder of carbohydrate metabolism.
- The child born with this disorder is deficient in the liver enzyme galactose 1-phosphate uridyl transferase.
- Normally, lactose is broken down into galactose and glucose; galactose is further broken down into additional glucose.
- Without the enzyme galactose 1-phosphate uridyl transferase, the conversion of galactose into glucose does not occur.
- Galactose then builds up in the blood stream (galactosemia) and spills into the urine (galactosuria).
- Symptoms of galactosemia appear when the child is begun on formula or breast-feeding.
- Untreated the child may die by 3 days of age.
- Children who are untreated but do survive have *mental retardation* and bilateral *cataracts*.
- Treatment of galactosemia consists of using a galactose-free diet or formula made with mild substitutes.
- Symptoms of the disease do not progress once the child is regulated on this diet.
- The duration of the diet is controversial; however it should be maintained at least past 8 years of age.

### ASSESSMENT FINDINGS

- Lethargy
- Hypotonia
- *Diarrhea*
- *Vomiting*
- Enlarged liver
- *Cirrhosis*
- Jaundice

- Bilateral *cataracts*
- Death

**NURSING IMPLICATIONS**
- Suggest genetic testing preferably before pregnancy in any family suspected of being carriers of the trait.
- Support the parents through analysis of the infant's cord blood, the Beutler test, if the child is known to be at risk for the disorder.
- Provide close follow-up to newborns who are discharged early from the hospital.
- Note any feeding or absorption problems, and be alert for any of the assessment findings.
- Immediately refer the infant and parents for measurement of levels of the affected enzyme in the infant's red blood cells.
- Explain to the parents the pathogenesis of the metabolic disorder and the subsequent complications associated with it.
- Promptly substitute the infant's formula or breast milk with galactose-free formula, such as casein hydrolysates (Nutramigen).
- Assist the parents in understanding that any neurologic or *cataract* damage that has already occurred is irreversible.
- Support the parents in coping with the loss of function or the loss of the child if death occurs.
- Explain to the parents of the child who survives about the dietary restrictions that need to be maintained.

## GASTROSCHISIS

**DESCRIPTION**
- Gastroschisis, a congenital defect, is characterized by incomplete closure of the abdominal wall with protrusion of the viscera.
- This defect represents an arrest in the development of the abdominal cavity at weeks 7 to 10 during intrauterine life.
- The child may have accompanying defects if the cause was secondary to a teratogen insult preventing normal intestinal growth.
- This is a condition similar to *omphalocele.*
- With gastroschisis, the abdominal wall defect is a distance from the umbilicus; the abdominal organs are

not contained by peritoneal membrane but instead spill from the abdomen freely.

- A greater amount of the intestinal contents tends to herniate, increasing the potential for *volvulus* and *intestinal obstruction*.
- Children with this disorder have decreased bowel motility leading to problems with nutrient absorption and stool passage even after surgical correction.

### ASSESSMENT FINDINGS

- Detection of abnormality on ultrasonography
- Protrusion of abdominal viscera

### NURSING IMPLICATIONS

- Help to prepare the parents during the pregnancy and explain the defect to them, supporting them through exceptance of a "less than perfect baby."
- Assess for the obvious defect at birth.
- Establish goals with the parents in terms of realistic expectations.
- Prevent infection of the exposed contents, keeping them moist with sterile saline-soaked gauze.
- Insert a nasogastric tube to prevent intestinal obstruction.
- Plan appropriate treatment for the child in conjunction with the parents about complications.
- Anticipate parenteral nutrition, which is adequate for the newborn.
- Encourage the parents to participate in the care of the child.
- Monitor the child's temperature so that the child maintains sufficient temperature and does not become hypothermic from cold saline.
- Discuss the surgical repair necessary depending on the child.
- Promote healing after surgery, and discuss measures that the parents can take to treat the complications of nutrient malabsorption and difficulty passing stool.

## GENU VALGUM (KNOCK-KNEES)

### DESCRIPTION

- Genu valgum is a deformity in which the legs are curved inward so that the medial surfaces of the knees touch.
- The medial surface of the ankles is widely separated.

- This is seen most commonly in children 3 to 4 years of age.
- No treatment is necessary for genu valgum.
- The deformity tends to correct itself as the child grows.

### ASSESSMENT FINDINGS
- Knocked-knee appearance
- Widely separated ankles

### NURSING IMPLICATIONS
- Assess the severity of the deformity at regular health maintenance visits.
- Approximate the medial aspects of the knees, and measure the distance between the medial malleoli of the ankles.
- Inform the parents that the abnormality tends to correct itself by school age.
- Evaluate if the abnormality is becoming more pronounced or correcting itself.
- Refer the child getting worse to an orthopedist for further evaluation.

## GENU VARUM (BOWLEGS)

### DESCRIPTION
- Genu varum is a deformity in which one or both legs are bent outward at the knee.
- The medial surface of the knees is widely separated, and the malleoli of the ankles are touching.
- A number of children develop this condition as part of normal development.
- This is seen most commonly in 2-year-old children.
- No treatment is usually necessary for genu varum.
- The deformity tends to correct itself as the child grows.

### ASSESSMENT FINDINGS
- Bowlegged appearance
- Ankles touching

### NURSING IMPLICATIONS
- Record the extent of the bowing at regular health maintenance visits.
- Approximate the medial malleoli of the ankles, and measure the distance between the patellas.
- Inform the parents that the abnormality tends to correct itself by 2 years of age or at the latest by school age.

- Evaluate if the abnormality is becoming more pronounced or correcting itself.
- Refer the child to an orthopedist for further evaluation if the condition rapidly worsens or is not corrected by school age.

## GLAUCOMA, CONGENITAL

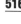

### DESCRIPTION

- Glaucoma refers to increased intraocular pressure in the eye globe because of inadequate or blocked drainage of aqueous humor.
- Congenital glaucoma is a developmental anomaly in the angle of the anterior chamber preventing proper drainage at the canal of Schlemm.
- This disorder, a rare condition caused by a recessive gene inheritance pattern occurring in about 1 in 30,000 live births, is usually bilateral in most infants.
- Congenital glaucoma accounts for vision impairment in 5% to 13% of children in schools for the visually impaired.
- The increased fluid content causes the globe of the eye to increase in size.
- Eventually the pressure in the eye globe continues to rise, compressing and destroying the optic nerve.
- Glaucoma, which means gray, gets its name from the color of the retinal or red reflex in the eye after the sight has been lost.
- A goniotomy, in which a new opening to the canal of Schlemm is constructed, is the surgical procedure required for congenital glaucoma; newer surgical techniques include laser surgery.
- Before surgical intervention, pharmacologic intervention with drugs that decrease aqueous humor may be used to reduce eye pressure temporarily.

### ASSESSMENT FINDINGS

- Enlarged, edematous, hazy cornea
- Tearing
- Pain
- Photophobia
- Tense eyeglobe on finger palpation
- Greater than 20 mm Hg eye pressure as measured by a tonometer

### NURSING IMPLICATIONS

- Regularly perform eye examinations on infants and children.
- Assess for congenital glaucoma in all infants.
- Aim to prevent the potential complications of congenital glaucoma through early recognition.
- Investigate for glaucoma in a newborn with a cornea measurement greater than 11 mm and in a 1-year-old with a cornea measurement greater than 12 mm.
- Assist with all measurements of eye pressure, and explain to the parents the potential need for anesthesia during this evaluation.
- Caution the child not to rub the eyes during the procedure if it is done under local anesthetic.
- Restrain an infant's arms to prevent eye rubbing for about 4 hours after an examination under local anesthetic to avoid corneal abrasion.
- Explain to parents why immediate surgery is necessary once diagnosis is confirmed.
- Discuss the surgical technique options, including laser surgery, with the parents.
- Manage the child's eye pressure temporarily before surgery with acetazolamide, which suppresses the formation of aqueous humor, or a miotic agent, which may increase aqueous humor drainage.
- Explain to parents that some infants may require 3 to 4 operations before the new opening for drainage of fluid is adequate to keep tension of the eye globe at a normal level.
- Do not administer any drugs (such as atropine sulfate) preoperatively that may dilate the child's pupil and potentially further occlude the canal of Schlemm.
- Place an eye patch over the operative eye postoperatively for protection.
- Maintain the child on bed rest to avoid any increases in intraocular pressure.
- Instruct the older child against any rough playing or contact sports for at least 2 weeks postoperatively to prevent potential increases in intraocular pressure.
- Support the parents and the child through the hospitalization, and encourage the parents to assist in caring for the child.

- Stress to parents the importance of follow-up visits to ensure the pressure within the eye globe is normal.

# GLOMERULONEPHRITIS, ACUTE POSTSTREPTOCOCCAL (APSG)

## DESCRIPTION

- APSG, the most common form of glomerulonephritis in children, is inflammation of the glomeruli of the kidney.
- APSG is an autoimmune disorder arising after an infection with untreated streptococcal pharyngitis.
- Group A beta-hemolytic bacteria are the most common causative organism.
- Damage occurs from a complement fixation reaction in the glomeruli activated by antigen-antibody reactions and obstruction of the glomeruli.
- Intravascular coagulation in minute renal vessels occurs.
- Ischemic damage leads to scar formation and decreases glomeruli formation.
- A reduction in the glomerular filtration rate leads to an accumulation of sodium and water.
- Increased glomeruli permeability secondary to inflammation leads to protein loss.
- APSG is generally self-limiting and resolves spontaneously within a few weeks.
- 2% of children do not completely recover from APSG but develop chronic nephritis.

**ASSESSMENT FINDINGS** (signs and symptoms of APSG occur 1 to 2 weeks after streptococcal infection)

- Sudden onset of hematuria
- Proteinuria
- Urine sediment with white blood cells; epithelial cells; and hyaline, granular, and red blood cell casts
- Oliguria
- Elevated urine specific gravity
- General malaise
- Anorexia
- Abdominal pain
- Weight gain
- *Hypertension*
- Headache
- Periorbital and peripheral edema

- Vomiting
- Low-grade fever
- If cardiac involvement occurs the child will have:
    Orthopnea
    Cardiac enlargement
    Enlarged liver
    Pulmonary edema
    Galloping heart rhythm
    T wave inversion
    PR interval prolongation
    Heart failure (may occur with extreme
        circulatory overload)
- Encephalopathy
- Cerebral symptoms
- Hypoalbuminemia secondary to massive
  proteinuria
- Low serum complement
- Mild anemia
- Elevated erythrocyte sedimentation rate
- Elevated blood urea nitrogen and creatinine levels
- Elevated antistreptolysin O (anti-DNase B) titer

## NURSING IMPLICATIONS

- Teach the parents and child about the disease and its
  progression, treatments and procedures to be performed, and their rationale.
- Offer support and guidance to parents, and explain
  that this is generally a self-limiting disease.
- With uncomplicated APSG, allow the child to engage
  in quiet play activities with gradual increase of level of
  activity.
- Monitor the child's cardiovascular and pulmonary
  status.
- Assess heart rate and respiratory rate and lung sounds
  every 4 hours.
- Evaluate the child's neurologic status and watch for
  increasing lethargy.
- To detect changes in fluid status, weigh the child
  everyday.
- Measure fluid intake and output.
- Monitor all signs of fluid status, such as edema.
- Prevent fluid retention by restricting dietary sodium.
- Maintain fluid restrictions secondary to oliguria.
- Treat accompanying complications of hypervolemia.

- Administer digoxin for cardiac decompensation.
- Administer antihypertensive medications as needed.
- Keep in mind that protein restriction may be necessary secondary to elevated blood urea nitrogen; however, a child losing large quantities of protein may need a high-protein diet. Most children do well on a normal diet.
- Administer antibiotics for active streptococcal infection.
- Position the child in a semi-Fowler's position if *congestive heart failure* occurs.
- Administer oxygen as prescribed.
- Limit competitive activity until kidney function has returned to normal.
- Be aware that proteinuria and impaired clearance of urea and creatinine may remain for as long as 2 months.
- Teach parents to be aware that increases in urine protein for 2 months do not indicate reinfection or the recurrence of the disease.
- Prepare parents for the small chance of APSG leading to a more chronic disease, and allow them to verbalize their fears and concerns.

## GLOMERULONEPHRITIS, BETA-HEMOLYTIC GROUP A STREPTOCOCCAL

### DESCRIPTION

- Glomerulonephritis (an inflammation of the glomeruli of the kidney) secondary to beta-hemolytic group A streptococci, is a rare disorder that occurs as a sequela to *scarlet fever* in only 2% to 3% of children.
- A reduction in the glomerular filtration rate leads to an accumulation of sodium and water; increased glomeruli permeability secondary to inflammation leads to protein loss.
- This occurs 1 to 3 weeks following the rash associated with *scarlet fever*.
- Beta-hemolytic group A streptococcus grows in children's bodies and produces a number of toxins.
- Erythrogenic toxin is the toxin responsible for the rash of *scarlet fever*.
- The occurrence of *acute glomerulonephritis* in children with *scarlet fever* is not related to the severity of the

*scarlet fever* but to the body's reaction to the toxins produced by the streptococci.

• There is no *immunization* available for *scarlet fever*.

**ASSESSMENT FINDINGS**

- Sudden onset of hematuria
- Proteinuria
- Oliguria
- Elevated urine specific gravity
- General malaise
- Anorexia
- Abdominal pain
- Weight gain
- *Hypertension*
- Headache
- Periorbital and peripheral edema
- *Vomiting*
- Low-grade fever
- Encephalopathy
- Signs and symptoms of heart failure (possible)
- Cerebral symptoms (possible)
- Hypoalbuminemia secondary to massive proteinuria
- Elevated erythrocyte sedimentation rate
- Elevated blood urea nitrogen and creatinine levels

**NURSING IMPLICATIONS**

- Stress to the parents the importance of giving the child a full course of antibiotic, usually a penicillin, for *scarlet fever* to prevent the complication of glomerulonephritis.
- Explain to the parents and child the potential for sequelae related to *scarlet fever*.
- Isolate the child for the first 24 hours of treatment for *scarlet fever* to prevent spread of infection.
- Be alert for signs and symptoms of glomerulonephritis 1 to 3 weeks after *scarlet fever* rash has occurred.
- Offer support and guidance to parents, and explain all treatments that the child requires.
- Monitor the child's cardiovascular and pulmonary status; assess heart rate and respiratory rate and lung sounds every 4 hours.
- Evaluate the child's neurologic status, and watch for increasing lethargy.

- To detect changes in fluid status, weigh the child everyday and measure fluid intake and output.
- Monitor for all signs of fluid status, such as edema.
- Prevent fluid retention by restricting dietary sodium.
- Maintain fluid restrictions secondary to oliguria.
- Treat accompanying complications of hypervolemia.
- Administer antihypertensive medications as needed.
- Keep in mind that protein restriction may be necessary secondary to elevated blood urea nitrogen; however, a child losing large quantities of protein may need a high-protein diet. Most children do well on a normal diet.
- Position child in a semi-Fowler's position if *congestive heart failure* occurs.
- Administer oxygen as prescribed.
- Limit competitive activity until kidney function has returned to normal.
- Keep in mind that proteinuria and impaired clearance of urea and creatinine may remain for as long as 2 months.
- Teach parents to be aware that increases in urine protein for 2 months do not indicate reinfection or the recurrence of the disease.
- Prepare parents for the small chance that the acute infection can become a chronic disease and allow them to verbalize their fears and concerns.

## GLOMERULONEPHRITIS, CHRONIC

### Description

- Chronic glomerulonephritis (chronic renal failure) is an irreversible disorder characterized by slow, progressive loss of renal function with nephron damage.
- This disorder is caused by anatomic abnormality, hereditary nephritis, or polycystic disease or may be idiopathic.
- It occasionally may follow *acute glomerulonephritis* or *nephrotic syndrome,* but it also occurs as a primary disease.
- Progression of the disease varies with the cause.
- Eventually, compensatory mechanisms fail, and chronic renal insufficiency or end-stage renal disease occurs.

- Treatment is aimed at symptomatic relief, with drugs such as hydralazine or diuretics to treat hypertension and corticosteroids to reduce inflammation.
- These patients have an increased susceptibility to infection, which is further aggravated when on corticosteroids.
- The prognosis is poor with the child eventually needing peritoneal dialysis, or hemodialysis to sustain life.
- Kidney transplantation is a viable option.

## ASSESSMENT FINDINGS
- Proteinuria
- Elevated blood urea nitrogen and serum creatinine
- Hyperphosphatemia
- *Hypocalcemia*
- Hyperkalemia
- *Metabolic acidosis*
- Edema with fluid and sodium retention
- Anemia
- Azotemia
- *Hypertension*
- Hematuria or oliguria

## NURSING IMPLICATIONS
- Refer any child found to have proteinuria on routine examination for further investigative workup.
- Educate the parents and the child regarding chronic glomerulonephritis, and support them in accepting this disease.
- Encourage the family to find alternative noncompetitive sports for the child who cannot engage in those activities.
- Promote the child's renal function by maintaining fluid and electrolyte balance.
- Monitor the child's weight daily and have the family notify the physician if greater than 2 kg weight gain in 1 day.
- Instruct the parents to keep track of urine output.
- Advise the family and child on dietary modifications that will be necessary; this may include a high-carbohydrate, moderate-fat, low-protein diet.
- Ensure adequate caloric intake.
- Teach the parents and child about vitamins and drugs necessary to limit effects of phosphorus and calcium

disturbances, such as vitamin D analogs and calcium supplements.
- Ensure that the family understands about all of the actions and potential side effects of drugs administered.
- Restrict sodium and fluid for a child with hypertension.
- Administer antihypertensives as prescribed, and evaluate family and child's understanding of the medications.
- Administer folic acid and iron supplements as prescribed for the anemic child.
- Explain the purpose and side effects of corticosteroid use, and help the child to accept the long-term side effects of this therapy.
- Monitor for and help the family to understand subtle signs of infection.
- Emphasize to the parents the importance of reporting the earliest signs of infection.
- Administer antibiotics as necessary, and adjust dose as prescribed according to renal function.
- Explain to the parents and child about different types of dialysis that may be required.
- Detect and manage complications of dialysis therapy.
- Support the family and child throughout this chronic disease.
- Honestly respond to questions regarding prognosis without renal transplantation.
- Help the family and child find ways to adapt to living with a chronic illness.

## GLUCOSE-6-PHOSPHATE DEHYDROGENASE (G6PD) DEFICIENCY

### DESCRIPTION
- G6PD is an inherited disorder characterized by red blood cells partially or completely deficient in G6PD, an enzyme critical in aerobic glycolysis and necessary for maintenance of red blood cell life.
- Lack of this enzyme results in destruction of red blood cells if the cells are exposed to an oxidant.
- Deficiency of the enzyme occurs most frequently in children of African, Asian, Sephardic Jewish, and Mediterranean descent.
- The disease is transmitted as a sex-linked recessive trait or on the genes of the X chromosome.

- G6PD deficiency may be diagnosed by a rapid enzyme screening test or electrophoretic analysis of red blood cells.
- Common forms of G6PD deficiency include congenital nonspherocytic hemolytic anemia and drug-induced G6PD deficiency.
- Congenital nonspherocytic hemolytic anemia causes hemolysis jaundice and splenomegaly and may cause aplastic crises.
- Drug-induced G6PD deficiency causes hemolysis approximately 2 days after exposure to fava beans or drugs such as antipyretics; it may cause fever and back pain, and Heinz bodies appear on blood smear; a newborn with the disorder may have marked hemolysis because the mother ingested an initiating drug during pregnancy.
- Drug-induced G6PD is self-limiting, and treatment with blood transfusions is rare.

### Nursing Implications

- Screen males of high-risk groups in infancy for this disorder.
- Tell both the parents and the child about the defect in the child's metabolism.
- Prepare the child and parents on how to live with this lifelong disorder.
- Educate the child and parents about how to avoid common drugs that may precipitate hemolysis.
- Provide parents with a list of the common drugs and foods to avoid, including acetylsalicylic acid, sulfonamides, antimalarials, baphthaquinolones, and fava beans.
- Teach the child and parents about the symptoms of hemolysis, and inform them to report these symptoms to their physician immediately.
- Administer transfusions if necessary, and monitor for any adverse reactions.

## GLYCOGEN STORAGE DISEASE

### Description

- Glycogen storage disease refers to a group of 13 genetically transmitted disorders characterized by altered production and use of glycogen.

- 12 of the disorders are inherited as autosomal recessive traits; 1 is a sex-linked disorder.
- Normally glycogen is stored in the liver as a reserve supply of glucose.
- The child with glycogen storage disease has glycogen deposited normally; however, an enzyme deficiency prevents retransformation of the glycogen back to glucose.
- The only source of readily available glucose is oral intake.
- Hypoglycemia can occur.
- The child's growth is stunted over time because there is not enough glucose for any function other than immediate energy.
- In one form of this disorder (type 11), glycogen is also stored in the muscle and the heart.
- With type 11 disorder, the child may have arrhythmias and usually dies of heart failure before reaching adulthood.
- There is a tendency toward *epistaxis* or hemorrhage in many affected children.
- Children with these disorders need to be maintained on a high-carbohydrate diet with snacks in between to prevent hypoglycemia.
- Liver transplantation may be a future answer for improving glucose regulation.

### Assessment Findings
- Hypoglycemia
- Brain damage if hypoglycemic episodes are severe
- Enlarged liver
- Protuberant abdomen
- Stunted growth

### Nursing Implications
- Assess for signs and symptoms of hypoglycemia.
- Take an in-depth history of the child's symptoms, diet history, and *growth and development.*
- Evaluate for the potential of these disorders, and explain the disorder to the parents and child.
- Teach the parents and child about glucose metabolism and liver function to help them understand about the disorder.
- Prepare the child for biopsy and chemical analysis to identify the missing enzyme and establish a definitive diagnosis.

- Begin teaching on necessary dietary modifications with the family and a dietitian.
- Stress the importance of avoiding hypoglycemic states.
- Teach the family about necessary continuous infusions of glucose via a nasogastric tube or gastrostomy feeding tube during the night to avoid hypoglycemia.
- Be aware that older children can use uncooked cornstarch in a water suspension every 6 hours to maintain serum glucose levels.
- Identify the specific disorder and any related complications, and honestly prepare the family for treatment of this chronic disorder.
- Monitor liver function tests for complications associated with a failing liver.
- Prepare the family for the potential for a needed liver transplant to control glucose metabolism, depending on the severity of the disorder.
- Ensure necessary follow-up to evaluate the child's dietary intake and progression of the disease and to monitor the child's *growth and development.*

## GROWTH AND DEVELOPMENT—INFANCY (1 MONTH–1 YEAR)

### DESCRIPTION

- Infancy is the period from 1 month to 1 year of age.
- Rapid growth and development occur during this period.
- The infant triples its birth weight and increases its length by 50%.
- Head circumference increases rapidly as the brain grows rapidly.
- All of the body systems continue to develop and grow during the first year:

  Cardiovascular: The heart becomes more efficient; the pulse and the blood pressure slightly increase.

  Hematologic: Physiologic anemia occurs but can easily be prevented, and fetal hemoglobin is converted to adult hemoglobin.

  Pulmonary: The respiratory rate slows, and the infant continues to be prone to *upper respiratory infections.*

  Gastrointestinal: The ability to digest food and mechanical action gradually mature during the first year.

  Hepatic: The liver remains immature.

Immune: This system becomes functional by 2 months of age with the infant able to produce both IgG and IgM antibodies by 1 year.

Renal: The kidneys remain immature and still are not very efficient in elimination of waste.

Endocrine: This system remains immature, and therefore the infant may not be able to react adequately to stress.

- The infant's ability to adjust to cold is mature by age 6 months.
- The first baby tooth usually erupts at age 6 months.
- The infant's developmental task, according to Erikson, is to acquire a sense of trust.

   Social relationships are initiated with attachment to primary caregivers.

   Proper stimulation, nutrition, and need gratification are essential during this period for an infant to trust and feel secure.

- Infancy is the stage of sensorimotor development, according to Piaget.

   Simple coordination is initiated to interact further with the infant's environment.

   The infant learns to engage others, solve problems, and manipulate the environment and gains motor ability.

- *Separation anxiety* comes full throttle during the 8th month; by 12 months, most children have overcome it.
- Object permanence begins at about 10 months.
- By 12 months, children are enjoying nursery rhymes and spending time with the family.
- Motor development control proceeds from head to trunk to lower extremities in progressive predictable sequence.
- By 3 months, the infant can reach for attractive objects in front of him or her, and can lift the head.
- By 4 months the infant brings his or her hands together and pulls at his or her clothes; the infant may begin to roll.
- By 5 months, the infant can accept an object handed to him or her or grasp it.
- By 6 months, the infant can hold an object in both hands, and the infant can sit leaning forward on hands.

- By 7 months, the infant can transfer a toy from hand to hand.
- By 10 months, the pincer grasp is evident; the child is sitting without support, creeps and crawls, and may be "cruising" from furniture to furniture.
- By 12 months, the infant can draw semistraight lines with a crayon, hold a cup and a spoon, and take socks off, and they may begin to stand unassisted and walk.
- During infancy, language development begins with cooing and crying and ends with the infant being able to say 2 words by 12 months.
- A range of devastating accidents can occur during infancy secondary to the infant's dependency.
- Accidents are the leading cause of death from 1 month to 24 years of age.
- Acute infections are the second cause of acute morbidity.

## Nursing Implications

- Facilitate an open environment for the parents to ask questions and receive anticipatory guidance.
- Encourage parents, especially first-time parents, to join clubs or network to help to increase their knowledge base and confidence level.
- Teach the parents about normal growth and developmental milestones, such as rolling and reaching for objects.
- Actively listen to the parents' concerns and provide guidance about infant care issues.
- Evaluate the infant according to the standardized schedule of evaluations and nutrition, growth, and development, and assess for any abnormalities or problems.
- Assess for effective breast-feeding and the maternal-infant bond.
- Ensure that the infant receives the first-year *immunizations.*
- Assess the family dynamics and for adequate stimulation of the infant.
- Examine the toys which the infant plays with and review the proper toys for each stage of infancy with the parents.
- Suggest that the parents spend a specific amount of time each night reading to the infant.

- Observe for any potential hearing or visual defects.
- Evaluate dental health every visit after teeth erupt.
- Assess for anemia, and do a lead screening at 9 months and tuberculosis testing at 12 months.
- Promote safety, and encourage the parents to become cognizant on preventive techniques to avoid aspiration, falls, motor vehicle injury, suffocation, drowning, animal bites, poisoning, and burns.
- Review the current recommendations for all safety and preventive measures with the parents and provide written literature to reinforce these.
- Examine the infant's environment and review childproofing measures.
- Address any specific parental concerns or problems related to normal infant development (i.e., teething, thumbsucking, use of pacifiers, head banging, sleep problems, *constipation*, loose stools, *colic*, spitting up, and *diaper dermatitis*).

# GROWTH AND DEVELOPMENT—TODDLER (1–3 YEARS)

### DESCRIPTION

- The toddler period is from age 1 to 3 years of age.
- The critical milestone during toddler development is being able to form two-word sentences by 2 years of age.
- The parental task during this period is to support the child's growing independence with patience and sensitivity.
- The parents must learn methods to handle effectively the child's frustrations that arise from the quest for autonomy.
- Physical growth slows in comparison to infancy, whereas developmentally the child makes great strides during this period.
- A child normally gains only 5 to 6 lbs per year and grows 5 inches per year during toddlerhood.
- Baby fat begins to disappear toward the end of the third year, and the child becomes leaner and more muscular.
- Head circumference becomes less than chest circumference by 2 years.
- The amount of sleep a child needs gradually decreases as they grow, with the norm being from 8 to 12 hours per day.

- Many toddlers are moved out of the crib during this period, and the parents need education about easing the adjustment.
- All body systems continue to mature during toddlerhood:

    Cardiovascular: The heart rate slows from 110 to 90 beats per minute and the blood pressure increases to about 99/64 mm Hg.

    Pulmonary: The respiratory rate slows slightly but continues to be mainly abdominal. The lumina of the pulmonary system increase in size, and the occurrence of lower respiratory system infections decreases.

    Gastrointestinal: Stomach capacity increases so that a child can eat 3 meals a day. Gastric juices increase in acidity, and gastrointestinal infections decrease. Anal sphincter control becomes possible.

    Immune: IgG and IgM antibody production becomes mature at 2 years of age, and passive immunity effects from intrauterine life are no longer operative.

    Renal: Urinary sphincter control becomes possible.

    Nervous system: The brain develops to about 90% of its adult size.

- Eight new teeth erupt during the second year of life, and all 20 deciduous teeth are generally present by 2 to 3 years of age.
- Erikson's developmental task during the toddler period is to form a sense of autonomy or independence versus shame or doubt.
- Parents view some of the independent behavior as being negative or difficult when really it is the parents misinterpreting the cues of positive expression of autonomy.
- Common concerns of parents during the toddler period are toilet training, ritualistic behavior, negativism, temper tantrums, discipline, and separation anxiety.
- Socialization is a major part of toddlerhood, and common routines are important to this population.
- A 15-month-old is still anxious to interact with people, but by 18 months, the toddler imitates what parents do, and by 2, the toddler recognizes gender differences.

- Play behavior during this period is side-by-side or parallel play.
- The toddler reaches 5th and 6th stages of Piaget's cognitive development, referred to as tertiary circular reaction stage and preoperational thought and assimilation.
- Child safety continues to be a concern with accidents being a major cause of death.
- Accidental ingestions, especially of cleaning products and prescription drugs, is not an uncommon occurrence.

### Nursing Implications

- Teach parents about the normal behaviors of toddlerhood, and encourage them to find healthy ways to cope with their child's frustrations.
- Plot the child's weight, height, and head circumference against standards to evaluate.
- Evaluate a child's dietary intake and ensure adequate nutrients.
- Evaluate all body systems and ensure normalcy of development.
- Evaluate dental health every visit, and teach parents appropriate care of teeth.
- Continue to maintain the child's *immunization* schedule according to current recommendations.
- Observe the parent-child relationship, and evaluate for any problems or health risks.
- Facilitate an open environment for the parents to ask questions and receive anticipatory guidance.
- Teach the parents about normal growth and developmental milestones of toddlerhood, such as language development and increased autonomy.
- Support the parent with their concerns during childhood, and educate them especially on appropriate responses with discipline and toilet training.
- Continue to promote toddler safety, screening for *lead poisoning*, and providing parents with information on poison and accident prevention.
- Ensure that the family has appropriately childproofed the house.
- Promote the toddler's independence by discussing issues around self-care, dressing, and eating with the parents.

- Promote autonomy in the toddler who is disabled or chronically ill by assisting the parents in creative planning.

# GROWTH AND DEVELOPMENT— PRESCHOOLER (3–5 YEARS)

## DESCRIPTION

- The preschool period is from 3 to 5 years of age.
- A major parental role during this time is to encourage the development of language.
- Physical growth slows dramatically during this period, with little weight gain.
- The child appears taller because their contour changes to more childlike proportions.
- Body systems continue to develop:
    Cardiovascular: Physiologic splitting of heart sounds may be present for the first time on auscultation. Nonpathologic heart murmurs may be heard owing to the changing size of the heart in reference to the thorax. Pulse rate decreases, and blood pressure holds at about 100/60 mm Hg.
    Immune: Lymphatic tissue begins to grow, particularly tonsils, and levels of IgG and IgA antibodies increase. Preschool illnesses tend to be more localized.
    Renal: The bladder remains palpable above the symphysis pubis, and voiding is frequent enough that play is interrupted and accidents may occur if the child becomes absorbed in an activity.
    Nervous system: At least 90% of brain growth is achieved.
- Children have all 20 of their deciduous teeth by age 3 and rarely do new teeth erupt during the preschool years. Deciduous teeth are generally present by 2 to 3 years of age.
- Gross motor, fine motor, and language development marks these years.
- Personality and cognitive growth is dramatic during this period.
- Erikson's developmental tasks for the preschool years include gaining a sense of initiative or learning how to do things.
    If children are criticized or punished for attempts at initiative, they develop a sense of guilt for wanting to try new activities.

The guilt developed during this period can create adults with difficulty making decisions.

- Freud explained the existence of the Oedipus complex and the Electra complex during these years.

    The Oedipus complex refers to the strong emotional attachment the preschool boy has to his mother.

    The Electra complex refers to the strong emotional attachment the preschool girl has to her father.

- Preschoolers determine right from wrong based on their parent's rules.
- Preschoolers usually have little understanding of the rationale for rules and therefore in a new situation have difficulty seeing how the same rules may apply.
- Preschoolers have some concept of religion and God and enjoy the rituals of the holidays.
- *Play* materials that stimulate creativity, such as modeling clay or colored markers, are ideal for this age group.
- Preschoolers' imaginations are keen, and they use imagination extensively in *play.*
- 4-year-olds divide their time between rough housing and imitative *play,* and imaginary friends often exist.
- *Play* for this age group is much more agreeable because they know how to share.
- By age 5, children develop "best friendships," perhaps based on who the child walks to school with.
- Language growth occurs, and the child asks many questions and is very concrete.
- Preschoolers are egocentric and have a difficult time seeing the other side of the problem.
- Preschoolers are still operating on a cognitive level.
- Promotion of childhood safety is essential for the preschooler because their imagination can lead them into dangerous situations.

### Nursing Implications

- Perform routine assessments obtaining both physical and developmental evaluations.
- Realize that preschoolers talk little during health assessments, and obtaining a detailed history of normal performance is necessary.
- Promote healthy family functioning, and educate parents about discipline, such as time-out for disciplining without extreme stress.
- Teach parents about the normal behaviors of preschoolers, and help them to separate those that the

preschooler can accomplish independently from those that still require some adult supervision.

- Assess the child's weight and height according to standard growth charts. Plot the child's weight, height, and head circumference against standards to evaluate.
- Evaluate a child's dietary intake and ensure adequate nutrients.
- Evaluate all body systems and ensure normalcy of development.
- Evaluate dental health every visit, monitor for cavities or dental complaints, and teach parents and children appropriate care of teeth.
- Continue to maintain the child's *immunization* schedule according to current recommendations.
- Observe the parent-child relationship and evaluate for any problems or health risks.
- Facilitate an open environment for the parents to ask questions and receive anticipatory guidance.
- Teach parents about normal growth and developmental milestones during the preschool years.
- Reassure parents that the Oedipal and Electra complex phenomena of competition and romance in preschoolers are normal.
- Help parents deal with their feelings of jealousy and anger, particularly if the child is vocal in expressing feelings toward that parent.
- Explain to parents the importance of exposure to the opposite gender so that the preschooler can become familiar with opposite gender roles.
- Support parents with their concerns during the preschool years, especially as related to "broken fluency," imaginary friends, difficulty sharing, and sibling rivalry.
- Educate parents on the importance of preparing a preschooler for the arrival of a sibling to help reduce sibling rivalry.
- Provide care for this age group that addresses and reduces the common fears of preschoolers (fear of the dark, mutilation, and abandonment).
- Provide good explanations to preschoolers on how procedures are done and how the procedures will benefit them in order for the preschoolers to agree to them.
- Educate parents on the importance of educating their child about potential threats:

Teach the child never to take rides from strangers.

Teach the child how and when to call 911.

Teach the child that a police officer is their friend, not their enemy.

Teach the child that if children or adults ask them to keep secrets, they should tell their parents.

Teach the child about his or her private parts and that only mom or dad during bath or the child himself or herself should be touching them.

Teach the child that it is always okay to talk to mom or dad about anything.

- Promote the child's independence by discussing issues around dressing, sleep, exercise, bathing, and care of teeth.
- Help the parent to begin to prepare the child for school.
- Promote special *play* times for the child who is disabled or chronically ill for stimulation and learning so that the child can begin to achieve a sense of initiative.

## GROWTH DEVELOPMENT—SCHOOL-AGE (6–12 YEARS)

### DESCRIPTION

- School age refers to children between 6 and 12 years old.
- Physical growth slows during this period, while cognitive and developmental growth proceed at a rapid rate.
- The annual average weight gain is 3 to 5 lbs, and increase in height is 1 to 2 inches.
- Deciduous teeth are lost and permanent teeth erupt during the school-age period.
- Posture becomes more erect.
- Brain growth is complete by age 10 years, and fine motor coordination becomes refined.
- Adult vision level is achieved.
- Immunoglobulins IgA and IgG reach adult levels, and there is a resultant abundance of tonsillar and adenoid tissue in the early school years.
- Frontal sinuses develop at age 6, and sinus-caused headaches become a possibility.
- The left ventricle of the heart enlarges to accommodate increasing cardiac requirements by the growing body.
- Innocent heart murmurs may be apparent secondary to the extra blood crossing the valves.

- The pulse rate decreases to 70 to 80 beats per minute, and the blood pressure rises to about 112/60 mm Hg.
- Increased ventilation perfusion allows for increases in exertion ability and stamina.
- Sexual maturation begins at age 10 to 14 with the hypothalamus transmitting an enzyme to the anterior pituitary gland to begin production of gonadotropic hormones, which activate changes in testes and ovaries.
- Changes in physical appearance can lead to problems and worries for both children and their parents.
- Changes in the sebaceous glands lead to acne.
- Vasomotor instability leads to blushing and perspiration increases.
- Girls begin puberty between ages 12 and 14, but it may start earlier.
- Girls are usually conscious of beginning breast development.
- Boys begin to have nocturnal emissions as seminal fluid is produced.
- Common health problems during this period are minor respiratory and gastrointestinal infections as well as dental caries and malocclusion.
- Gross motor development varies from the 6- to 12-year-old child.
- The 6-year-old child is in constant motion; the 8-year-old improves coordination; the 9-year-old does all activities with the "gang" and is on the go constantly; the 11-year-old is active but ungainly and awkward; and the 12-year-old's coordination improves, and the child is intense with concentrating on the activity.
- Fine motor development ranges from the 7-year-old "eraser year" to the older child beginning to evaluate his or her teachers' ability and performing at varying levels, with reading becoming a fulfilling activity.
- Psychosocial development varies greatly during these years as the child develops friendships, conquers insecurities, becomes awkward with members of the opposite sex, and develops a real sense of humor.
- Erikson's developmental task for the school-age child is to gain a sense of industry or of how to do things well.
    An important part of developing a sense of industry is learning how to solve problems.

- *Play* is initially rough at the beginning of school-age years and continues to be; however, it becomes interspersed with the "collecting period," reading as a quiet pastime, and expanding interest in music.
- Rules continue to be important as the school-age child forms "best friendships," becomes part of a social group, and continues to play hard.
- Common parental concerns during this period include language development; fears and anxieties; and behavior problems, such as stealing and use of drugs.
- Language development and cognitive growth are an important part of the school-age years.
- Cognitively the child ends the school years able to focus on others' views, adapt thought processes to fit what is perceived, appreciate that a change in shape does not necessarily mean a change in size, and understand that objects can belong to more than one classification.
- The school-age child begins to make truly independent judgments.
- The child is in the concrete stage of operational thought and may have limited understanding of concepts he or she actually sees.
- The school-age child thrives on set rules and becomes confused when the rules are changed unless good explanations are given.
- The school-age child is influenced by the attitudes of friends.
- 90% of school-age parents are dual-earner families, implying problems with latch-key children.
- Promotion of school-age safety to avoid accidents and addressing the use of recreational drugs are important issues during this period.
- A national health goal for this group is to increase to at least 30% the proportion of people age 6 and older engaging in regular, daily physical activity for at least 30 minutes per day.

### Nursing Implications

- Perform yearly health visits and address history, physical examination, school activities and progress, and behavioral issues or conflicts.
- Interview the child over 10 years of age at least in part without the parents.

- Show your awareness of and respect for the child's modesty by having the child use a cover gown.
- Evaluate all body systems and ensure normalcy of development.
- Ensure an adequate and nutritionally balanced diet of the school-age child by taking a detailed dietary intake history.
- Perform and evaluate yearly vision examination.
- Assess dental history and evaluate for malocclusion.
- Prepare the parents and the 10-year-old child for the beginning development of secondary sex characteristics.
- Advocate to parents the importance of their discussing sexual responsibility with children and the importance of reinforcing previous teaching.
- Inform girls of the potential beginning of vaginal secretions as part of the preparation for menstruation.
- Prepare boys for the common occurrence of nocturnal emissions, which begin as seminal fluid is produced.
- Address any parental concerns relevant during this period.
- Discuss safety issues with the parents and explain that school-age children do not always use common sense and still require adult supervision.
- Teach the parents and child points on how to avoid *sexual abuse:*

    Your body is your property.

    Secrets are fun; however, secrets about things that were done to you are not okay, and it is okay to tell about it.

    Do not go anywhere with a stranger.

    Do not be fooled by someone wanting to show you something.

    If you report someone that is touching your private parts and that person does not believe you, keep telling people until someone believes you.

- Promote development of school-age child daily activities and discuss dress, sleep, exercise, hygiene, and care of teeth with the parents and child.
- Openly discuss behavioral difficulties, including teaching on use of recreational drugs and discussing stealing.
- Counsel families on how to make the child who returns home before the parents feel safe and how this can be a positive experience.

- Use concrete examples to increase the level of health education teaching in this population.
- Address the needs of the chronically ill or disabled school-age child, including loss of school time and ways to achieve the growth and developmental tasks within the boundaries of the disability or illness.

## GROWTH AND DEVELOPMENT—ADOLESCENT (13 TO 18 YEARS)

### DESCRIPTION

- The major milestones of this period are the onset of puberty and cessation of body growth.
- Adolescent physiologic growth is rapid; the development of adult coordination is slow.
- Physical growth initially occurs with an increase in weight and later in height.
- Girls grow 2 to 8 inches and gain 15 to 55 pounds; they generally stop growing 3 years after menarche.
- Boys generally grow 4 to 12 inches and gain 15 to 65 pounds.
- The increase in body size does not occur in all organ systems at the same rate, which leads to a lack of coordination, possibly poor posture, and insufficient energy for various activities.
- Throughout adolescence, androgen stimulates sebaceous glands to extreme activity, resulting in acne.
- The apocrine sweat glands are formed shortly after puberty.
- Adolescents gain their second molars at about 13 years and their third molars between 18 and 21 years of age.
- Male secondary sex changes include body hair growth, increased size of sex organs, and voice changes.
- Female secondary sex changes include body hair growth, breast growth, and menstruation.
- Developmental milestones are achieved through sports, peer relationships, quiet alone time, part-time jobs, and inclusion in charitable activities.
- Erikson describes the emotional tasks of this time as:
  Accepting their changed body image.
  Establishing a value system.
  Making a career decision.
  Becoming emancipated from parents.
  Achieving a sense of intimacy.
- The final stage of cognitive development occurs and includes formal operations.

- Moral and spiritual development is included as part of the adolescent's identity and formation of his or her value system.

NURSING IMPLICATIONS
- Assess the adolescent's physical and emotional state.
- Urge parents to encourage involvement in sports for health, well-being, and companionship.
- Encourage communication between parents and the adolescent, and allow both time to ventilate concerns and frustrations.
- Use the J. M. Tanner scale for assessing sexual maturity.
- Support the adolescent and parents through changes experienced during this period.
- Encourage parents to acknowledge the importance of the adolescent's peer group and become acquainted with friends to promote open communications.
- Advise parents to give their child privacy and ignore moodiness.
- Advise parents and the adolescent on health-related matters, including nutrition, safety, and sexuality.

# GUILLAIN–BARRÉ SYNDROME (INFLAMMATORY POLYRADICULONEUROPATHY)

DESCRIPTION
- Guillain-Barré syndrome is a perplexing syndrome involving the motor and sensory portions of peripheral nerves.
- Inflammation of the nerve fibers causes temporary demyelinization of the nerve sheaths.
- 10% to 20% of children develop severe respiratory involvement, necessitating *assisted ventilation.*
- The course of Guillain-Barré syndrome is paralysis peaking at 3 weeks, followed by a gradual but slow recovery.
- Guillain-Barré syndrome affects both sexes and occurs most often in school-age children and adolescents.
- The cause of Guillain-Barré syndrome is not known, but an immune-medicated response following upper respiratory and gastrointestinal illnesses and *immunizations* is suspected.
- The aim of therapy for this disorder is supportive until the process runs its course.
- 95% of all children recover completely without any residual effects of the syndrome with conscientious nursing care that wards off complications.

### ASSESSMENT FINDINGS
- Peripheral neuritis several days after the primary infection
- Decreased or absent tendon reflexes
- Muscle paralysis and paresthesia beginning in the legs and ascending upward
- Cranial nerve involvement, such as facial weakness and difficulty swallowing
- Respiratory muscle involvement, including cessation of spontaneous respirations
- Elevated cerebrospinal fluid protein level
- Denervation and decreased nerve conduction velocity on electroencephalogram

### NURSING IMPLICATIONS
- Explore any complaints of peripheral neuritis, especially following upper respiratory infection, gastrointestinal infection, or *immunization.*
- Assist the family as the diagnosis of Guillain-Barré syndrome is confirmed through an understanding of the disorder, the testing, the course of the disease, and the prognosis.
- Administer prednisone to halt the autoimmune response as prescribed.
- Perform plasmapheresis or transfuse immune serum globulin potentially to shorten the course of the illness.
- Prepare the child and parents for the potential need for *assisted ventilation* to support the child through peak paralysis.
- Explain to the child before insertion of an indwelling urinary catheter that it is necessary to monitor urine output.
- Ensure adequate nutrition either parenterally or enterally.
- Administer an analgesic if the child has pain from the neuritis.
- Include the parents in the care of the child and encourage their participation.
- Prevent against all effects of immobilization, and prevent respiratory infection with meticulous nursing care.
- Prevent muscle contracture by performing passive range of motion every 4 hours.
- Turn, reposition, and inspect the child's skin every 2 hours.

- Provide adequate stimulation for the child during the long weeks of immobility.
- Encourage the parents to read to the child, and continually reassure the child and the parents that recovery will occur.

# HEARING IMPAIRMENT

## DESCRIPTION

- Hearing impairment refers to any condition in which there is an interference with sound transmission.
- Hearing impairment occurs in many different degrees and is rated by levels of severity.
- The usual classifications are as follows:

  Slight: Unable to hear whispered words, no speech impairment, achieves well in school by leaning forward and speaking loudly.

  Mild: Difficulty hearing if not facing speaker, beginning speech impairment, difficulty with normal conversation.

  Moderate: Difficulty with normal conversation, speech impairment present, and requires speech therapy.

  Severe: Difficulty with any but nearby loud noises, hears vowels better than consonants, requires speech therapy for clear speech.

  Profound: Hears almost no sound.

- 1 in 1000 children are profoundly hearing-impaired in the United States.
- 50% of severe hearing impairment is inherited.
- Congenital hearing impairment is transmitted by autosomal dominant inheritance.
- Prenatal *rubella* accounts for a large portion of the other percentage.
- Causes of slight hearing impairments are serous *otitis media,* trauma, and untreated *acute otitis media* with rupture of the tympanic membrane.
- Hearing impairment also can include hearing loss.
- Hearing loss is termed a conduction loss if there is interference with sound reaching the inner ear.
- Conduction loss occurs with difficulty with the external canal (obstruction with cerumen or a foreign object), the tympanic membrane (damaged or immobile), or the middle ear filled with fluid (serous *otitis media*).

- Hearing loss is termed nerve or sensorineural loss if the inner ear or the nerve is affected.
- Sensorineural loss occurs from disease that affects the transmission of sound sensation to the cerebral cortex.
- Sensorineural loss also occurs with pathology of the cochlea, a condition that is usually congenital in children but may be secondary to drug therapy, infection from an illness such as *meningitis,* or exposure to loud sounds.

## NURSING IMPLICATIONS

- Assess hearing and evaluate any signs of hearing impairment in the child that the parents may bring to the health visit.
- Refer the child with suspected hearing impairment to a specialist for evaluation.
- Encourage parents of children with congenital hearing impairments to enroll their children in special programs for the hearing-impaired as soon as the hearing loss is discovered.
- Educate parents that early exposure to speech and hearing therapy can assist the child in learning effective speech.
- Discuss the potential introduction of sign language with parents of hearing-impaired children to offer another option at communication from an early age, especially for the profoundly hearing-impaired.
- Advise parents of children with conductive losses that improvement can occur with the use of hearing aids.
- Assist children to become comfortable with hearing aids and to discuss any feelings of being self-conscious.
- Encourage a healthy view of needing the device by presenting it positively.
- Teach the parents and children use and care of the hearing aid.
- Educate parents of children with neural deafness that there is a difference between types of hearing loss and that nerve deafness does not improve with hearing aids.
- Examine the use of cochlear transplants with parents of children with neural deafness to replace the non-functioning inner ear.
- Inform parents that after transplant surgery, hearing is adequate but muffled.

- Educate parents that children who spoke with a speech impediment before surgery require speech therapy afterward to restore their speech pattern.
- Encourage parents with a child who has an inherited hearing impairment to seek genetic counseling to discover the chance of the same condition in siblings.
- Prepare parents who have one child with congenital hearing impairment that future siblings will probably also be impaired.

# HEMOLYTIC-UREMIC SYNDROME

## DESCRIPTION

- Hemolytic-uremic syndrome is a renal disorder that causes hemolytic anemia.
- Hemolytic-uremic syndrome is most common in white children from 6 months to 3 years.
- The cause of the syndrome is not known; however, it usually follows an infection, suggesting it is the result of an antigen-antibody reaction.
- The lining of the glomerular arterioles becomes inflamed, swollen, and occluded with particles of platelets and fibrin.
- Red blood cells and platelets continue to be damaged as they flow through the partially occluded blood vessels.
- The damaged cells return to the circulation and are destroyed by the spleen.
- This leads to hemolytic anemia.
- Treatment is with peritoneal dialysis for the oliguria and transfusions of red blood cells for the anemia.
- 95% of children with this syndrome heal completely, with the other 5% continuing to have chronic renal involvement.

## ASSESSMENT FINDINGS

- Oliguria
- Proteinuria
- Hematuria
- Urinary casts
- Lethargy
- Anorexia
- Pallor
- Easy bruising
- Increased creatinine and blood urea nitrogen

- Fibrin-split products in serum
- Thrombocytopenia
- Increased reticulocyte count

#### NURSING IMPLICATIONS

- Obtain a thorough history and physical examination to establish a baseline.
- Investigate all symptoms and refer to physician for continued care; carefully monitor all vital parameters, including vital signs and cardiovascular, pulmonary, gastrointestinal, urinary, and neurologic status.
- Educate the parents on the pathology of hemolytic-uremic syndrome.
- Inform parents that 95% of children with this syndrome recover completely.
- Administer fluid and transfusions of red blood cells if necessary.
- Answer all questions and prepare the parents and child for the invasive procedures required to initiate peritoneal dialysis.
- Support the parents and child through all procedures, and encourage them to ask questions and verbalize their fears.
- Encourage parents to assist in caring for the child and let them know it is good to hold the child even during the dialysis.
- Provide the parents with information about results of all procedures, as appropriate.
- Evaluate the child's progress and whether the child's renal function is improving.
- Provide the child with stimulating activities, such as a play board, while on dialysis.
- Prepare the parents and child for discharge by reviewing all medications and ensuring that they have a follow-up appointment.
- Assess the child's growth and development at subsequent health visits, and ensure that the family is viewing the child as well again.

## HEMOPHILIA A

#### DESCRIPTION

- Hemophilia A is the classic form of hemophilia, an inherited interference with blood coagulation, caused by deficiency of factor VIII, the antihemophilic factor.

- This form affects 1 in 1000 white males with severity of the disease dependent on varying levels of factor VIII.
- The female carrier has slightly lower levels of factor VIII but sufficient enough not to manifest a bleeding disorder.
- Factor VIII is an intrinsic factor of coagulation, and in deficient amounts thromboplastin formation is incomplete.
- The child's extrinsic coagulation remains intact, allowing eventual coagulation after an injury.
- This hemophilia may often reveal itself first with excessive bleeding after *circumcision.*
- Repeated bleeding into the joints can lead to hemarthrosis and result in severe loss of joint mobility.
- Severe gastrointestinal, peritoneal cavity, or central nervous system bleeding may occur.
- Even minor abrasions require administration of factor VIII to control bleeding.
- As with all hemophilia, this disorder has no cure, and prevention of symptoms is the goal of therapy.

### ASSESSMENT FINDINGS

- Prolonged bleeding
- Bruising, especially in lower extremities when child begins to walk and bump into things
- Painful swollen, warm joints, from soft tissue bleeding and hemorrhage into joints
- Gastrointestinal and central nervous system bleeding
- *Epistaxis*
- Whole blood clotting times prolonged or normal depending on level of factor VIII present
- Abnormal thromboplastin generation test
- Decreased partial thromboplastin time

### NURSING IMPLICATIONS

- Obtain a thorough history from the parents prenatally to screen for the possibility of this disorder.
- Observe all male infants carefully after *circumcision.*
- Note and evaluate any complaints or signs of bruising or painful joints.
- Evaluate the child for potential coagulation abnormality to assess which type of hemophilia is present.
- Ensure that the parents and child have an adequate understanding of the pathology of factor VIII disease.

- Ensure that the child and parents are evaluated for bleeding after any traumatic injury.
- Administer fresh whole blood, fresh frozen plasma, or cryoprecipitate to provide repletion of factor VIII, as prescribed.
- Administer plasma in no more than 30 minutes to maintain the potency of factor VIII at room temperature.
- As prescribed, administer epsilon aminocaproic acid, a fibrinolytic enzyme that stabilizes clot formation and promotes wound healing if antibodies to factor VIII develop.
- Consider administration of factor IX concentrate to halt bleeding if antibodies to factor VIII have developed.
- Assist parents and the child in adapting to the condition and the need for long-term monitoring.
- Teach parents and the child (over 10 years of age) how to self-administer replacement factor intravenously to prevent immediate bleeding after injury.
- Advise immobilization and ice packs to the injured area to halt bleeding and relieve pain.
- Help parents to cope with this frightening disease, and suggest support groups and organizations that would help.
- Institute preventive teaching for children who are known hemophiliacs:

    Teach parents and child prevention of injuries.

    Suggest safeguards for the house, such as removal of sharp objects and keeping chairs away from counters to prevent the child from climbing and falling.

    Pad crib sides for active infants.

    Advise supervision for outside *play*.

    Emphasize that contact sports are prohibited.

    Teach the child to use a soft toothbrush.

    Teach an adolescent to use an electric shaver versus a razor.

    Advise against taking any over the counter medications that contain aspirin or ibuprofen.

    Teach parents and child how to minimize active bleeding with firm pressure to site for 10 to 15 minutes, elevation of the injured area above the

level of the heart, and application of ice to area
for 24 hours.

Teach parents and child to assess for hidden signs
of bleeding, including joint pain and stiffness,
hematuria, black stools, severe headache, slurred
speech, and lethargy.

- Assess the child's self-esteem as related to living with a
chronic disease.
- Encourage the family to allow the child to lead a normal life with toys and bicycle riding.
- Promote independence to assist the school-age child
to monitor his or her own activities.

# HEMOPHILIA B, FACTOR IX DEFICIENCY (CHRISTMAS DISEASE)

### DESCRIPTION
- Christmas disease is a clotting disorder in which factor
IX is either defective or lacking.
- Dysfunctional or deficient clotting factors prevent
normal coagulation and cause inappropriate, pro-
longed bleeding.
- Christmas disease is transmitted by an X-linked reces-
sive inheritance pattern.
- Only 15% of hemophiliacs have this form.
- Christmas disease is treated with a concentrate of fac-
tor IX.

### ASSESSMENT FINDINGS (usually asymptomatic unless injury, trauma, or surgery occurs)
- Prolonged bleeding from any significant injury
- *Epistaxis*
- Abnormal partial thromboplastin time

### NURSING IMPLICATIONS
- Ensure that the parents and child have an adequate
understanding of the disease.
- Help the parents to cope with this frightening disease
and suggest support groups and organizations that
would help.
- Institute preventive teaching for children who are
known hemophiliacs:
  Teach parents home administration of factor IX.
  Teach parents and child about the need for
  preventing injuries.

> Suggest safeguards for the house, such as removal of sharp objects and keeping chairs away from counters to prevent the child from climbing and falling.
>
> Advise supervision for outside *play*.
>
> Emphasize that contact sports are prohibited.
>
> Teach the child to use a soft toothbrush.
>
> Teach the adolescent to use an electric shaver versus a razor.
>
> Advise against taking any over-the-counter medications that contain aspirin or ibuprofen.
>
> Teach the parents and the child how to minimize active bleeding with firm pressure to site for 10 to 15 minutes, elevation of the injured area above the level of the heart, and application of ice to area for 24 hours.
>
> Teach the parents and child to assess for hidden signs of bleeding, including joint pain and stiffness, hematuria, black stools, severe headache, slurred speech, and lethargy.

- Assess the child's self-esteem as related to living with a chronic disease.
- Provide potential alternative activities that could have a positive impact on the child's self-esteem.

## HEMOPHILIA C, FACTOR XI DEFICIENCY

### DESCRIPTION

- Hemophilia C, a clotting disorder, is genetically transmitted as an autosomal recessive trait and therefore occurs in both sexes.
- Plasma thromboplastin precursor is deficient secondary to factor XI deficiency.
- The symptoms associated with this hemophilia are mild compared with those children with factor VIII or IX deficiencies.
- Bleeding episodes are treated with the transfusion of fresh blood or plasma.
- As with all hemophilia, this disorder has no cure, and prevention of symptoms is the goal of therapy.

### ASSESSMENT FINDINGS (usually asymptomatic unless injury, trauma, or surgery occurs)

- *Epistaxis*
- Bruising

- Minor pain and joint stiffness with hemarthrosis—bleeding into the joints
- Spontaneous bleeding

**NURSING IMPLICATIONS**

- Ensure that the parents and child have an adequate understanding of the disease.
- Assist the parents and child in adapting to the condition and the need for long-term monitoring.
- Help the parents to cope with this frightening disease and suggest support groups and organizations that would help.
- Initiate preventive teaching for children who are known hemophiliacs:

   Teach parents and child prevention of injuries.

   Suggest safeguards for the house, such as removal of sharp objects and keeping chairs away from counters to prevent the child from climbing and falling.

   Advise supervision for outside *play*.

   Emphasize that contact sports are prohibited.

   Teach the child to use a soft toothbrush.

   Teach the adolescent to use an electric shaver versus a razor.

   Advise against taking any over-the-counter medications that contain aspirin or aspirin-like substances.

   Teach parents and child how to minimize active bleeding with firm pressure to site for 10 to 15 minutes, elevation of the injured area above the level of the heart, and application of ice to area for 24 hours.

   Teach parents and child to assess for hidden signs of bleeding, including joint pain and stiffness, hematuria, black stools, severe headache, slurred speech, and lethargy.

- Ensure that the child is evaluated for bleeding after any traumatic injury.
- Administer fresh blood or plasma if needed to treat spontaneous or traumatic bleeding.
- Assess for signs of transfusion reaction and treat appropriately.
- Evaluate all body systems for signs of bleeding, and ascertain that the child returns for a follow-up visit.

- Assess the child's self-esteem as related to living with a chronic disease.
- Provide potential alternative activities that could have a positive impact on the child's self-esteem.

## HEPATITIS A

### DESCRIPTION

- Hepatitis A (infectious hepatitis), an inflammation of the liver, is one type of hepatitis; it is caused by the hepatitis A virus.
- It has an incubation period of 25 days with a period of communicability digest during the 2 weeks preceding the onset of jaundice.
- It is transmitted by ingestion of fecally contaminated water or shellfish, sexual transmission from anal intercourse, or day care center spread from changing tables.
- Hepatitis A is highly contagious and affects children and overly crowded populations.
- One episode of hepatitis A provides lifetime immunity; passive artificial immunity is acquired through immune globulin.
- All types of hepatitis begin with an incubation period and are followed by three phases of the disease: the symptomatic preicteric phase, the symptomatic icteric phase, and the recovery phase.
- Although hepatitis specifically affects the liver, the entire body suffers from the infection.
- Liver cell destruction, leading to elevated liver enzyme levels, decreased albumin synthesis, and impaired bile formation and excretion, occurs.
- Hepatitis A virus usually leaves children without any long-term affects.

### ASSESSMENT FINDINGS (abrupt onset)

- Headache
- *Vomiting*
- Generalized aching
- Right upper quadrant pain
- Low-grade fever
- Sore throat
- Nasal discharge
- Irritability
- Pruritus
- Dark urine secondary to the excretion of bilirubin (3 to 7 days after onset of symptoms)

- Scleral jaundice
- Generalized jaundice
- White or gray stool
- Malaise, fatigue
- Anorexia
- Increased urine bilirubin
- Elevated liver enzymes
- Elevated serum bilirubin
- Elevated white blood count

## Nursing Implications

- Obtain a thorough history and physical examination to determine mode of, and therefore type of, hepatitis.
- Explain the disease process and likely course to the parents and child, and inform them that the child can be cared for at home.
- Teach the parents how the virus is transmitted and the importance of proper hand washing before meals and after toileting; instruct in proper disposal of feces because type A may be cultured from feces.
- Use universal precautions to prevent cross-contamination.
- Administer immune globulin as appropriate for people who may have contact with the specific virus.
- Insist that parents understand the importance of providing rest to the child for recovery.
- Review with parents the importance of maintaining an adequate dietary intake for the child.
- Obtain information from the child as to which foods in particular create nausea and avoid these foods if possible.
- Teach parents to provide mouth care before each meal to encourage eating.
- Inform parents that because children are usually hungrier in the morning, encourage a big breakfast.
- Teach parents how to manage the pruritus with tepid water baths with emollients.
- Discourage parents from using soap and hot showers.
- Encourage the child that must scratch to use his or her knuckles instead of fingernails.
- Educate parents regarding the complications of hepatitis, and make them aware of signs of hepatic coma (mental aberrations, changing level of consciousness).

- Insist that parents call the physician with any concerns regarding treatment as well as with any symptoms of a change in awake state.
- For the child in hepatic coma, administer lactulose to prevent absorption of ammonia in the colon or administer neomycin to decrease the production of ammonia by the intestinal bacteria.
- Inform parents of children cared for at home that the child cannot return to school until the jaundice has completely disappeared and the liver enzymes are no more than twice normal.
- Ensure adequate follow-up for the child and provide a home health care referral if necessary.
- Educate all health care professionals and high-risk populations to obtain passive immunity.

## HEPATITIS B

### DESCRIPTION

- Hepatitis B (serum hepatitis), an inflammation of the liver, is one type of hepatitis; it is caused by the hepatitis B virus.
- It has an incubation period of 120 days (on average) with a period of communicability from the later part of the incubation period and during the acute stage.
- Hepatitis B is spread via transfusion of contaminated blood and plasma or semen, accidental inoculation by a needle, or spread to the fetus during the third trimester if the mother is infected.
- Hepatitis B affects all age groups.
- Adolescents are at risk for hepatitis B following intimate contact or use of contaminated syringes for drug injection or contaminated ear piercing or tatooing.
- Hepatitis B has a high incidence in the Asian population and in immunosuppressed children.
- One episode of hepatitis B induces natural immunity for the specific virus; active artificial immunity is acquired through vaccine for the B virus; passive artificial immunity is acquired through specific hepatitis B immune serum globulin.
- All types of hepatitis begin with an incubation period and are followed by three phases of the disease: the symptomatic preicteric phase, the symptomatic icteric phase, and the recovery phase.

- Although hepatitis specifically affects the liver, the entire body suffers from the infection.
- Liver cell destruction, leading to elevated liver enzyme levels, decreased albumin synthesis, and impaired bile formation and excretion, occurs.
- For children with hepatitis B, 90% recover completely, whereas 10% develop chronic hepatitis and become hepatitis carriers.
- Infants who contract hepatitis B at birth have an increased risk of developing liver carcinoma later in life.

**ASSESSMENT FINDINGS** (abrupt onset)
- Headache
- *Vomiting*
- Generalized aching
- Right upper quadrant pain
- Low-grade fever
- Sore throat
- Nasal discharge
- Irritability
- Pruritus
- Dark urine secondary to the excretion of bilirubin (3 to 7 days after onset of symptoms)
- Scleral jaundice
- Generalized jaundice
- White or gray stool
- Malaise, fatigue
- Anorexia
- Increased urine bilirubin
- Elevated liver enzymes
- Elevated serum bilirubin
- Elevated white blood count

**NURSING IMPLICATIONS**
- Obtain a thorough history and physical examination to determine mode of, and therefore type of, hepatitis.
- Explain the disease process and likely course to the parents and the child, and inform them that the child can be cared for at home.
- Teach parents how the virus is transmitted and the importance of infection control measures.
- Use universal precautions to prevent cross-contamination; instruct staff, child, and parents in the proper disposal of needles and syringes.

- Administer hepatitis B immune globulin as appropriate for people who may have contact with the specific virus.
- Insist that parents understand the importance of providing rest to the child for recovery.
- Review with parents the importance of maintaining an adequate dietary intake for the child.
- Obtain information from the child as to which foods in particular create nausea and avoid these foods if possible.
- Teach parents to provide mouth care before each meal to encourage eating.
- Inform parents that because children are usually hungrier in the morning, encourage a big breakfast.
- Teach parents how to manage the pruritus with tepid water baths with emollients.
- Discourage parents from using soap and hot showers.
- Encourage the child that must scratch to use his or her knuckles instead of fingernails.
- Educate parents regarding the complications of hepatitis, and make them aware of signs of hepatic coma (mental aberrations, changing level of consciousness).
- Insist that parents call the physician with any concerns regarding treatment as well as with any symptoms of a change in awake state.
- For the child in hepatic coma, administer lactulose to prevent absorption of ammonia in the colon or administer neomycin to decrease the production of ammonia by the intestinal bacteria.
- Inform parents of children cared for at home that the child cannot return to school until the jaundice has completely disappeared and the liver enzymes are no more than twice normal.
- Ensure adequate follow-up for the child and provide a home health care referral if necessary.
- Educate all health care professionals and high-risk populations to obtain passive immunity.
- Screen all women during pregnancy for hepatitis B.

## HERNIA, DIAPHRAGMATIC

### DESCRIPTION

- A diaphragmatic hernia is a protrusion of an abdominal organ through a defect in the diaphragm into the chest cavity.

- The organ protruding is usually the stomach or intestine.
- The protrusion is usually through the left diaphragm displacing the heart to the right of the chest and collapsing the left lung.
- This defect can be detected during intrauterine life on ultrasonography, occurring in 1 in 3000 live births.
- The incidence of occurrence among males and females is the same.
- Normally during intrauterine life, the chest and abdominal cavity are one until week 8, when the diaphragm forms to separate them.
- If incomplete diaphragm growth occurs, the intestine or stomach herniates through the opening into the chest cavity.
- Correction in utero can be done to remove the bowel from the chest.
- Newborns with extensive diaphragmatic hernias have impaired pulmonary functioning from birth.
- These children are at risk for developing persistent pulmonary hypertension secondary to resistance of blood flow through the unexpanded lung.
- The heart is subsequently involved with right-to-left shunting through the *patent* foramen ovale or *ductus arteriosus.*
- The mortality rate of children with diaphragmatic hernias is 25% to 50%, with death secondary to an associated anomaly of the heart, lung, or intestine.
- The immediate goal of treatment is surgical repair of the diaphragm and replacement of the herniated intestine.

### ASSESSMENT FINDINGS
- Decreased breath sounds on at least one side
- Cyanosis
- Intercostal or subcostal retractions
- Sunken abdomen

### NURSING IMPLICATIONS
- Educate pregnant couples as to the positive results of an ultrasonogram revealing a diaphragmatic hernia.
- Discuss the potential for in utero surgical repair with a fetoscopy.
- Evaluate all options, keeping the couple fully informed and supporting their educated decision.

- Prepare the parents who opt to wait until after delivery for the potential respiratory problems their child will have as well as how the child may initially appear.
- Inform the parents of the importance of early surgical correction.
- Maintain the infant with the head elevated for easier breathing.
- Keep the infant with the compressed lung down for optimal expansion and aeration with the good lung.
- Place a nasogastric tube to decompress the herniated intestine and promote pulmonary function.
- Ensure that the pressure on the nasogastric tube is set low suction to avoid injury to the stomach lining.
- Educate the parents and support them through the surgical experience, encouraging their assistance in caring for the child.
- Provide the parents with information regarding the use of a synthetic patch if the defect is large.
- Provide the parents with information regarding potential complications of repair, including the removal of a hypoplastic lung, need for extracorporeal membrane oxygenation postoperatively, or the potential need to return for closure of the abdominal wound.
- Prepare the parents for the thoracic incision and the need for chest tubes postoperatively.
- Keep the infant in a semi-Fowler's position postoperatively to keep pressure of the replaced intestine off the repaired diaphragm.
- Keep the infant in a warm humidified environment to encourage lung fluid drainage; suction as necessary.
- Institute positive pressure ventilation to encourage lung expansion.
- Maintain $PO_2$ no greater than 100 mm Hg and $PCO_2$ at no lower than 30 to 35 mm Hg to prevent vasoconstriction of the arteries of the hypoplastic lung and increase lung function.
- Provide intravenous fluids for hydration postoperatively.
- Provide total parenteral nutrition postoperatively for 1 to 2 weeks to improve nutritional status.
- Bubble the infant well after feeding to reduce the amount of swallowed air and limit bowel expansion.
- Prepare the parents for the transition to home with the infant.

- Discuss appropriate care, and teach the parents about any discharge medications.
- Elicit any concerns the parents may have.
- Provide a home health care nurse visit if necessary as well as a phone number to call with any questions regarding the child's care.
- Ensure that the parents have a follow-up checkup scheduled.

# HERNIA, HIATAL

## DESCRIPTION

- A hiatal hernia is the intermittent protrusion of the stomach through the esophageal opening in the diaphragm.
- The volume of the stomach is suddenly restricted when this occurs, leading to periodic *vomiting*.
- Ultrasonography or barium swallow definitively diagnoses hiatal hernia.
- By 6 months if the condition has not corrected itself, surgery may be done to reduce the size of the esophageal opening in the diaphragm.

## ASSESSMENT FINDINGS

- Periodic *vomiting* accompanied by pain
- Shortness of breath if the lung is compressed by the herniated stomach

## NURSING IMPLICATIONS

- Educate the parents as to the pathology of hiatal hernia, and help them to understand associated symptoms.
- Keep the infant in an upright position to prevent reflux.
- Help the parents to understand the importance of maintaining the child in an upright position most of the day.
- Inform the parents that by 6 months if the hiatal hernia has not corrected itself, surgical correction may be necessary.
- Prepare the parents and child for the surgical procedure.
- Teach the parents how to monitor for any signs of infection postoperatively.
- Educate the parents on care of the child and medication teaching.

# HERNIA, INGUINAL

## DESCRIPTION

- An inguinal hernia is a protrusion of a section of the bowel into the inguinal ring.
- This occurs in males as the testes descend from the abdominal cavity into the scrotum late in fetal life.
- A fold of parietal peritoneum descends forming a tube from the abdomen to the scrotum.
- In most infants, this tube closes completely; however, failure to close causes a descent of the intestine into the inguinal ring whenever increased intra-abdominal pressure occurs.
- In female infants, an inguinal hernia may occur owing to a weakness of the muscle surrounding the round ligament.
- 60% of hernias are on the right side.
- Definitive diagnosis of inguinal hernias is with history and physical examination.
- Surgical correction is the treatment of choice and is done by sealing the inguinal ring after returning the bowel to the abdominal cavity.
- Surgical correction is recommended for the newborn before discharge or at 1 to 2 months of age.
- Pneumoperitoneum during surgery may be performed to reveal the presence of an enlarged inguinal ring on the opposite side and therefore need for surgical repair.
- Incarcerated inguinal hernias are a painful, emergent complication requiring immediate surgical intervention to prevent bowel obstruction or ischemia.

## ASSESSMENT FINDINGS

- Painless lump in the groin
- Lump apparent with crying secondary to an increase in abdominal pressure

## NURSING IMPLICATIONS

- Inform parents of the presence of an inguinal hernia in the newborn.
- Advise parents on the importance of early surgical intervention to avoid the serious complication of incarcerated bowel.
- Prepare the parents of the newborn for the surgical procedure and answer all of their questions supporting them through the entire experience.

- Allow the parents to hold, nurture, and care for the newborn as much as possible.
- Keep the suture line as dry as possible and free from urine to prevent infection.
- Use collodion to cover the incision instead of a dressing.
- Encourage the parents to provide frequent diaper changes and good diaper area care.
- Assess the incision and circulation in the leg on the side of the surgical repair to be certain that edema of the groin is not compressing vascular supply to the leg.
- Prepare the parents for care of the newborn at home, and teach them what signs of infection to monitor for.
- Answer all questions the parents may have before discharge to alleviate some of their concerns.
- Provide the parents with a follow-up surgical appointment.

## HERNIA, UMBILICAL

### DESCRIPTION
- An umbilical hernia is the protrusion of a portion of the intestine through the umbilical ring, the muscle, and fascia surrounding the umbilical cord.
- The bulging protrusion under the skin at the umbilicus is rarely noticeable at birth while the cord is still present.
- Umbilical hernias become noticeable at health care visits during the first year.
- Umbilical hernias are found most frequently in African-American children.
- They occur more often in girls than in boys.
- If the fascial ring is less than 2 cm in size, closure usually occurs spontaneously without needing to repair the defect surgically.
- If the fascial ring is greater than 2 cm in size, surgical repair is indicated.
- Surgical repair of the umbilical hernia is usually done close to school age.
- Home remedies for nonsurgical correction of umbilical hernias include taping a penny over it or taping the umbilical hernia.
- These remedies not only are ineffective, but also may cause bowel strangulation.

### ASSESSMENT FINDINGS

- Bulging protrusion under the skin at the umbilicus
- Varying size, usually 1 to 2 cm

### NURSING IMPLICATIONS

- Advise parents of children with umbilical hernias not to tape them or to put pennies over them in an attempt to reduce or correct them because it may be dangerous.
- Prepare the parents and the school-age child for ambulatory setting, surgical correction of the umbilical hernia if indicated.
- Use age-appropriate developmental preoperative teachings with the child.
- Inform the child that he or she may be groggy after surgery but that the parents will be allowed to see him or her as soon as possible.
- Allow the parents to be in the recovery room with the child if possible.
- Assess the pressure dressing for bleeding, and inform the parents to keep the pressure dressing on the area for 7 days.
- Administer a nonnarcotic analgesic if the child is having pain.
- Remind the parents to sponge bathe the child until the postoperative visit.
- Answer any questions the parents may have regarding the child's care.
- Encourage the parents to report any fever or other signs of infection to the physician.
- Ensure that the parents have a return follow-up visit for 1 week.

## HERPESVIRUS INFECTIONS

### DESCRIPTION

- Herpesvirus infections cause childhood infections of the skin, eyes, and genitalia (considered integumentary).
- Integumentary system infections with the herpesvirus are responsible for a number of infections in children.
- The causative agent is herpes simplex or herpes type 1 or type 2 virus.

- The incubation period is 2 to 12 days, with the period of greatest communicability earliest in the course of the infection.
- Direct contact is the mode of transmission.
- Immunity to primary herpes response is gained after one incident.
- No immunity exists for recurrent herpes infections because the virus lies dormant in the body until it is activated.
- The virus remains latent in the neurons of local sensory ganglia, and children become permanent carriers of herpes simplex.
- Activation of the dormant virus is by stress, sun exposure, fever, other illness, or menstruation.
- Acute herpetic gingivostomatitis is the most common form of herpes simplex in children, occurring in children 1 to 4 years of age.
    - This is an example of primary not recurrent response.
    - The disease runs its course in 5 to 7 days.
- Herpes simplex virus, herpes labialis, is better known as a cold sore or fever blister.
    - Herpes simplex virus represents the recurrent form of type 1 herpesvirus.
    - This remains dormant in the trigeminal or 5th cranial nerve.
    - Herpes simplex appears on the lip or skin surrounding the mouth.
- Acute herpetic vulvovaginitis, genital herpes, is caused by herpesvirus hominis type 2 (HSV-2), which remains dormant in the ganglia of the sacral nerves.
    - This is one of four similar herpesviruses: cytomegalovirus, Epstein-Barr, varicella zoster, and herpes type 1 and 2.
    - Genital herpes occurs in epidemic proportions in the United States, and its incidence is growing.
    - No known cure exists for acute herpetic vulvovaginitis.
    - This virus is a *sexually transmitted disease.*
    - Newborns infected by mothers with the virus can become systemically infected, and it can be fatal.
    - The incubation period is 3 to 14 days.

After the first exposure to the virus, extensive primary lesions occur.

The virus lingers in latent form after the primary stage.

Flare-ups with genital herpes occur during infection, premenstrual syndrome, fever, overexposure to sunlight, or stress.

A cesarean section is required if the mother has active genital herpes.

- Eczema herpeticum is a generalized reaction of a child with *atopic dermatitis* after contact with the herpes infection.

    Lesions associated with this may occur at different times during the course of the disease, which is 7 to 9 days.

    By day 10, eczema herpeticum lesions have crusted.

    Fluid loss from oozing vesicles can be severe.

    Depending on the extent of involvement with eczema herpeticum, the child may be gravely ill.

- Herpes *conjunctivitis* is from the herpes simplex virus and may occur along with development of a facial herpes lesion.

    Herpes *conjunctivitis* can spread easily and become a corneal infection with resultant opacity and permanent scarring.

- *Exanthem subitum (roseola infantum)* is a childhood rash caused by herpesvirus 6 (HSV-6).

- Herpes zoster is caused by the varicella zoster virus, the virus of *chickenpox.*

    After the episode of *chickenpox,* subsequent symptoms of herpes zoster may appear owing to reactivation of a latent virus or possibly owing to a second or third exposure.

    Herpes zoster tends to occur in older children but can occur in infants.

### Assessment Findings

#### *Acute herpetic gingivostomatitis*

- High fever—104°F
- Restlessness
- Anorexia
- Sore mouth
- Swollen, red gumline that bleeds easily

- White plaques or shallow ulcers with red areolae on the buccal mucosa, tongue, palate, and tonsillar fauces
- Enlarged, tender anterior cervical lymph nodes

***Herpes simplex virus***
- Painful, grouped vesicles
- Crusting after 2 to 3 days

***Acute herpetic vulvovaginitis (genital herpes)***
- Pinpoint vesicles on an erythematous base, ulcerating and becoming moist, draining open lesions
- Flulike symptoms with first exposure
- Vaginal discharge
- Intense pain with any contact with clothing or acid urine

***Eczema herpeticum***
- Painful, oozing, lesions

***Herpes conjunctivitis***
- Pinpoint vesicles on the conjunctiva

***Exanthem subitum (roseola infantum)***
- High fever
- Irritable
- Anorexia
- Slightly inflamed pharynx
- Enlargement of occipital, cervical, and postauricular lymph nodes

***Herpes zoster***
- Pruritus

**NURSING IMPLICATIONS**
- Address all herpes infections with the parents and explain to them the viral and dormant nature of the disease.
- Administer topical acyclovir to reduce pain and increase healing on the blisters associated with herpes simplex virus.
- For *acute herpetic gingivostomatitis:*
    Administer antipyretics to reduce fever.
    Apply local anesthetic to lesions to relieve pain (ensure that the child does not swallow this).
    Administer soft acid-free food.
    Monitor for signs of *dehydration* because intake can be poor.
- For *genital herpes* infection:

Administer acyclovir to destroy the herpes 2 virus of acute herpetic vulvovaginitis (genital herpes).

Encourage clients with this to take soothing sitz baths 3 times a day.

Inform an adolescent with genital herpes of the pathology of the disease.

Inform the female adolescent of the increased incidence of cervical cancer associated with genital herpes and the need to follow up with Pap smears.

Provide the adolescent with information on this *sexually transmitted disease*, and educate him or her on prevention and use of condoms.

Question any parent of a child with genital herpes about *sexual abuse*.

Report any child with genital herpes to the department of human services to evaluate fully the child's home environment and potential of child *abuse*.

- For *eczema herpeticum:*

  Inform parents of children with infantile eczema of the risk associated with herpetic exposure, eczema herpeticum, in this population.

  Assess eczema herpeticum lesions, and evaluate the child's level of hydration.

  Treat the pain associated with eczema herpeticum.

- For **herpes conjunctivitis:**

  Treat with idoxuridine or trifluorothymidine, drugs specific to herpesvirus to limit corneal involvement.

  Withhold all steroids in treatment of herpes conjunctivitis.

- For **roseola infantum:**

  Provide symptomatic relief of rash discomfort and fever.

- For **herpes zoster:**

  Provide symptomatic relief of associated itching.

  Administer acyclovir to limit herpes zoster.

  Administer varicella zoster immune globulin to minimize the symptoms of herpes zoster.

# HIP DYSPLASIA

### DESCRIPTION

- Developmental hip dysplasia is improper formation and function of the hip socket.
- It may be evident as subluxation or dislocation of the head of the femur.
- The cause of the defect is unknown, but it may be from a polygenic inheritance pattern or from uterine position.
- Hip dysplasia is found in females more requently than in males.
- It is usually of unilateral development.
- Hip dysplasia occurs most often in children of Mediterranean ancestry.
- Hip dysplasia is difficult to detect at birth in an infant who delivered from a footling or frank breech presentation because the knees are stiff and do not flex readily.
- Early recognition in newborns is necessary for proper correction to occur.
- Some newborns may have proper hip abduction at birth, but by age 4 to 6 weeks a secondary shortening of the adductor muscles occurs and the defect becomes evident.
- Therapeutic management to correct subluxated and dislocated hips involves positioning the hip into a flexed, abducted (externally rotated) position to press the femur head against the acetabulum and deepen its contour by pressure.
- Splints, halters, or casts may be used to treat the hip dysplasia.
- Often splint correction to rotate the legs externally is begun during the newborn's initial hospital stay by placing 2 to 3 diapers on the infant.
- Some children require surgery and a pin inserted to stabilize the hip.

### ASSESSMENT FINDINGS

- One leg shorter than the other
- One knee appearing lower than the other when the thighs are flexed to a 90 degree angle toward the abdomen

- Increased number of skin folds present on the posterior thighs
- Inability of affected hip to abduct fully because the femoral head cannot rotate fully
- Ortolani's sign
- Barlow's sign
- X-ray study or ultrasonography revealing shallow acetabulum and a more lateral placement of the femur head than normal

### Nursing Implications

- Examine all newborns and follow up at well-baby visits to evaluate for hip dysplasia.
- Once hip dysplasia is confirmed, explain the deformity to the parents and the need to initiate the treatment proposed right away.
- Ensure that the parents are comfortable in holding their infant before discharge and familiar with how to use the splinting technique recommended.
- Inform parents that swaddling the newborn and thereby bringing the legs together should be avoided.
- Tell parents from the beginning that the double diapering may not work and prepare them for the other potential devices.
- Spend time with the parents and teach them how to stimulate their child.
- Assess the parent-child bond at each health care visit.
- Monitor for diaper rash with the Frejka splint if used and teach the parents to wash the infant with water after every voiding or defecation and apply an ointment to protect the skin from irritation.
- Teach the parents that the Frejka splint must be kept in place at all times.
- Provide the parents with a telephone number for any questions that they may have regarding the application of the splint.
- Teach parents how to use the Pavik harness and about the need to be worn continually.
- Teach the parents to assess the skin under the straps daily for irritation or redness.
- Teach parents of children with severe hip dysplasia that their child will need to be placed in a Spica cast.

- Inform the parents of the importance of evaluating and how to evaluate the neurocirculation of their child's extremities.
- Apprise parents that although the cast will be changed as the child grows, the child will need to have it on for 6 to 9 months.
- Assure parents that once the cast is removed, the child will quickly catch up to this developmental level of physical mobility.
- Prepare the parents of the child not successfully treated with splints or cast that surgical intervention is necessary to stabilize the hip with the insertion of pins.
- Support and prepare the parents and child for the surgical procedure.

# HIRSCHSPRUNG'S DISEASE (AGANGLIONIC MEGACOLON)

## DESCRIPTION

- Hirschsprung's disease, aganglionic megacolon, is absence of ganglionic innervation to the smooth muscle wall of the colon.
- This disorder is more common in males than in females.
- The incidence is approximately 1 in 5000 live births.
- The lower portion of the sigmoid colon just above the anus is most commonly affected.
- The passage of fecal material through that segment of intestine does not occur because no peristaltic waves occur with the absence of the nerve cells.
- Intestinal contents accumulate proximal to the affected bowel areas, causing abdominal distention.
- Chronic *constipation* also results in the passage of ribbonlike stools.
- Failure to pass meconium after 24 hours with accompanying abdominal distention is highly suspect of this defect.
- A barium enema reveals dilatation of the proximal colon and narrowing of the distal colon.
- A rectal biopsy reveals lack of ganglia.
- A temporary colostomy is necessary with resection of the affected bowel.
- Reanastomosis of the distal and proximal bowel can occur between 12 and 18 months of age.

### Assessment Findings

#### *Older infant, 6–12 months*
- Chronic *constipation*
- Foul-smelling stool
- Intermittent *constipation* and *diarrhea*
- Ribbonlike stools
- Palpable fecal masses
- Distended abdomen
- Anemia
- Hypoproteinemia secondary to malabsorption
- *Failure to thrive*

#### *Neonate*
- Poor feeding
- Bile-stained vomitus
- Abdominal distention

### Nursing Implications

- Educate the parents on the pathology of aganglionic megacolon once a definitive diagnosis is made.
- Teach the parents how to perform daily enemas to achieve bowel movement before surgical correction.
- Prepare the parents for the two-stage surgical procedure and the need to establish a temporary colostomy.
- Inform the parents that the stoma is not painful, and prepare them for the appearance of the infant's colostomy.
- Preoperatively administer a diet of clear fluids for 24 to 48 hours, encourage bowel emptying with enemas and oral solutions, and administer systemic antibiotics to eliminate normal bowel flora.
- Postoperatively, fit the child for a colostomy appliance, and educate the parents on caring for a child with a colostomy.
- Monitor the stoma and ensure that it is red and protruding.
- Once bowel sounds return, provide a diet of clear fluid, then advance as tolerated and appropriate for the child's age.
- Monitor nutritional intake and weight gain carefully in these children and provide low-residue diet, vitamin, and stool softener information to the parents.
- Prepare the parents for reanastomosis of the colon.
- Postoperatively, maintain nasogastric tube patency and assess for abdominal distention.

- Monitor intake and output, and maintain the urinary catheter patency.
- Assess for bowel sounds, and observe for the passage of flatus and stools.
- Remove the nasogastric tube after peristalsis has returned.
- Begin the child on small frequent feedings of fluid and advance diet as tolerated.
- Prepare the child and parents for the necessary postoperative barium enema to be certain that the bowel empties well and the anastomosis site is not leaking.
- Inform the parents that the child may be a fussy eater for a while and to diminish the importance of meals gradually.
- Evaluate the child's growth and development carefully at all subsequent health care visits.

## HOOKWORM

### DESCRIPTION

- Hookworm is a helminthic infection and refers to the pathogenic or parasitic worms.
- Most helminths begin life when the eggs or larvae are eliminated in feces or urine of humans.
- The infection is transmitted to the oral cavity by unclean foods or hands.
- Children are prone to these infections because they are careless about hand washing before eating.
- Hookworms are found in human feces.
- Hookworms enter a child's body through the skin and then migrate to the intestinal tract, where they attach themselves onto the intestinal villi.
- Hookworms suck blood from the intestinal wall to sustain themselves.
- Severe anemia may result if enough hookworms are present.
- Treatment is aimed at destroying the worms.

### NURSING IMPLICATIONS

- Perform preventive health teaching regarding the need for frequent hand washing, especially after going to the bathroom.
- Evaluate the sequelae of hookworm and treat appropriately.

- Advise parents on how to administer the anthelmintic and monitor for signs of anemia.
- Treat anemia if severe.

# HYDROCELE

### DESCRIPTION

- Hydrocele refers to the collection of fluid in the space that occurs as the testes descends in utero preceded by a fold of tissue, the processus vaginalis.
- Hydrocele is present at birth.
- If the hydrocele is uncomplicated, the fluid is gradually reabsorbed into the body, and no treatment is necessary.
- A hydrocele may form later in life secondary to an inguinal hernia with accompanying fluid.
- The hernia needs to be repaired for the hydrocele to be reabsorbed.

### ASSESSMENT FINDINGS

- Enlarged scrotum

### NURSING IMPLICATIONS

- Reassure the parents that the hydrocele is only excess fluid and the scrotal enlargement is not due to an abnormal testis, tumor, or hernia.
- Instruct the parents that no treatment usually is necessary because the fluid is reabsorbed.

# HYDROCEPHALUS

### DESCRIPTION

- Hydrocephalus is an excess of cerebrospinal fluid (CSF) in the ventricles and subarachnoid spaces of the brain.
- Hydrocephalus occurs in 3 to 4 per 1000 live births.
- Hydrocephalus is commonly classified as congenital or acquired.
- The excess fluid causes enlargement of the head.
- An imbalance between production and absorption of CSF exists.
- Overproduction of CSF by the choroid plexus is rare and usually caused by a tumor in the choroid plexus.
- Obstruction of the passage of fluid somewhere between the point of origin and the point of absorption is the most frequent cause of hydrocephalus.

- Hydrocephalus secondary to an obstruction of the passage is called obstructive hydrocephalus or intraventricular hydrocephalus.
- Obstructive hydrocephalus is usually the result of congenital atresia or may be secondary to infections such as *meningitis,* which leave adhesions that obstruct flow.
- Hemorrhage or a growing tumor may obstruct the passage of CSF.
- An *Arnold-Chiari deformity* may also lead to obstruction.
- Passage of fluid between the ventricles and the spinal cord is called communicating hydrocephalus or extraventricular hydrocephalus.
- Another cause of hydrocephalus is interference with the absorption of fluid from the subarachnoid space.
- Interference with absorption may occur after extensive subarachnoid hemorrhage when portions of the membrane absorption surface are obscured.
- Symptoms of hydrocephalus may develop rapidly depending on the underlying cause.
- Hydrocephalus results in *increased intracranial pressure* causing brain displacement, and motor and mental damage.
- The prognosis for a child with hydrocephalus depends on the underlying cause, rate of development, and duration of *increased intracranial pressure.*
- Prompt surgical intervention improves prognosis.
- Central nervous system infections worsen the prognosis.
- Medical management of hydrocephalus depends on the cause but generally requires surgical intervention.
- With overproduction hydrocephalus, destruction of a portion of the choroid plexus is attempted.
- With disorders for obstructive lesions, the lesion is removed.
- A drainage catheter is often placed within the obstructed ventricle and threaded into the extracranial compartment—a ventriculoperitoneal shunt—to allow excess CSF to drain from the obstructed ventricle into the peritoneum.
- Valves within the catheter respond to a preset intracranial pressure and open if needed to drain CSF.

- Potential complications of ventriculoperitoneal shunts include infection such as *meningitis* developing 1 to 2 months after placement or peritonitis and malfunction allowing accumulation of CSF.
- Prognosis for hydrocephalus has improved with better ventriculoperitoneal shunting procedures.

## Assessment Findings

- Widened, tense fontanelles
- Dilated prominent scalp veins
- Separation of cranial sutures
- Displaced frontal area of the skull
- "Setting sun" sign
- Hyperactive reflexes
- Strabismus
- Optic atrophy
- Lethargy
- Irritability
- Shrill, high-pitched cry
- Opisthotonos
- Lower limb spasticity
- Difficulty breathing and swallowing
- *Vomiting*
- *Seizures*
- Ultrasonography, computed tomography and magnetic resonance imaging of the head positive for hydrocephalus
- Separating sutures and thinning of the skull bones on skull x-ray film
- Transillumination revealing a skull filled with fluid rather than solid brain matter

## Nursing Implications

- Perform a thorough physical examination to ensure prompt detection of hydrocephalus.
- Record head circumference in all children under age 2 years and plot this at health care visits.
- Measure the head circumference of all infants at birth and within an hour of discharge.
- Measure head circumference on all children who have suffered *head trauma* severe enough to be seen at a health care facility.
- Note any asymmetry that is occurring.

- Assess motor function and signs of neurologic impairment.
- Discuss the underlying cause with the parents, and prepare the parents and the child for surgery.
- Maintain the child (NPO) nothing by mouth.
- Administer acetazolamide as prescribed to decrease the production of CSF.
- Discuss the postoperative period with the child and parents.
- Position the child on the side opposite the shunt insertion site to prevent pressure on the shunt valve and injury to the incision site postoperatively.
- Keep the head of the bed flat to prevent rapid drainage of CSF, which could cause the cortex to tear away from the dura resulting in a *subdural hematoma.*
- Administer prophylactic antibiotics as prescribed.
- Monitor intravenous therapy and intake and output carefully.
- Monitor for signs of *increased intracranial pressure.*
- Encourage the parents to assist in care of the infant when possible, especially with calming the infant or offering a pacifier.
- Assess bowel function, and when bowel sounds are audible begin oral intake of clear fluids and advance as tolerated.
- Monitor nutritional intake and ensure adequate calories.
- Note any changes in sucking or beginning *vomiting* because this may indicate increased intracranial pressure.
- Monitor skin integrity, washing the child's head daily and assessing pressure points.
- Begin teaching with the parents on how to care for a child with a shunt immediately to encourage them being comfortable with it by discharge.
- Encourage the parents to verbalize any fears they have connected with the hydrocephalus, surgery, and care of the child postoperatively.
- Instruct the parents to watch for signs of shunt malfunction or central nervous system infection and to report the signs to the physician immediately.
- Ensure that the parents help the child to understand that the pumping device implanted behind an ear is

not to be felt continually because the child could accidentally evacuate cerebrospinal fluid from the ventricles at too rapid a rate.

- Be sure the parents have ample opportunity to care for and feed the child before discharge.
- Teach the parents signs to observe for that would indicate *increased intracranial pressure* and have them report them immediately.
- Be certain that parents have a telephone number to call if they have a question or concern regarding the child's condition or care.
- Continue to evaluate the child as an outpatient and ready the school-age child for school by making the school nurse aware that the child has a shunt in place.
- Inform the school nurse and the parents that the child may need special head protection with sports activities.

## HYDRONEPHROSIS

### DESCRIPTION

- Hydronephrosis is an enlargement of the pelvis of the kidney with urine as a result of back pressure in the ureter.
- Hydronephrosis is a serious disorder because elevated back pressure on the kidney interferes with tubular function or causes destruction of nephrons.
- The cause of the back pressure is usually secondary to obstruction.
- The point of obstruction is either at the ureter or at the point where the ureter joins the bladder, such as with vesicoureteral reflux.
- Hydronephrosis most often occurs in the first 6 months of life.
- Hydronephrosis may be revealed by fetal ultrasonography.
- Surgical correction of the obstruction is required to avoid the sequela of glomerular or tubular destruction.

### ASSESSMENT FINDINGS (if present)

- Repeated urinary tract infections secondary to urine stasis
- General irritability and crying
- Increased blood pressure secondary to elevated tubular pressure (which activates the angiotensin response)

- Flank or abdominal pain if severe
- Abdominal palpation revealing a mass, which is the dilated kidney pelvis
- Intravenous pyelogram revealing the enlarged pelvis and the point of obstruction

### NURSING IMPLICATIONS
- Obtain a thorough history and physical examination to establish a baseline and identify possible symptoms to be reported to the physician.
- Anticipate intravenous pyelography to establish a definitive diagnosis.
- Educate the parents on the dangers intrinsic to the pathology of this disorder.
- Prepare the child and the parents for surgical intervention.
- Encourage the parents to be with the child and participate in his or her care as much as possible.
- Monitor intake and output postoperatively to ensure adequate kidney function.
- Prepare the parents and child for discharge, and advise them on how to assess for signs of infection and to notify the physician if any signs are present.

## HYPERLIPIDEMIA

### DESCRIPTION
- Hyperlipidemia is an increased fatty acid level in the blood.
- There is an association between total cholesterol and low-density lipoprotein (LDL) and the incidence of coronary artery disease.
- Total cholesterol can be measured without the child fasting; LDL requires a 12-hour fasting period for accuracy.

### ASSESSMENT FINDINGS
- Total cholesterol level above 170 mg/dL
- LDL cholesterol level above 110 mg/dL

### NURSING IMPLICATIONS
- Screen all children of parents with premature coronary artery disease or with a family history of hypercholesterolemia for total serum cholesterol.
- Be aware that screening must be done especially if the child smokes, is obese, or has a sedentary lifestyle.

- Assess the nutritional value of the diet of any child with elevated fatty acid level, cholesterol, or LDL.
- Encourage a discussion with the child and the parents on exercise and diet modification.
- Discuss the risk of hyperlipidemia with the parents to stress the need for a change in the child's diet and lifestyle.
- Inform parents not to place children on a total low-fat diet because they need the fat calories for growth.
- Be aware that infants under age 2 are rarely placed on low-fat diets because it would interfere with myelinization of the nerves and neurologic development.
- Encourage parents to follow a low-cholesterol diet and discuss the entire diet with them.
- Encourage parents to evaluate their eating habits and to maintain a good role model for their child.
- Be alert to the possibility of cholestyramine being prescribed for children over 10 years of age who have not been successful in reducing their cholesterol levels with diet or exercise.
- Advise parents and children on cholestyramine of its side effects, which include large bulky stools and gastrointestinal discomfort.
- Continue to address the issues of hypercholesterolemia with children and parents at all subsequent health care visits to maintain their compliance with the diet and exercise modifications established.
- Remember that hypercholesterolemia has no symptoms and requires vigilance on the part of the health care professional to keep the family and child motivated with the prescribed regimen.

## HYPERSPLENISM

### DESCRIPTION

- Hypersplenism refers to an enlargement of the spleen; almost any underlying splenic condition can cause hypersplenism.
- The spleen appears to be relatively important in early infancy with its function decreasing as the child grows older.
- Normally, blood is filtered rapidly through the spleen; when the spleen is enlarged and functioning abnor-

mally, the blood cells pass through more slowly, and more are destroyed in the process.

- A splenectomy may be required to treat the underlying disorder.
- No decrease in general immunity, gamma globulin formation, or antibody formation exists with the removal of the spleen.
- An increased susceptibility to *meningitis* caused by pneumococci may exist with the removal of the spleen's filtering function.
- A splenectomy is usually delayed until age 2 years old when the risk of *meningitis* decreases.

### Assessment Findings
- *Anemia*
- Pancytopenia

### Nursing Implications
- Assess for signs of anemia in children and obtain a hematocrit if required to establish diagnosis.
- Monitor for hypersplenism and refer to the physician to establish the underlying cause.
- Explain to the parents the role of the spleen in the body and why removal after the age of 2 may be warranted with hypersplenism.
- Prepare and support the parents and child through the hospital and surgical experience, encouraging the parents to stay with the child as much as possible.
- Administer *immunization* against pneumococci postoperatively.
- Assess the incision and monitor for signs of infection.
- Monitor intake and output and establish oral fluids when bowel functioning returns.
- Administer prophylactic penicillin, and instruct the parents that the child must take this for 2 years after the splenectomy.
- Prepare the parents and the child for discharge with instructions for dressing changes and medications.

## HYPERTELORISM

### Description
- Hypertelorism is a congenital deformity represented by abnormally wide-spaced eyes.

- The true condition is revealed when the distance is measured between the pupils and compared with normal standards for that age.
- Hypertelorism is associated with chromosomal abnormalities, most notably Waardenburg's syndrome.
- This syndrome also involves congenital *hearing impairment.*

### ASSESSMENT FINDINGS
- Abnormally wide-spaced eyes
- White forelock of hair
- Different-colored irises
- Eyebrows growing together in a straight line
- Inability to hear sound

### NURSING IMPLICATIONS
- Obtain a thorough history and physical examination to establish a baseline.
- Refer child to a *hearing impairment* specialist to assess specific *hearing impairment.*
- Explain to parents the congenital nature of this disorder.
- Refer parents planning to have more children to a genetic counselor.

## HYPERTENSION

### DESCRIPTION
- Hypertension refers to the criterion of a systolic blood pressure reading greater than 2 standard deviations above the mean for a given age.
- Primary hypertension is rare in children.
- Hypertension in children occurs more often as a secondary manifestation of another disease, such as a kidney disorder.
- There is a high incidence among African-American children.
- Hypertension occurs in 1% to 2% of school-age children and 11% of adolescents.
- Underlying conditions that can lead to hypertension include cardiac disease, renal disease, *Cushing's syndrome*, primary aldosteronism, *adrenogenital syndrome*, pheochromocytoma, and brain tumors.
- Treatment of hypertension depends on the underlying cause.

## Assessment Findings

- Red blood cells in urine (indicate *glomerulonephritis*)
- White blood cells in urine (indicate pyelonephritis)
- Proteinuria (may indicate nephron disease)
- Abdominal bruit (suggest renal vascular disease)
- Papilledema, spasm, or hemorrhage with chronic elevated blood pressure

## Nursing Implications

- Assess blood pressure measurements at health care visits beginning at 3 years of age.
- Obtain the blood pressure reading while the child is relaxed and after at least 1 to 2 minutes after rest.
- Evaluate elevated blood pressure readings at subsequent visits to establish the norm for the child and compare with the normal blood pressure for his or her age group.
- Discuss hypertension with the child and the parents and inform them of the need to perform additional studies to discover underlying disease processes.
- Evaluate blood pressure in the lower extremities to rule out *coarctation of the aorta*.
- Obtain a urine specimen for analysis.
- Auscultate the abdomen for an abdominal bruit.
- Perform a funduscopic examination of the child's eyes to evaluate the effects of chronic elevated blood pressure.
- Establish the normal diet and exercise of the individual child.
- Place the child who is obese with idiopathic hypertension on a reducing diet and continue to counsel on dietary modification and an exercise program.
- Limit salt intake in this population if it has been excessive.
- Encourage adolescent girls with hypertension and on oral contraceptives not to use oral contraceptives because they elevate blood pressure.
- Educate children and parents of children who require a diuretic or an antihypertensive medication of the importance of taking the medication as well as any associated side affects.
- Educate children with hypertension of the long-term effects of the condition—increased risk of heart and blood vessel disease.

- Continue to reinforce educational and medication information at each health care visit along with monitoring the effects of the dietary, exercise, and medication regimen.

# HYPERTHYROIDISM

## DESCRIPTION

- Hyperthyroidism, thyrotoxicosis, or Graves' disease is an oversecretion of thyroid hormones by the thyroid gland.
- Thyrotoxicosis is the body's response to excessive production of thyroid hormones.
- In children, thyrotoxicosis usually presents at the time of puberty or during adolescence.
- This disorder is more common in girls than in boys.
- The oversecretion may be secondary to overstimulation by the thyrotropic hormone of the pituitary as a result of a pituitary tumor.
- More often the hyperthyroidism and thyrotoxicosis in children is caused by an autoimmune reaction that results in production of IgG class immunoglobulins that stimulate the thyroid gland.
- Graves' disease often follows a viral illness or a period of stress.
- A genetic predisposition to this disorder may exist.
- The child has an advanced bone age, which means the child will not be able to reach normal adult height because the epiphyseal lines of long bones will close before normal height is reached.
- Medical management is aimed at controlling the antibody response first with a beta-adrenergic medication and then suppressing the formation of thyroxine with an antithyroid medication.

## ASSESSMENT FINDINGS

- Exophthalmos
- Nervousness
- Loss of muscle strength
- Fatigue
- Increased basal metabolic rate
- Increased blood pressure and heart rate
- Hunger
- Increased perspiration
- Eat constantly without weight gain
- Advanced bone age on x-ray film

- Prominent thyroid gland on neck confirmed by ultrasonography
- Fine tremors of extremities
- Elevated thyroxine and triiodothyronine levels
- Increased uptake of radioactive iodine
- Low thyroid-stimulating hormone levels secondary to stimulation by the antibodies not by the pituitary gland

## NURSING IMPLICATIONS

- Identify any signs of hyperthyroidism in children early to prevent complications.
- Refer the family to an endocrinologist for management.
- Explain to the family the function of the thyroid gland and the pathophysiology of the disease process.
- Educate the family on appropriate therapy for hyperthyroidism.
- Administer a beta-adrenergic blocking agent, such as propranolol, as prescribed to decrease the antibody response.
- Introduce an antithyroid drug, such as propylthiouracil or methimazole, as prescribed to suppress the formation of thyroxine.
- Explain to parents and the child that it can take up to 2 weeks to see an effect from these drugs.
- Advise the family that the child needs to take the antithyroid medication for several years before the condition "burns itself out."
- Inform the family that the exophthalmos may not recede, but it will not become worse from the time therapy is instituted.
- Monitor for decreased white blood cell level, which is a side effect of the antithyroid medication.
- Isolate the child and discontinue the medication if serious leukopenia occurs.
- Educate the family of the child with a toxic reaction to the antithyroid medication or the child who is noncompliant that radioiodine ablative therapy can be used to reduce the size of the thyroid gland.
- Inform the family that surgical removal of part or all of the thyroid gland may be necessary in a young adult.
- Teach the family and child that if radioiodine ablative therapy or a thyroidectomy is required, the child will need to be on supplemental thyroid hormone therapy for life.

# HYPOCALCEMIA

## DESCRIPTION

- Hypocalcemia refers to a lowered blood calcium level.
- Calcium levels are regulated by the parathyroid gland, which controls the rate of bone metabolism by the secretion of parathyroid hormone.
- A negative feedback system of the circulatory serum levels of calcium controls the parathyroid hormone.
- Low calcium levels increase the secretion of parathyroid hormone.
- Vitamin D is necessary for calcium absorption from the gastrointestinal tract into the blood stream, and it influences the secretion of parathyroid hormone.
- Calcitonin (thyrocalcitonin) is secreted by the thyroid gland and opposes the action of parathyroid hormone and therefore decreases blood calcium levels.
- Hypocalcemia occurs in infants with birth anoxia, immature infants (with the parathyroid gland being immature), and infants of diabetic mothers (because it tends to follow hypoglycemia).
- An indirect relationship exists between the balance of calcium and phosphorus in the blood stream.
- An imbalance of calcium and phosphorus in milk can cause hypocalcemia.
- Hypocalcemia secondary to cow's milk occurs at about the 7th day of life.
- The neuromuscular irritability associated with this electrolyte imbalance can be life-threatening.
- Therapeutic management of hypocalcemia is aimed at increasing the serum level of calcium to the point above the level that leads to latent tetany.

## ASSESSMENT FINDINGS

- Neuromuscular irritability—latent tetany
- Crying
- Muscle twitching
- Carpopedal spasms
- Positive Chvostek's sign
- Positive Trousseau's sign
- Positive Erb's sign
- Positive peroneal sign
- Laryngospasm
- *Seizures*

#### NURSING IMPLICATIONS

- Assess the newborn carefully and note any signs of neuromuscular irritability.
- Determine if the irritability is secondary to hypocalcemia, a central nervous system problem, or some other cause.
- Assess the newborn at home and ensure proper milk intake.
- Educate the general public on why cow's milk cannot be used with the infants.
- Refer any child with signs of hypocalcemia for medical treatment.
- Administer 10% calcium chloride by mouth as prescribed if the infant can suck.
- Administer 10% solution of calcium gluconate intravenously as prescribed if the tetany has progressed to the point at which the child does not have the muscular strength to take an oral fluid safely.
- Do not administer calcium gluconate intramuscularly or subcutaneously because it can cause necrosis at the injection site.
- Administer sodium phenobarbital as prescribed in addition to the calcium gluconate for infants having *seizures.*
- Evaluate the need for emergency intubation to relieve laryngospasm.
- Educate the parents of children treated emergently for complications of hypocalcemia that the child requires oral calcium therapy until the calcium level has been regulated.
- Administer vitamin D to increase absorption of calcium from the gastrointestinal tract.

## HYPOGAMMAGLOBULINEMIA

#### DESCRIPTION

- Hypogammaglobulinemia is an immunodeficiency disorder resulting in abnormally low levels of all immunoglobulins.
- Hypogammaglobulinemia is an X-linked inherited defect in the maturation of B lymphocytes.
- This is usually first recognized at about age 6 months, when passively transferred maternal antibodies begin to fade.

- The male infant begins to show an increased susceptibility to bacterial infections.
- Autoimmune disorders, such as *rheumatoid arthritis* and *systemic lupus erythematosus,* occur in later life.
- Cellular and T lymphocyte response remains adequate with hypogammaglobulinemia, allowing the child to resist viral, fungal, and parasitic infections.
- Treatment of this disorder is with monthly gamma globulin injections.
- *Bone marrow transplantation* may be successful in restoring immune competency.

### ASSESSMENT FINDINGS
- Frequent respiratory, digestive, and throat infections

### NURSING IMPLICATIONS
- Note any trends in increasing bacterial infections in male infants over 6 months of age.
- Refer the family to an immunologist for definitive diagnosis of hypogammaglobulinemia.
- Educate the family on the role of the immune system and the specific indications related to this disorder.
- Prepare the child and the family for monthly gamma globulin injections.
- Support the family and the child with this disorder, and discuss potential treatment with a *bone marrow transplantation.*
- Encourage the family to verbalize their concerns, and educate the family on the need for protection against bacterial infection.

## HYPOPITUITARY DWARFISM

### Description
- Hypopituitary dwarfism, hypopituitary gland dysfunction, can lead to a decrease in production of human growth hormone (somatotropin).
- The cause of hypopituitarism in most children is unknown.
- Some causes of hypopituitarism include nonmalignant cystic tumors of embryonic origin, which causes pressure on the pituitary gland, or *increased intracranial pressure* from another cause; a history of loss of vision, headache, increased head circumference, nausea, and *vomiting* is suggestive of pituitary tumor.

- A history that reveals a well child except for abnormal lack of growth typically represents hypopituitary dwarfism.
- When this hormone is deficient, it causes a child to remain short in stature.
- The child will be well proportioned but simply miniature in size.
- The eventual height that the child who is untreated grows to is individualized and difficult to predict.
- Without treatment, the child will not reach a height over 3 to 4 feet.
- With advances in recombinant DNA synthesis, synthetic growth hormone needed to treat hypopituitary dwarfism is readily available.
- Accompanying treatment depends on accompanying pituitary dysfunctions and may include supplements of gonadotropin or other hormones.
- Often, these children have delayed epiphysial closure and are able to grow to normal heights with supplemental treatment.

### Assessment Findings

- Lower than standard height and weight on growth charts after 2 to 3 years of life.
- Recessed mandible
- Small nose
- High-pitched voice
- Delayed onset of pubic, facial, and axillary hair and genital growth
- Decreased level of circulating growth hormone

### Nursing Implications

- Evaluate height and weight of all children at each health care visit and plot it against the national standard.
- Note any variation along the curve and investigate family history for traits of short stature.
- Detect if the main problem is constitutional delay (innocent late development).
- Obtain estimates of the parents' height and siblings' height and weight during periods of growth.
- Assess the child's prenatal and birth history to find a source of pituitary injury.
- Assess past health history for signals of chronic illness, such as heart, kidney, or intestinal disorders, that could contribute to the decreased level of growth.

- Take a 24-hour nutritional history to evaluate intake, and ask about urinary and bowel function.
- Rule out the presence of a pituitary tumor, such as is suggested with sudden halt in growth.
- Prepare the parents and the child for tests needed to determine the cause, such as funduscopic and neurologic testing.
- Obtain blood studies to rule out hypothyroidism, hypoadrenalism, and hypoaldosteronism because these conditions can influence growth.
- Obtain information regarding bone age from x-ray films.
- Prepare the family for necessary scans to detect possible enlargement of the sella turcica, which would suggest pituitary tumor.
- Test the child for growth hormone response to hypoglycemia.
- Carefully monitor the child to avoid extreme hypoglycemia.
- Encourage the use of an intermittent venous access device, such as a heparin lock, for blood sampling to avoid frequent venipunctures.
- Provide diversional and enjoyable activities during the testing period.
- Explain the normal functioning of the pituitary gland and growth hormone to the parents and child.
- Educate the family on the need to replete the child with hypopituitary dwarfism by administration of intramuscular human growth hormone injections 2 to 3 times per week.
- Teach the parents and eventually the child how to administer this intramuscular injection.

## HYPOSPADIAS

### DESCRIPTION

- Hypospadias is a urethral defect in which the urethral opening is not at the end of the penis but on the ventral aspect of the penis.
- The meatus may be near the glans, midway, or back at the base of the penis.
- The degree of hypospadias may be minimal or maximal.
- Many newborns with hypospadias have an accompanying short chordae causing the penis to curve downward.

- This is a common anomaly occurring in 1 in 300 male newborns.
- Hypospadias may be familial and may occur from a multifactorial genetic focus.
- Surgical intervention, meatotomy, to establish better urinary function is done in the newborn.
- At 12 to 18 months of age, the infant may have the adherent chordae released.
- Extensive plastic surgery is usually delayed until the child is 3 to 4 years of age.
- Pharmacologic intervention to encourage penis growth and make future plastic surgeries easier can be done by applying testosterone cream.
- Surgical interventions should be done before school age to allow the child to appear normal to his classmates.
- Later in life a repair of the meatal opening is necessary to avoid infertility.
- After surgical intervention for hypospadias, a child is expected to be normal in both urinary and reproductive function unless accompanying anomalies of the penis are present.

### ASSESSMENT FINDINGS
- Penile opening on ventral surface
- Downward penile curvature

### NURSING IMPLICATIONS
- Inspect all male newborns at birth for hypospadias.
- Inspect newborn boys with hypospadias for *cryptorchidism,* undescended testes, which is often found with this defect.
- Establish sex determination with a Barr body analysis from a buccal cell smear or full sex cell karyotyping if the penis defect is extensive.
- Assist parents in accepting the medical diagnosis of hypospadias and reassure them that eventually the child will have normal urinary and probably reproductive function.
- Explain to parents that a *circumcision* is not done on a child with this defect because the foreskin may need to be used in the future with plastic reconstruction.
- Openly discuss the defect with the parents to ease their ability in discussing it.
- Encourage the parents to verbalize their feelings regarding the defect.

- Inform the parents of the initial surgical procedure necessary to establish better urinary function.
- Help parents to become familiar with the urinary catheter placed after this surgery to keep tension off the urethral sutures.
- Administer an antispasmodic as prescribed for painful bladder spasms while the catheter is in place, usually 1 to 10 days.
- Prepare the parents for future surgical procedures to release the chordae and potentially extensive plastic surgery.
- Teach the parents how to apply the testosterone cream, if prescribed.
- Prepare the parents and child for each surgical procedure and encourage them to verbalize any of their concerns.

## HYPOTHYROIDISM, CONGENITAL

### DESCRIPTION

- Congenital hypothyroidism, an inborn error of metabolism, occurs as a result of an absent or nonfunctioning thyroid gland.
- Thyroid hypofunction results in reduced production of both thyroxine ($T_4$) and triiodothyronine ($T_3$).
- This disorder occurs in 1 in 4000 live births.
- Females are affected twice as often as males.
- Congenital hypothyroidism may not initially be noted because of the maternal thyroid hormones circulating in the fetus during pregnancy.
- During the first 3 months of life in a formula-fed infant and at about 6 months of life in a breast-fed infant, the symptoms become noticeable.
- All children delivered in American hospitals undergo a mandatory screening test for hypothyroidism at birth.
- If the condition goes unrecognized, both *mental retardation* and physical developmental retardation occurs.
- Medical management of the child with congenital hypothyroidism is aimed at maintaining an adequate level of circulating thyroid hormone accomplished by administering daily thyroid hormone replacement in the form of levothyroxine sodium.
- To avoid delays in cognitive development, the child is begun on full-dose therapy immediately.

## Assessment Findings

- Sleepy
- Enlarged tongue, which may cause respiratory difficulty, noisy respirations, or obstruction
- Trouble feeding because of sluggishness or choking
- Cold skin
- Subnormal body temperature secondary to slow basal metabolic rate
- Slow pulse
- Slow respiratory rate
- Prolonged jaundice secondary to immature liver's inability to conjugate bilirubin
- *Anemia*
- Short, thick neck
- Dull facial expression
- Short, fat extremities
- Hypotonic muscles
- Slow deep tendon reflexes
- Obesity
- Dry, brittle hair
- Delayed dentition or defective teeth
- Chronic *constipation*
- Enlarged abdomen secondary to poor muscle tone
- Large posterior fontanelle
- *Umbilical hernia*
- Dry, scaly skin
- Low radioactive iodine uptake
- Low serum $T_4$ and $T_3$ levels
- Elevated thyroid-stimulating factor
- Increased serum lipids
- No femoral epiphyseal line or delayed bone growth on x-ray film

## Nursing Implications

- Establish a definitive diagnosis of congenital hypothyroidism by evaluating the $T_4$ and thyroid-stimulating hormone levels.
- Discuss the disorder with the parents and the necessity to begin medical therapy immediately for life.
- Teach the parents appropriate home-management skills.
- Educate the parents and child about the purpose and type of medication to be taken.

- Teach the parents always to have a supply on hand for vacations, summer camp, and holidays.
- Involve the child as soon as possible in administering the medication.
- Ensure that the family and child understand the importance of adequate thyroid hormone levels.
- Remind the parents and the child that periodic monitoring of $T_3$ and $T_4$ helps to ensure appropriate medication dosage.
- Teach the parents and child to be alert to signs of underdosage and overdosage and to alert the physician at once.
- Remind parents that they must consider all medicine a potential poison and keep it out of children's reach.
- Help the family adapt to this chronic condition and have it become a normal part of their lifestyle.

## IDIOPATHIC THROMBOCYTOPENIC PURPURA (ITP)

### DESCRIPTION

- ITP is the result of a decrease in the number of circulating platelets, although adequate megakaryocytes (precursors to platelets) are present.
- The cause is unknown, but it probably results from an increased rate of destruction of platelets owing to an antiplatelet antibody that destroys platelets (making this an autoimmune illness).
- In most instances, ITP occurs approximately 2 weeks following a viral infection such as *rubella, rubeola,* or an upper respiratory tract infection; congenital ITP may occur in the newborn of a woman who has had ITP during pregnancy.

### ASSESSMENT FINDINGS

- History of a viral infection such as *rubella, rubeola,* or an upper respiratory tract infection.
- Miniature petechiae or large areas of asymmetric ecchymosis most predominately over legs.
- *Epistaxis*
- Marked thrombocytopenia (platelets as low as 20,000/mm$^3$)

### NURSING IMPLICATIONS

- Perform a complete history and physical assessment to establish a baseline and identify any possible history of recent viral infection.

- Administer oral predisone, as prescribed.
- Prepare the child with central nervous system bleeding for splenectomy, as prescribed.
- Caution the parents that salicylates should not be given to relieve joint pain from bleeding because salicylates interfere with blood clotting by preventing the aggregation of platelets at wound sites.

- Be prepared to administer immunosuppressive drugs, as prescribed, if the chronic state of ITP persists.
- Administer intravenous gamma globulin, as prescribed to improve the platelet count.
- Prepare for plasmapheresis, as prescribed.
- Advise the parents to be certain that siblings are up to date with immunizations against *rubella* and *rubeola,* which can lead to this defective coagulation process.
- Instruct parents in safety measures to prevent injury and subsequent bleeding.
- Advise the parents to watch for and report signs of intracranial hemorrhage, such as persistent headache, nuchal rigidity, and lethargy.
- Advise the parents to pad surfaces where the child plays to avoid a serious bleeding injury.
- Reassure the parents that this illness, although lengthy, is not *leukemia* and does not develop into *leukemia.*
- Know that these children are sometimes initially diagnosed as abused children because of the amount of bruises present.
- Allow the parents time to express their anger at the suspicion of abuse and regain their confidence in the health care team.
- Explain all procedures to the parents and try to answer their questions.
- Provide support and reassurance to the parents during this illness.

## IMMUNIZATIONS

### Description

- Immunizations refer to substances (vaccines) used for health promotion and disease prevention to confer immunity (ability to destroy a particular antigen).
- Vaccines, the solutions used to immunize children, provide artificially acquired active or passive immunity.
- They are prepared in a number of forms.
- Attenuated vaccines are made from live organisms that have been reduced in virulence to a point at which

they do not cause active disease but ensure a good antibody response.
- Toxoids are vaccines made from an extract of a toxin produced by some bacteria, such as diphtheria, reduced in virulence.
- Antitoxins, the antibodies for toxin-producing bacteria, are solutions given for passive immunity.
- Gamma globulin is a serum obtained from the pooled blood of many people and contains the antibodies of many people and probably has antibody protection against *measles, rubella, poliomyelitis,* and infectious *hepatitis* among other infectious diseases and offers passive immunity.
- Immune serum is serum removed from horses that have been given a disease.
- The schedule of immunizations for children to receive is recommended by the American Academy of Pediatrics.

### NURSING IMPLICATIONS
- Review the schedule from the American Academy of Pediatrics for routine immunizations for healthy infants and children.
- Know that children who are seriously ill should not receive immunizations; however, a slight runny nose or an upper respiratory infection is not a contraindication.
- Assess the immunization status of all ill children at clinic or hospital admission to identify those who need their immunizations updated.
- Assess each child's health status before administering any vaccine because children who are immunosuppressed, receiving corticosteroids, or have *chemotherapy* or *radiation therapy* cannot receive live vaccines.
- Know that the live attenuated viruses (*measles, rubella,* oral polio, and *mumps*) should not be given to girls who are pregnant because these vaccines could cross the placenta and cause actual disease in the fetus.
- Be sure to ask the child or the parents if the child is allergic to horses before administering an immune serum because it is removed from horses.

- Know that side effects of the *diphtheria,* pertussis, *tetanus* (DPT) vaccine may include drowsiness, fretfulness, low-grade fever, and redness and pain at the injection site.
- Advise the parents that they have a right to refuse immunizations for their children; however, advise them that the child may be refused admission into preschool or kindergarten.
- Know that pertussis vaccination is contraindicated in children who have a progressive or unstable neurologic disorder or who have had a severe allergic reaction to pertussis in a previous DPT vaccination.
- Know that oral polio vaccine (OPV) should not be administered to children who are immunosuppressed because it could cause a rare form of paralytic poliomyelitis.
- Advise the parents of a child who has received OPV that the child should not come in contact with a person who is immunosuppressed because the OPV is shed in the child's stool.
- Know that it is not recommended that the *measles* vaccine be administered to children younger than 15 months because children receive a great deal of passive immunity to this disease from maternal placental transfer.
- Know that side effects of the *measles* vaccine may include rashes and a fever.
- Skin test children for tuberculosis before *measles* vaccine administration because *measles* virus can cause *tuberculosis* to become systemic.
- Know that *tuberculosis* skin tests may show false-negative reactions if given shortly after *measles* immunization.
- Fully inform parents about what immunizations are being given and what side effects may be expected.
- Tell the parents to report any untoward symptoms of immunization.

## IMPERFORATE ANUS

### DESCRIPTION

- Imperforate anus is stricture of the anus occurring when the two sections of bowel fail to meet in utero or if the membrane between them is not absorbed.

- The defect can be relatively minor, requiring just surgical incision of the persistent membrane, or much more serious, involving sections of the bowel that are many inches apart with no anus.
- There may be an accompanying fistula to the bladder in males and to the vagina in females.
- This problem occurs in 1 in 5000 live births, more commonly in males than females.
- It may occur as an additional complication of spinal cord defects because both the external anal canal and the spinal cord arise from the same germ tissue layer.

### Assessment findings

- No anal formation visible
- Anal formation visible but defect further beyond inspection
- Membrane filled with meconium visible protruding from anus
- Inability to insert a rectal thermometer
- No passage of stool
- Abdominal distention
- Absent "wink" reflex at the rectum

### Nursing Implications

- Obtain vital signs and assess for the ability to insert a rectal thermometer.
- Assess the infant's intake and output, observing ability to pass stools.
- Perform a follow-up assessment of infants born in birthing centers as to whether they are passing stools.
- Examine the urine of all infants diagnosed with imperforate anus for the presence of meconium to determine whether the child has a fistula.
- Place a urine collection bag over female infants with imperforate anus to reveal a meconium-stained discharge.
- Administer intravenous fluid therapy to maintain fluid and electrolyte balance.
- Keep the infant NPO (give nothing by mouth).
- Prepare the infant and parents for impending surgery.
- Teach the parents about colostomy care if the infant returns from surgery with a colostomy.
- Provide support and encouragement to the parents during this time.

- Obtain axillary or tympanic temperature, not rectal, after surgery.
- Irrigate the suture line after the infant has a bowel movement to prevent infection.
- Do not place the infant on the abdomen because at this age infants tend to pull their legs up to their knees placing pressure on the suture line.
- Demonstrate to the parents the importance of and how to perform rectal dilatation once or twice a day using a lubricated finger cot to prevent constriction.
- Explain to the parents how to administer stool softeners, as prescribed, and the importance of adhering to the correct times and dosage.

## IMPETIGO

### DESCRIPTION

- Impetigo is a superficial infection of the skin usually caused by beta-hemolytic streptococcus, group A or possibly staphylococcus.
- Impetigo is only mildly infectious because it seems to be transmitted only by direct contact.
- Impetigo is often seen as secondary infections of insect bites or in children who have pierced ears.
- Although rare, complications of *rheumatic fever* or *acute glomerulonephritis* may occur following impetigo as they may after other streptococcal infections.

### ASSESSMENT FINDINGS

- Papulovesicular lesions surrounded by erythema, most commonly on face and extremities
- Vesical becoming purulent, oozing, and forming honey-colored crusts
- Local adenopathy

### NURSING IMPLICATIONS

- Assure the parents that streptococcal organisms are so numerous that the cleanest child can contact this disease.
- Assure the parents that the presence of the infection reflects on the number of organisms available, not the child's care.
- Caution parents to seek health supervision for any lesion that appears reddened or filled with pus (infected) because the causative agent may be a particularily virulent form of streptococcus.

- Advise the parents about the administration of oral penicillin or erythromycin or the application of mupirocin (Bactroban) ointment for a full 10-day period.
- Inform the parents and child that the lesions heal most quickly if the crusts are washed daily with soap and water.
- Instruct the parents and child to avoid touching or scratching the lesions and to wash hands after applying the ointment.

## INFANTILE AUTISM

### DESCRIPTION

- Infantile autism is a category of pervasive developmental disorders that is marked by serious distortions in psychological functioning.
- There may be deficits in language, perceptual, and motor development; defective reality testing; and an inability to function in social settings.
- There is a lack of responsiveness to other people, gross impairment in communication skills, and bizarre responses to various aspects of the environment, all developing within the first 30 months of age.
- It is a rare condition occurring in only 2 to 4 children out of 10,000; it occurs about 3 times more often in males than in females.
- The cause is unknown, but it is linked with cerebral and limbic system anomalies that probably occurred in utero.
- Infantile autism has been associated with maternal *rubella* or *phenylketonuria, meningitis,* and *encephalitis* in the child.
- As many as 75% of children with the disorder also suffer from *mental retardation.*

### ASSESSMENT FINDINGS

- Social isolation
- Stereotyped behaviors
- Resistance to any change in routine
- Abnormal responses to sensory stimuli
- Insensitivity to pain
- Inappropriate emotional expressions
- Disturbances of movement
- Poor development of speech

- Specific, limited intellectual problems
- Failure to cuddle or make eye contact (infants)
- Inability to play cooperatively or form friendships
- Absent language (possible)
- Attachment to odd objects
- Rocking and rhythmic body movements
- Intensely preoccupied by moving objects
- Excellent long-term memory
- Labile mood (crying occurs suddenly followed immediately by giggling or laughing)

### Nursing Implications

- Obtain a thorough history and physical examination to establish a baseline and rule out other pathologies.
- Provide emotional support and encouragement to the parents so that they do not reject the child because he or she is rejecting them; assist them with measures to cope with the child's behavior.
- Advise the parents that behavior modification therapy may be effective in controlling some of the bizarre mannerisms that accompany autism.
- Suggest to the parents that day care programs can help to promote social awareness.
- Tell the parents that some children are eventually able to lead independent lives, although social ineptness and awkwardness are apt to remain, especially if *mental retardation* accompanies autism.
- Offer ongoing support and guidance.

## INFECTIOUS MONONUCLEOSIS

### Description

- Infectious mononucleosis is also known as glandular fever or, because it was first discovered as a disease that is transferred readily from one person to another by kissing, the kissing disease.
- It occurs most commonly in adolescents, although it may occur in any age child.
- The causative agent is the Epstein-Barr virus, and apparently one episode gives lasting immunity; no vaccination is available.

### Assessment Findings

- Chills, fever
- Headache
- Anorexia and malaise

- Cervical lymph nodes tender to touch
- Enlarged and erythematous tonsils
- Thick white membrane covering tonsils
- Petechiae on the palate
- Abdominal pain
- Enlarged spleen
- *Lymphocytosis*
- Positive monospot test

### Nursing Implications
- Perform a thorough history and physical assessment to establish a baseline.
- Obtain vital signs and be alert for abnormal findings.
- Obtain a monospot test or additional ordered laboratory specimens; instruct the child about all laboratory tests ordered.
- Be extremely gentle while palpating the spleen to avoid possible rupture.
- Know that the child with this disease is kept on bed rest during the acute stage of the illness (7 to 10 days) because with the splenomegaly, there is a danger of *splenic rupture* with any trauma to that area.
- Be careful in helping the child with this disease turn in bed so that no pressure is placed over the splenic area.
- Teach the parents and child the importance of maintaining a good fluid intake despite the sore throat, emphasizing the use of cool and nonacidic fluids, which are better tolerated.
- Administer corticosteroids, as prescribed to reduce inflammation.
- Caution the child to avoid contact sports as long as the spleen is enlarged.
- Advise the parents and child that he or she may notice weakness and general fatigue for up to 6 weeks following the illness.
- Help the child to voice frustration with this illness.
- Offer support and help the child through this interruption in school life.

## INTESTINAL OBSTRUCTION

### Description
- Intestinal obstruction refers to a blockage in the intestines.

- If canalization of the intestine does not occur in utero at some point in the bowel, an atresia (complete closure) or stenosis (narrowing) of the bowel can occur, the most common site being the duodenal bowel portion.
- Intestinal obstruction can occur because of a twisting (rotation) of the mesentery of the bowel as the bowel reenters the abdomen after being contained in the base of the umbilical cord early in intrauterine life or because of severe twisting of the mesentery owing to the looseness of the intestine in the abdomen of the neonate (this continues to be a problem for the first 6 months of life).
- Obstruction can also occur because of thicker than usual meconium formation.

## ASSESSMENT FINDINGS

- Maternal history of hydramnios during pregnancy
- Presence of more than 30 mL of stomach contents aspirated from stomach at birth
- Absence of meconium or passage of one stool and then cessation
- Distended abdomen
- *Vomiting* (bile stained or black)
- Increased bowel sounds
- Visible waves of peristalsis over abdomen
- Crying, especially while drawing legs up against abdomen
- Increased respiratory rate

## NURSING IMPLICATIONS

- Obtain a thorough history and physical assessment to establish a baseline and identify any possible maternal contributing factors.
- Obtain maternal labor and birth history.
- Obtain vital signs and report any deviations from normal ranges.
- Insert an orogastric or nasogastric tube and attach to intermittent low suction to prevent further distention.
- Administer intravenous therapy to restore fluid balance.
- Prepare the infant for immediate surgery, as prescribed.
- Obtain the necessary laboratory specimens and send for analysis.

- Maintain the infant on NPO (nothing by mouth) status.
- Know that the infant may return from surgery with a temporary colostomy if the repair was anatomically difficult or if the infant had other anomalies that interfered with health.
- Advise the parents that if the infant returns from surgery with a colostomy, follow-up surgery to re-connect will probably be rescheduled for age 3 to 6 months.
- Teach the parents about caring for the infant's colostomy.
- Provide support and encouragement to the parents during this time; allow them to verbalize their fears and anxieties.

## INTRACRANIAL PRESSURE, INCREASED

### DESCRIPTION

- Increased intracranial pressure is not a single dis-order but a syndrome arising with many neurologic disorders.
- Increased intracranial pressure may occur when there is an increase in the cerebrospinal fluid volume, when blood enters the cerebrospinal fluid, when cerebral edema is present, or when there are space-occupying lesions, such as tumors.
- Examples that lead to increased intracranial pressure in the newborn are birth trauma or *hydrocephalus;* in the infant or preschooler, *head trauma* or infection; in the school-age child or adolescent, *brain neoplasm* or *Guillain-Barré syndrome.*
- The rate at which symptoms develop depends on the cause and on whether the child's skull can expand to accommodate the increased pressure; children with open fontanelles can withstand more pressure without brain damage than older children, whose suture lines and fontanelles are already closed.

### ASSESSMENT FINDINGS

- Increased head circumference >2 cm/month in first 3 months of life, >1 cm/month in second 3 months of life, and >0.5 cm/month for the next 6 months
- Tense and bulging anterior fontanelle

- Late closing of fontanelles
- *Vomiting* in the absence of nausea, on awakening in the morning or after a nap, becoming projectile
- Vision changes (diplopia, "sunset eyes," limited visual fields, papilledema)
- Elevated temperature and blood pressure
- Decreased pulse and respiratory rate
- Headache
- Irritability, altered consciousness

### Nursing Implications

- Perform a thorough history and physical assessment, including neurologic assessment to establish a baseline and ongoing to identify changes.
- Obtain vital signs, and evaluate pupillary response, level of consciousness, and motor and sensory function.
- Be aware that changes in neurologic status may occur gradually; therefore, compare new neurologic assessment recordings against recordings taken in the last 24 hours or since the child's hospital admission.
- Ask questions that are appropriate to the age level of the child when assessing level of consciousness.
- Explain to the parents that you are frequently asking the child questions to assess level of consciousness not knowledge and remind the parents not to respond for the child.
- Test deep tendon reflexes, which decrease in intensity with decreased level of consciousness.
- Observe the child for any *seizure* activity because this is a late sign of increased intracranial pressure.
- Perform intracranial pressure monitoring per hospital protocol.
- Explain to the parents about the brain's anatomy and that the intracranial monitoring catheter does not puncture or tear brain tissue.
- When bubbling (burping) infants with increased intracranial pressure, do not put pressure on the jugular veins because this increases the intracranial pressure.
- Administer steroids, such as dexamethasone (Decadron), as prescribed to help reduce intracranial pressure.
- Insert indwelling urinary catheter as prescribed; before intravenous administration of mannitol to prevent bladder distention from rapid diuresis.

# INTUSSUSCEPTION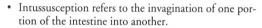

## DESCRIPTION

- Intussusception refers to the invagination of one portion of the intestine into another.
- This generally occurs in the second half of the first year.
- In infants younger than age 1 year, intussusception generally occurs for idiopathic reasons.
- In infants older than age 1 year, a "lead point" on the intestine likely cues the invagination and may be due to a *Meckel's diverticulum,* a polyp, hypertrophy of Peyer's patches, or bowel tumors.
- This condition is a surgical emergency; reduction of the intussusception must be done promptly by barium enema or surgery before necrosis of the invaginated portion of the bowel results.

## ASSESSMENT FINDINGS

- Legs drawn up when crying
- Cry as if with severe pain
- *Vomiting* (may contain bile)
- Peristaltic wave bringing severe pain, possibly occurring every 15 minutes
- Blood in stool ("currant jelly" appearance)
- Bowel distention
- Increased temperature, rapid pulse
- Peritoneal irritation (child guards abdomen during attempt to palpate)
- Increased white blood cell count

## NURSING IMPLICATIONS

- Perform a thorough history and physical assessment to establish a baseline.
- Ask the parents to describe the child's pain: the duration, intensity, and frequency.
- Ask the parents if the child is sick in any other way.
- Know that infants need to be held and rocked and comforted in an attempt to relieve their frustration at this pain that returns and then goes away only to return again.
- Arrange for necessary x-ray films, blood work, and laboratory specimens as prescribed.
- Maintain the child on NPO (nothing by mouth) status until surgery.
- Offer the infant a pacifier to help relieve discomfort through sucking.

- Administer intravenous fluids to reestablish electrolyte balance and to supply adequate fluid to hydrate the child.
- Keep the parents informed of the status of their child.
- Provide support and encouragement to the parents; prepare the parents and child physically and psychologically for surgery and include all aspects of preoperative and postoperative care.

## IODINE DEFICIENCY

### DESCRIPTION
- An iodine deficiency usually occurs as a result of a diet deficient in iodine; it may lead to hyperplasia of the thyroid gland (goiter).
- In the United States, areas where goiter is endemic are mainly the states bordering Canada, especially the Great Lakes area and those states between the Rocky Mountains and the Appalachians.
- When the thyroid gland does not have adequate iodine to make thyroxine, its chief hormone, the gland is overstimulated by the pituitary gland; the overstimulation leads to hyperplasia.
- Goiter tends to occur most frequently in girls at puberty and during pregnancy.

### ASSESSMENT FINDINGS
- Enlarged thyroid gland
- Goiter present or palpable
- Difficulty breathing
- Symptoms of *hypothyroidism*

### NURSING IMPLICATIONS
- Perform a physical assessment, especially palpating the thyroid if iodine deficiency is suspected.
- Obtain a dietary history to ascertain intake.
- Administer supplemental iodine or synthetic thyroxine, as prescribed.
- Teach the child and parents how to maintain a diet that is adequate in iodine, including foods high in iodine.

## IRRITABLE BOWEL SYNDROME

### DESCRIPTION
- Irritable bowel syndrome is the presence of either intermittent episodes of loose stools or recurrent abdominal pain.

- It appears slightly more often in females than in males and has an increased incidence at ages 5 to 6 years and again at ages 10 to 11 years.
- The cause is unknown, but it is associated with low fat intake (without fat slowing absorption, stool passes rapidly through the bowel) or excessive fluid intake.

### Assessment Findings

- *Diarrhea* or pain several times a week or as infrequently as once a month
- Generally mild or "annoying" pain rather than colicky or severe
- Pain radiating to bizarre sites
- Nausea, pallor, dizziness, headache, and faintness preceding or accompanying episodes of pain
- History of family problems (possible)
- Symptoms of stress or sleep disturbances

### Nursing Implications

- Perform a thorough health history, including a history of any family problems.
- Perform a thorough physical assessment to establish a baseline and rule out any other underlying problems.
- Be certain that during history taking, in light of family problems, a physical basis for the pain is not overlooked.
- Prepare the child for any diagnostic procedures that may be ordered to rule out organic disease.
- Explain to the parents the reason for any diagnostic tests.
- Obtain a complete blood count, as prescribed, to rule out infection and anemia.
- Obtain a stool sample for ova, parasites, and occult blood, as prescribed.
- Obtain a urine specimen for analysis to rule out *urinary tract infection.*
- Perform a perineal examination and observe for *pinworms.*
- Arrange for the child and the parents to receive counseling regarding the underlying cause of the problem.

## JUVENILE RHEUMATOID ARTHRITIS (JRA)

### Description

- JRA is a disorder that primarily involves the joints of the body, although it also affects blood vessels and other connective tissue.

- Peak incidence occurs at two times in childhood: 1 to 3 years and 8 to 12 years.
- The cause is unknown, although it is probably an autoimmune process or the child has developed circulating antibodies (immunoglobins) against his or her own body cells.
- T lymphocytes may also be involved in the process or changed to attack and destroy body cells, or ineffective lymphocytic-inhibition cells are unable to halt lymphocyte production.
- A genetic predisposition may make it apt to happen in some people more than others.
- Three separate types of JRA exist, and the types differ mainly by the type of joint affected and the severity of systemic effects: polyarticular JRA, monarticular or pauciarticular JRA (most common form), and systemic JRA.
- Therapy includes a balanced program of exercise, rest, and medication administration.
- Aspirin is the drug of choice for children with JRA, and other nonsteroidal anti-inflammatory drugs also may be used as well as steroids, intramuscular gold injections, and immunosuppressants.

### ASSESSMENT FINDINGS

Symptoms occur before age 16 and last 3 months.

#### Polyarticular
- Stiffness and minimal swelling in multiple joints, especially fingers and toes, leading to limited movement
- IgM antibodies present
- Antinuclear antibodies present
- Elevated white blood cell count, complement, and sedimentation rate

#### Monarticular or pauciarticular
- Painless swelling of one to four major joints of knees, ankles, and elbows
- Joint stiffness in morning and refusal to bear weight on leg
- Joints warm to touch
- Presence of HLA-B27 (more in males)
- Normal white blood cell count (elevated with septic JRA)
- Uveitis

### Septic
- *Elevated body temperature* (103°F twice daily for 3 to 4 weeks)
- Multiple joint swelling
- Pale, red, macular rash on trunk and extremities
- Enlarged lymph nodes
- Elevated white blood cell count
- Enlarged liver or spleen
- Fluid-filled joints

#### Nursing Implications
- Assess child not only for signs and symptoms of the disease, but also for the effect the disease is having on self-care.
- Assess the child and the parents' understanding of the illness and planned therapy.
- Aid the parents in creating alternative activities to help the child avoid those motions he or she should not do.
- Teach the parents and child how to perform full range-of-motion exercises.
- Advise the parents and child to perform full range-of-motion exercises twice daily.
- Encourage the child to do as much self-care activities as he or she is capable.
- Teach the child and parents how to perform isometric exercises during acute phases of inflammation.
- Teach the child and parents the importance of good body alignment.
- Teach the parents how to perform warm water soaks and paraffin soaks, as prescribed.
- Encourage adequate nutrition, and teach the parents to plan mealtimes for the child's best time of the day.
- Stress the importance of not wearing a splint past a period of inflammation because the splint can cause a contracture and deformity with extended use.
- Educate parents that aspirin should not be given on an empty stomach and to have the child drink a glass of milk before taking the medication.
- Teach the parents that they should give the aspirin even though the child does not have any noticeable pain because the anti-inflammatory effects of the aspirin are equally important as the pain relief.
- Help the parents and child schedule exercise and medication programs around school and other activities.
- Perform ongoing evaluation of the child's self-image.

# KAWASAKI DISEASE

### DESCRIPTION

- Kawasaki disease (mucocutaneous lymph node syndrome) is a febrile, multisystem disorder that occurs almost exclusively in children before the age of puberty.
- Peak incidence is in boys under 4 years of age, with Asian Pacific children being the most at risk.
- Vasculitis is the principal and life-threatening finding, leading to formation of aneurysm and myocardial infarction.
- The cause is unknown, but it apparently develops in genetically predisposed individuals after exposure to an as yet unidentified infectious agent resulting in altered immune function.

### ASSESSMENT FINDINGS (To be diagnosed with Kawasaki disease, the child must manifest fever and four of the typical symptoms listed below.)

- Fever of 5 or more days (38.9° to 41.4°C) that does not respond to antipyretics
- Bilateral congestion of ocular conjunctiva
- Changes of the mucous membrane of the upper respiratory tract, such as reddened pharynx; red, dry, fissured lips; or protuberance of tongue papillae (strawberry tongue)
- Changes of the peripheral extremities, such as peripheral edema, peripheral erythema, desquamation of the palms and soles
- Rashes, primarily truncal and polymorphous
- Cervical lymph node swelling

### NURSING IMPLICATIONS

- Perform a detailed history and physical assessment.
- Administer salicylic acid (aspirin) to decrease inflammation and block platelet agglutination.
- Arrange for sequential echocardiograms to monitor if aneurysms are developing.
- Obtain necessary laboratory specimens, as prescribed.
- Administer dipyridamole, as prescribed, to increase coronary vasodilatation and decrease platelet accumulation.
- Administer intravenous gamma globulin, as prescribed, to reduce the antigen-antibody reaction and the possibility of coronary artery disease.

- Administer warfarin (Coumadin) or heparin or fibrinolytic therapy, such as streptokinase, urokinase, or tissue plasminogen activator, as prescribed.
- Provide emotional support to the parents during this disease.
- Provide the parents with ongoing information about the status of their child; allow parents to verbalize their feelings and fears.

## KERATITIS

### DESCRIPTION

- Keratitis is inflammation and infection of the superficial layers of the cornea.
- It may accompany or be a complication of *conjunctivitis* and may result when a foreign body strikes the cornea.
- The invading organism may be bacterial, fungal, or viral in origin.

### ASSESSMENT FINDINGS

- Pain
- Tearing
- Redness
- Photophobia (intolerance to light)

### NURSING IMPLICATIONS

- Make sure that the child with keratitis is referred to an ophthalmologist for therapy because the infection could lead to scarring of the cornea, resulting in vision impairment when light rays are no longer able to enter the eye normally.
- Teach the parents how to give eye medications.
- Teach the parents and the child how to use good hygiene to prevent spreading eye infection to other siblings.

## KIDNEY AGENESIS

### DESCRIPTION

- Kidney agenesis describes a condition in which there was a lack of growth or no kidney(s) was formed in utero.
- Absence of kidneys in a newborn is suggested when the volume of amniotic fluid on sonogram or at birth is less than normal (oligohydramnios) because urine usually adds to the volume of amniotic fluid in utero.
- The infant with kidney agenesis usually has Potter's syndrome.

- Bilateral kidney agenesis is obviously incompatible with life unless a renal transplant can be accomplished but usually it is not successful because of the newborn's inoperative lungs.

### ASSESSMENT FINDINGS
- Oligohydramnios
- Misshapen, low-set ears
- Hypoplastic lungs (stiff, inflexible)
- Absence of voided urine

### NURSING IMPLICATIONS
- Obtain a thorough labor and birth history, especially the amount of amniotic fluid present on sonogram or at rupture of membranes.
- Assess the newborn for voiding, observing the amount voided.
- Perform a physical assessment of the newborn, observing the placement of the ears.
- Assess vital signs on the newborn, assessing respiratory status.
- Provide support and understanding to the parents and inform them of the status of their newborn; allow the parents to verbalize their feelings about the newborn's condition.

## KWASHIORKOR

### DESCRIPTION
- Kwashiorkor is a disease caused by protein deficiency.
- It occurs most frequently in children ages 1 to 3 years because this is an age group requiring a high protein intake.
- It tends to occur after weaning when children change from breast milk to a diet consisting mainly of carbohydrates.
- Kwashiorkor is fatal without treatment using a diet rich in protein.

### ASSESSMENT FINDINGS
- Growth failure
- Edema (may obscure light weight)
- Severe wasting of muscles (masked by edema)
- Irritability and disinterest in surroundings
- Delayed motor development
- Zebra sign (hair shafts striped brown and white)
- *Diarrhea*

- *Iron deficiency anemia*
- Hepatomegaly

### NURSING IMPLICATIONS
- Perform a thorough history and physical assessment, including a dietary history.
- Teach the parents about a diet and foods that are rich in protein.
- Teach the parents ways to encourage the child to eat to increase protein intake.
- Explain to the parents the importance of adhering to the diet regimen.
- Educate the child and parents about the need for follow-up to evaluate improvement in condition.

## LARYNGEAL STRIDOR, CONGENITAL

### DESCRIPTION
- Congenital laryngeal stridor (laryngomalacia) results when the child's laryngeal structure is weaker than normal and collapses more than usual on inspiration.
- The stridor is generally present from birth; it may be intensified when the child is in the supine position.

### ASSESSMENT FINDINGS
- Sternal retractions on inspiration
- Stridor (raucous sound) most noticeable during sucking

### NURSING IMPLICATIONS
- Reassure the parents that although the sound of stridor is raucous, they may care for their child at home.
- Show the parents a growth chart to assure them that their child is growing and thriving despite this problem.
- Assess at health care visits that the parents are getting adequate rest and not becoming too exhausted to care for their child because some parents sleep with their hands on the infant's chest to ensure that they are breathing.
- Instruct the parents that no routine therapy is necessary except to feed the child slowly, providing periods of rest as needed.
- Advise the parents that the condition improves as the child matures because cartilage in the larynx becomes stronger at about 1 year of age.

- Caution the parents to bring the child in for early care if signs of an upper respiratory tract infection develop.
- Advise the parents that anytime the stridor becomes more intense they should have their child seen by a physician.
- Know that as parents become more used to the sound their infants make while breathing, they become astute reporters of change in their infant's condition; listen to them carefully when they report a change so as not to miss this important information.

## LARYNGITIS

### DESCRIPTION
- Laryngitis is inflammation of the larynx, which results in brassy, hoarse voice sounds or inability to make audible voice sounds.
- It may occur as a spread of *pharyngitis* or from excessive use of the voice.

### ASSESSMENT FINDINGS
- Brassy, hoarse voice sounds
- Complaints of annoying tickling sensation
- History of recent *pharyngitis*

### NURSING IMPLICATIONS
- Instruct the parents to offer the child sips of fluid (either cold or warm) to offer relief from the annoying tickling sensation often present.
- Tell the parents that the most effective measure is to instruct the child not to talk for at least 24 hours until the inflammation subsides.
- Advise the parents to try and meet the infant's needs before they have to cry for things; older children simply need to be cautioned not to speak.
- Tell the parents that it is not necessary to have the child on bed rest, and the child will probably use the voice to ask for things if restricted to bed.

## LEGG-CALVE-PERTHES DISEASE (COXA PLANA)

### DESCRIPTION
- Legg-Calve-Perthes disease is avascular necrosis of the proximal femoral epiphysis.
- It occurs more often in males than in females; the peak age of incidence is between 4 and 8 years of age.

- Legg-Calve-Perthes disease passes through four stages: synovitis stage (painful inflammation), necrotic stage (bone in femur becomes smaller with increased density), fragmentation stage (resorption of dead bone), and reconstruction stage (final healing with deposition of new bone).
- Treatment includes the use of containment braces or casting, which contains the femur head in the acetabulum socket by abducting the leg.
- A reconstructive surgery technique (an osteotomy to center the femur head in the acetabulum followed by cast application) is available that limits the time of containment to 3 to 4 months.

### ASSESSMENT FINDINGS
- Hip joint pain
- Muscle spasm
- Limited motion
- Previous diagnosis of synovitis of hip joint

### NURSING IMPLICATIONS
- Obtain a thorough history and physical examination to establish a baseline.
- Prepare the parents and child for treatment modalities, including possible surgery.
- Assess the extremity for possible circulation impairment caused by brace or cast application.
- Help the parents plan how they will care for the child at home.
- Help the parents arrange for transportation (large cast may not fit in some cars), and plan for possible tutoring of child if he or she cannot attend school.
- Offer support and encouragement to the parents as they try to cope with caring for a child with long-term therapy.
- Provide cast care and instruct the parents and the child about cast care; instruct the parents in measures to care for braces if used.
- Provide instructions about crutches to the child.
- Instruct the parents and the child about the long-term consequences of this therapy.
- Know that most children seen for synovitis of the hip joint should be seen in 3 to 4 weeks for a repeat x-ray film to rule out Legg-Calve-Perthes disease, which begins with the same symptoms.

## LIVER RUPTURE

### DESCRIPTION

- Liver rupture or laceration is a medical emergency, and such children require immediate surgery because the liver is a highly vascular organ, and blood loss from it is acute and damaging.
- Occasionally a communication between an artery and a bile duct occurs at the time of trauma, which delays symptoms.

### ASSESSMENT FINDINGS

- Severe abdominal pain (most marked on inspiration)
- Tachycardia
- Hypotension
- Anxiety
- Pallor
- Low or falling hematocrit
- Colicky upper abdominal pain relieved by emesis
- Hematemesis or melena

### NURSING IMPLICATIONS

- Perform a thorough history, including the events that led to the accident or the trauma.
- Obtain vital signs frequently and report any abnormal findings.
- Obtain necessary laboratory specimens and be alert for any abnormal values.
- Arrange for a liver arteriogram, as prescribed.
- Be alert for signs and symptoms of shock from excessive bleeding.
- Keep the parents informed as to the status of their child and the reason for any ordered tests.
- Offer support and understanding to the parents during their child's hospitalization.
- Prepare the child for emergency surgery and obtain necessary consent forms.

## LYME DISEASE

### DESCRIPTION

- Lyme disease is caused by a spirocete *Borrelia burgdorferi* that is transmitted by a tick often carried on deer.
- The disease is the most frequently reported vectorborne infection in the United States.

- It occurs most often in the summer and early fall.
- Lyme disease includes systemic involvement that leads to cardiac, musculoskeletal, and neurologic symptoms.
- Cardiac involvement can be so severe that it leads to heart block from atrioventricular conduction abnormalities.

### ASSESSMENT FINDINGS

- Erythematous papule noticeable at tick bite site that spreads over the next 3 to 30 days to become a large, round ring with a raised swollen border
- Stiff neck
- Headache
- Cranial nerve palsy
- Painful, swollen arthritic joints (usually knee)

### NURSING IMPLICATIONS

- Perform a thorough history and physical assessment to establish a baseline and identify possible tick exposure.
- Administer oral penicillin to younger children and tetracycline to those older than age 8.
- Administer anti-inflammatory agents and daily prednisone to reduce the cardiac and arthritic effects, as prescribed.
- Caution parents to inspect the skin of children who have been playing in wooded areas for possible tick bites.
- Advise parents that their children (and they themselves) should wear protective clothing, such as long sleeves, long slacks, and high necklines when hiking in wooded areas.
- Teach parents that they and their children should wear light-colored clothing so that any tick present on clothing can be readily observed.
- Teach parents to report any inflammation that might be a tick bite to a health care provider for early diagnosis.
- Provide support and encouragement to the child and parents because this is a long-term illness.

## LYMPHOCYTOSIS

### DESCRIPTION

- Lymphocytosis refers to an increase in lymphocytes; it occurs normally in the preschool period when there

is a marked predominence of lymphocytes in relation to neutrophils.
- Disorders characterized by an increase in the number of white blood cells or specific white blood cell components occur in response to other disease (often infection or an allergic reaction) in the body.

### Assessment Findings
- Elevated lymphocyte count (laboratory values of white blood cell count aid in specific diagnosis)

### Nursing Implications
- Obtain a thorough history and physical examination to establish a baseline and rule out specific diseases.
- Know that abnormally elevated lymphocytes may indicate childhood illnesses, such as pertussis, *infectious mononucleosis,* and lymphoblastic *leukemia.*
- Monitor the child's differential white blood cell count for changes.

## MALOCCLUSION

### Description
- Malocclusion refers to a condition in which the upper teeth do not overlap the lower teeth by a small amount and the teeth are not evenly spaced and in good alignment.
- It may be congenital and related to conditions such as *cleft palate,* a small lower jaw, or familial traits tending toward malocclusion.
- The condition can result from constant mouth breathing or abnormal tongue position (tongue thrusting) or from the loss of teeth because of extraction or accident if not properly treated to maintain alignment.
- The upper jaw in children mature rapidly in early childhood along with skull growth; the lower jaw forms more slowly, which forces teeth to make a prolonged series of changes until they reach their final adult alignment and position.
- Good tooth occlusion is necessary for optimum formation of teeth, health of the supporting tissue, optimum speech development, and pleasant physical appearance.

- Malocclusion may be crossbite (sideways), anterior, or posterior.

### ASSESSMENT FINDINGS
- Upper teeth not overlaping lower teeth by a small amount
- Teeth not evenly spaced and in good alignment

### NURSING IMPLICATIONS
- Perform a physical assessment and observe the oral cavity and the teeth for possible malocclusion.
- Obtain a health history and assess any factors that may predispose the child to malocclusion.
- Suggest that children with a malocclusion be evaluated by an orthodontist to determine if braces or other orthodontic work is necessary.
- Know that braces are not only expensive, but also they cause pain for children when they are first applied and at periodic visits when they are tightened to maintain pressure for further straightening.
- Encourage the child to rub dental wax over the wires to dull the surface and possibly prevent the shallow ulcerations (canker sores) of the buccal membrane from friction of a metal wire.
- Suggest the use of over-the-counter aids such as Oragil rubbed on the ulceration to help give relief.
- Tell the child that he or she will have to have teeth assessed frequently to ensure that the child is brushing properly around the braces.
- Know that following the removal of braces, many children need to wear retainers to help maintain the correction the braces achieved.
- Show appropriate sympathy to the child and help the child problem solve if he or she is bothered by the appearance of braces or a retainer.

## MAPLE SYRUP URINE DISEASE

### DESCRIPTION
- Maple syrup urine disease, an inborn error of metabolism, is a rare disorder, inherited as an autosomal recessive trait.
- There is a defect in amino acid metabolism leading to cerebral degeneration similar to that of *phenylketonuria.*

- The infant appears well at birth but quickly begins to show symptoms.
- The maple syrup odor of urine is due to the presence of ketoacids, the same phenomenon that makes the breath of diabetic children with severe acidosis smell sweet.
- Cerebral degeneration can be prevented (just as it can be prevented in *phenylketonuria*) if the disease is diagnosed in the first day or two of life and the child is placed on a well-controlled diet high in thiamine and low in the amino acids leucine, isoleucine, and valine.
- Hemodialysis can be used to reduce abnormal serum levels temporarily at birth or during a childhood infection.

### ASSESSMENT FINDINGS
- Feeding difficulty
- Loss of Moro reflex
- Irregular respirations
- Opisthotonus
- Generalized muscular rigidity
- Convulsions
- Urine with odor of maple syrup by first or second day of life

### NURSING IMPLICATIONS
- Assess the newborn's wet diapers for the color, amount, and odor of urine.
- Report any findings of urine with characteristic odor of maple syrup.
- Provide or arrange for the parents to receive intensive dietary counseling.
- Offer support and encouragement to the parents.
- Provide frequent, ongoing information about the status of the child.
- Teach the parents the importance of adhering to the dietary regimen and follow-up.

## MARASMUS

### DESCRIPTION
- Marasmus is a nutritional disease caused by deficiency of all food groups.

- It is basically a form of starvation, and although it is seen most commonly in developing countries where food supplies are short, it is seen in grossly neglected children in the United States.
- This condition generally results from poor maternal-infant bonding in the United States.

### ASSESSMENT FINDINGS
- Child less than 1 year of age with growth failure
- Wasting of muscles
- Irritability
- *Iron deficiency anemia*
- *Diarrhea*
- Starving (sucks at any object offered)

### NURSING IMPLICATIONS
- Perform a thorough health history and obtain vital signs.
- Perform a thorough physical and nutritional assessment, including height and weight to establish a baseline, and compare with standards to identify the degree of condition.
- Teach the parents about the importance of a healthy diet; offer suggestions and guidelines for proper nutrition based on the child's nutritional needs; arrange for dietitian to talk with parents about appropriate food choices for the child.
- Inform the parent(s) of possible assistance for which they may be eligible, such as food stamps and welfare assistance, if finances are a problem.
- Encourage the maternal-infant bonding process.
- Suggest that the parent(s) seek counseling to understand the reason for a poor maternal-infant bonding.

## MECKEL'S DIVERTICULUM

### DESCRIPTION
- Meckel's diverticulum is a small pouch off the ileum, approximately 18 inches from the ileum-colon junction, that remains in about 2% or 3% of all infants when the omphalomesenteric (vitelline) duct becomes a vestigial ligament as the infant reaches term.
- In this structure, there may be some misplaced gastric mucosa, which secretes gastric acids that flow into the intestine and are irritating to the bowel wall resulting in ulceration and bleeding.

- In some instances, Meckel's diverticulum may act as a lead point and cause an *intussusception* or a fibrous band extending from the diverticulum pouch to the umbilicus, which acts as a constricting band, causing bowel obstruction.

### ASSESSMENT FINDINGS
- Painless, tarlike (black) stools
- Grossly bloody stools

### NURSING IMPLICATIONS
- Perform a thorough physical assessment and history, including information about the appearance of the infant's stool.
- Test the infant's stool for occult blood.
- Prepare the infant for possible surgery.
- Provide the parents with support and encouragement during this time, including explanations about all preoperative and postoperative events, procedures, and care.

## MECONIUM ILEUS

### DESCRIPTION
- Meconium ileus (obstruction of the intestinal lumen by hardened meconium) is a specific phenomonen that occurs most commonly in the infant with *cystic fibrosis.*
- With *cystic fibrosis,* the enzyme that moistens and makes all body fluids free and flowing is absent; therefore, all body fluids are thick and tenacious, affecting intestinal and pancreatic secretions (as well as lung) signaled at birth by hardened obstructive meconium at the ileus level (from lack of trypsin secretion from the pancreas) resulting in meconium ileus.

### ASSESSMENT FINDINGS
- No meconium passage
- Abdominal distention
- *Vomiting* of bile-stained fluid

### NURSING IMPLICATIONS
- Perform a thorough newborn physical assessment, including measurement of abdominal girth.
- Obtain newborn vital signs.
- Perform ongoing abdominal girth measurements to determine the progression of abdominal distention.
- Observe the newborn for passage of meconium stool.

- Prepare the newborn for possible x-ray or appropriate diagnostic test as prescribed.
- Administer enemas to attempt to reduce the obstruction, as prescribed.
- Maintain the newborn's NPO (nothing by mouth) status.
- Prepare the newborn for impending surgery.
- Provide emotional support and encouragement to the parents during this time, including explanations of preoperative and postoperative events, procedures, and care.
- Advise the parents that because newborns do not sweat freely owing to immaturity of their temperature regulating system, a sweat test to determine a diagnosis of *cystic fibrosis* may not be done until 4 to 6 weeks of age.

# MECONIUM PLUG SYNDROME

### DESCRIPTION
- A meconium plug is an extremely hard portion of meconium that completely obstructs the intestinal lumen, causing bowel obstruction.
- Why this occurs is unknown, but it probably reflects normal variations of meconium consistency.
- If a meconium plug has formed, it is usually present in the lower end of the bowel because this is the meconium that formed early in intrauterine life and has the best chance to become dry and inspissated.

### ASSESSMENT FINDINGS
- Infant past 24 hours of age
- No meconium passage
- Presence of hardened stool on rectal examination (but may be too far removed to be palpable)

### NURSING IMPLICATIONS
- Assess the family history for *cystic fibrosis* or aganglionic megacolon.
- Assess the newborn for signs of hypothyroidism, such as large protruding tongue, lethargy, or subnormal body temperature.
- Obtain a hypothyroid screening, as prescribed in any newborn with a meconium plug.
- Record and report the passage of any plug of hardened meconium.

- Observed the newborn that has passed a hardened meconium plug for continued defecation to rule out the presence of another larger and truly obstructing plug.
- Prepare the infant for a barium enema, as prescribed, to determine the extent of the obstruction and possibly to loosen the plug.
- Administer acetylcysteine proteolytic enzyme (Mucomyst) rectally, as prescribed, to dissolve the plug.
- Administer a saline enema, as prescribed (never use tap water in newborns because it leads to water intoxication), which may cause enough peristalsis to expel the plug.
- Instruct the parents about the importance of observing for meconium after the infant is discharged and the need to telephone the pediatrician should the child have no further defecation at home.
- Know that the infant needs further assessment for aganglion megacolon and *cystic fibrosis* (illnesses that present with constipation or *meconium ileus*) during health care visits during the first year of life.

# MENINGITIS, BACTERIAL

## DESCRIPTION

- Meningitis, an infection of the cerebral meninges, occurs between the ages of 1 month and 5 years; half of the cases occur in children less than 1 year; peak incidence is during the winter.
- In the United States (except in newborns), meningitis is most commonly caused by *Haemophilus influenzae* type B; in newborns, group B streptococcus is the most common cause; in children with myelomeningocele who develop meningitis, *Pseudomonas* infection is the most common cause.
- Children who have had a splenectomy are susceptible to meningococcal meningitis.
- Organisms spread to the meninges from an upper respiratory infection via the lymphatic drainage through the mastoid or the sinuses or by direct introduction via lumbar puncture or skull fracture.
- Once in the meningeal space, the organism multiplies rapidly spreading throughout the cerebrospinal fluid.
- Organisms invade brain tissue, and an inflammatory response may lead to thick, fibrinous exudate that blocks cerebrospinal fluid flow.

- Brain abscesses or invasion of the infection into the cranial nerves may result in blindness, deafness, or facial paralysis.
- Exudate that obstructs flow in the narrow aqueduct of Sylvius leads to hydrocephalus.
- Brain tissue edema can increase pressure on the hypopituitary gland causing increased production of antidiuretic hormone, which leads to further edema secondary to the body's inability to excrete urine.
- Immunization with *H. influenzae* vaccine has limited the number of children who contract meningitis.
- Meningococcal vaccine is recommended for children over 5 who have been exposed to someone with this form of meningitis or for children who have had a splenectomy.

ASSESSMENT FINDINGS (can be insidious or sudden)
- 2 to 3 days of upper respiratory infection
- Fever
- Chills
- *Vomiting*
- Increasing irritability
- Headache
- Behavioral or intellectual changes
- Positive Kernig's and Brudsinski's signs
- *Seizures* or shock
- Nuchal rigidity and opisthotonus
- Cranial nerve paralysis
- Bulging, tense fontanelles (if they are open)
- Papilledema (if fontanelles are closed)
- Septic arthritis (with meningitis secondary to *H. influenzae*)
- Papular or purple petechial skin rash (with *Neisseria meningitidis*)
- Febrile *seizures*
- Increased white blood cells, increased protein, decreased glucose level in cerebrospinal fluid analysis
- Leukopenia

*In newborns:*
- Poor sucking
- Weak cry
- Lethargy
- Cardiovascular shock

## NURSING IMPLICATIONS

- Prepare the child suspected of this disorder for a lumbar puncture for definitive analysis of cerebrospinal fluid.
- Treat all children with febrile convulsions as if they had meningitis until proved otherwise.
- Place the child on respiratory precautions for at least 24 hours after antibiotics have begun.
- Assess cerebral functioning and evidence of *seizures,* and institute *seizure* precautions.
- Explain to the parents and child the nature of the symptoms and the probable cause. Also, explain the rationale for all therapeutic interventions, and support the parents so that they know they are not responsible for their child's illness.
- Assure parents that the signs of meningitis are insidious and that they could not predict the extent of the disease from early symptoms.
- Educate parents about the illness and help them to learn isolation techniques.
- Encourage parents to care for the child during the illness both to make the child more comfortable and to help them manage their own anxiety.
- Identify any persons who had contact with this child because the disease has a high risk for transmission; treat identified persons appropriately.
- Institute medical treatment for the child with bacterial meningitis as indicated: intravenous antibiotics, measures to reduce intracranial pressure, measures to control *seizures,* fluid management, and pain management.
- Always give antibiotics on time to ensure adequate blood levels.
- Monitor blood urea nitrogen and creatinine because the antibiotics needed to control bacterial meningitis are potent.
- Monitor intake and output, weight, and fluid balance carefully to prevent overhydration.
- Avoid flexing the child's neck because it will cause pain.
- Administer acetaminophen for fever and irritability.
- Keep the child's room quiet and dark and minimize environmental stimuli and sudden position changes.
- Keep painful procedures, such as blood sampling, to a minimum.

- Explain to the parents that the child's irritability is part of the illness.
- Allow time for the parents to discuss their concerns.
- For infants with group B beta-hemolytic streptococcal meningitis, help the parents to understand how their infant suddenly became so ill.
- Support the parents of infants and children left neurologically disabled, and refer them to the appropriate consultations.

## MENINGOCELE

### DESCRIPTION

- A meningocele, a *neural tube defect,* occurs if the meninges covering the spinal cord herniate through formed vertebrae and appear as a protruding mass, usually the size of an orange.
- A meningocele occurs at the center of the back generally at the lumbar region, although it might be present anywhere along the spinal canal.
- The protrusion may be covered by a layer of skin or only the clear dura mater.
- When infants are detected as having meningocele, they are usually delivered by cesarean birth to avoid pressure and injury to the spinal cord.

### ASSESSMENT FINDINGS

- Visible protruding mass at birth or during ultrasonography, fetoscopy, amniocentesis, or analysis of alpha-fetoprotein in maternal serum.

### NURSING IMPLICATIONS

- Obtain a thorough history and physical examination to establish a baseline and identify any visible defect.
- Observe and record spontaneous movements of the extremities and the pattern of voiding and defecating to differentiate between meningocele and *myelomeningocele.*
- Place the infant in a prone position or supported on his or her side to prevent pressure on the neural sac.
- Place a sterile, wet compress of saline, antiseptic, or antibiotic gauze over the lesion to keep the lesion moist.

- Use caution when placing the infant under a radiant heat warmer for warmth so that the lesion does not become dry and crack.
- Encourage the mother to hold the infant in as normal a feeding position as possible, making sure that no pressure is exerted on the defect.
- Measure the child's head circumference once daily or more frequently if prescribed, and assess for signs of *increased intracranial pressure.*
- Prepare the child and parents for possible surgery.
- Observe the child postoperatively for signs of *increased intracranial pressure,* such as a change in vital signs, neurologic signs such as pupillary changes, or an increase in head circumference or bulging fontanelles, as well as behavioral changes, such as irritability or lethargy.
- Turn the infant's head every 2 hours if *hydrocephalus* has developed to prevent pressure areas at the temples.
- Offer support and guidance to the parents to alleviate their fears and anxieties; allow parents to verbalize their feelings.

## MENSTRUAL IRREGULARITIES

### DESCRIPTION

- Menstrual irregularities refer to menstruation that is infrequent or too frequent.
- Menstrual irregularities are the most frequent of the reproductive disorders in females.
- Menstrual irregularities include menorrhagia and metrorrhagia.
- Menorrhagia refers to an abnormally heavy menstrual flow resulting from anovulatory cycles. Without ovulation, subsequent progesterone and estrogen secretion continues and causes extreme proliferation of the endometrium. A heavy flow can indicate endometriosis; a systemic disease; blood dyscrasia, such as a clotting defect; or a uterine abnormality, such as a myoma (fibroid) tumor. It can be a symptom of infection, such as pelvic inflammatory disease, or an indication of an early pregnancy loss that is coincidentally occurring at the time of an expected menstrual flow.
- Metrorrhagia refers to bleeding between menstrual periods. It may be normal in some adolescents who have spotting at the time of ovulation; it may also occur in

females taking oral contraceptives for the first 3 to 4 months or from vaginal irritation from an infection.

- Because menstruation is an ongoing process throughout half a woman's life greatly affecting her self-image, irregularities can be extremely upsetting.

## ASSESSMENT FINDINGS

### *Menorrhagia*
- Abnormally heavy flow, saturating a pad or tampon in less than 1 hour
- Anemia (possible from excessive iron loss)

### *Metrorrhagia*
- Midcycle spotting or bleeding

## NURSING IMPLICATIONS

- Obtain a thorough history and physical examination to establish a baseline and rule out any possible underlying disorders.
- Obtain a thorough menstrual history from the adolescent, including the date of her last menstrual period, length of usual cycle, amount of usual flow, and use of oral contraceptives or intrauterine devices (IUDs).
- Keep in mind that there is often an unusual amount of flow in girls using IUDs and that with oral contraceptives the flow is often light but may seem alarmingly heavy once the pills are discontinued.
- Be aware that with metrorrhagia, breakthrough bleeding can occur for the first 3 to 4 months when using oral contraceptives.
- Question the adolescent about amount of flow; ask her to describe the number of pads or tampons used per day and how long it takes to saturate a pad or tampon.
- Monitor the adolescent's hemoglobin and hematocrit for changes indicating anemia from excessive blood loss.
- Be aware that the adolescent who is losing excessive blood because of anovulatory cycles may receive progesterone during the luteal phase to prevent proliferative growth during this phase.
- If the ability to conceive is unimportant, anticipate the use of a low-dose oral contraceptive to decrease the flow.
- Instruct the adolescent to see her physician if metrorrhagia occurs for more than one menstrual cycle and

she is not on oral contraceptives because vaginal
bleeding is an early sign of uterine carcinoma or ovarian cysts.
- Provide support and health promotion teaching to the
adolescent regarding menstruation.

# MENTAL RETARDATION

## DESCRIPTION

- The DSM-IV defines mental retardation based on two
criteria: significantly subaverage intellectual functioning—an intelligence quotient (IQ) of 70 or below—
and concurrent deficits in adaptive functioning.
- Approximately 1% to 3% of children in the United
States are mentally retarded, with the incidence being
twice as high in males than in females.
- A biologic cause for retardation can be documented in
only about 25% of retarded children.
- Fragile X syndrome is the most common inherited
cause of mental retardation.
- Common causes of mental retardation also include
chromosomal abnormalities, such as *Down syndrome*
and fragile X syndrome; infection in utero, such as
*rubella* or cytomegalic inclusion disease; anoxia at
birth, such as from *umbilical cord compression; fetal alcohol syndrome;* inherited metabolic disorders, such as
*phenylketonuria;* lead poisoning; *hypothyroidism;* brain
malformations, such as *anencephaly; prematurity;* and
infection, such as *measles encephalitis.*
- Mental retardation can be classified as mild (IQ between 70 and 50), moderate (IQ between 55 and 35),
severe (IQ between 40 and 20), and profound (IQ below 20).

## ASSESSMENT FINDINGS

- History and IQ testing revealing a degree of mental retardation

## NURSING IMPLICATIONS

- Perform a thorough history and physical assessment to
establishment a baseline.
- Arrange for the child's intelligence to be tested using
standardized tests, notably the Wechsler Intelligence
Scale for Children (WISC) or Stanford-Binet.
- Help the parents gain a realistic prognosis for their
child.

- Consider the individual circumstances of the family before giving advice about where the child should be raised.
- Be certain to consider the feelings of each family member and how adequately they are coping when planning with them.
- Know that it is more difficult to detect illness in a mentally retarded child than in child of normal intelligence.
- Explain everything that you are about to do to the child before you do it because he or she may not be able to know ahead of time what you will be doing unless you explain your intentions.
- Make sure that the parents know the signs and symptoms of illness because they will be more difficult to determine in a child with mental retardation.
- Offer support and guidance to the parents; allow them time to discuss their feelings and arrive at a decision regarding care for the child.

## METABOLIC ACIDOSIS

### DESCRIPTION

- Metabolic acidosis occurs when there is a rapid loss of base (cations) through intestinal secretions, as in *diarrhea,* or from an accumulation of acids, as when ketone bodies (acids or anions) accumulate in *diabetes mellitus.*
- The child develops hyperpnea (the body attempts to "blow off" carbon dioxide ($CO_2$) to prevent it from combining with water ($H_2O$) and releasing hydrogen ($H^+$) ions as hydrogen ($H^+$) and carbonic acid ($HCO_3$).
- There is increased chloride ion ($CL^-$) and ammonia formation in the urine as the kidney attempts to remove excess $H^+$.
- The blood $CO_2$ level is low, reflecting the large number of cations that have been lost.

### ASSESSMENT FINDINGS

- Rapid, deep respirations (Kussmaul's respirations)
- Weakness, lethargy
- Confusion, coma
- Decreased plasma pH (less than 7.35)
- Decreased urine pH (less than 6)
- Decreased plasma $CO_2$ (less than 40 mEq/L)

- Decreased plasma bicarbonate (less than 20 mEq/L)
- Base deficit (a negative number such as $-8$)
- Potassium excess (possible [more than 5.5 mEq/L])

**NURSING IMPLICATIONS**
- Obtain a health history, especially how long the *diarrhea* has occurred and the amount.
- Obtain vital signs.
- Obtain a stool culture on admission to determine the causative organism for the severe *diarrhea.*
- Administer antibiotic therapy as prescribed.
- Administer intravenous fluid replacement to replace fluid losses.
- Obtain blood samples for white blood cell count, differential counts, and hemoglobin; obtain arterial blood gases as prescribed to identify changes.
- Before administering potassium replacement solution, if prescribed, ensure that the child is voiding adequately to assess that the kidneys are functioning.
- Maintain the child on NPO (nothing by mouth).
- Give the infant a pacifier to suck if this seems to comfort him or her.
- Apply petroleum jelly (Vaseline) to the infant's lips if they appear to be dry and cracking.
- Record fluid intake and output to evaluate fluid balance status.
- Offer the child small sips of clear fluid, an oral rehydration solution, or breast milk, when prescribed.
- Gradually increase the child's diet as prescribed to a soft diet (sometimes called a BRAT diet because it comprises bananas, rice cereal, applesauce, and toast).
- Do not use a rectal thermometer to assess temperature because this could initiate more *diarrhea.*

## METABOLIC ALKALOSIS

**DESCRIPTION**
- Metabolic alkalosis can occur when there is excessive loss of chloride ion ($Cl^-$), such as occurs with persistent *vomiting,* or it can occur when there is potassium deficiency owing to inadequate intake or excessive loss in stools or urine.
- To increase the number of hydrogen ($H^+$) ions in the blood, $H^+$ ions are released from cells in exchange for sodium ($Na^+$) or potassium ($K^+$).

- The kidneys excrete $K^+$ into urine to reduce the intracellular load, resulting in low $K^+$ levels that invariably accompany alkalosis.
- The child develops hypopnea (slowed respirations) as the body attempts to retain carbon dioxide ($CO_2$) in the lungs to increase $H^+$ ions further.
- Tetany may also occur with alkalosis because the increased carbonate ions ($HCO_3^-$) may combine with calcium ions ($Ca^{++}$).

## ASSESSMENT FINDINGS
- Slowed respirations
- Twitching or tremors of muscles
- Confusion
- Elevated plasma pH (more than 7.45)
- Elevated urine pH (more than 7)
- Elevated plasma bicarbonate (more than 25 mEq/L)
- Normal or elevated plasma $CO_2$ (more than 40 mEq/L)
- Base excess (a positive number, such as $+8$)
- Decreased plasma potassium (less than 3.6 mEq/L)

## NURSING IMPLICATIONS
- Perform a thorough physical assessment and dietary history.
- Obtain information about the length of time the child has been *vomiting* (the amount and type) or if there has been any change in the child's eating habits or appetite.
- Maintain the child on NPO (nothing by mouth).
- Obtain necessary blood samples for analysis, including arterial blood gases and electrolyte levels.
- Administer intravenous fluid replacement therapy, as prescribed.
- Offer the child ice chips, as prescribed, and then water in small amounts: approximately 1 tablespoon every 15 minutes, 4 times, then 2 tablespoons every ½ hour, 4 times.
- Gradually increase the child's diet as prescribed to clear liquids, such as tea or ginger ale, and then clear broth, clear soup, and skimmed milk in addition to the clear liquids.
- Teach the parents the importance of following these slow routines of increasing fluids at intervals.

- Assure the parents that if the child receives a small amount of fluid and does not vomit, he or she can ultimately receive more fluid than if he or she takes a large amount and then, because of gastroenteritis, vomits that amount.
- Caution the parents not to give the child over-the-counter preparations for *vomiting;* instead they should control *vomiting* by dietary management to protect the child's electrolyte balance.
- Know that prochlorperazine (Compazine) may result in bizarre behavior symptoms (toxicity) if used in children who have not reached adolescence.

# MICROCEPHALY

### DESCRIPTION

- Microcephaly is a disorder involving brain growth so slow that it falls more than 3 standard deviations below normal on growth charts.
- The cause might be a defect in brain development associated with maternal *phenylketonuria* or an intrauterine infection, such as *rubella,* cytomegalovirus, or toxoplasmosis, and is apparent at birth in these instances.
- Microcephaly may also result from severe malnutrition or anoxia in early infancy.
- Microcephaly generally results in *mental retardation* because of the lack of functioning brain tissue.
- True microcephaly must be differentiated from *craniosynostosis* (normal brain growth but premature fusion of the cranial sutures), which also causes decreased head circumference.
- The prognosis for a normal life is guarded in children with microcephaly and depends on the extent of restriction of brain growth and on the cause.

### ASSESSMENT FINDINGS

- Decreased head circumference
- Maternal history of an intrauterine infection or *phenylketonuria*
- History of severe malnutrition or anoxia

### NURSING IMPLICATIONS

- Perform a thorough newborn physical assessment, including head circumference.

- Obtain maternal health history and observe for evidence of an intrauterine infection, such as *rubella,* cytomegalovirus, or maternal *phenylketonuria.*
- Observe the child's fontanelles for abnormally closed fontanelles and possible bulging (bossing of the forehead and signs of *increased intracranial pressure*), which may indicate *craniosynostosis* (which also causes decreased head circumference) rather than microcephaly.
- Perform head circumference evaluations during health care visits after the child is discharged.
- Provide education for the parents about signs and symptoms to watch for indicating *increased intracranial pressure.*
- Offer support and guidance to the parents; allow the parents to verbalize their feelings about the prognosis for the child.

## MILIARIA

### DESCRIPTION

- Miliaria, or prickly heat rash, occurs most often in warm weather or when infants are overdressed or sleep in overheated rooms.
- It is a common skin problem in the infant.

### ASSESSMENT FINDINGS

- Clusters of pinpoint, reddened papules with occasional vesicles and pustules surrounded by erythema.
- Rash appearing on neck first and spreading upward to around the ear and onto the face or down onto the trunk.

### NURSING IMPLICATIONS

- Obtain a thorough history and physical examination to establish a baseline and rule out other possible skin disorders.
- Perform a thorough inspection of the child's skin to identify the characteristic rash.
- Suggest to the parents that they bathe the infant twice a day during hot weather and attempt to keep the infant free of perspiration.
- Tell the parents to add a small amount of baking soda to the bath water to improve the rash.
- Tell the parents that to help eliminate perspiration, they should reduce the amount of clothing on the in-

fant or lower the room temperature, which should bring about immediate improvement and prevent further eruption.

# MUMPS (EPIDEMIC PAROTITIS)

### Description

- Mumps is an infectious disorder that is caused by the mumps virus and is transmitted by direct and indirect contact.
- Contracting the disease seems to give lasting natural immunity; active and passive artificial immunity can be accomplished with attenuated live mumps vaccine and mumps immune globulin.
- Mumps is now a rare disease because of successful *immunization* programs.
- Between 20% and 30% of males older than the age of puberty who develop mumps develop complication of orchitis (inflammation of the testes), which, fortunately, is generally unilateral.
- Meningoencephalitis may occur in a small number of children.
- Severe *hearing impairment* is a rare complication of mumps that occurs because of neuritis of the auditory nerve and is permanent.

### Assessment Findings

- Fever
- Headache
- Anorexia
- Malaise
- Complaints of an earache (pain site is jawline just in front of earlobe)
- Swollen parotid gland (in front of earlobe)
- Ear displaced upward and backward

### Nursing Implications

- Perform a history and physical assessment to establish a baseline.
- Obtain vital signs to identify changes.
- Place a hand along the child's jawline to differentiate between mumps and maxillary adenitis; major swelling below the handline signifies adenitis and above the handline signifies mumps.
- Advise the parents that the child needs to be kept on soft or liquid foods until the major portion of the

swelling recedes because chewing movements are painful.
- Assure the parents that the child can get the mumps only once and that if they believe the child had mumps on only one side, the diagnosis was probably confused with cervical adenitis one of the two times.
- Teach the parents the importance of maintaining the child's *immunization* schedule.

# MURINE TYPHUS

### DESCRIPTION
- Murine typhus is an infectious disorder that is seen almost exclusively in the southern United States.
- It is transmitted by mites and fleas that live on rats.

### ASSESSMENT FINDINGS
- Fever
- Severe headache
- Measleslike rash

### NURSING IMPLICATIONS
- Perform a thorough history and physical assessment to establish a baseline.
- Obtain vital signs.
- Assess the presence of any recent flea infestations or any rat-infested areas in the environment.
- Administer tetracycline or a third-generation antibiotic, such as ciprofloxacin, as prescribed.

# MUSCULAR DYSTROPHY

### DESCRIPTION
- Muscular dystrophy is progressive degeneration of skeletal muscles from an as yet unknown biochemical defect within the muscle.
- It is not a single disorder but a group of inherited disorders that lead to gradual degeneration of muscle fibers.
- Muscular dystrophy may present as congenital muscular dystrophy, facioscapulohumeral muscular dystrophy, or pseudohypertrophic muscular dystrophy (Duchenne's disease).

### ASSESSMENT FINDINGS
- History of meeting motor milestones later than other children (sitting, walking, standing) with symptoms becoming acute and obvious at age 3

- Difficulty in lifting the child under the axillae (child slips through your hands because of lax shoulder muscles)
- Hypertrophied calf muscles (measure larger than normal)
- Waddling gait
- Difficulty climbing stairs
- Positive Gower's sign when attempting to stand
- Walking on toes
- Speech and swallowing difficulty
- *Scoliosis* of spine and fractures of long bones as disease progresses
- Tachycardia as heart muscle weakens and enlarges
- *Pneumonia* as cough reflex becomes ineffective

### Nursing Implications

- Perform a thorough history and physical assessment to establish a baseline.
- Obtain a blood specimen for serum creatine phosphokinase, as prescribed.
- Prepare the child for muscle biopsy, as prescribed, to demonstrate fibrous degeneration and fatty deposits.
- Encourage the child to remain ambulatory as long as possible.
- Help the child plan a program of both active and passive range-of-motion exercises to do daily.
- Help the child to make reminder sheets so that the exercises are done daily.
- Teach the child and parents about splinting and bracing if they become necessary to maintain lower extremity stability and avoid contractures.
- Encourage the overweight child to remain ambulatory as it becomes more difficult for them.
- Be certain that when making goals for the child that they are realistic goals.
- Encourage a low-calorie, high-protein diet to help the child avoid becoming overweight.
- Prevent constipation by encouraging a high-fiber, high-fluid diet.
- Advocate for a stool softener, if necessary.
- Help the parents locate a parent support group.
- Offer support and guidance to the child and parents to help alleviate their fears and anxieties; allow the child and parents to verbalize their feelings.

# MYASTHENIA GRAVIS

### DESCRIPTION

- Myasthenia gravis is a disorder of skeletal muscles.
- Myasthenia gravis interferes with the release of a neurotransmitter, acetylcholine, at synaptic junctions not allowing muscles to contract and inhibiting nerve conduction.
- The defect is probably a motor end plate insufficiency (a decreased number of acetylcholine receptors present) probably occurring from an autoimmune process.
- There is some evidence that a tendency for the condition may be inherited; the thymus gland is usually enlarged in persons with the condition, suggesting that thymopoietin may be overproduced leading to neuromuscular block.

### ASSESSMENT FINDINGS

- "Floppy" appearance of newborns with poor sucking, weak respiratory effort, and ptosis (drooping eyelids)
- Blurred or double vision (diplopia), ptosis, extreme fatigue (at age 10)
- Increased symptoms with emotional stress, fatigue, menstruation, respiratory infections, and alcohol intake
- Poor motor function
- Enlarged thymus gland

### NURSING IMPLICATIONS

- Perform a thorough history and physical assessment to establish a baseline.
- Ask the child to perform repetitive movements observing for deviations from normal.
- Prepare the child for electromyography to document poor muscle function.
- Prepare the child for a chest x-ray and computed tomography scan to demonstrate an enlarged thymus gland.
- Prepare the child for the administration of edrophonium chloride (Tensilon), which increases muscle strength and demonstrates positive diagnosis of myasthenia gravis.

- Administer anticholinesterase drugs, such as neostig-mine (Prostigmine), as prescribed, which prolong acetylcholine action.
- Assess the child for side effects of anticholinesterase drugs, such as bradycardia, increased peristalsis, ab-dominal cramping, sweating, and miotic pupils.
- Have atropine, an antidote for an overdose of anti-cholinesterase drugs, at the bedside before administer-ing these drugs.
- Prepare the child for plasmapheresis as prescribed to attempt to remove immune complexes from the blood stream.
- Teach both parents and children that symptoms be-come worse under stress.
- Tell the parents to prepare the child well for new ex-periences, such as menstruation, high school, parental divorce, or surgery, to help keep stress at a minimum.
- Advise the parents to allow rest periods before meals if chewing and swallowing are difficult.
- Advise the parents that the child may need a soft diet.
- Teach the child to learn to chew slowly and cautiously to avoid choking and aspiration.
- Tell the parents to schedule medication administra-tion for about an hour before mealtime.
- Caution the parents that if symptoms of muscle weak-ness suddenly become severe, the child should be seen at a health care facility because paralysis of intercostal muscles may lead to respiratory arrest.
- Provide emotional support and guidance to the par-ents about all aspects of the child's care.

# MYELOMENINGOCELE

### DESCRIPTION

- Myelomeningocele is a *neural tube defect* in which the spinal cord and the meninges protrude through the vertebral defect and the spinal cord often ends at the point of the defect so that motor and sensory function is absent beyond this point.
- The child has flaccidity and lack of sensation of the lower extremities and loss of bowel and bladder control.
- Children often have accompanying *talipes (clubfoot)* defects and subluxated hip.

- *Hydrocephalus* may accompany myelomeningocele in as many as 80% of infants; the higher the myelomeningocele occurs on the cord, the more likely *hydrocephalus* will accompany it.
- When infants are detected as having myelomeningocele or *meningocele*, they are usually delivered by cesarean *birth* to avoid pressure and injury to the spinal cord.

### ASSESSMENT FINDINGS

- Defect visible at birth or during ultrasonography, fetoscopy, amniocentesis, or analysis of alpha-fetoprotein in maternal serum
- Accompanying motor and sensory deficits

### NURSING IMPLICATIONS

- Obtain a thorough history and physical examination to establish a baseline.
- Observe and record spontaneous movements of the extremities and the pattern of voiding and defecating to differentiate between myelomeningocele and *meningocele.*
- Place the infant in a prone position or supported on his or her side to prevent pressure on the neural sac.
- Place a sterile, wet compress of saline, antiseptic, or antibiotic gauze over the lesion to keep the lesion moist.
- Use caution when placing the infant under a radiant heat warmer for warmth so that the lesion does not become dry and crack.
- Encourage the mother to hold the infant in as normal a feeding position as possible making sure that no pressure is exerted on the defect.
- Measure the child's head circumference once daily or more frequently if prescribed, and assess for signs of *increased intracranial pressure.*
- Prepare the child and parents for possible surgery.
- Observe the child postoperatively for signs of *increased intracranial pressure,* such as a change in vital signs; neurologic signs, such as pupillary changes; or an increase in head circumference or bulging fontanelles as well as behavioral changes, such as irritability or lethargy.
- Turn the infant's head every 2 hours if *hydrocephalus* has developed to prevent pressure areas at the temples.
- Provide the parents with support and encouragement because their child will have a multiple disability.

# NASOPHARYNGITIS, ACUTE (COMMON COLD)

## DESCRIPTION

- Acute nasopharyngitis, the most frequent infectious disease in children, is caused by one of several viruses.
- The most common causative organisms are rhinovirus, coxsackievirus, respiratory syncytial virus, adenovirus, parainfluenza, and influenza viruses.
- Children are commonly exposed to colds at school from other children; toddlers average 10 to 12 colds a year; school-age children and adolescents have 4 to 5 colds a year.
- The incubation period for a cold is 2 days.
- Children who are in ill health from some other cause are more susceptible to the cold viruses than are well children.
- Stress factors appear to play a role in developing a cold.
- Other possible factors associated with increasing the susceptibility to colds include exposure to drafts, cold feet, and chilling.

## ASSESSMENT FINDINGS

- Nasal congestion
- Watery rhinitis
- Low-grade fever (infants and toddlers may develop fevers of 102° to 104°F)
- *Dehydration*
- Reddened, swollen nasal mucous membrane
- Difficulty in breathing secondary to nasal edema and congestion
- *Pharyngitis* secondary to posterior rhinitis and local irritation
- Cough secondary to draining pharyngeal secretions
- Swollen and palpable cervical lymph nodes
- Thick, purulent nasal discharge secondary to bacteria, such as streptococci, causing a secondary infection

## NURSING IMPLICATIONS

- Monitor vital signs.
- Monitor fluid and electrolytes in infants and toddlers.
- Be aware that there is no specific treatment unless secondary bacterial infection requires the administration of antibiotics.

- Keep in mind that symptoms persist for approximately 1 week and then subside.
- Control fever greater than 101°F with antipyretics, such as acetaminophen.
- Teach the parents how to monitor young children for dehydration.
- Teach the parents that acetaminophen is for fever reduction and does not reduce cold symptoms.
- Teach the parents to instill saline nose drops to liquefy nasal secretions and help them drain.
- Teach the parents correct use of bulb suction to clear nasal mucous by compressing the bulb before insertion into the child's nostril.
- Administer phenylephrine nose drops to free the airway by constricting the mucous membranes.
- Teach the parent that it is not necessary to suppress the cough because this mobilizes secretions and prevents pooling and subsequent infection.
- Encourage the parents to use a vaporizer to loosen secretions.
- Teach the parents about the safe use of vaporizers, such as cleaning, and safe placement to prevent burn injury to the child from the steam.
- Teach the parents the signs of *otitis media,* elevated temperature, and ear pain because this can be a complication of the common cold and requires treatment.

## NEAR DROWNING

### DESCRIPTION

- Near drowning is the term used to describe the person with a submersion injury who requires emergency treatment and who survives the first 24 hours postinjury.
- Drowning is defined as death caused by suffocation from submersion in liquid when inhaled water fills and therefore blocks the exchange of oxygen in the alveoli.
- Toddlers and preschool children who cannot swim are the most frequent victims of drowning and neardrowning accidents, although children (and adults) of all ages and swimming abilities are at risk.
- If children hyperventilate before swimming under water, excess carbon dioxide is blown off; during an extended period of underwater swimming, carbon

dioxide levels rise but not adequately to cause the child to experience distress, resulting in decreased oxygen levels with drowsiness and listlessness.

- If treatment is given at the point that the child has not inhaled much water because the larynx has gone into spasm and closed, treatment is effective; if the child remains in the water and the larynx relaxes, allowing water to enter the lungs, the alveoli fill with water, hypoxia deepens, and cardiac arrest occurs.
- Additional changes that occur when water enters the lungs depend on whether the water is fresh or salt; salt water is hypertonic, which causes fluid to diffuse from the blood stream and enter the alveoli; fresh water is hypotonic, and fluid in the lungs is absorbed into the blood stream.
- Very young children display a mammalian diving reflex when they plunge under cold water; immediately a life-saving bradycardia and shunting of blood away from the periphery of their body to their brain and heart occur.

### Assessment Findings
- History of water submersion
- *Cardiopulmonary arrest*

### Nursing Implications
- Institute mouth-to-mouth resuscitation at once.
- Determine if the child was submerged in fresh or salt water and the temperature of the water.
- Determine the length of time that the child was submerged.
- Obtain vital signs and appropriate blood specimens.
- Perform and maintain *assisted ventilation*, as prescribed.
- Administer isoproterenol, albuterol, or racemic epinephrine by aerosol as prescribed to prevent bronchospasm.
- Administer intravenous aminophylline as prescribed to discourage inflammation.
- Provide gradual warming to increase the child's body temperature if he or she were submerged in cold water.
- Administer prophylactic antibiotics as prescribed to prevent *pneumonia*.
- Assess vital signs and auscultate lung sounds for adventitious sounds, such as rales or fine rhonchi.
- Turn the child every 2 hours if on bed rest, and encourage deep breathing every hour to aerate the lungs

fully and prevent the accumulation of fluid, which invites infection.
- Provide the child with frequent reassurance that he or she is all right if he or she should wake with a nightmare.
- Allow the child and parents to verbalize their fears.

## NECROTIZING ENTEROCOLITIS (NEC)

### DESCRIPTION
- NEC is a condition that develops in approximately 5% of all infants in intensive care nurseries.
- In NEC, the bowel develops necrotic patches interfering with digestion and possibly leading to a paralytic ileus; perforation and peritonitis may follow.
- The necrosis appears to result from ischemic or poor perfusion of blood vessels in sections of bowel.
- The ischemic process may occur when, owing to shock or hypoxia, there is vasoconstriction of blood vessels to nonessential organs, such as the bowel.
- The entire bowel may be involved, or it may be a localized phenomenon.
- The incidence of NEC is highest in immature infants and those who have suffered anoxia or shock.
- Infants with infection may develop NEC as a further complication of their already stressed state.
- There seems to be a lower incidence of NEC in infants who are breast-fed probably because intestinal organisms grow more profusely with cow's milk than breast milk because cow's milk lacks the antibodies; the response to the foreign protein in cow's milk may be a mechanism that starts the necrotic process.

### ASSESSMENT FINDINGS
- Distended and tense abdomen
- Aspiration of more than 2 mL of undigested milk before gavage feeding
- Stool positive for occult blood (possible)
- Periods of apnea
- Signs of blood loss from intestinal bleeding (lowered blood pressure and inability to stabilize temperature)
- X-ray film positive for areas of air invading the intestinal wall if perforation has occurred

#### Nursing Implications

- Discontinue bottle or gavage feedings as soon as NEC is recognized.
- Administer intravenous or total parenteral nutrition, as prescribed to maintain nutrition and to rest the gastrointestinal tract.
- Administer antibiotic therapy, as prescribed.
- Test the infant's stool for occult blood.
- Prepare the child and the parents for impending surgery to remove the necrotic bowel.
- Teach the parents about colostomy care if their infant should return from surgery with a colostomy.
- Provide support and guidance to the parents to help alleviate their fears and anxieties.

## NEPHROTIC SYNDROME (NEPHROSIS)

### Description

- Nephrotic syndrome, also called nephrosis, is altered glomeruli permeability caused by fusion of the glomeruli membrane surfaces; it causes abnormal protein in the urine.
- Immunologic mechanisms are involved in instigating the process; the cause may be hypersensitivity to an antigen-antibody reaction or an autoimmune process; a T cell dysfunction may be responsible.
- Nephrotic syndrome in children occurs in three forms: (1) congenital; (2) secondary, as a progression of glomerulonephritis or in connection with systemic diseases, such as *sickle cell anemia* or *systemic lupus erythematosus;* or (3) idiopathic (primary).
- Minimal change nephrotic syndrome is the type most often seen in children; with this, as the name implies, little scarring of glomeruli occurs.
- Age of peak incidence of the idiopathic nephrotic syndrome is 2 to 3 years; the syndrome occurs more often in males than in females.

### Assessment Findings

- Proteinuria (single dipstick of $1^+$ to $4^+$ and 24-hour up to 15 g of protein)
- Periorbital edema
- Ascites (parents note child's clothes do not fit around middle)

- Pale, stretched, taut skin
- Marked scrotal or labial edema
- Anorexia and vomiting (from extensive ascites)
- Diarrhea
- Irritability
- Elevated sedimentation rate
- Low serum albumin (hypoalbuminemia)
- Hyperlipidemia (increased blood lipid level)

## NURSING IMPLICATIONS

- Perform a thorough history and physical assessment to establish a baseline.
- Obtain necessary blood and urine samples, as prescribed.
- Obtain vital signs.
- Administer oral prednisone, as prescribed, to reduce proteinuria rapidly and consequently edema.
- Teach the parents first to test the child's urine for protein with a dipstick method and to keep an accurate chart showing the pattern of protein loss.
- Tell the parents that approximately once a week they need to collect a 24-hour urine specimen from the child to measure total protein loss.
- Assure the parents that prednisone therapy administered every other day is best for the child to prevent them from changing the schedule from every day or giving twice the calculated dose by adding extra tablets on alternate days.
- Help the parents design a reminder chart for the refrigerator or the bathroom door to help them remember when to administer the medication.
- Be certain that the parents and child know that the prednisone causes a cushingoid appearance (moon face, extra fat at the base of the neck, and increased body hair).
- Caution the parents to plan ahead when getting refills of the prescriptions so that the prednisone therapy is not stopped abruptly because they ran out of the medication, causing adrenal insufficiency.
- Obtain frequent blood studies on children receiving long-term diuretic therapy, as prescribed.
- Be sure to administer a rapidly acting diuretic, as prescribed, after an albumin infusion to prevent fluid overload and congestive heart failure.

- Caution the parents of a child receiving cyclophosphamide (Cytoxan) not to be misled into believing that their child has cancer because he or she is receiving a chemotherapeutic drug.
- Perform frequent position changes to prevent skin breakdown of edematous skin.
- Check the child's clothing to make sure that the elastic band around the waist is not too tight.
- Check a boy's scrotum and apply soft gauze between skin surfaces to prevent skin irritation and breakdown.
- Position the child with the head elevated in a semi-Fowler's position to reduce periorbital edema.
- Be aware that medication should be administered orally if possible, and intramuscular injections should be kept at a minimum because medications are poorly absorbed from edematous skin.

## NEURAL TUBE DEFECTS

### DESCRIPTION

- The neural tube is the embryonic structure that matures to form the central nervous system.
- Because the neural tube forms in utero first as a flat plate and then molds to form the brain and the spinal cord, it is susceptible to malformation, known as a neural tube defect.
- The term spina bifida (Latin for "divided spine") is most often used as a collective term for all spinal cord defects, but there are well-defined degrees of spina bifida involvement and not all neural defects involve the spinal cord, but all of these disorders, however, occur because of lack of fusion of the posterior surface of the embryo in early intrauterine life.
- The incidence is approximately 1 to 3 in 1000 live births.
- There is no specific cause for many such deformities that can be isolated, but poor nutrition, especially a diet deficient in vitamins, appears to be a contributing factor.
- Some disorders may occur as a polygenic inheritance pattern.
- Neural tube defects include *anencephaly, microcephaly,* dermal sinus, *spina bifida occulta, meningocele, myelomeningocele,* and *encephalocele.*

### Assessment Findings

- Defect visible at birth or during ultrasonography, fetoscopy, amniocentesis, or analysis of alpha-fetoprotein in maternal serum

### Nursing Implications

- Obtain a thorough history and physical examination to establish a baseline.
- Observe and record spontaneous movements of the extremities and the pattern of voiding and defecating to differentiate between *meningocele* and *myelomeningocele.*
- Place the infant in a prone position or supported on the side to prevent pressure on the neural sac.
- Place a sterile, wet compress of saline, antiseptic, or antibiotic gauze over the lesion to keep the lesion moist.
- Use caution when placing the infant under a radiant heat warmer for warmth so that the lesion does not become dry and crack.
- Encourage the mother to hold the infant in as normal a feeding position as possible, making sure that no pressure is exerted on the defect.
- Measure the child's head circumference once daily or more frequently if prescribed, and assess for signs of *increased intracranial pressure.*
- Prepare the child and parents for possible surgery.
- Observe the child postoperatively for signs of *increased intracranial pressure,* such as a change in vital signs; neurologic signs, such as pupillary changes; or an increase in head circumference or bulging fontanelles as well as behavioral changes, such as irritability or lethargy.
- Turn the infant's head every 2 hours if *hydrocephalus* has developed to prevent pressure areas at the temples.
- Advise the woman who has a child with a spinal cord defect to have a maternal serum assay or amniocentesis to determine if such a defect is present in a second pregnancy.
- Provide emotional support and guidance to parents to help alleviate their anxieties and fears; allow parents to discuss their feelings about their "defective child."

# NEUROFIBROMATOSIS (VON RECKLINGHAUSEN'S DISEASE)

## DESCRIPTION

- Neurofibromatosis is a neurocutaneous syndrome in that it involves skin or pigmentation along with central nervous system involvement.
- Neurofibromatosis is the unexplained development of subcutaneous tumors; it is inherited as an autosomal dominant trait occurring in approximately 1 in 4000 live births.
- The 8th cranial nerve is usually involved, leading to hearing loss; involvement of the optic nerve causes vision loss.
- About 15% of all children develop neurologic complications, such as *seizures.*
- About 10% develop *mental retardation* from cerebral deterioration.
- Prenatal diagnosis is available, and the disease is invariably fatal.

## ASSESSMENT FINDINGS

- Excessive pigmentation in childhood
- Pigmented nevi or café-au-lait spots that follow paths of cutaneous nerves
- Presence of 5 or more spots larger than 1 cm in diameter (diagnostic)
- Multiple soft cutaneous tumors forming in puberty along nerve pathways

## NURSING IMPLICATIONS

- Perform a complete history and physical assessment, including a neurologic assessment.
- Perform hearing and vision tests to determine possible losses secondary to 8th cranial nerve or optic nerve involvement.
- Administer a mast cell blocker such as ketotifen, as prescribed to slow the growth rate of the tumors.
- Provide emotional support and encouragement for the parents and child.
- Arrange for counseling for the parents and child to help all of them deal with the effects of a fatal disease.
- Advise the parents that prenatal testing and diagnosis is available.

# NEUTROPENIA

### DESCRIPTION

- Neutropenia refers to a reduced number of white blood cells, which may occur as a transient phenomenon with pyrogenic infections, such as viral disease.
- It also may be predictable as a response to therapy with some drugs, such as 6-mercaptopurine or nitrogen mustard.
- It may also occur as a side effect from drugs such as phenytoin sodium (Dilantin), chloramphenicol, or chlorpromazine.

### ASSESSMENT FINDINGS

- Decreased white blood cell count
- History of drug therapy with nitrogen mustard or 6-mercaptopurine
- Recent history of phenytoin use (or other drug that may cause this side effect)

### NURSING IMPLICATIONS

- Administer prophylactic antibiotics, as prescribed.
- Administer white blood cell transfusions, as prescribed, to restore a functioning cell level.
- Know that a white cell count of less than 1500/mm$^3$ is always serious because absence of neutrophils lessens the child's protection against overwhelming infection (opportunistic infection); institute appropriate isolation precautions to prevent possible infection.

# NEUTROPHILIA

### DESCRIPTION

- Neutrophilia refers to an increased number of circulating white blood cells, primarily neutrophils, which occurs in the presence of infection or inflammation.
- The total number of cells not only increases, but also the proportion of mature neutrophils changes with an increase in immature cells.
- The presence of many banded or immature forms is sometimes referred to as a "shift to the left."

### ASSESSMENT FINDINGS

- Increased number of white blood cells and immature cells

#### NURSING IMPLICATIONS
- Know that disorders characterized by an increase in the number of white blood cells or specific white blood cell components occur in response to other disease (often infection or an allergic reaction) in the body.
- Obtain a thorough history and physical examination to establish a baseline and identify any contributing factors for other diseases.

## NUTRITIONAL NEEDS, ADOLESCENT

#### DESCRIPTION
- Nutritional needs of adolescence vary with the timing of growth spurts.
- Nutrient needs peak during growth spurts, and poor nutrition during this time may slow growth and sexual maturation.
- Adolescents are frequently involved in sports activities, which increases nutrient and energy needs.
- Most adolescents always feel hungry, but frequently they skip meals and supplement their diets with low-nutrition snacks.
- Factors affecting nutritional intake in an adolescent include time spent away from the family, participation in sports, and skipping meals.
- Adolescents require the upper limits of ranges for the basic food groups.
- Girls between 11 and 14 years old need 33 to 66 cal/kg/day, 1.2 g/kg/day of protein, and 55 ml/kg/day of fluid.
- Boys between 11 and 14 years old need 44 to 81 cal/kg/day, 1.2 g/kg/day of protein, and 55 ml/kg/day of fluid.
- Girls and boys between 15 and 18 have decreased fluid requirements of 45 ml/kg/day.
- Adolescents who are obese may begin low-calorie or starvation diets to lose excess weight. Weight-loss diets may be appropriate but must be supervised to ensure sufficient calories and nutrients for growth.
- Athletic adolescents need more carbohydrates or energy than do adolescents not as engaged in strenuous activity.
- Glycogen loading, a procedure used to ensure adequate glycogen to sustain energy, is not recommended for adolescents, who need various nutrients for growth.

- Eating disorders, such as *anorexia nervosa, bulimia,* and obesity, typically begin in adolescence and may persist into adulthood.

### Nursing Implications

- Assess nutritional health through history and physical examination.
- Plot height and weight measurements on growth curve to see if they remain within normal limits.
- Evaluate the adolescent's diet, lifestyle, and food preferences preferably without a parent present.
- Support an adolescent in his or her diet and consider cultural variations and budgetary restrictions when developing a food plan.
- Identify any adolescent with a change in food intake or potential for eating disorder and refer them appropriately.
- Promote adequate nutritional intake in varied diets, such as with the vegetarian adolescent.
- Be aware that any weight reduction diet should be carefully evaluated before the adolescent follows it for any length of time.
- Keep in mind that adolescents who are vegetarians need to increase consumption to fulfill caloric intake requirements.

## NUTRITIONAL NEEDS, INFANT

### Description

- The entire first year of life is one of rapid growth in which the infant requires high-protein and high-calorie intake.
- During the year, caloric requirements decrease from 120 calories per kg to 100 calories per kg by the end of the year.
- If calories are not gradually reduced over the first year, the infant can become overweight.
- An infant who is overweight during the first year of life is more likely to become an obese adult.
- Overfeeding produces large numbers of excess fat cells used to store fat.
- These cells are permanent and remain filled with fat; once they are present, weight regulation can become difficult throughout life.

- The infant receives a majority of his or her nutrition through milk, either through breast-feeding or formula feeding.
- Breast-feeding can provide certain physiologic benefits to both the mother and the infant.
- For the infant, breast milk contains secretory immunoglobulin A to assist the infant in fighting infection and ideal electrolyte and mineral composition for human infant growth; also, breast milk is higher in lactose than cow's milk, which provides ready glucose for rapid brain growth.
- Although breast milk is lower in protein than cow's milk, it is more readily digested, and therefore the infant receives more of the protein.
- Breast milk contains nitrogen in other compounds than proteins so that cell building from sources other than just protein is available.
- Breast milk contains linoleic acid for skin integrity.
- Infants who receive breast milk have less difficulty with regulation of calcium-phosphorus levels than those who are bottle-fed.
- The introduction of solid foods usually begins around 6 months of age; an infant is considered physiologically ready for solid food when he or she is taking more than 32 oz (960 ml) of formula per day and does not seem satisfied or is nursing vigorously every 3 to 4 hours and does not seem satisfied.

#### Nursing Implications

- Encourage and assist first-time mothers with breast-feeding.
- Inform the mother that this is the most beneficial food for the child; however, it may be difficult for the first month as the child learns to suck and the mother and child develop a routine and a "natural comfort" with the technique.
- Recommend an iron-fortified infant formula for the mother who chooses not to breast-feed.
- Evaluate the water supply available to the child and determine if fluoride supplements are required.
- Recommend that the mother continue to provide breast milk or infant formula until the child is 12 months old.

- Instruct the parents and caregivers to hold the baby during bottle-feeding to avoid aspiration, dental caries, and promotion of middle ear infections.
- Emphasize that bottle propping is not conducive to important close human contact, which the infant needs to mature physically and emotionally.
- Evaluate the infant's nutritional intake; weigh the child at each health maintenance visit.
- Discuss feeding schedules with the mother, and recommend demand feeding but not more than every 2 hours.
- Instruct the parents to use a pacifier to soothe the infant.
- Recommend that solid foods be introduced between 4 and 6 months of age.
- Teach the parents to introduce solid foods one food at a time with a period of 5 to 7 days before introducing another to help ensure that no allergy to the food exists.
- Keep in mind that the first solid food usually given is cereal mixed with just enough fluid to make it a liquid consistency.
- Encourage the parents to use a positive attitude when introducing new foods.
- Instruct the parents about appropriate food selections because chewing movements do not begin until 7 to 9 months; thus, food requiring chewing should not be given until this age.
- Discuss any problems the parents may have with spoon feeding the child.
- Instruct parents not to add salt or sugar to infant foods.
- Educate the parents on how to wean an infant from the breast or from the bottle, beginning with the elimination of one feeding or bottle at a time.
- Instruct parents who wish to wean the infant from breast-feeding before 6 months of age to use a bottle not a cup, to encourage the infant's sucking needs and maintain nutrition.
- Continue to monitor the infant's height and weight at each health care visit, and compare with standards for the age group.
- Evaluate carefully for any indication of lactose intolerance or food *allergy,* and recommend changes appropriately.

# NUTRITIONAL NEEDS, PRESCHOOLER

### Description

- The preschool years are not a time of fast growth, so the child is not likely to have a ravenous appetite.
- Experiences with eating can help the preschooler reinforce his or her own sense of initiative.
- The preschooler may have intense food preferences.
- The preschooler usually requires approximately 1800 kcal/day.

### Nursing Implications

- Educate the parents as to the nutritional needs and recommendations for the preschooler.
- Inform the parents that the preschool diet should include the following:
    - 6 to 11 bread servings
    - 2 to 4 fruit servings
    - 3 to 5 vegetable servings
    - 2 meat servings
    - 2 to 3 dairy servings
- Offer the preschooler small servings so as not to overwhelm the child and allow successful feeling of cleaning a plate and asking for more.
- Encourage parents to offer varied sources of calcium to ensure bone growth.
- Advise the parents to continue to offer a variety of foods but caution them not to force food on the child.
- Continue to evaluate the preschooler's height, weight, and growth and compare with standards in that age group.
- Caution parents about using vitamins, not giving more than the recommended daily amount, or else poisoning from high doses of fat-soluble vitamins and iron can result. Instruct parents to store them out of the reach of children because children often think of them as candy because of their attractive shapes and colors.

# NUTRITIONAL NEEDS, SCHOOL-AGE CHILD

### Description

- During the school-age period, caloric needs continue to decrease relative to body size.
- Nutritional requirements for the school-age child resemble those for other children; only the serving size increases.

- For the 6-year-old, the caloric requirement is 90 cal/kg/day, and the fluid requirement is 95 ml/kg/day.
- The 7- to 10-year-old requires 70 calories/kg/day and 80 ml/kg/day of fluid.
- At 11, the recommended daily requirements are separated into categories for girls and boys because boys require more calories than other nutrients at this time.
- The 11- to 12-year-old boy requires 55 calories/kg/day and 55 ml/kg/day of fluid.
- The 11- to 12-year-old girl requires the same fluid, however, only 47 calories/kg/day.
- All school-age children require 1.2 g/kg/day of protein.
- Both boys and girls require more iron in prepuberty than they did between the ages of 7 to 10 years of age.
- Adequate calcium and fluoride intake remain important to ensure good teeth.

### Nursing Implications
- Encourage the parents to provide a variety of foods in both snacks and meals.
- Advise parents to educate their children on good nutrition because as the child enters school, eating patterns and habits become increasingly independent of parental control.
- Provide nutritional counseling to the child as well as the parents.
- Inform the child and parents that the child's diet should consist of the following:
    - 6 to 11 bread servings
    - 2 to 4 fruit servings
    - 3 to 5 vegetable servings
    - 2 meat servings
    - 2 to 3 dairy servings
- Continue to evaluate the child's weight, growth, and height, and compare with children of the same age group.
- Evaluate the need for iron supplements in this group, and educate the child on how to take this medication.

## NUTRITIONAL NEEDS, TODDLER

### Description
- During the toddler years, physical growth slows, and the toddler has lower nutritional requirements than an infant.

- The toddler has a smaller appetite than the infant.
- The toddler may suddenly become a picky eater, refusing all but one or two certain favorite foods.
- Food preferences are frequently established at this time.
- After 12 months, the toddler should be able to take most types of adult foods slightly modified for the toddler.
- Toddlers love finger foods.
- Weaning from the bottle completely begins during the early toddler period and should be accomplished by 36 months.
- The infant can tolerate cow's milk and no longer requires breast milk or infant formula.
- Whole milk is recommended for brain cell development.
- After the age of 2, the toddler can drink 2% milk to reduce fat intake but should not be given 1% or skim milk because the protein concentration is too high for the toddler's immature kidneys.
- A toddler requires 100 calories/kg, 1.2 g/kg of protein, and 115 ml/kg of fluid each day.
- Children under 3 are at risk for iron deficiency anemia from inadequate iron intake.

NURSING IMPLICATIONS
- Monitor weight, height, and growth at all toddler health maintenance visits.
- Inform parents to put small amounts of food on a plate and allow the child to eat it and ask for more.
- Educate parents that toddlers have erratic eating patterns and this is normal.
- Counsel parents to avoid forcing food, and reassure them that a toddler will eat when hungry.
- Encourage parents to offer a variety of foods.
- Advise parents that toddlers do not like food mixed up and that they usually love finger foods, which they can eat independently.
- Caution the parents not to add salt or pepper to the toddler's food.
- Advise parents to limit milk intake to 18 to 24 oz; otherwise the child will reduce solid food consumption.
- Educate the parents on giving whole milk until after 2 years of age and then 2% milk but not 1% or skim milk.

- Inform parents of the average daily caloric, protein, and fluid requirement for this age group.
- Discuss with parents the food groups and daily necessary intake from each group for the toddler, which should include:
  - 6 to 11 bread servings.
  - 2 to 4 fruit servings.
  - 3 to 5 vegetable servings.
  - 2 meat servings.
  - 2 to 3 dairy servings.
- Screen for *iron deficiency anemia* in low-risk toddlers at age 18 months.
- Inform parents of children who require iron supplements that it may darken the child's stools and cause constipation.
- Encourage increased intake of fluid with iron supplements to avoid constipation.
- Educate parents to have the child drink water or juice after taking the iron preparation because it can otherwise cause tooth staining.

## OMPHALOCELE

### Description

- An omphalocele is a protrusion of abdominal contents through the abdominal wall at the point of the junction of the umbilical cord and the abdomen.
- The herniated organs are usually the intestines, but they may include the stomach and liver.
- There is usually a thin layer of transparent peritoneum covering the organs.
- The omphalocele is obvious at birth and reflects an arrest of development of the abdominal cavity at weeks 7 to 10 of intrauterine life.
- The incidence of omphalocele is rare—1 in 5000 live births.
- A child with an omphalocele may have accompanying defects that also were caused by the teratogenic insult that prevented normal intestinal growth.
- An omphalocele is detectable on ultrasonography.
- There is no difference on the outcome of the child with omphalocele with vaginal delivery or cesarean birth.
- Small defects require immediate surgery to replace the bowel.

- Large defects are managed by topical application of silver sulfadiazine, which prevents infection of the sac, followed by delayed surgical closure.
- It is not possible to replace the entire bowel immediately owing to the unusually small abdomen.
- The bowel may be contained by a Silastic pouch that is suspended over the infant's bed and gradually decreased in size as more bowel is returned to the abdomen.
- The infant requires total parenteral nutrition during this time.
- After the final surgical repair, the child with an omphalocele is the perfect child the parents once envisioned except for a large abdominal scar.

## Nursing Implications

- Explain the defect that has occurred to the parents and support them through the initial shock of acceptance.
- Discuss the options that may be available to the child depending on the size of the defect.
- Record the general appearance and size of the omphalocele at birth.
- Prevent infection by application of topical antibiotics as prescribed.
- Monitor for infection and assess for erythema or foul drainage.
- Do not allow the lining of the peritoneum to be ruptured or to dry out.
- Keep the sac moist with saline-soaked gauze.
- Insert a nasogastric tube as prescribed to prevent intestinal distention.
- Continue to monitor nutritional status explaining to the parents why the child cannot be fed until the surgical repair is complete.
- Begin oral feedings gradually, once complete bowel repair and healing have occurred.
- Prepare the parents of the newborn for the possibility of a long hospitalization, 1 to 2 months, while the child awaits the second and third stages of repair.
- Encourage the parents to visit and hold the baby as much as possible.
- Assign a primary nurse to the infant to minimize the number of and exposure to caregivers.

- Provide stimulation for the infant with mobiles and toys.
- Continue to provide support to the frustrated parents throughout the long hospitalization, and help them to verbalize their feelings and accept the situation.
- Prepare the parents of the baby to be cared for at home on home parenteral nutrition about all aspects of the baby's care.
- Evaluate the readiness of the family to take the sick child home, and recommend home health nurses if appropriate.
- Prepare the parents ready to take the healed child home for continued monitoring and provide a phone number they may call with any questions.
- Ensure that the parents have a follow-up appointment and understand all instructions before the child's discharge.

# OSGOOD-SCHLATTER DISEASE

### Description
- Osgood-Schlatter disease is an incomplete separation of the epiphysis of the tibial tubercle from the tibial shaft.
- This can occur secondary to thickening and enlargement of the tibial tuberosity; it is an overuse injury secondary to repeated traction or pull on the patellar tendon.
- This injury is most common in boys 10 to 16 years of age.
- Osgood-Schlatter disease is self-limiting and resolves once the epiphyseal growth plates close.
- Therapy is usually directed at limiting the strenuous physical exercise or immobilization of a leg in a walking cast or immobilizer for 6 weeks.

### Assessment Findings
- Pain, tenderness, and swelling over the anterior portion of the knee
- Pain subsiding with rest and worsening with activity, which causes stress or pressure on the knee or tibial tubercle

### Nursing Implications
- Evaluate complaints of knee pain and swelling and correlate with specific activities.
- After definitive diagnosis, advise the parents and child about supportive treatment used.

- Educate the parents and the child on use of ibuprofen, if prescribed, to relieve inflammation and discomfort.
- Advise the child to engage in physical activities when free of pain.
- Caution the child on the need to take short rest periods when the pain occurs and to avoid activities that cause pain.
- Prepare the child and the parent about the potential need for casts, braces, or immobilization if physical activity modification is not enough.
- Identify physical activities in which the child can participate comfortably, such as swimming or bicycle riding.

## OSTEOGENESIS IMPERFECTA

### DESCRIPTION
- Osteogenesis imperfecta is characterized by the formation of brittle bones.
- This occurs in two forms: a severe form that is recognized at birth, *osteogenesis imperfecta congenita,* and a form that occurs later in life, *osteogenesis imperfecta tarda.*
- *Osteogenesis imperfecta congenita* is an autosomal recessive disorder.
- Children with the congenital form are born with countless fractures, and more fractures develop during childhood.
- *Osteogenesis imperfecta tarda* is an inherited dominant trait disorder.
- Administration of growth hormones may stimulate growth.
- Therapy is aimed at protecting the child from trauma and treating and aligning fractures.

### ASSESSMENT FINDINGS
#### *Osteogenesis imperfecta congenita*
- Numerous fractures at birth
- Fragile bones
- Fractures continuing during childhood owing to poor collagen formation
#### *Osteogenesis imperfecta tarda*
- Fractures
- Associated deafness, dental deformities, and unusual blueness of the sclera because of poor connective tissue formation

- Ribbonlike or mosaic pattern in bones on x-ray film (aids in diagnosis)
- Limb and spinal cord deformities (eventually develop after multiple breaks and interfere with alignment and growth)

### NURSING IMPLICATIONS

- Explain to the parents of the child diagnosed with osteogenesis that the disorder is chronic and requires attention throughout the child's life.
- Treat associated medical disorders.
- Assist the parents and child in adapting their lifestyle, which is necessary to maintain a productive but trauma-free life.
- Evaluate growth hormone and leg braces or intermedullary rods, which may be helpful in strengthening bones.
- Carefully assess the hospital environment to ensure that all safety precautions, such as side rails, are maintained.
- Lift a child with this disorder gently and never by a single arm or leg.
- Educate parents on appropriate care for the child, and support them in adapting their home and lifestyle.
- Recommend diversional activities that keep the child stimulated and safe.

## OSTEOMYELITIS

### DESCRIPTION

- Osteomyelitis is infection of the bone, most often caused by *Staphylococcus aureus* in older children and by *Haemophilus influenzae* (which is carried to the bone site by septicemia) in younger children.
- Osteomyelitis results from local trauma, or it may be a complication of extensive *impetigo, burns, otitis media, tonsillitis,* tooth abscesses, or skin abscesses.
- Children with *sickle cell anemia* have a special susceptibility to *Salmonella* invasion in the long bones.
- During blood sampling via a heel puncture, strict aseptic technique must be used to avoid osteomyelitis.
- Osteomyelitis can be acute or chronic.
- The acute form, which is blood borne, affects rapidly growing children.

- The chronic form, characterized by multiple open draining sinus tracts and metastatic lesions, lasts more than 4 weeks and is refractory to therapy.
- With osteomyelitis, the bacterial invasion of bone causes an inflammatory response.
- An abscess forms, and pus may drain into the metaphysis.
- Bony tissue within the abscessed area becomes necrotic.
- An abscess spreads and forms along the shaft of the bone, under the periosteum.
- The abscess can extend to the bone marrow or between the infected bone and the skin above.
- If the epiphyseal plate is infected, altered bone growth may result.
- Therapy for acute osteomyelitis calls for a 3- to 4-week course of high-dose intravenous antibiotic therapy and limitation of weight bearing on the affected part.
- A child with chronic osteomyelitis requires additional therapy with an alternate antibiotic.
- Some children require surgical intervention to evacuate the pus from the metaphyseal space and prevent rupture of the periosteum.

## ASSESSMENT FINDINGS

- Fever
- Irritability
- Sharp pain at bone metaphysis
- Edematous, warm area of skin covering infected bone
- Increased white blood cell count
- Increased sedimentation rate
- Soft tissue swelling and movement of the periosteum away from the bone and its vascular supply on x-ray film
- Aspiration of the bone and culture positive for causative organism

## NURSING IMPLICATIONS

- Obtain a thorough history and physical examination to establish a baseline and identify any recent history of trauma or previous infection.
- Detect signs and symptoms of osteomyelitis early to administer prompt treatment.

- Educate parents and children on what osteomyelitis is and how it must be treated.
- Explain to parents and children that immobilization is necessary to protect the bone from injury.
- Teach the child to avoid weight bearing on the affected limb.
- Assess the child's pain and administer analgesics as needed.
- Support the family in the lifestyle changes that are required of them in the next several weeks so as to be with the child as much as possible in the hospital and then stay with the child for an extended period at home.
- Evaluate the child's response to the antibiotics by assessing temperature, monitoring blood levels, and assessing pain.
- Monitor carefully for adverse affects of antibiotics, such as renal toxicity and ototoxicity.
- Handle the extremity gently when giving care because the child will have pain.
- Offer a diet high in calcium, calories, and protein to enhance bone healing.
- Suggest diversional activities to distract the child.
- Investigate with the parents the possibility of home intravenous antibiotics.
- Educate the family and the child on antibiotics, adverse effects, intravenous therapy, intake and output, and need for compliance with the antibiotic therapy before discharge.
- Evaluate the need and availability of a home health care nurse.
- Educate the parents of the child discharged on oral antibiotics on the importance of giving medication even though the child's symptoms have completely disappeared.
- Explain to parents that if the infection is not entirely eradicated with the initial treatment, it returns and results in chronic osteomyelitis, which may result in bone deformity.

## OTITIS MEDIA, ACUTE

### DESCRIPTION

- Acute otitis media is an inflammation of the middle ear.

- It is the most prevalent disorder of childhood after respiratory tract infections.
- It occurs most often in the child 6 to 36 months of age and again at 4 to 6 years.
- It occurs more frequently in males.
- There is a higher incidence in formula-fed infants than those who are breast-fed because of the more slanted position that formula-fed infants are held while feeding, allowing milk to enter the eustachian tube.
- The incidence is highest in winter and spring and in homes in which a parent smokes.
- If acute otitis media is not treated and cured, permanent damage can occur to middle ear structures, leading to *hearing impairment.*

## ASSESSMENT FINDINGS

- History of a recent respiratory infection
- Red, bulging tympanic membrane
- Fever
- Sharp, constant pain in one or both ears
- Pulling on the ear(s)
- Irritability
- Purulent drainage in external ear canal
- Loss of appetite
- Nasal congestion
- Positive culture and sensitivity for organism

## NURSING IMPLICATIONS

- Administer antipyretics as prescribed to reduce fever.
- Administer analgesics as prescribed to relieve pain.
- Help the child limit chewing to reduce pain by offering liquids or soft foods.
- Apply local heat or cool compress over the affected ear to minimize pain; encourage the child to prevent pressure on the affected ear by lying on the opposite side.
- If the tympanic membrane has ruptured, place the child on the side of the affected ear with the affected ear in a dependent position to facilitate drainage.
- Keep the external ear clean and dry to prevent skin breakdown.
- Assess for *hearing impairment* and refer for audiometric testing if indicated.
- Administer antibiotics, such as ampicillin, gentamicin, amoxicillin, erythromycin, or sulfonamide, as prescribed.

- Administer decongestant nose drops as prescribed to relieve nasal congestion and open up the eustachian tube allowing air to enter the middle ear; caution the parents to administer the nose drops for no more than 3 days because a rebound effect may occur, causing edema and increasing the mucous membrane size.
- Instruct the parents in the medication regimen, importance of completing entire prescription of antibiotics, signs of hearing loss, and need for follow-up.
- Instruct the parents in preventive measures, such as holding the child upright during feeding, gentle nose blowing, blowing games, and chewing sugarless gum.
- Educate the parents to recognize the signs and symptoms for early diagnosis and treatment.
- Anticipate the possibility of surgical intervention if *chronic otitis media* occurs.

## OTITIS MEDIA, CHRONIC

### DESCRIPTION

- Otitis media is inflammation or infection of the middle ear.
- Chronic otitis media is usually caused by gram-negative bacteria, such as *Proteus, Klebsiella,* and *Pseudomonas.*
- Chronic otitis media causes serous otitis media.
- The source of air to the middle ear is cut off, and the epithelial cells become secretory cells.
- The middle ear fills with secretions, which are a good medium for infection.
- The fluid becomes thick and tenacious.
- There may be a drop of 20 to 40 decibels in hearing secondary to the fluid.
- Children aged 3 to 10 years of age are most commonly seen with this disorder.

### ASSESSMENT FINDINGS

- History of chronic ear infections following recent upper respiratory infection
- Red, bulging tympanic membrane
- Sharp, constant pain in one or both ears
- Purulent drainage in external ear canal
- Fever
- Gradual loss of hearing

#### NURSING IMPLICATIONS

- Maintain careful records and evaluate a child's history for recent ear infections and treatment.
- Educate the parents to recognize the symptoms of *acute otitis media* and to seek medical attention early for this serious disorder.
- Refer the child to an ear specialist for further evaluation.
- Administer antibiotics as prescribed, and educate the parents on administering a full dose for pain and fever.
- Administer analgesics/antipyretics as prescribed for pain and fever.
- Encourage the child to lie on the opposite side of the infected ear to decrease pressure.
- Assess hearing and evaluate for any *hearing impairment.*
- Instruct the parents on the potential need for a myringotomy to allow purulent drainage and to prevent rupture from the bulging ear drum.
- Prepare the parents and child for the surgical procedure, usually done in day surgery and requiring general anesthesia.
- Educate the parents on postoperative care, continued antibiotics or eardrops (or both), and the need to keep water out of the ear during swimming and bathing.
- Ensure the child and parents have a follow-up appointment.

## OVERANXIOUS DISORDER

### Description

- Overanxious disorder is a psychiatric disorder that manifests as excessive or unrealistic anxiety or worry.
- Overanxious disorder is not limited to any particular object or event.
- Overanxious disorder is more common in eldest children of small families in upper socioeconomic groups.
- Within the family, there is often concern about achievement even though the child is functioning at average and higher levels.
- Overanxious disorder is found equally in both males and females.
- Impairment with this disorder is unusual unless the disorder is severe enough to result in the child's inability to meet the demands of home and school.

- The child with this disorder may have it persist into adult life as an anxiety disorder.
- Family therapy may help the child and family gain insight into the problem and focus on the real concern.
- Antianxiety medication may be used.

### Assessment Findings

- Sudden or gradual onset of excessive worrying for a period of 6 months or longer
- Exacerbations during periods of stress
- Gastrointestinal distress, duodenal ulcer, headache, or dizziness
- Extremely self-conscious, perfectionist behavior, appearing mature because of their seriousness about various circumstances
- Shy, self-deprecating behavior often with a nervous habit, such as thumb sucking or nail biting
- Preoccupations with the object of the worry taking up a lot of the child's time

### Nursing Implications

- Carefully evaluate any complaints of excessive worry made by the child or the parent.
- Assess the child within the family system and evaluate the family dynamics.
- Consider somatic complaints and assess the need for medical evaluation.
- Refer the entire family to a family therapist for further assessment so as to gain insight into the problem.
- Use antianxiety medications as prescribed, and educate the family and the child about the medication.
- Explain to the family that the medications make the child more amenable to therapy, especially if the child's anxiety is high.

## OVERHYDRATION

### Description

- Overhydration is a serious fluid imbalance in a child generally occurring in children receiving intravenous fluid.
- Normally the body is able to maintain control of fluids and electrolytes and would inhibit the release of antidiuretic hormone and aldosterone, thereby increasing kidney excretion of excess water.
- Situations that can cause overhydration include tap water enemas.

- The body transfers water from the extracellular space into the intracellular space to restore normal osmotic relationships.
- Intracellular edema occurs.
- Excess fluid from the extracellular space may result in cardiovascular overload, cardiac failure, and respiratory failure.
- Electrolyte imbalances also occur in states of overhydration.

### ASSESSMENT FINDINGS
- Headache
- Nausea/*vomiting*
- Blurred vision
- Cramps
- Muscle twitching
- *Seizures*

### NURSING IMPLICATIONS
- Monitor intake and output with all hospitalized children, especially those receiving intravenous therapy.
- Evaluate daily electrolytes and assess for associated symptoms, especially hyponatremia and hypokalemia with overhydration.
- Be aware of potentially dangerous treatments that may cause overhydration, such as tap water enemas in a child with aganglionic disease of the intestines.
- Report any symptoms of intracellular edema, especially monitoring for changes in level of consciousness.
- Assess cardiac and respiratory function carefully in at-risk patients.
- Note signs of tachypnea, dyspnea, tachycardia, and cardiac failure.
- Aggressively treat any child with overhydration or electrolyte imbalance as prescribed by the health care team.

## PARASITIC INFESTATIONS, PEDICULOSIS

### DESCRIPTION
- Pediculosis is a parasitic infectious process that occurs with the infestation of bloodsucking lice.
- Two forms of pediculosis are pediculosis capitis (head lice infestation) and pediculosis pubis (lice infestation of the pubic hair region).
- Pediculosis capitis commonly occurs with the school-age child.

- Pediculosis pubis is mostly found with adolescents and is spread by physical contact.
- The lice are rarely visible; however, the eggs are seen as white flecks on hair shafts.
- The itching from the pediculosis can cause secondary infection.
- Lindane (Kwell shampoo) or pyrethrin is effective in killing head lice.

### ASSESSMENT FINDINGS
- Intense pruritus
- Excoriation of skin from itching
- Lice visible behind ears and at the base of hairline (possible)

### NURSING IMPLICATIONS
- Inspect all schoolchildren regularly for head lice.
- Evaluate any complaints of scalp itching or intense pubic area itching and assess for lice.
- Explain to the child and parents that lice infestation can occur to any child regardless of the cleanliness of the child.
- Inspect all family members for infestation.
- Educate the family and child that lice do not fly from person to person; however, they may crawl from one place to another.
- Explain to adolescents with pediculosis pubis that this is spread via physical contact, and all intimate partners need to be evaluated.
- Educate sexually active adolescents on the dangers of *sexually transmitted disease,* and encourage them to use protection if they are going to be sexually active.
- Refer all children with pediculosis pubis for further evaluation of possible sexual abuse.
- Explain to parents the need to do this is to protect the child and that it is not an accusation against them.
- Teach parents and children with pediculosis about the treatment with Lindane (Kwell shampoo [contraindicated in children under 2]) or pyrethrin.
- Inform the parents that they will need to comb the hair after application with a fine-tooth comb to remove the parasitic eggs (nits).
- Have parents remove the shampoo according to the manufacturer's directions to avoid neurotoxicity.

- Tell the parents and the adolescent child to continue treatment for 7 days.
- Educate the parents on the need also to launder the child's linens and clothes worn recently because lice spread easily.
- Do not allow the child to share combs or towels after gym or to share hair ornaments or hats so as to discourage parasitic spread further.
- Inform parents of the need to spray rugs and upholstered furniture with special spray, such as R and C spray.

## PARASITIC INFESTATIONS, SCABIES

### DESCRIPTION
- Scabies is a parasitic skin disorder caused by a female mite, *Acarus scabei*.
- The mite burrows into the skin and deposits eggs in areas that are thin and moist, particularly the areas between fingers and toes, palms, in the axilla, and in the groin, although in the young child, the sites may be much more scattered in location.

### ASSESSMENT FINDINGS
- Black-colored burrows, contaminated by mite feces, approximately 1/2 inch in length visible
- Severe itching
- Secondary infections
- Breaks in the skin

### NURSING IMPLICATIONS
- Thoroughly inspect the skin to identify burrows and rule out other skin disorders.
- Wash the child thoroughly with soap and warm water using a rough washcloth, and towel dry.
- Apply lindane (Kwell lotion) or permethrin to child's body as prescribed.
- Instruct parents in good hygiene measures and to change bed linens, towels, and clothing after bathing and lotion application.
- Anticipate treating close family and personal contacts if indicated because the parasite is transmitted by close personal contact and through clothing or linens.
- Provide emotional support to the parents and child because the infestation can be traumatic.

## PATENT URACHUS

### DESCRIPTION

- Patent urachus is a fistula that develops between the bladder and the umbilicus.
- Normally, during embryonic development, the umbilicus and the bladder are joined by a narrow tube called the urachus; failure of this to close in utero leads to patent urachus.
- Patent urachus occurs more commonly in males than in females.
- The urachus remnant is seen on ultrasonography.
- Some patent urachus abnormalities heal spontaneously; however, it frequently requires surgical correction to prevent pathogens from entering the fistula site and causing persist bladder infection.
- This is done in the immediate neonatal period using only a small subumbilical incision.

### ASSESSMENT FINDINGS

- Clean, odorless fluid draining from the base of the cord
- pH of the specimen positive for urine

### NURSING IMPLICATIONS

- Explain to the parents all the medical terminology and the condition of patent urachus.
- Allow the parents time to accept this condition, and help them to realize it is surgically correctable.
- Answer any questions the family may have regarding the condition, surgery, and how it may affect the care of the child.
- Support the parents during surgery, and encourage them to hold and care for the child as much as possible.

## PECTUS EXCAVATUM

### DESCRIPTION

- Pectus excavatum refers to an indentation of the lower portion of the sternum.
- This is a congenital deformity, but it also may occur following chronic obstructive lung disease or rickets.
- Surgical intervention is used for cosmetic purposes or to expand the lung volume.

### ASSESSMENT FINDINGS
- Indentation of lower sternum
- Decreased lung volume
- Displacement of the heart to the left

### NURSING IMPLICATIONS

- Obtain a thorough history and physical examination to establish a baseline.
- Prepare the child and parents for surgical correction; include information about all aspects of preoperative and postoperative care.
- Provide emotional support and guidance to the child and parents to help alleviate their anxieties and fears.

## PEPTIC ULCER

### DESCRIPTION
- A peptic ulcer is a shallow excavation formed in the mucosal wall of the stomach, the pylorus, or the duodenum.
- Children usually have duodenal peptic ulcers.
- Peptic ulcers occur secondary to excess gastric acid or failure of the mucosa to neutralize gastric secretions.
- The acid is irritating to the mucosa, and a small ulceration of the gastric or duodenal lining leads to symptoms.
- Peptic ulcers may also be associated with infection, such as *C. jejuni*.
- Medications such as corticosteroids and salicylates cause gastric irritation and may lead to ulceration.
- Neonates may suffer peptic ulcers with the stress of prolonged labor, sepsis, or the trauma of intubation.
- Neonatal peptic ulcers are usually superficial and heal rapidly, although rupture can occur, leading to respiratory distress, abdominal distention, *vomiting,* and cardiovascular collapse.
- Secondary ulcers occur in children with *burn trauma.*
- There may be a genetic association, with many children with peptic ulcers having positive family histories.
- Untreated peptic ulcers can lead to bowel or stomach perforation with acute hemorrhage or pyloric obstruction.
- Chronic peptic ulcers cause constant blood loss and lead to *anemia.*

- 2% to 18% of people with chronic duodenal ulcers date the onset of their symptoms to childhood.
- Peptic ulcers in children are increasing in frequency, which may be a reflection of increased societal stress.
- Peptic ulcers occur more frequently in males than in females.
- Whites more than any other race and urban more than rural populations suffer from peptic ulcers.
- The dangers of peptic ulcers are perforation and intestinal obstruction.
- Children with peptic ulcer disease are treated with medications to suppress gastric acidity, and antibiotics may be prescribed for infection.
- Uncomplicated peptic ulcers heal rapidly with therapy.
- Surgical intervention may be required to remove part of the stomach or denervate the stomach.
- The long-term data, however, reveal the likelihood of developing ulcers again later in life.

### Assessment Findings
#### *In neonates*
- Hematemesis
- Melena

#### *In toddlers*
- Feeding problems
- *Vomiting*
- Hematemesis and melena
- Pain on arising in the morning not relieved by ingestion of food or milk

#### *In older children and adolescents*
- Gnawing or aching pain in the epigastric area before meals
- Pain relieved by eating
- *Vomiting* secondary to spasm and edema of the pylorus
- Epigastric region tenderness on palpation

### Nursing Implications
- Assess children with symptoms of peptic ulcer disease and refer for further evaluation.
- Educate the child and parents on what peptic ulcers are and how they may be treated.
- Prepare the child and parents for x-ray study or endoscopy to establish a definitive diagnosis.

- Establish goals with the child, and ensure that the parents and the child realize the importance of taking the prescribed medication.
- Help the parents and child understand that the medication will take a while to heal the ulcer and that is why pain may persist.
- Administer small feedings or slow continuous nasogastric drip of combined formula and an antacid to infants to provide pain relief and healing.
- Advise the older child to eat a regular diet but to avoid spicy foods.
- Advise parents to give the child in school a less conspicuous antacid tablet instead of the elixir.
- Monitor all children for signs and symptoms of complications, and teach the parents and child about these symptoms.
- Periodically monitor children who have had peptic ulcer disease for hypochromic, microcytic *anemia.*
- Explore with children any situational or family stress and encourage the family and the child to discuss this openly.
- Help the child to learn appropriate coping mechanisms and teach age-appropriate stress reduction techniques to the child.

## PHARYNGITIS

### DESCRIPTION
- Pharyngitis is an infection and inflammation of the throat, bacterial or viral in origin.
- Pharyngitis frequently accompanies the common cold.
- The peak incidence of pharyngitis is between 4 and 7 years of age.
- Chronic *allergies* may cause pharyngitis with the constant postnasal discharge and resultant secondary irritation.
- Treatment for viral pharyngitis is directed to comfort interventions, such as acetaminophen for pain and fever or gargling with warm water.
- Group A beta-hemolytic streptococcus is the organism most frequently involved in bacterial pharyngitis, usually affecting children age 6 and older.
- Treatment for streptococcal pharyngitis is a full 10-day course of antibiotic, such as clindamycin or amoxicillin.

- Children not fully treated can develop a hypersensitivity reaction resulting in *rheumatic fever* (rare).
- Symptoms of *acute glomerulonephritis* may appear in 1 to 2 weeks after streptococcal pharyngitis regardless of a full course of antibiotics.
- If the bacterial strain was a nephrogenic one, the chances are as high as 50% that the kidney disease will develop.

### Assessment Findings

#### *Viral pharyngitis*
- Sore throat
- Fever
- General malaise
- Enlarged lymph nodes
- Erythematous pharynx and palatine arch
- Increased white blood cell count

#### *Streptococcal pharyngitis*
- Erythematous and enlarged palatine and tonsils
- White exudate in the tonsilar crypts
- Petechiae present on the palate (possible)
- High fever
- Extreme sore throat
- Lethargy
- Difficulty swallowing
- Headache
- Enlarged abdominal lymph nodes and abdominal pain
- Throat cultures positive for streptococcus bacteria (which can be virulent causing necrosis of tissue and extensive damage)

### Nursing Implications

- Encourage parents always to have a child with pharyngitis seen at a health care facility.
- Tell parents that the child needs to have a throat culture because it is impossible to discriminate between pharyngitis from a virus or streptococcal pharyngitis, which requires treatment to prevent life-threatening illness.
- Educate parents on the importance of administering a full 10-day course of antibiotic therapy to ensure that the streptococci are completely eradicated.
- Instruct the parents on appropriate comfort measures for the child.

- Inform the parents that the child with streptococcal pharyngitis is infectious until the 24 hours after antibiotics have begun.
- Ensure that the child returns to the health care facility 2 weeks after treatment to obtain a urine specimen and evaluate for *poststreptococcal glomerulonephritis.*

# PHENYLKETONURIA (PKU)

## DESCRIPTION

- PKU is an inborn error of metabolism inherited as an autosomal recessive trait.
- The absence of liver enzyme phenylalanine hydroxylase prevents conversion of phenylalanine, an essential amino acid, which would normally convert into tyrosine, a precursor of epinephrine, thyroxine, and melanin.
- The results from this lack of conversion is an excessive buildup of phenylalanine in the blood stream and tissues.
- This causes irreversible brain damage and severe *mental retardation.*
- A strong association exists between *atopic dermatitis* and PKU.
- All children with *atopic dermatitis* are rescreened for PKU.
- PKU is found in 1 in 10,000 live births in the United States.
- Untreated the child with PKU will have an IQ of 20.
- Complications associated with PKU include recurrent *seizures,* muscular hypertonicity, and spasticity.
- PKU is not detected by amniocentesis or percutaneous umbilical cord blood analysis because the phenylalanine level does not rise in utero.
- Recombinant DNA techniques can be used for carrier detection and prenatal diagnosis.
- Early identification of this disorder is essential to prevent *mental retardation.*

## ASSESSMENT FINDINGS

- Mousy or musty odor to urine or child
- Fair-skinned
- Eczema
- Blue eyes
- Small size
- *Seizure* disorder

### Nursing Implications

- Ensure that all children are screened for PKU, usually 2 days after birth.
- Request that children that go home early or are born at home have a home health nurse in after 2 days of feeding to evaluate for PKU.
- Initiate a diet of extremely low phenylalanine formula right away if this disorder is found.
- Explain to parents the need to maintain the child on a low-phenylalanine diet to prevent permanent brain damage.
- Answer all the parents' questions, and assure them that following this diet can prevent *mental retardation.*
- Consult with a dietitian and promote discussion and education with the dietitian and the parents.
- Realistically explain to parents of the child with PKU not detected early that the damage done thus far cannot be reversed.
- Educate the family and the child on the importance of maintaining the child on a diet that keeps the blood level of phenylalanine below 9 mg/100 ml.
- Monitor this child's blood and urine frequently and assess hemoglobin levels to ensure that the child is not becoming anemic.
- Inform the parents that the child needs to remain on this diet until at least 5 years of age, when 90% of brain growth has occurred.
- Explain to the parents that controversy over the length of time the child needs to be maintained on this diet exists, and some believe the child needs this modified diet indefinitely.
- Instruct women with PKU who wish to become pregnant that they must maintain a diet low in phenylalanine for 3 months before conception and then through the pregnancy, or the fetus will be born mentally retarded from exposure to high levels of phenylalanine.

## PHIMOSIS

### Description

- Phimosis describes a foreskin that remains tight that interferes with voiding.
- Normally after birth, the tight foreskin is held by adhesions, which generally cannot be retracted.

- After a few months, the adhesions should dissolve, and the foreskin becomes retractable.
- With phimosis, the foreskin remains tight.
- Phimosis can lead to balanoposthitis because the foreskin cannot be retracted for cleaning.
- True phimosis is rare.
- A circumcision, commonly performed in the United States on male babies, corrects phimosis.

### NURSING IMPLICATIONS
- Inform the parents of the condition and explain to them that it is correctable with circumcision.
- Describe the technique to be used, and educate the parents on postcircumcision incision care.
- Evaluate the incision for signs of infection at the infant's 1- to 2-week checkup.
- Teach the parents what signs of infection to be aware of and to report.

## PINWORM

### DESCRIPTION
- Pinworm is a benign but highly contagious parasitic infection caused by *Enterobius vermicularis.*
- It is transmitted via stool through the person to oral to fecal route.
- The incubation period of this infection is 3 to 6 weeks.
- Pinworm infection is named for the small, white, threadlike worms that live in the cecum.
- At night, the female pinworm travels down the intestinal tract and out the anus to deposit eggs in the anal and perianal region.
- The anal itching from the parasite causes the child to scratch, and some of the eggs are carried from their fingernails to their mouths.
- The cycle is then repeated.
- Treatment for pinworm is with mebendazole (Vermox) or with pyrantel pamoate (Antiminth): both drugs effectively destroy the pinworm.

### ASSESSMENT FINDINGS
- Perianal pruritus, especially at night
- Restlessness during sleep
- Ova or threadlike worms appear near rectum on awakening

### Nursing Implications

- Educate parents on administration of mebendazole tablets, 100 mg immediately and 100 mg 10 days later.
- Tell the parents that the mebendazole may be chewed or crushed and mixed with food.
- Inform the family that all nonpregnant members need to be treated as well because the parasite is easily spread.
- Educate the family on the potential side effects from the drug, such as abdominal cramps and *diarrhea.*
- Emphasize the need for compliance and the importance of administering the second dose of the drug.
- Advise parents to give the child warm baths and to apply ointment such as Desitin to relieve rectal irritation.
- Stress the importance of good personal hygiene to prevent autoinfection.
- Educate the child on handwashing after toileting and before food preparation or eating.
- Tell the parents to keep the child's fingernails short.
- Have the child change underwear twice a day.
- Direct the parents to wash bedding, towels, and nightclothing before reuse.

## PITUITARY GIGANTISM

### Description

- Pituitary gigantism is generally caused by an overproduction of growth hormone, usually a result of a tumor of the anterior pituitary.
- Excessive growth can be caused by an overproduction of growth hormone before the epiphyseal lines of the long bones close.
- Weight also is excessive but proportional to the height.
- This excessive growth becomes evident at puberty.
- Acromegaly may accompany the excessive growth in stature, becoming more pronounced after the epiphysial lines of the long bones close and linear growth is no longer possible.
- Untreated the child can reach a height of 8 feet.
- Surgical removal of the tumor or cryosurgery is required if the increased growth hormone is from an adenoma.
- Irradiation or radioactive implants to reduce the growth hormone is required if no tumor is found.

### Assessment Findings

- Increased skull circumference
- Fontanelles closing late or not at all
- Enlarged thick tongue

### Nursing Implications

- Carefully monitor height and weight at all health maintenance visits and compare with standard for the age group.
- Note any changes that continue to reveal increasing height and weight.
- Refer the child for further evaluation of pituitary function.
- Explain to parents what the pituitary gland does and how a tumor is affecting the child's growth.
- Discuss the treatment options available to the child and prepare the family and child for surgical intervention if necessary.
- Be aware that other hormones may be affected and need to be evaluated.
- Explain to the parents and child that the child may require thyroid extract, cortisol, and gonadotropin hormones if the treatment eradicates pituitary functioning.
- Inform the parents and child that the increased height and weight cannot be reversed but can be controlled now that a diagnosis has been made and treatment initiated.
- Encourage the parents and child to verbalize their feelings about the child's increased size.

## PITYRIASIS ROSEA

### Description

- Pityriasis rosea is a skin disorder, probably a viral infection with an unknown causative organism.
- The incubation period is unknown, and no evidence exists to suggest it is contagious.
- Pityriasis rosea occurs in school-age and older children.
- The rash usually lasts 6 to 8 weeks.
- Treatment for pityriasis rosea is directed toward comfort measures, such as oral antihistamines.
- No immunity from the virus exists.
- No sequelae or complications from the virus are known.

- This is simply a baffling rash of childhood and should be differentiated from serous exanthems.

### Assessment Findings
- Fever (prodromal period)
- Sore throat (prodromal period)
- Herald patch and erythematous round lesion with a scaly border usually appearing on the trunk (the first obvious lesion)
- Generalized christmas tree like configuration rash of papules, vesicles, or urticaria, usually confined to the trunk one week following the first lesion
- Pruritus

### Nursing Implications
- Assess and evaluate any complaints of rash and refer to the physician for definitive diagnosis.
- Obtain a thorough history and physical examination to differentiate this disorder and ensure the child does not have a more serious exanthem.
- Explain to the parents that although this may appear like the ringworm rash, it is not and they simply need to tolerate the rash for the duration.
- Educate the parents that the virus does not have any serious sequela or complications.
- Direct the parents to administer antihistamines to increase the child's comfort.
- Ensure a follow-up visit to assess the rash.

## PLAY

### Description
- Play may be defined as any voluntary activity engaged in for the purpose of enjoyment.
- Play varies greatly from child to child and among different age groups.
- The work of play actually allows a child to develop increasing cognitive, psychomotor, and social capabilities.
- The repetitive acts involved in most games encourage the musculoskeletal skills of a child.
- Play is a task of childhood that provides security because it is an activity that has continuity with home life.
- Hospitalized children may not feel well enough for play; however, once the acute period is over, the interest in play usually returns.

- Monitoring a child's interest in play is an indicator of the child's health.
- Toys that the child uses at play are a good indication of growth and development and of emotional state.
- There are four basic types of play: observational, parallel, associative, and cooperative play.
- Observational play occurs during the infant period.
    With observational play, the child watches particular play intently but is not actively engaged in it.
- Parallel play occurs during the toddler period.
    Toddlers are egocentric and concerned with their own world; two toddlers play side by side; however, seldom does interaction between the two occur.
    With parallel play, the play activity serves to bring the children in contact with each other, yet they are not yet able to share attitudes, feelings, or activities with others.
- Associative play also occurs during childhood.
    Associative play is nonsocial primarily because of the egocentric nature of toddlers; however, there is interaction and socialization.
    This is normal play in which a group of children participate in similar or identical activities without formal organization, group direction, group interaction, or a definite goal.
    Children borrow or lend toys, but overall they act independently.
    Associative play is seen at preschool playgrounds or among a group of riding bicycles or tricycles.
- Cooperative play occurs among school-age children.
    Children partaking in cooperative play have an organized structure or compete for a desired goal or outcome.
    Cooperative play encourages a child to share materials as well as rules; it also helps children to understand and operate in groups.

### Nursing Implications

- Question the parents at health maintenance visits about the type of play the child participates in.
- Evaluate any changes in play and assess that the play is developmentally appropriate.
- Help the parents to understand the meaning and the importance of play during childhood.

- Encourage the parents of hospitalized children to bring in favorite games or toys and to play them with the child.
- Provide instructions to the parents about age-appropriate toys for the child.

##  PLAY THERAPY

### DESCRIPTION

- Play therapy is a psychoanalytic technique used by professionals to help children to understand their feelings, thoughts, and motivations.
- Play is the universal language of children.
- Children who have difficulty voicing their thoughts in words can often speak clearly through *play*.
- Hospital environments and ambulatory care settings are new and different environments that can cause a great deal of anxiety for children; using toys and *play* can help to reduce some of this anxiety.
- The basis for play therapy is to help a child to confront and gain insight into their fears.
- During play therapy, a therapist attempts to interpret a child's verbal and nonverbal cues using therapeutic play.
- Therapeutic play is a play technique used by a play therapist or nurse to understand children's thoughts and feelings better.
- Therapeutic play can be divided into three forms: energy release, dramatic play, and creative play.
- Energy release is based on the premise that any time people feel anxious, action feels good; it allows children to release anxiety by pounding, hitting, running, punching, or shouting.
- Dramatic play is acting out an anxiety-producing situation; it is an effective intervention for preschool children, who have wonderful imaginations.
- Instruments used during dramatic play include those that may be making them anxious, such as hospital equipment.
- Anatomically correct dolls are used to help children act out their feelings about sexual abuse.
- 9- to 10-year-old children may find playing with dolls too childish but benefit from handling medical equipment before use.

- If a child is too angry, he or she may not be able to use dramatic play to act out feelings.
- An extremely angry child may be able to draw a picture that expresses his or her emotions or knowledge, and this is considered creative play.
- Interpretation of drawings needs to be done carefully and using common sense.
- Analysis of all therapeutic play must be guarded, remembering that all children may treat a doll cruelly at times.
- Continuous signs of anger and hostile feelings seen through therapeutic play are more important than a single event.

### Nursing Implications

- Understand that many situations, including hospitalizations, create anxiety in children.
- Use play therapy to help the child to identify, confront, and verbalize fears and anxieties.
- Realize that preschoolers may have the most difficult time with a hospital experience because they have so many fears.
- Prepare and promote therapeutic play to reduce trauma to a tolerable level.
- Include the parents in the care of the child in a hospital to alleviate further some of the child's anxieties.
- Allow a child to choose the article(s) with which to play.
- Allow play to be unstructured, or let the child use the materials however he or she wishes.
- Sit and play with the child if the child seems too anxious to handle certain objects, to help alleviate some of the anxiety and make the child more amenable to handle the items.
- Ask the child what he or she would like you to do with certain items, especially if the child is not able to manipulate the item himself or herself (cast on arm).
- Reflect only what the child expresses.
- Do not criticize play because it may inhibit further expression.
- Use therapeutic responses, such as, "Are you worried that will happen?"

- Always supervise therapeutic play, not only to analyze it, but also to maintain the child's safety.

# PNEUMONIA

## DESCRIPTION

- Pneumonia is an acute inflammation of the lungs, including the alveoli.
- The cause of pneumonia may be viral or bacterial in origin.
- Aspiration of lipid or hydrocarbon substances also causes pneumonia.
- Pneumonia is the most common pulmonary cause of death in infants under 48 hours of age.
- The causative organism of pneumonia frequently depends on the season and the age of the patient.
- *Escherichia coli, Klebsiella, Staphylococcus,* and group A streptococcus pneumonias typically occur in children from birth to age 3.
- Ruptured amniotic membranes in newborns can make them prone to pneumonia in the first few days of life.
- Chlamydial pneumonia is most often seen in newborns up to 12 weeks of age.
- Streptococcal and *Haemophilus influenzae* pneumonias occur in children age 3 months to 5 years of age.
- Respiratory syncytial virus and other viruses are common causes of pneumonia in children 2 months to 5 years of age during the winter and spring.
- *Haemophilus parainfluenzae* virus causes pneumonia in children age 5 to 12 years old, especially in the fall.
- *Mycoplasma pneumoniae* affects children 5 to 12 years of age in the fall and winter.
- *Pneumocystis carinii* pneumonia is seen almost exclusively with HIV syndrome.
- In all types of pneumonia, the airway is inflamed, and exudate accumulates in the alveoli.
- Pneumonia is frequently classified by the portion of the lung affected: lobar, disseminated lobular, and interstitial.
- Viral pneumonias can be treated at home, with symptomatic relief provided by antipyretics, fluids, cool-mist vaporizer, and rest.
- Bacterial pneumonia may require inpatient treatment depending on the degree of respiratory distress or hypoxia in the child.

- Hospital treatment for bacterial pneumonia is with antipyretics, intravenous antibiotics, intravenous fluids, chest physiotherapy, oxygen, and rest.
- Home management of bacterial pneumonia is with antipyretics, fluid, cool-mist vaporizer, rest, and oral antibiotics.
- Mycoplasmal pneumonia is treated with antibiotics and symptomatic relief measures and can usually be managed at home.

### ASSESSMENT FINDINGS

#### Pneumococcal pneumonia
- Sudden onset of symptoms
- High fever
- Nasal flaring
- Chest retractions
- Chest pain
- Chills
- Dyspnea
- Febrile *seizures*
- Tachypnea, tachycardia
- Bronchial breath sounds

#### Chlamydial pneumonia
- Gradual onset
- Nasal congestion
- Sharp cough
- Failure to gain weight
- Tachypnea, wheezing, rales
- Elevated IgG and IgM antibodies
- Antibodies to *Chlamydia trachomatis*

#### Viral pneumonia
- Low-grade fever
- Nonproductive cough
- Malaise
- Tachypnea
- Diminished breath sounds
- Fine rales
- Apnea (with respiratory syncytial virus)

#### Mycoplasmal pneumonia
- Insidious or sudden onset
- Fever
- Chills
- Headache
- Cervical lymph node enlargement

- Persistent rhinitis
- Malaise
- Upper airway congestion
- Sore throat
- Nonproductive cough
- Fine crackles

### Lipid pneumonia
- Coughing spell at time of aspiration
- Chronic cough
- Dyspnea
- General respiratory distress

### Hydrocarbon pneumonia
- Gastrointestinal symptoms, such as nausea and *vomiting*
- Drowsiness
- Increasing dyspnea

### NURSING IMPLICATIONS
- Assess level of respiratory distress with the child, and evaluate the need for home or hospital management.
- Obtain a thorough history and physical examination to help identify the type and severity of the pneumonia.
- Educate parents on home management, including antibiotic education and administration instructions for bacterial or mycoplasmal pneumonia.
- Ensure that the child is adequately hydrated and teach the parents to administer 8 to 10 glasses of clear fluids daily.
- Educate the parents on signs of increasing respiratory distress, and direct them that the child will need hospital admission for further intensive care.
- Support the parents and help them to understand that antibiotics are not effective with viral pneumonias.
- Answer all procedural questions for the family and support them through the hospitalization.
- Direct the parents to visit or stay with the child, if possible, to help allay the child's fears.
- Institute primary nursing for the child to decrease the number of strangers caring for the child.
- Explain all procedures to the child in terms that are developmentally appropriate.
- Encourage oral intake, and maintain a patent intravenous line if hospitalized.
- Promote airway clearance and gas exchange.
- Perform chest physiotherapy as prescribed.

- Reposition the child every 2 hours to prevent *atelectasis* and encourage lung expansion.
- Administer supplemental oxygen as required.
- Administer intravenous fluid to maintain hydration and thin pulmonary secretions.
- Decrease the child's work of breathing with comfortable positioning and encouraging rest periods.
- Administer antipyretics for fever above 101.3°F.
- Inform parents of children with lipid pneumonia that surgical resection of a lung portion may be done to remove a lobe or segment if the pneumonitis does not heal by itself.
- Do not induce *vomiting* in children with hydrocarbon pneumonia because aspiration of the poison can occur.
- Instruct parents to administer olive oil or mineral oil to delay gastric absorption of the hydrocarbon; once at the hospital, perform stomach lavage.
- Observe the child for signs of increasing drowsiness or central nervous system involvement.
- Administer cool, moist air with supplemental oxygen to decrease lung inflammation.
- Support the parents and let them know that you realize they did not mean for this to happen.
- Advise the parents after the illness to store poisons in a safe place.

## PNEUMOTHORAX

### DESCRIPTION

- A pneumothorax, a serious respiratory problem, refers to the presence of air in the pleural space.
- The presence of air causes the alveoli of the lungs to collapse.
- The extent of symptoms and the outcome depend on the cause of the entry of air and the initiation of prompt treatment.
- Pneumothorax in children usually occurs when air seeps from ruptured alveoli and collects in the pleural cavity.
- Pneumothorax can also occur when puncture wounds allow air to enter the chest from the outside.
- Pneumothorax occurs in 1% of newborns, occurring secondary to the extreme intrathoracic pressure needed to initiate the first inspiration.
- Children require oxygen therapy if respiratory distress is present.

### Assessment Findings
- Tachypnea
- Grunting with respirations
- Flaring of the nares
- Cyanosis
- Absent or decreased breath sounds
- Shift of the apical pulse away from the site of pneumothorax
- *Atelectasis*
- Darkened area of the air-filled pleural space

### Nursing Implications
- Carefully evaluate all newborns for respiratory distress and assess for pneumothorax.
- Initiate prompt treatment for pneumothorax.
- Assist with insertion of a needle or chest tube for thoracotomy.
- Set up the low pressure suction and water seal and ensure adequate functioning.
- Tape all chest tube connections to avoid complications.
- Keep in mind that pneumothorax symptoms are relieved within 24 hours after suction has begun.
- If the air in the pleural space is secondary to a puncture wound, cover the chest wound immediately with impervious material, to prevent further entering of atmospheric air into the space.
- Use petroleum gauze or a gloved finger to cover a puncture wound until the thoracotomy can be performed.
- Continue to monitor respiratory status and administer supplemental oxygen.
- Support the child and parents and explain all procedures to them.
- Alleviate anxiety in the child, and medicate with anxiolytics and analgesics if necessary.
- Ensure that the parents understand the nature of the pneumothorax, and update them on the child's respiratory status and improvement frequently.

## POISONING, HYDROCARBON

### Description
- Hydrocarbons are substances contained in products such as kerosene and furniture polish.

- Fumes rise from these products because they are volatile and therefore cause respiratory irritation.
- These products are a common cause of childhood poisonings and can result in hydrocarbon *pneumonia.*

## ASSESSMENT FINDINGS
- History of ingesting poison
- Nausea
- Drowsiness
- Increased respirations
- Dyspnea
- Increased percussion sound (from presence of air trapped in alveoli from inflammation)
- Rales, diminished breath sounds
- Cyanosis

## NURSING IMPLICATIONS
- Perform a thorough history and physical assessment to establish a baseline.
- Obtain vital signs and blood samples for laboratory analysis.
- Ask the parents or caregiver if they know what type of poison that they suspect the child took.
- Ask the parents to describe the type of bottle the poison was in if they do not know the name of the product.
- Ask the parents to bring any vomited material with them to the hospital for analysis.
- Be aware that hydrocarbon aspiration may occur when children initially swallow the fluid; do not induce vomiting because they may aspirate at the time of vomiting.
- Assist with gastric lavage to empty the stomach of the poison.
- Instruct the parents to administer an oily substance, such as olive oil or mineral oil, to delay gastric absorption.
- Teach the parents about poison prevention and treatment.
- Advise the parents to keep syrup of ipecac in the house for possible poisoning.
- Teach the parents to call the emergency number in their community used by the poison control center.
- Tell the parents to have ready the child's name, telephone number, address, weight, and age.

- Advise the parents that they should be prepared to tell the poison control center when the poisoning occurred, what was the route of the poisoning (oral, inhaled, sprayed on the skin), and how much of the poison the child took.
- Teach the parents how to poison-proof their house.
- Provide opportunities for *play therapy* to help alleviate the child's guilt and anger over handling substances that they should not have been.

## POISONING, INSECTICIDE

### DESCRIPTION

- Children can be poisoned by insecticides by accidental ingestion or through skin or respiratory tract when playing in an area that has recently been sprayed with one.
- Long-term exposure may result from exposure to a parent's clothing if he or she comes home covered with insecticide spray.
- Many insecticides have an organophosphate base that leads to an accumulation of acetylcholine at neuro-muscular junctions.

### ASSESSMENT FINDINGS

- History of ingestion or exposure to an insecticide
- Nausea and *vomiting*
- *Diarrhea*
- Excessive salivation
- Weakness of respiratory muscles
- Confusion
- Depressed reflexes
- *Seizures*

### NURSING IMPLICATIONS

- Perform a thorough history and physical assessment to establish a baseline.
- Obtain vital signs and blood samples for laboratory analysis.
- Ask the parents or caregiver if they know what type of poison that they suspect the child took or was exposed to.
- Ask the parents to describe the type of container the poison was in if they do not know the name of the product.

- Ask the parents if either of them work with insecticides or have recently had the lawn sprayed.
- Ask the parents to bring any vomited material with them to the hospital for analysis.
- Assist with gastric lavage to empty the stomach of the poison.
- Administer activated charcoal, as prescribed either through lavage tube or orally.
- Wear gloves to protect your skin and remove any contaminated clothing from the child, and then bathe the child and wash his or her hair to remove any insecticide left on the skin and hair.
- Administer intravenous atropine or Pralidoxime, as prescribed, as an antidote to reverse symptoms.
- Warn the parents that the child will have black stool for several days if he or she receives activated charcoal.
- Know that activated charcoal should never be administrated before syrup of ipecac because it inactivates the ipecac.
- Teach the parents about poison prevention and treatment.
- Advise the parents to keep syrup of ipecac in the house for possible poisoning.
- Teach the parents to call the emergency number in their community used by the poison control center.
- Tell the parents to have ready the child's name, telephone number, address, weight, and age.
- Advise the parents that they should be prepared to tell the poison control center when the poisoning occurred, what was the route of the poisoning (oral, inhaled, sprayed on the skin), and how much of the poison the child took.
- Teach the parents how to poison-proof their house.

# POISONING, IRON

## DESCRIPTION
- Iron is frequently swallowed by small children because it is an ingredient in vitamin preparations, particularly prenatal vitamins.
- Iron poisoning occurs frequently because parents do not think of iron pills as real medicine.
- Initially the child may have symptoms, but they disappear and after 6 hours the child may appear fine, but

hemorrhagic necrosis of the lining of the gastrointestinal tract has occurred.

**ASSESSMENT FINDINGS** (symptoms may disappear after 6 hours)

- Nausea
- *Vomiting*
- *Diarrhea*
- Abdominal pain

*Then after 12 hours*

- Melena (blood in stool)
- Hematemesis (blood in emesis)
- Lethargy
- *Coma*
- Cyanosis
- Vasomotor collapse
- Coagulation defects
- Shock
- Serum iron levels greater than 500 μg/ml (significant); 20 to 30 mg/kg (toxic); 60 to 80 mg/kg (potentially lethal).

**NURSING IMPLICATIONS**

- Perform a thorough history and physical assessment to establish a baseline.
- Obtain vital signs and blood samples for serum iron and iron binding concentration.
- Know that the initial symptoms of iron poisoning may fade after 6 hours and the child may appear fine; after 12 hours, the symptoms return as lethargy and coma.
- Administer syrup of ipecac as prescribed to remove any iron not yet absorbed by the stomach.
- Administer a gastric lavage as prescribed with bicarbonate solution to convert the remaining ferrous iron to a less absorbable carbonate compound.
- Administer a cathartic as prescribed to help the child pass enteric-coated iron pills.
- Know that activated charcoal has no effect on iron poisoning.
- Administer a chelating agent, such as intravenous or intramuscular feroxamine, as prescribed to allow the metal to be excreted by the body.
- Advise the parents that feroxamine turns the child's urine orange as the iron is excreted.

- Assist with an exchange transfusion, if necessary.
- Arrange for liver studies and upper gastrointestinal series 1 week after ingestion.
- Test the child's stool for occult blood for the next 3 days to assess for stomach irritation.
- Teach the parents about poison prevention and treatment.
- Advise the parents to keep syrup of ipecac in the house for possible poisoning.
- Teach the parents to call the emergency number in their community used by the poison control center.
- Tell the parents to have ready the child's name, telephone number, address, weight, and age.
- Advise the parents that they should be prepared to tell the poison control center when the poisoning occurred, what was the route of the poisoning (oral, inhaled, sprayed on the skin), and how much of the poison the child took.
- Stress to the mother taking supplemental iron that overdoses in small children can be fatal.

# POISONING, LEAD

## DESCRIPTION

- Lead poisoning most often occurs with the ingestion of paint chips or paint dust.
- In the body, lead interferes with red blood cell function by blocking the incorporation of iron into the protoporphyrin compound that makes up the heme portion of hemoglobin in red blood cells, resulting in hypochromic, microcytic *anemia.*
- Kidney destruction may occur, causing excess excretion of amino acids, glucose, and phosphate in the urine.
- The ultimate result is lead *encephalitis* or inflammation of brain cells from the toxic lead content.
- Lead poisoning occurs most frequently in the summer and is largely a preventable disease.

## ASSESSMENT FINDINGS

- Lethargy
- Impulsiveness
- Learning difficulties
- *Seizures*
- *Mental retardation*

- Basophilic stippling on blood smear
- Lead lines near the epiphyseal line of long bones on x-ray film
- Proteinuria
- Ketonuria
- Glycosuria
- Cerebrospinal fluid positive for increased protein level (possible)
- Blood lead level (2 on successive occasions) greater than 10 µg/dl

### NURSING IMPLICATIONS

- Perform a thorough history and physical assessment to establish a baseline.
- Obtain vital signs and blood samples for laboratory analysis.
- Ask the parents if they have recently started to remodel an old house in which the air might be saturated with lead paint dust.
- Ask the parents if the child has possibly been teething on an old crib or a window sill.
- Cleanse the child's finger thoroughly before obtaining a finger stick for free erythrocyte protoporphyrin because there may be enough lead in the dust on a child's finger to contaminate the sample.
- Know that the child with a blood lead level between 10 and 14 µg/dl needs to be rescreened to confirm the level.
- Advise the parents that simply wallpapering or repainting does not remove a source of peeling paint adequately; paneling or masonite must be applied, or plastic-covered contact paper may be used temporarily.
- Administer chelating agents such as dimercaprol (BAL) or edetate calcium disodium (CaEDTA), as prescribed to remove lead from the soft tissue and bone (although not from red blood cells).
- Combine procaine with chelating agents (pull them into the syringe last so they enter the child first) to make them less painful.
- Measure serum calcium to determine calcium loss from the use of chelating agents.
- Measure intake and output to ensure adequate kidney function.

- Obtain specimens for blood urea nitrogen, serum creatinine, and protein in urine, as prescribed.
- Advise the parents who live in homes built before 1940 that their children should be screened yearly for possible lead poisoning.
- Teach the parents about lead poisoning, the sources, and how to make the home and their children safe from lead poisoning.

## POISONING, PLANT

### DESCRIPTION

- Plant poisoning (ingestion of a growing plant) occurs because parents do not think of plants as being poisonous.
- Common plants to which children may be exposed are holly (berries), English ivy, hydrangea, lily of the valley, mistletoe, morning glory (seeds), philodendron, poinsettia, rhubarb (leaves), and rhododendron.

### ASSESSMENT FINDINGS (depend on the plant ingested but may include the following)

- Nausea
- *Vomiting*
- *Diarrhea*
- Abdominal pain
- Muscle weakness
- *Seizures*
- Dyspnea
- Hallucinations
- Swelling of the tongue and lips
- Irritation of the gastrointestinal tract
- Limb paralysis

### NURSING IMPLICATIONS

- Perform a thorough history and physical assessment to establish a baseline.
- Obtain vital signs and blood samples for laboratory analysis.
- Ask the parents or caregiver if they know what type of plant or berries that they suspect the child ate.
- Ask the parents to describe the plant or berries if they do not know the name of the plant.
- Ask the parents to bring any vomited material with them to the hospital for analysis.

- Teach the parents about poison prevention and treatment.
- Advise the parents to keep syrup of ipecac in the house for possible poisoning.
- Teach the parents to call the emergency number in their community used by the poison control center.
- Tell the parents to have ready the child's name, telephone number, address, weight, and age.
- Advise the parents that they should be prepared to tell the poison control center when the poisoning occurred, what was the route of the poisoning (oral, inhaled, sprayed on the skin), and how much of the poison the child took.
- Teach the parents how to poison-proof their house and to avoid potentially poisonous plants.
- Teach the child not to eat attractive berries on a bush unless a parent or trusted adult has deemed them acceptable for eating.

## POISONING, RECREATIONAL DRUG

### DESCRIPTION
- Adolescents (and more frequently grade-school children) are brought to health care facilities by parents or friends because of a drug overdose or a "bad trip" caused by an unusual reaction of the effect of an unfortunate combination of drugs.

### ASSESSMENT FINDINGS
- Disorientation
- Hallucinations

### NURSING IMPLICATIONS
- Perform a thorough physical assessment and history even though it may be difficult to obtain from the child.
- Obtain vital signs and note any changes.
- Obtain blood samples for electrolytes and a toxicology scan.
- Know that it may be difficult to determine what the child took because he or she may only be able to describe the color of the pill as a "red one" or a "yellow one."

- Know that the child may also be reluctant to tell you what kind of pill he or she took especially if the child knows the drug was illegal.
- Ask the friends of the child if they know if someone might have slipped their friend "a mickey" or put something in his drink.
- Explain to the child's friends that you are not a law enforcer but that you need to ask these questions only to try and help their friend.
- Ask the parents or friends to have someone at home check the child's room for any possible drugs that he or she may have taken.
- Try to determine if the ingestion was an accident (a child is unaware that two drugs would react this way or took a wrong dose) or whether the child was actually attempting *suicide.*
- Know that all drug ingestions in children over 7 years of age should be considered potential *suicides* until established otherwise.
- Administer oxygen, as prescribed.
- Provide intravenous fluid administration, as prescribed to replace electrolytes or to dilute the drug.
- Provide emotional support to the parents and offer to arrange for counseling for the child and the parents.

## POISONING, SALICYLATE

### DESCRIPTION
- About 25% of childhood poisonings are salicylate (aspirin) poisonings.
- This percentage is decreasing, however, because of safety packaging and less use of aspirin for childhood fever (to prevent *Reye's syndrome*).

### ASSESSMENT FINDINGS
- History of ingesting a poison
- Tachycardia
- Tachypnea
- Hypoglycemia
- Fever
- *Vomiting*
- *Diarrhea*
- Restlessness

- Stupor
- *Seizures*
- *Coma*
- Areas of purpura
- Tinnitus (ringing of the ears—specific toxic effect of salicylate overdose)

### Nursing Implications

- Perform a thorough history and physical assessment to establish a baseline.
- Obtain vital signs and blood samples for laboratory analysis.
- Test a urine specimen with a diagnostic strip such as Phenistix and evaluate the results to determine salicylate poisoning.
- Ask the parents or caregiver if they know what type of poison the child took.
- Ask the parents to describe the type of bottle the poison was in if they do not know the name of the product.
- Ask the parents to bring any vomited material with them to the hospital for analysis.
- Assist with gastric lavage to empty poison from the stomach.
- Administer activated charcoal, as prescribed either through lavage tube or orally.
- Warn the parents that the child will have black stools for several days if he or she receives activated charcoal.
- Know that activated charcoal should never be administrated before syrup of ipecac because it will inactivate the ipecac.
- Never administer activated charcoal if acetylcholine (mucomyst, the specific antidote for acetaminophen poisoning) is used because the charcoal inactivates it.
- Teach the parents about poison prevention and treatment.
- Advise the parents to keep syrup of ipecac in the house for possible poisoning.
- Teach the parents to call the emergency number in their community used by the poison control center.
- Tell the parents to have ready the child's name, telephone number, address, weight, and age.
- Advise the parents that they should be prepared to tell the poison control center when the poisoning oc-

curred, what was the route of the poisoning (oral, inhaled, sprayed on the skin), and how much of the poison the child took.
- Teach the parents how to poison-proof their home.

# POLIOMYELITIS (INFANTILE PARALYSIS)

## DESCRIPTION
- Poliomyelitis is an infectious disease caused by the poliovirus, which is transmitted by direct and indirect contact; contracting the disease causes active immunity against one strain of the virus causing the illness.
- Poliovirus may be caused by any of the three strains of poliovirus, which is why children must be immunized with trivalent (three-strain) vaccine.
- Paralysis is generally asymmetric, and children's legs seem to be more susceptible than the arms.
- Respiratory paralysis can occur when there is damage to the cells of the cervical and thoracic segments of the spinal cord.

## ASSESSMENT FINDINGS
- Fever
- Headache
- Nausea
- *Vomiting*
- Abdominal pain
- Slight erythema of throat
- Pain and stiffness of the neck, back, and legs
- Cerebrospinal fluid positive for increased protein and lymphocytes
- Intense pain and tremors of extremities
- Paralysis
- Positive Kernig's sign
- Deep tendon reflexes hyperactive then diminishing

## NURSING IMPLICATIONS
- Instruct parents about the need for routine *immunizations* at health maintenance visits.
- Perform a thorough history and physical assessment to establish a baseline.
- Observe the child for Kernig's sign, which is indicated when the child assumes a tripod position when sitting because they are unable to sit without placing both their arms and hands behind them to brace themselves.

- Assess for the presence or absence of deep tendon reflexes.
- Assist with spinal fluid analysis and send the specimen to the laboratory for analysis.
- Provide emotional support and encouragement to the parents.
- Help the parents to understand the importance of complete bed rest for their child.
- Teach the parents about moist, hot packs to help with the pain.
- Teach the parents how to perform passive movements and muscle therapy as soon as the pain and spasm are gone.
- Help the parents and the child deal with the use of braces to strengthen atrophied muscles.

## POLYCYSTIC KIDNEY

### DESCRIPTION

- Polycystic kidney refers to a condition in which large, fluid-filled cysts have formed in place of normal kidney tissue.
- The most frequent type of polycystic disease seen in children is inherited as an autosomal recessive trait resulting in abnormal development of the collecting tubules.
- The treatment for polycystic formation is the surgical removal of a kidney if only one kidney is cystic; if both are involved, a renal transplant is a consideration but difficult because few infant kidneys are available.

### ASSESSMENT FINDINGS

- Kidneys large, soft, and spongy on palpation
- No passage of urine if condition is bilateral
- Decreased urination if unilateral
- Maternal oligohydramnios
- *Hypertelorism* (wide-spaced eyes), epicanthal folds, flattened nose, micrognathia (small jaw)—a Potter facies
- Cysts evident on ultrasonography or transillumination

### NURSING IMPLICATIONS

- Perform a thorough history and physical assessment to establish a baseline.

- Observe the newborn for voiding, which should occur within the first 24 hours of birth, to help establish a diagnosis and prognosis.
- Obtain a maternal labor and pregnancy history and assess for oligohydramnios.
- Make the parents aware of the availability of genetic counseling to inform them fully that future children also may have this problem.
- Prepare the child and parents for surgery; include information about all aspects of preoperative and postoperative care.

## POLYCYTHEMIA

### DESCRIPTION

- Polycythemia refers to an increase in the number of red blood cells that results as a compensatory response to insufficient oxygenation of the blood.
- With this disorder, erythropoiesis is increased to attempt to supply enough red blood cells to supply oxygen to cells.
- Chronic pulmonary disease and cyanotic *congenital heart disease* are the usual causes of polycythemia in childhood.
- It also may occur from twin transfusion at birth (one twin receives excess blood and the second is anemic).

### ASSESSMENT FINDINGS

- Plethora (marked reddening of the skin)
- Elevated mean corpuscular hemoglobin
- Normal mean corpuscular hemoglobin concentration
- Red blood cells elevated as high as 7.0 million/mm$^3$
- Increased hemoglobin as high as 23 g/100 ml

### NURSING IMPLICATIONS

- Perform a thorough history and physical assessment to establish a baseline.
- Assess the history for any chronic pulmonary disorders or a cyanotic *congenital heart disease.*
- Obtain blood samples as prescribed and send to the laboratory.
- Know that the child with polycythemia is particularly in danger of a cerebrovascular accident or of an embo-

lus developing if he or she becomes dehydrated, as occurs with fever or during surgery.
- Assist with exchange transfusion, as prescribed to reduce the red blood cell count.

# POSTURAL DRAINAGE

## DESCRIPTION

- Postural drainage refers to the simple changing of the child's position to help mucus to move, to initiate the cough reflex, and to help expel mucus.
- Postural drainage is performed on children with obstructive respiratory disease, when mucus blocks the airways preventing proper oxygen exchange and contributing to the development of bronchial infections.
- When the child is positioned so that the chest is lower than the abdomen, gravity aids the removal of mucus from the lower lobes and bronchi.
- When the child sits upright, gravity aids drainage from the upper lobes and bronchi.
- When lying supine, anterior bronchi drain; when prone, posterior bronchi drain.
- Frequent changing of position is important, therefore, to prevent pools of mucus from forming in a certain lung area.
- In addition to postural drainage, cupping (percussion against the chest using a cupped or curved palm) and vibration (pressing a vibrating hand against the child's chest during exhalation) helps mechanically to loosen and move tenacious secretions.

## NURSING IMPLICATIONS

- Assist the child in lying predominantly in one position to encourage drainage of that lung segment for a localized mucus problem.
- Perform postural drainage before meals or at least an hour after a meal because the coughing this initiates may cause *vomiting* if the stomach is full.
- Position an infant on your lap to perform postural drainage.
- Perform postural drainage on an older child using a slant board, if available, or position the bed so that the lobe of the lung to be drained is in a superior position.

- Perform clapping and vibrating following each position of postural draining and then encourage the child to cough and remove the loosened secretions.
- Teach the child to cough by telling him or her to take in a deep breath and blow out, to take in another deep breath and blow out, and to take in a third breath and then cough because the irritation of the mucus in the major airway by the third breath makes a cough happen almost spontaneously.
- Teach at least one parent how to perform postural drainage with cupping and vibrating before the child is discharged.

# PRECOCIOUS PUBERTY

### DESCRIPTION

- Precocious puberty or sexual development is the development of breasts or pubic hair before age 8 years or menses before age 9 years.
- Often, such development is expressed as isolated breast or pubic hair growth but can proceed to complete spermatogenesis and menstrual function.
- It occurs more often in girls than in boys and is caused by the early production of gonadotropins by the pituitary gland: Gonadotropins stimulate the ovaries or testes to produce sex hormones.
- This stimulation of gonadotropin can occur because of a pituitary tumor, cyst, or traumatic injury to the third ventricle next to the pituitary gland.
- It can also occur because of estrogen-secreting cysts or tumors of the ovary or testosterone-secreting cysts of the testes.
- In rare instances, it occurs because of an estrogen-secreting or testosterone-secreting adrenal tumor or, in girls, ingestion of oral contraceptives.

### ASSESSMENT FINDINGS

- Increased breast development
- Accelerated skeletal maturation
- Vaginal bleeding
- Little pubic or axillary hair
- Increased androgen or estrogen serum to adult levels

### Nursing Implications

- Perform a thorough history and physical assessment to establish a baseline.
- Assess for recent traumatic injury or ingestion of medication, such as oral contraceptives.
- Assist with preparation for diagnostic tests to rule out a hormone-secreting tumor.
- Administer a synthetic analog to luteinizing hormone–releasing hormone, as prescribed, subcutaneously daily.
- Offer support and encouragement to the parents as they worry that their child is different and may become sexually active and possibly pregnant.
- Reassure the parents that once the child reaches normal puberty age, he or she will again be the same as other children.
- Assure the parents that although their child's sexual maturity started early, their genitals will not be out of proportion to the rest of their body.
- Explain to the parents that their child is fully fertile and able to conceive when early puberty occurs.
- Know that oral contraceptives are not recommended for girls this young because the increased load of estrogen hastens the closing of the epiphyseal lines of the long bones too early and stunts their growth prematurely.
- Parents may need to be reminded that, although their child seems older, the changes are only in their sexual characteristics and, therefore, household tasks, responsibilities, and expectations must be geared to their chronologic age, not to outward appearance.

## PRUNE BELLY SYNDROME

### Description

- Prune belly syndrome is severe urethral obstruction in utero from abnormal urethral valves.
- Occurring mostly in males, it causes severe back pressure and destruction of the kidneys.
- There is massive dilation of the ureters and possibly *patent urachus.*
- Accompanying disorders, such as undescended testicles, cardiac abnormalities, malrotation of the bowel, and abnormal limbs, are common.

- Without therapy, the prognosis is poor because of end-stage renal disease; however, with surgery to correct the obstruction in the ureters, the prognosis is good.

### ASSESSMENT FINDINGS
- Abdomen wrinkled like a prune
- Oligohydramnios
- Pulmonary dysplasia
- Presence of accompanying common abnormalities, such as malrotation of the bowel, cardiac abnormalities, undescended testicles, and abnormal limbs

### NURSING IMPLICATIONS
- Perform a thorough history and physical assessment to establish a baseline.
- Observe the maternal labor and pregnancy history and assess for oligohydramnios.
- Advise the parents to protect the abdomen of the child from trauma that could be caused by lap belts or baby walkers because their child lacks abdominal support.
- Offer emotional support and encouragement to the parents.
- Prepare the parents and child for surgery to repair the obstructed ureters.

## PTOSIS

### DESCRIPTION
- Ptosis is the inability to raise the upper eyelid normally so that it always remains slightly closed.
- The condition may be congenital or acquired.
- The congenital type is frequently inherited and tends to be bilateral.
- Acquired ptosis is generally unilateral, and it may have a neurogenic origin (injury to the 3rd cranial nerve) or be caused by injury to the lid or levator muscle.
- When the cause is neurogenic, there is generally paralysis of one or more of the other muscles supplied by the 3rd cranial nerve.
- *Myasthenia gravis,* which produces generalized muscle weakness, must always be ruled out as the cause of bilateral ptosis.

### ASSESSMENT FINDINGS
- Inability to keep the upper eyelid open
- Dilated pupil
- Inability to rotate the eye globe upward, medially, or downward
- Weakness of accommodation
- Wrinkling of forehead (on attempt to raise the eyelid)
- Head cocking backward (on attempt to see under the eyelid)

### NURSING IMPLICATIONS
- Perform a thorough history and physical assessment to establish a baseline.
- Help the parents to understand the necessity of early surgery to prevent the development of *amblyopia.*
- Prepare the parents and the child for surgery.
- Teach the parents how to perform eye care after surgery.
- Provide support and understanding to the parents and the child.

## PULMONARY STENOSIS

### DESCRIPTION
- Pulmonic stenosis is a narrowing of the pulmonary valve or the pulmonary artery just distal to the valve.
- Pulmonary stenosis accounts for 25% to 35% of congenital heart anomalies.
- The inability of the right ventricle to evacuate blood easily by way of the pulmonary artery may lead to right ventricular hypertrophy.
- If the stenosis is severe, the increased pressure in the right side of the heart may reopen the foramen ovale, and blood flowing from the right to left chambers of the heart may produce mild cyanosis.
- Management depends on the severity of the stenosis and the child's age.

### ASSESSMENT FINDINGS
- Systolic ejection murmur, grade IV or V crescendo-decrescendo, heard lowest in the upper left sternal border possibly radiating to the suprasternal notch
- Thrill in upper left sternal area or at suprasternal notch

- Widely split second heart sound (possible)
- Right ventricular hypertrophy on ECG

### Nursing Implications

- Perform a thorough history and physical assessment to establish a baseline.
- Obtain vital signs, paying close attention to heart sounds.
- Provide oxygen, as prescribed.
- Assist with ECG, as prescribed.
- Provide emotional support to the parents to alleviate anxieties and fears.
- Prepare the parents and the child for surgery, if necessary.
- Teach the parents to watch for signs of increased cyanosis or difficulty in breathing and to report these signs to the physician.

## PYLORIC STENOSIS

### Description

- Pyloric stenosis is a condition involving difficulty emptying the stomach occurring with hypertrophy or hyperplasia of the muscle surrounding the pylorus (the valve between the stomach and the beginning portion of the intestine).
- This condition tends to occur most frequently in first-born white male infants.
- The cause is unknown, but multifactorial inheritance is likely.
- It occurs less frequently in breast-fed infants, but breast-fed infants demonstrate symptoms later than bottle-fed infants because the breast milk curd is smaller and it passes through a hypertrophied muscle more easily.
- Surgical procedure for pyloric stenosis is pyloromyotomy (a Fredet-Ramstedt operation), in which the muscle of the pyloris is split, allowing for a larger lumen.

### Assessment Findings

- *Vomiting* almost immediately after each feeding (at 4 weeks of age), extremely forceful until projectile, sour smelling, and without bile
- Infant usually hungry after *vomiting*

- Signs of *dehydration,* such as lack of tears, dry mucous membranes of the mouth, sunken fontanelles, fever, decreased urine output, poor skin turgor, loss of weight
- Alkalosis, hypokalemia, and hypochloremia
- Hypopnea
- Tetany

## NURSING IMPLICATIONS
- Perform a thorough history and physical assessment to establish a baseline.
- Ask the parents to describe the vomitus: how much, how frequent, is it projectile, sour smelling, does it contain bile.
- Palpate the child's right upper quadrant of the abdomen for a pyloric mass before the child drinks; as the child drinks, observe the peristaltic waves pass from right to left across the abdomen as the mass becomes more prominent resulting in projectile vomiting.
- Obtain a baseline weight to determine the extent of dehydration.
- Explain to the parents that the child cannot go to surgery until electrolyte imbalance is improved.
- Prepare the child for a surgical procedure to remove the stenosis.
- Administer intravenous fluid, as prescribed to correct the electrolyte imbalance before surgery.
- Administer calcium with the intravenous solution, as prescribed if tetany is present.
- Know that potassium should not be administered before it is established that the child's kidneys are functioning.
- Provide the child with small, frequent feedings after surgery, as prescribed not to overwhelm the newly operated-on pyloris.
- Obtain daily weights after surgery to confirm adequate intake.
- Encourage the parents to room in during the child's hospitalization, if possible, so that they can grow comfortable with caring for their child.
- Allow the parents to verbalize their feelings and provide emotional support.

# RABIES

## DESCRIPTION

- Rabies is an infectious disorder resulting in central nervous system disease caused by the rabies virus.
- It has an incubation period of 2 to 6 weeks, possibly as long as 12 months with a period of communicability of 3 to 5 days before the onset of symptoms through the course of the disease.
- Rabies is transmitted through the bite of rabid animals and rarely through saliva from infected animals being transferred to open lesions on the child's skin.
- Contracting the disease apparently offers active immunity; active artificial immunity is acquired through human diploid cell rabies vaccine; passive artificial immunity is acquired through human rabies immune globulin.
- Wild animals, such as skunks, squirrels, and bats, constitute the most important sources of infection from rabies in the United States. Children receive more bites, however, and, therefore, more treatments for rabies from bites of dogs or cats.
- When a child is bitten by an infected animal, the virus migrates from the bite area to the central nervous system; cranial nerve and spinal cord nuclei become acutely damaged.
- Once the disease process begins, rabies is invariably fatal; hope lies in preventing the active process.

## ASSESSMENT FINDINGS

- History of an animal bite
- Malaise
- Fever progressing to high fever
- Anorexia
- Nausea
- Sore throat
- Drowsiness progressing to *coma*
- Irritability and restlessness progressing to hyperexcitability
- Slight leukocytosis
- Slight numbness or hyperesthesia at area of bite and along the course of involved nerves
- Involuntary twitching movements
- Generalized *seizures*

- Violent contractions of the mouth muscles
- Total body paralysis
- Peripheral vascular collapse and death (quickly in only 5 or 6 days)
- Positive Negri bodies in brain cells (on post-mortem examination)

### Nursing Implications

- Instruct the parents to bring the child who has been bitten to see the physician to evaluate the circumstances and decide whether rabies prevention measures are necessary.
- Obtain a thorough history and physical examination to establish a baseline and identify the type of animal bite; question the child about the animal's behavior because a rabid animal usually does not act normally.
- Reassure the child that he or she is not going to be punished if he or she was provoking an animal.
- Locate the animal and confine it for 5 to 10 days to determine whether the animal shows signs of rabies; if it does, the animal is destroyed and the brain examined for evidence of rabies.
- Check the immunization status of the animal; an animal that has been properly immunized against rabies rarely transmits the virus.
- Inspect the wound carefully to see whether it was caused by teeth marks or scratch marks because a bite mark is much more serious than a scratch mark.
- Wash the wound well with soap and water and an antiseptic; be aware that a puncture wound is not sutured closed.
- If the animal is found to be rabid, prepare to administer rabies vaccine and antirabies serum as prescribed.
- Provide emotional support and guidance to the child and parents; explain all procedures and treatments, including the possibility of active *immunization*.

## RADIAL HEAD DISLOCATION

### Description

- Radial head dislocation is a musculoskeletal disorder in which the head of the radius escapes the ligament surrounding it, becoming dislocated.
- It commonly occurs when a small child is lifted by one hand, as happens when a parent pulls on one arm to lift the child over a curb or up a step.

### Assessment Findings
- Holding arm flexed at elbow
- Pronated forearm
- Pain on palpation of radial head

### Nursing Implications

- Obtain a thorough history and physical examination to establish a baseline and identify the cause of the injury.
- Assist the physician with reducing a simple dislocation using gentle pressure on the radial head while the arm is flexed and supinated.
- Following the simple reduction, assess the child for immediate relief of pain and ability to use the arm.
- Allow the parents to verbalize their feelings of guilt over having caused the injury.
- Assure the parents that this is a common injury in small children.
- Be aware that this injury can occur from extremely rough handling as seen in child *abuse;* investigate the situation thoroughly and carefully.

## RADIATION THERAPY

### Description
- Radiation therapy refers to a method of treatment used for a child with a malignancy.
- Radiation therapy acts to change the DNA component of a cell nucleus to a point at which the cell cannot replicate DNA material and so cannot divide and grow further.
- Radiation is not effective on cells that have a low oxygen content (a proportion of cells in every tumor mass); it is effective at the time of cell division (mitosis).
- Therefore, radiation therapy schedules are designed to take place over 1 to 6 weeks so that cells that are not in a susceptible stage on one day are in a susceptible stage on another.
- Radiation therapy has both systemic and local effects; radiation sickness (anorexia, nausea, and *vomiting*) is the most frequently encountered systemic effect occurring if the gastrointestinal tract was irradiated and from the release of toxic substances from destroyed tumor cells; extreme fatigue is also common.

- Radiation therapy also has long-term effects, which are becoming more apparent as increasing numbers of child who have had intense radiation survive.
- Because radiation damages all cells in its path, any body tissue can be affected.
- Long-term effects may include asymmetric bone growth, easy fracturing, *scoliosis,* kyphosis; thyroid, hypothalamic, and pituitary gland dysfunction resulting in hormone deficiencies, such as growth hormone, thyroid hormone, estrogen, and testosterone; demyelinization and necrosis of the white matter of the brain resulting in lethargy, sleepiness, and *seizures;* gray matter effects resulting in learning disabilities, abnormal electroencephalogram tracings, low-intensity headaches, *cataracts,* salivary gland damage, and chronic change in or loss of taste; chronic pneumonitis and pulmonary fibrosis or thickening; pericardial thickening and reduced heart expandability; chronic malabsorption, hepatic fibrosis resulting in reduced liver function; nephritis and chronic cystitis; and secondary malignancies from oncogenic changes in cells.

### Nursing Implications

- Explain all aspects of radiation therapy and necessary care to the child and parents.
- Provide emotional support and guidance to the child and parents; allow them to verbalize their feelings and fears; answer questions honestly and directly.
- Prepare the child for skin markings.
- Assure the child and parents that during the treatment the child will experience no sensation from radiation exposure.
- Premedicate infants as prescribed to ensure that they lie still during the procedure; keep the child active early in the day and introduce calming activities after the sedative is administered.
- Assist the older child in planning activities to think about during radiation because he or she has to lie still for about 20 minutes on an uncomfortable table in a room away from personnel or parents.
- Prepare the child receiving radiation therapy to the head for alopecia.
- Monitor leukocyte and platelet counts frequently because radiation to bone marrow may cause decreased production.

- Institute measures to promote skin integrity, including:
    Keeping radiation area exposed to the air as much
        as possible.
    Avoiding exposing the area to direct heat or sun.
    Not washing off the markings that designate the
        radiation area.
    Using only mild shampoo (if head is being
        radiated).
    Using a soft toothbrush to prevent excoriation of
        gumline.
    Providing frequent sips of water and mouthwash
        rinse 3 to 4 times daily to compensate for
        decreased salivary gland secretions.
    Avoiding the use of creams or lotions to the
        radiated area.
- Assist the child with maintaining nutrition by:
    Administering an antiemetic as prescribed to
        prevent nausea.
    Encouraging adequate calories for breakfast and
        before treatment when the child is less apt to be
        nauseated.
    Allowing the child to have as much choice about
        food as possible; encouraging parents to bring in
        favorite foods or beverages from home.
    Praising the child for eating, keeping mealtime a
        positive experience.
- Institute measures to prevent fluid loss, including:
    Providing good perianal skin care if *diarrhea* is a
        problem.
    Reducing fresh fruit and vegetables concentrated in
        cellulose.
    Eliminating apple juice.
    Administering antidiarrheal medications as
        prescribed.
    Monitoring intake and output and administering
        intravenous fluid replacement as prescribed.
- Institute infection control measures to prevent
    infection.
- Provide adequate rest periods and balance with activi-
    ties to prevent fatigue; allow activities that do not tire
    the child.
- Provide *play therapy* to assist the child in coping with
    treatment and promote self-esteem.
- Encourage the use of scarves or caps to deal with
    alopecia.

- Assess the child at health maintenance visits for possible abnormalities resulting from long-term effects of radiation therapy.

# RAPE

## DESCRIPTION

- Rape is sexual activity that occurs under actual or threatened force of one person by another.
- Forcible rape is legally defined in most states as intercourse or penetration of a body orifice by a penis or other object.
- Statutory rape is sexual activity with a person under the age of consent (in most states, 18 years of age) and is considered to have occurred despite the apparent willingness of the underage person.
- Sexual assault is used to refer to other forced sexual acts, such as oral-genital or anal-genital intrusion.
- A growing phenomenon is date rape, in which a man forces a date or casual friend into having coitus despite her voiced unwillingness.
- Both rape and sexual assault represent deviant behavior—acts of violence, not passion, lacking the components of privacy and mutual consent.
- The average rape victim is an adolescent girl, although victims can be any age, and they can be male.
- In more than half of reported rapes, the rapist is a stranger; the average rapist is a young man with a background of aggressive behavior with motivation relating to the expression of power or anger.
- Rape tends to be a repetitive, planned activity, rather than an isolated event.
- Many rape victims demonstrate immediate physical and emotional symptoms; this is termed rape trauma syndrome generally occurring in two stages: disorganization and reorganization.

## ASSESSMENT FINDINGS

- Injuries such as bruising, lacerations, teeth marks or abrasions
- Torn or stained clothing
- Bleeding
  ### Disorganization phase
- Feelings of humiliation, shame, guilt, embarrassment, anger, and vengefulness

- Trembling from fear
- Complaints of pain from perineal lacerations
- Easily startled at the sound of anyone approaching or touching her

*Reorganization phase*
- Recurring nightmares
- Sexual dysfunction (possible)
- Continuing inability to relate to men or face new and surprising situations
- Continuing difficulty discussing the rape

### NURSING IMPLICATIONS

- Obtain a thorough history and physical assessment to establish a baseline; describe the physical appearance and quote the client's words exactly.
- Approach the client in a calm, nonthreatening manner and provide privacy.
- Question the client if she bathed or washed before coming for care because this can obscure evidence and obliterate the presence of sperm.
- Follow institution's rape protocol for gathering evidence, and prepare the client for any procedures and treatments, photographs, gynecologic examination, specimens and cultures, and interviews with police.
- Obtain a vaginal culture for gonorrhea and Pap test and obtain blood specimens for a pregnancy test and VDRL for syphilis and possibly HIV.
- Begin prophylactic administration of antibiotics against gonorrhea and syphilis as prescribed.
- Thoroughly document all care given.
- Allow the client to talk about what happened; explore with the client about the event, the assailant, the details of the assault, and the resistance to assault.
- Contact a rape counselor for assistance and support.
- Give the client the number of a counseling service before leaving the emergency room.
- Instruct the client to return for a repeat VDRL and HIV testing in 6 weeks.
- Be certain that the client has a support person to accompany her home; assure the client that if her distress becomes acute, she can return as needed to the health care facility for additional care and counseling.
- Inform the client of any local support groups that may provide follow-up counseling for victims of rape.

- Provide support to the victim's parents or sexual partner and arrange for counseling if appropriate.

# RENAL HYPOPLASIA

## DESCRIPTION

- Renal hypoplasia refers to kidneys that contain fewer lobes than normal.
- The kidneys are underdeveloped and small.

## ASSESSMENT FINDINGS

- Poor renal function
- *Hypertension* (possible from stenosis of renal arteries)

## NURSING IMPLICATIONS

- Obtain a thorough history and physical examination to establish a baseline.
- Obtain any diagnostic tests, as prescribed to evaluate kidney function.
- Prepare the child and parents for all diagnostic tests.
- Carefully assess the child's renal function, including urine output and specific gravity.
- Monitor the child's blood pressure for changes possibly indicating *hypertension.*
- Prepare the child and parents for possible renal transplant later in life to maintain kidney function.
- Provide emotional support and guidance to the parents and child to alleviate fears and anxieties.

# RENAL INSUFFICIENCY, ACUTE

## DESCRIPTION

- Acute renal insufficiency is one form of kidney failure, usually due to a sudden body insult that leads to renal ischemia, ultimately leading to acute renal insufficiency.
- Children who undergo prolonged anesthesia, hemorrhage, shock, severe *diarrhea* leading to *dehydration,* or sudden traumatic injury may develop acute renal insufficiency.
- It also can occur in a child who is placed on a pump oxygenator while undergoing heart surgery or who receives common antibiotics, such as aminoglycosides, penicillin, cephalosporins, and sulfonamides.

- Children who swallow poisons, such as arsenic, or are exposed to industrial wastes, such as mercury, may develop acute renal insufficiency.
- The active course of acute *group A hemolytic poststreptococcal glomerulonephritis* may also cause acute renal insufficiency.

### Assessment Findings

- Oliguria
- Azotemia
- Uremia
- Increased blood urea nitrogen level
- Decreased urine creatinine level
- Elevated serum potassium levels (hyperkalemia), evidenced by weak irregular pulse, abdominal cramps, lowered blood pressure, and muscle weakness
- Increased serum phosphorus levels (hyperphosphatemia)
- Decreased serum calcium levels (hypocalcemia); if severe, leading to muscle twitching and convulsions
- Fixed specific gravity
- Lack of kidney function on intravenous pyelogram or radioactive uptake scan

### Nursing Implications

- Support the child's body systems while correcting the underlying cause.
- Administer intravenous fluids as prescribed, slowly, to replace plasma volume and avoid *congestive heart failure.*
- Avoid administering potassium in intravenous fluids until kidney function is adequate.
- Anticipate using calcium gluconate or an oral cation exchange resin, such as Kayexalate, or prepare for dialysis, as prescribed, if serum potassium level is above 6 mEq/L.
- Administer sodium bicarbonate or intravenous glucose and insulin, as prescribed to help reduce serum potassium levels.
- Monitor serum laboratory values, such as electrolyte levels, for changes.

- Administer a diuretic, such as furosemide or mannitol, as prescribed to increase urine production.
- Provide a diet low in protein, potassium, and sodium and high in carbohydrate to supply adequate calories for metabolism while limiting urea production.
- Limit fluid intake to prevent *congestive heart failure.*
- Obtain daily weights and monitor intake and output frequently for changes indicating possible fluid overload.
- Assess for the onset of diuresis, as an indication of recovery.
- Note increase in urine output, and administer additional fluids as necessary to prevent hypovolemia.
- Provide information to the parents about the child's status and treatment.
- Reassure the parents about the child's status once recovery has begun.
- Inform the parents that the urine output is remaining at a normal level.
- Encourage interaction of the parents with the child to relieve anxiety.

## RENAL INSUFFICIENCY, CHRONIC

### DESCRIPTION

- Chronic renal insufficiency results when acute renal failure becomes long-term or when chronic kidney disease has caused extensive nephron destruction.
- The nephrons available are inadequate in number to sustain kidney function.
- Kidney function diminishes after 50% of glomeruli are destroyed.
- Kidneys no longer concentrate the urine.
- Chronic osteodystrophy occurs.
- To compensate for *hypocalcemia,* the parathyroid gland becomes hyperactive, and further osteodystrophy occurs.
- Bone growth eventually halts.
- Anemia develops from decreased erythropoietin production.

### ASSESSMENT FINDINGS

- Polyuria
- Enuresis
- *Dehydration*

- Oliguria
- Anuria
- *Metabolic acidosis* secondary to inability to secrete H+ ions
- *Hypocalcemia*
- Hyperphosphatemia
- Anemia
- Pruritus
- Elevated blood urea nitrogen
- Elevated serum creatinine

## Nursing Implications

- Educate the family and child with chronic renal insufficiency about the disease and the normal role of kidneys.
- Place the child on a low-protein, high-carbohydrate, and low-phosphorus diet.
- Explain to the parents the need to administer aluminum hydroxide gels with the child's meals to help bind phosphorus.
- Assist the preparer of the child's meals on how to select low-protein foods.
- Let the child choose the low-protein food he or she wishes to increase compliance.
- Monitor the child's electrolytes and fluids, and teach the parents the importance of monitoring weight and urine output.
- Be aware that fluid and sodium may or may not be restricted according to the individual situation.
- Provide educational information to the parents and the child about supplemental calcium.
- Assess the child's growth and encourage verbalization regarding insufficient growth with altered calcium absorption.
- Facilitate communication about feelings of depression, chronic fatigue, and unappetizing diet.
- Encourage the child and family to express their feelings, and support the family in caring for a child with a chronic disease.
- Recommend age-appropriate activities, such as school work or collections.
- Advocate peer communications through letter writing or telephone calls for the isolated child.
- Provide opportunities for *therapeutic play.*

- Help the parents contact a support group.
- Administer and teach the parents about the potential need for antihypertensive medications.
- Cautiously administer blood if needed, monitoring for fluid overload.
- Explain to the family and child regarding the potential need for dialysis or renal transplant (or both).

## REYE'S SYNDROME

### DESCRIPTION

- Reye's syndrome is acute *encephalitis* with accompanying fatty infiltration of the liver, heart, lungs, pancreas, and skeletal muscle.
- It occurs in children from 1 to 18 years of age.
- There is no difference in sex distribution; a sibling has increased risk of developing the disease, perhaps because of a genetic susceptibility.
- The cause is unknown, but it generally occurs after a viral infection, such as varicella (*chickenpox*) or an upper respiratory infection, so it may be caused by viral invasion of the tissues or specific toxic reactions to a virus.
- Research has confirmed the association of acetylsalicylic acid (aspirin) intake during the viral infection with the onset of Reye's syndrome afterward.
- If left untreated, Reye's syndrome is rapidly fatal.
- The child is not infectious at the onset of Reye's syndrome.
- Treatment is directed toward supporting respiratory function, controlling hypoglycemia, and reducing brain edema.

### ASSESSMENT FINDINGS (appearing 1 to 3 weeks after recovery from a viral illness)

- Lethargy
- Severe *vomiting* possibly leading to *dehydration*
- Agitation
- Anorexia
- Confusion progressing to stupor to deep coma, *seizures*
- Combativeness
- Hypoglycemia
- Elevated serum ammonia levels
- Elevated serum glutamic-oxaloacetic transaminase
- Elevated serum glutamic-pyruvic transaminase

- Normal direct bilirubin
- Delayed prothrombin time
- Delayed partial thromboplastin time
- Elevated blood urea nitrogen
- Elevated serum amylase
- Elevated short-chain fatty acids
- Elevated white blood cell count
- Slightly elevated opening cerebrospinal fluid pressure; otherwise normal
- Cerebral edema and decreased ventricle size on skull computed tomography (later)
- Fatty infiltration on liver biopsy
- Respiratory arrest

## NURSING IMPLICATIONS

- Advise all parents to give children acetaminophen for fever instead of aspirin.
- Start an infusion of 10% to 15% dextrose solution as prescribed to reduce cerebral edema and correct hypoglycemia; anticipate using mannitol or a corticosteroid to reduce cerebral edema.
- Keep in mind that Reye's syndrome is categorized by stages of involvement from 1 to 5 depending on the amount of the child's lethargy or presence of *coma*.
- Perform frequent neurologic assessments to identify changes indicating deterioration.
- Monitor blood studies closely for changes.
- Monitor the child's fluid status carefully, and regulate fluid intake to prevent overload and increase cerebral edema; monitor output and insert an indwelling urinary catheter if necessary to monitor urine output more closely.
- Monitor intracranial and central venous or arterial pressure line for changes.
- Insert a nasogastric tube as prescribed to prevent *vomiting* and aspiration.
- Keep emergency equipment, such as endotracheal tube and ventilatory support, at the bedside in case of respiratory arrest.
- If *assisted ventilation* is used, administer pancuronium as prescribed to paralyze respiratory muscles, allowing maximum ventilation.
- Orient the child to surroundings when the child awakens.

- Provide emotional support and guidance to the parents because of the seriousness of the disease following such a common infection.
- Provide the parents with frequent updates on their child's status, explaining all events and treatments; allow the parents to verbalize their feelings and fears.

## RHEUMATIC FEVER

### DESCRIPTION

- Rheumatic fever is an autoimmune disease that occurs as a reaction to a group A beta-hemolytic streptococcus infection.
- It often follows an attack of *pharyngitis, tonsillitis, scarlet fever,* strep throat, or *impetigo.*
- It occurs most often in children 6 to 15 years of age, with a peak incidence at 8 years.
- Because streptococcal infections recur, rheumatic fever can also recur.
- It is seen most often in socioeconomically depressed urban areas.
- The course of rheumatic fever is 6 to 8 weeks.

### ASSESSMENT FINDINGS

#### *Major:*
- Carditis with systolic murmur and prolonged P-R and QT intervals on electrocardiogram
- Chorea (involuntary limb movement) along with dysfunctional speech, weak or spasmodic hand grasp, and facial expression changes
- Subcutaneous nodules by the joints
- Polyarthritis with swollen and tender joints.
- Erythema marginatum (macular rash primarily on trunk)

#### *Minor:*
- Fever
- Arthralgia
- History of previous rheumatic fever
- Elevated sedimentation rate and C-reactive protein levels

### NURSING IMPLICATIONS

- Maintain bed rest during the acute phase of illness until the erythrocyte sedimentation rate decreases and the C-reactive protein level and pulse rate return to normal.

- Frequently assess the child's vital signs, including apical pulse while awake and sleeping, for changes.
- Administer penicillin as prescribed to treat the infection; give as a single intramuscular injection of benzathine penicillin; use erythromycin in children who are sensitive to penicillin.
- Administer oral salicylates to reduce inflammation and pain; monitor for symptoms of aspirin toxicity that may result from the high dosage, including tinnitus, nausea, vomiting, headache, and blurred vision.
- Be alert for petechiae if the aspirin dosage interferes with prothrombin synthesis.
- Anticipate administering corticosteroids as prescribed for the child who is not responding to salicylate therapy, and monitor for possible side effects of corticosteroid therapy.
- Administer phenobarbital as prescribed to reduce the purposeless movements of chorea.
- Keep in mind that the prognosis depends on the extent of myocardial involvement; permanent valve destruction, especially of the mitral valve, may occur; there are no aftereffects of joint or chorea involvement.
- Offer support and guidance to the parents and child to help alleviate their fears and anxieties.
- If chorea is present, provide toys and games for children that do not require fine coordination to minimize the frustrations of not being able to use the hands meaningfully; assist with feeding as necessary; pad the bed rails as necessary to prevent injury from thrashing movements.
- Emphasize that chorea is transitory and the lack of coordination will pass without permanent effects.
- Administer appropriate antibiotic treatment as prescribed for streptococcal infections to help prevent the occurrence of rheumatic fever.
- Inform parents to bring the child with an upper respiratory infection in to see the physician to evaluate for the possibility of a streptococcal infection and ensure prompt treatment.
- Instruct parents of a child with a streptococcal infection receiving antibiotic therapy in all aspects of the medication regimen, including the dosage, frequency, and duration, and to continue the course of therapy for the full 10 to 14 days as prescribed.

- For the child who has had rheumatic fever, instruct parents in the need to maintain prophylactic antibiotic therapy for at least 5 years after the initial attack, or until the child is 18 years old, or as long as the physician may prescribe.
- Educate the child and parents about extra prophylactic measures when dental or tonsillar surgery is planned; because most children have streptococci in their throats, an open incision in the mouth increases the risk of streptococcal invasion into the blood stream.

# RICKETTSIALPOX

### DESCRIPTION
- Rickettsialpox is a rickettsial disease carried by a mouse mite.
- It is a disease of crowded urban areas.

### ASSESSMENT FINDINGS
- Local lesion at site of bite
- Generalized rash over entire body except for palms and soles

### NURSING IMPLICATIONS
- Obtain a thorough history and physical examination, including any living conditions and possible mouse bite, to establish a baseline.
- Administer tetracycline as prescribed.
- Provide support and education to the parents regarding all aspects of the child's care.

# ROCKY MOUNTAIN SPOTTED FEVER

### DESCRIPTION
- Rocky Mountain spotted fever is a rickettsial disease (rickettsiae are organisms that resemble viruses both in size and in their ability to reproduce except inside the cells of a host organism) caused by *Rickettsia rickettsii.*
- It has an incubation period of 3 to 12 days, and it is not communicable from one person to another.
- It is transmitted by wood, dog, or rabbit tick.
- Active artificial immunity is acquired with the Rocky Mountain spotted fever vaccine.
- Rocky Mountain spotted fever is the most common rickettsial disease seen in the United States.
- It is transmitted by a tick, so it is seen most often during the spring and early summer when ticks are most commonly seen.

- Untreated, the disease is fatal.

**ASSESSMENT FINDINGS**
- History of tick bite
- Fever
- Severe headache
- Measleslike rash beginning as bright red macules on the ankles and wrists, spreading as a hemorrhagic rash to the palms, soles, back, arms, thighs, and chest

**NURSING IMPLICATIONS**
- Obtain a thorough history and physical examination, including any recent trips to wooded areas, to establish a baseline.
- Immediately after the tick bite, remove the tick slowly and steadily and cleanse the wound with soap and water.
- Administer tetracycline as prescribed.
- Provide support and education to parents regarding all aspects of the child's care.

## ROSEOLA INFANTUM

**DESCRIPTION**
- Roseola infantum (exanthem subitum) is a childhood skin disorder caused by the herpesvirus 6 (HHV-6).
- It has an incubation period of approximately 10 days with a period of communicability during the febrile period.
- Its mode of transmission is unknown.
- Contracting the disease offers lasting natural immunity; no artificial immunity is available.
- Roseola is a disease whose symptoms are out of proportion to its severity (appears more severe than it really is).
- It generally occurs in children ages 6 months to 3 years, mainly in the spring and fall, although it can occur at any time of the year.

**ASSESSMENT FINDINGS**
- High fever (104° to 105°F [40.0° to 40.6°C])
- Irritability
- Anorexia
- Slightly inflamed pharynx (possible)
- Enlarged occipital, cervical, and postauricular lymph nodes (possible)

- Decreased white blood cell count with increased proportion of lymphocytes
- Discrete rose-pink macules (darker in color than *rubeola* or *rubella*) approximately 2 to 3 mm in size, appearing after abrupt fall in fever, occurring most prominently on trunk and fading under pressure; often reported as a heat rash
- No accompanying coryza, cough, or conjunctivitis

## NURSING IMPLICATIONS
- Obtain a complete history, including the child's *immunization* history and the onset and duration of the child's symptoms to establish a baseline.
- Thoroughly inspect the child's skin for characteristics of the rash to identify the disorder and rule out other disorders.
- Be aware that the most frequent complication is febrile convulsion with the onset of the disease.
- Administer antipyretics, such as acetaminophen, for fever; be aware that fever responds to antipyretics, but, after 4 hours, it rises again; encourage the parents to use other measures, such as cool compresses and tepid sponge baths, to reduce fever
- Provide comfort measures, such as cool compresses, cool light clothing, and avoidance of itching, for the rash.

# ROUNDWORM (ASCARIASIS)

## DESCRIPTION
- Roundworm is a pathogenic worm (helminthic) infection.
- The roundworm parasite lives in the intestinal tract; eggs are excreted in the feces.
- If children eat food that is improperly washed or with hands that are improperly washed, eggs may be ingested by them along with soil.
- Larvae, which hatch from the ingested eggs, penetrate the intestinal wall and enter the circulation; from there, they may migrate to any body tissue.

## ASSESSMENT FINDINGS
- Loss of appetite
- Nausea (possible)
- *Vomiting* (possible)

- Intestinal obstruction (possible from mass of roundworms in intestinal tract)

**NURSING IMPLICATIONS**
- Obtain a thorough history and physical examination to establish a baseline and rule out the possibility of other disorders.
- Question the parents and child about food intake, including where and when, and the community's sanitary disposal system; investigate the possibility of other cases.
- Instruct the parents and child in the need for good hygiene measures, including washing hands after going to the bathroom and before eating.
- Be aware that ascariasis can be prevented by sanitary disposal of feces so this does not contaminate soil.
- Administer single dose of anthelmintics, such as pyrantel pamoate (Antiminth), as prescribed to control the infection.

# RUBELLA

**DESCRIPTION**
- Rubella is a childhood skin disorder caused by the rubella virus.
- It has an incubation period of 14 to 21 days with a period of communicability from 7 days before to approximately 5 days after the rash appears.
- Rubella is transmitted by direct and indirect contact with droplets.
- Contracting the disease offers lasting natural immunity; active artificial immunity is acquired through attenuated live virus vaccine; passive artificial immunity is acquired through immune serum globulin (considered for pregnant women).
- Rubella is a disease of older school age and adolescent children, occurring most commonly during the spring.

**ASSESSMENT FINDINGS**
### *Prodromal period*
- Low-grade fever
- Headache
- Malaise
- Anorexia
- Mild *conjunctivitis*

- Sore throat (possible)
- Mild cough (possible)
- Lymphadenopathy of suboccipital, postauricular, and cervical nodes (possible)
- Discrete pink-red maculopapular rash (occurring 1 to 5 days after prodromal signs) beginning first on the face then spreading downward to the trunk and extremities, disappearing by the 3rd day
- Arthritic joint pain (in some children on 2nd or 3rd day of rash)

### NURSING IMPLICATIONS

- Obtain a complete history, including the child's *immunization* history and the onset and duration of child's symptoms, to establish a baseline.
- Thoroughly inspect the child's skin for characteristics of the rash to identify the disorder and rule out other disorders.
- Administer antipyretics for fever.
- Provide comfort measures, such as cool compresses, cool light clothing, and avoidance of itching, for the rash.
- If arthritis occurs, administer acetaminophen to control joint pain as prescribed; encourage bed rest for 2 to 3 days until the discomfort subsides.
- Be aware that if rubella occurs during pregnancy, it can cause extensive congenital malformations.

## RUBEOLA

### DESCRIPTION

- Rubeola is a childhood skin disorder caused by the measles virus.
- It has an incubation period of 10 to 12 days with a period of communicability from the 5th day of the incubation period through the first few days of the rash.
- Rubeola is spread by direct or indirect contact with droplets.
- Contracting the disease offers lasting natural immunity; active artificial immunity is acquired through the attenuated live measles vaccine; passive artificial immunity is acquired through the immune serum globulin.
- Rubeola is sometimes called brown or black, regular, or 7-day measles to differentiate it from *rubella* (German or 3-day measles).

- It formerly occurred most frequently in children ages 5 to 10 years; because most children of preschool and school age have now been immunized, outbreaks currently most often occur in the college-age population.
- Incidence is highest in winter and spring months.

### ASSESSMENT FINDINGS

#### *Prodromal period*

- Enlarged lymphoid tissue, particularly postauricular, cervical, and occipital lymph nodes
- High fever (103° to 104°F [39.5° to 40.0°C])
- Malaise
- Ill appearance
- Coryza (sore throat and rhinitis) by 2nd day with nasal congestion and mucopurulent discharge
- Conjunctivitis with photophobia, watery eyes
- Deep brassy, bronchial cough
- Koplik's spots (small, irregular bright red spots with blue-white center point) on buccal membrane with drop in fever on the 5th day (diagnostic of measles)
- Deep red macular pruritic rash on 4th day of fever (lasting 5 to 6 days) beginning at the hairline of the forehead, behind the ears, and at the back of the neck spreading to include the face, neck, upper extremities, trunk, and lower extremities
- Red rash fading on pressure progressing to a brown color

### NURSING IMPLICATIONS

- Obtain a complete history, including the child's *immunization* history and the onset and duration of the child's symptoms to establish a baseline.
- Thoroughly inspect the child's skin for characteristics of the rash to identify the disorder and rule out other disorders.
- Administer antipyretics for fever.
- Provide comfort measures, such as cool compresses, cool light clothing, and avoidance of itching, for the rash.
- Apply a lubricating jelly or emollient to the child's skin below the nose, which may become excoriated from the constant nasal drainage.
- Administer a cough suppressant as prescribed to control the cough.

- Institute measures, such as drawing the shades or curtains, wearing dark glasses, and avoiding bright lights, to minimize photophobia.
- Instruct the parents in all aspects of the child's care.
- Reassure parents that usually on the 3rd or 4th day of the rash, when the temperature falls, the other symptoms clear quickly, and the child will begin to feel better.
- Be aware that fever that lasts beyond the 3rd or 4th day of the rash generally suggests that a complication of measles has occurred.
- Monitor the child closely for possible complications, such as *otitis media, pneumonia,* airway obstruction, and acute *encephalitis.*

## SCALDED SKIN DISEASE

### Description

- Scalded skin disease (Ritter's disease) is a staphylococcal infection seen primarily in newborns.
- It is an extreme infection requiring intensive therapy with antibiotics.

### Assessment Findings

- Rough texture skin
- General erythema
- Large bullae filled with clear fluid
- Separation of epidermis in large sheets, leaving a red, glistening, scalded-looking surface

### Nursing Implications

- Inspect the skin of the newborn closely for signs of the disorder.
- Administer penicillinase-resistant antibiotics, such as methicillin and flucloxacillin, as prescribed.
- Provide emotional support and guidance to the parents to minimize their fears and anxieties; allow the parents to verbalize their feelings.
- Monitor the infant closely for changes.

## SCARLET FEVER

### Description

- Scarlet fever refers to a streptococcal infection caused by group A beta-hemolytic streptococci.
- It has an incubation period of 2 to 5 days, with a period of communicability being greatest during the acute phase of the respiratory illness.

- It is transmitted by direct contact and large droplets.
- One episode of scarlet fever gives lasting immunity to the scarlet fever toxin.
- Scarlet fever occurs most commonly in the 6- to 12-year-old age group, although it may be seen in the preschooler.
- The incidence is highest in temperate climates, and it occurs usually in late winter or early spring months.
- *Rheumatic fever* and *acute glomerulonephritis* occur as sequelae to scarlet fever in only approximately 2% to 3% of children, occurring 1 to 3 weeks following the rash; the occurrence seems to be related not to the severity of the scarlet fever but to the body's reaction to the toxins produced at the time of the illness.

**ASSESSMENT FINDINGS** (begin abruptly with the onset of streptococcal pharyngitis)

- Extremely high fever (103° to 104°F [39.5 to 40.0°C]) on 1st day and again on day of rash, falling gradually to normal
- Increased pulse rate out of proportion to fever
- Sore throat
- Headache
- Chills
- Malaise
- Exanthematous and enanthematous rash appearing 12 to 48 hours after onset of pharyngeal symptoms; pinpoint lesions blanching on pressure, most dense on trunk and skin folds
- Circumoral pallor
- Hyperpigmentation in folds of joints
- Desquamation of rash after 1 week
- Inflamed, enlarged tonsils covered with white exudate
- Beefy red uvula and pharynx
- Pinpoint lesions and scattered petechiae on hard palate
- White furry tongue (during first 2 days), progressing to white strawberry appearance (by day 3), progressing to strawberry red appearance (by day 4 or 5)
- Throat culture positive for streptococcus

**NURSING IMPLICATIONS**

- Obtain a thorough history and physical examination to establish a baseline; question the child and parents about any recent sore throat and appearance of a rash.

- Obtain a throat culture as prescribed to confirm the diagnosis.
- Offer the child a soft or liquid diet to minimize throat discomfort.
- Administer analgesics, such as acetaminophen for pain and an antipyretic for fever, as prescribed.
- Institute comfort measures to alleviate itching from the rash, such as cool compresses and lotions; encourage the child not to scratch the rash.
- Administer penicillin as prescribed for the complete course of therapy.
- Instruct the parents about the medication; caution them to give the full amount prescribed for the full course to prevent complications.
- Be aware that children who are administered penicillin do not have the typical extreme rash and obviously do not have as severe a systemic illness (commonly referred to as scarlatina) as those who do not receive penicillin.
- Caution parents that no matter what name is applied to the problem, the consequences can be grave and penicillin therapy is necessary.

## SCOLIOSIS, FUNCTIONAL

### DESCRIPTION
- Functional scoliosis refers to the lateral (sideways) curvature of the spine occurring as a compensatory mechanism in children who have unequal leg lengths and sometimes in those children with ocular refractive errors that cause them constantly to tilt their head sideways.
- The pelvic tilt caused by unequal leg length or the neck tilt results in a spinal deviation for the child to stand upright.
- The curve that occurs tends to be C-shaped.

### ASSESSMENT FINDINGS
- C-shaped curvature of the spine
- Little change in vertebral shape on x-ray film

### NURSING IMPLICATIONS
- Obtain a thorough history and physical examination to establish a baseline.
- Prepare the child for corrective devices, such as lift inserted into a shoe to correct unequal leg length or corrective ocular lenses to improve vision problems.

- Instruct the parents and child in ways to maintain good posture in everyday activities.
- Teach the child about exercises, such as chinning themselves, walking with a book on the head for 10 minutes, sit-ups, push-ups, and swimming, to stretch the spine.
- Assure the parents and child that the condition can be corrected to help alleviate concerns and maintain a positive body image.
- Caution parents about nagging the child about exercises and using good posture to prevent possible rebellion by the child.

## SCOLIOSIS, STRUCTURAL

### DESCRIPTION

- Structural scoliosis refers to an idiopathic, permanent curvature of the spine with damaging vertebral changes.
- The spine assumes a primary lateral curvature, and to allow children to hold their head level, a compensatory second curve develops giving an S-shaped appearance.
- The primary curve is often a right thoracic curve; as it becomes severe, rotation and angulation of the vertebrae occur; the thoracic rib cage rotates to become protuberant on the convex curve.
- Vertebral growth may halt because of extreme pressure changes; as long as children are growing, the spinal curves become more severe, explaining why the symptoms become most marked at prepuberty, a time of rapid growth.
- Structural scoliosis is 5 times more common in females than males and the age of peak incidence is 8 to 15 years.

### ASSESSMENT FINDINGS

- S-shaped appearance of spine
- Shoulder elevated on convex side of scoliotic curve
- Scapula higher on convex side of curve
- Hump on back on convex side of curve
- Elbows at the level or closer to the iliac crest on one side
- Leaning to one side
- One hip higher than the other

### Nursing Implications

- Assess all children over 10 years of age for scoliosis at all health assessment visits.
- Obtain a thorough physical examination:

  Observe the child from a posterior view when undressed except for underpants.

  Ask the child to hold arms at sides and inspect for unequal shoulder or hip level, prominence of one scapula, or a curved spinal column.

  Compare the level of the elbows in relation to the iliac crest.

  Ask the child to bend over and touch the toes, continuing to observe the back.

- Anticipate x-rays to estimate the extent of the deformity and serve as a baseline description.
- Be aware that if the spinal curve is less than 20 degrees, no therapy is usually required except for close observation until the child reaches about 18 years of age.
- If the curve is greater than 20 degrees, anticipate the use of braces, traction, surgery, or a combination.
- Provide support to the child to help alleviate concerns about body image and spinal curve correction, which may take years.
- If a brace is used:

  Instruct the child and parents about how to apply the brace correctly, the length of time the brace is to be worn, the need for frequent follow-up, the use of mild analgesics and rest to relieve muscle aches, prescribed exercises, and activity level.

  Advise the parents that they must be firm about insisting that the child wear the brace continuously.

  Be aware that the brace will be worn until the child's spinal growth stops; wean the child gradually from the brace because some demineralization of vertebrae may have occurred.

- If Halo traction is used:

  Explain the apparatus to the child to minimize fear about the device.

  For the first 24 hours following application, administer analgesia to reduce headache and pain at pin insertion sites.

Frequently shampoo the scalp to keep the pin sites clean.

Wash around the pins daily with half-strength peroxide or other prescribed solution to remove crusting.

Encourage the child to be as self-sufficient as possible.

Give the parents a telephone number that they can call for help or questions as to what activity will be safe after the child returns home.

Allow the child to verbalize feelings about the device to minimize fears and promote a healthy body image.

- If surgical correction is necessary, prepare the child and parents physically and psychologically for the surgery, including deep breathing exercises, use of rods, expected degree of pain, and mobility level.
- Following surgery:

Do not gatch the bed; anticipate using a Stryker frame.

Keep the child flat and log roll to a side-lying position every 2 hours.

Perform neurovascular checks on lower extremities to detect neurologic impairment.

Monitor intake and output carefully, including any wound drainage system, urinary catheter, and nasogastric tube used.

Maintain NPO status (nothing by mouth) until bowel sounds return; then advance diet as tolerated; allow moderate calcium intake to prevent renal calculi, but replace the rapid release of calcium from the bones following surgery.

Administer analgesics as prescribed to relieve pain.

Encourage parents to touch and comfort the child.

Allow the child out of bed as prescribed, usually on the 2nd to 4th postoperative day; allow the child to dangle before getting out of bed.

Instruct the child and parents about gradual resumption of activity; warn them to avoid extremely active gymnastics or trampoline work.

Be aware that the rods do not interfere with other sports or childbearing.

Allow the child to readjust to the freedom of normal body movement because he or she has been in some type of restraining device for probably a long time; reassure the child that with the surgery, the problem finally is corrected and that no further curvature can occur after this point.

- Instruct the child and family in all aspects of care following the child's discharge, including the need for follow-up and compliance with devices.

## SEIZURES

### DESCRIPTION

- Seizures, also known as convulsions, are a type of paroxysmal disorder (one that occurs suddenly and recurrently) involving an involuntary contraction of muscle caused by abnormal electrical brain discharges.
- Although seizures may have an unknown cause, they can also be attributed to infection, trauma, tumor growth, or familial or polygenic inheritance.
- Seizures are not so much a disease as a symptom of an underlying disorder that needs close investigation.
- Seizures are classified as partial (involving only one hemisphere of the brain) and generalized (involving the entire brain and loss of consciousness).
- Partial seizures can involve motor, sensory, cognitive, affective, psychosensory, or compound symptoms; they are further classified as simple or complex depending on the degree of symptoms.
- Generalized seizures are further classified as *absence*, myoclonic, atonic, clonic, or *tonic-clonic*.
- The types and causes of seizures vary according to the child's age.
- Seizures in the newborn may be caused by perinatal injury, effects of anoxia, or a metabolic disorder.
- Seizures in the infant and toddler periods may be from an unknown cause, such as infantile spasms, or result from a high fever, poisoning, or drugs.
- Seizures in children over 3 years of age may be idiopathic or occur from organic diseases that result from focal or diffuse brain injury that has left residual damage. Types of seizures commonly seen in children over 3 include psychomotor seizures (*simple partial seizures*); focal seizures, previously called jacksonian seizures (*complex partial seizures*); absence seizures (more common in girls, usually 6 to 7 years of age); and tonic-clonic seizures.

**ASSESSMENT FINDINGS** (vary with the type of seizure)
    *Simple partial seizures*
- Motor changes, such as change in posture or twitching of head, arms, or eyes
- Sensory changes, such as hallucinations
- Circumoral pallor
- Flushing
- Tachycardia
- Normal electroencephalogram (EEG)

    *Complex partial seizures*
- Seizure beginning in fingers and spreading to wrist, arm, and face in a clonic contraction
- Jacksonian march

    *Absence seizures*
- Staring spell lasting a few seconds; daydreaming
- Rhythmic blinking and twitching of mouth or extremity
- EEG positive for typical 3 wave second spike and slow wave discharge

    *Tonic-clonic seizures*
- Prodromal stage involving drowsiness, dizziness, malaise, lack of coordination or tension
- Aura, such as flashing lights, hallucinations, numbness of an extremity, or "Cheshire cat grin"
- Muscle contraction accompanied by facial distortion, cyanosis, guttural cry
- Rapid muscle contraction and relaxation (quick jerky movements) accompanied by foaming saliva, jaw spasms, and stool or urine incontinence
- Postictal sleep of 1 to 4 hours, arousing only to painful stimuli followed by severe headache on awakening and no memory of seizure
- Abnormal EEG

**NURSING IMPLICATIONS**
- Obtain a thorough history and physical examination, including a full neurologic evaluation, to establish a baseline and rule out metabolic or infectious processes.
- Question the child and parents about events immediately before the seizure; include an accurate description of the seizure itself.
- Assess the child's overall behavior over the last few weeks to determine any changes and help to detect

possible signs of small seizures occurring in school or at night.

- Obtain blood studies as prescribed to rule out metabolic or infectious causes.
- Prepare the child for diagnostic testing, including lumbar puncture to rule out *meningitis* or bleeding into the cerebrospinal fluid, computed tomography or skull x-ray to rule out trauma or tumors, and EEG.
- Be aware that seizure activity in the newborn period may be difficult to recognize because it may consist only of twitching of head, arms, or eyes; slight cyanosis; and respiratory difficulty or apnea, with the infant appearing flaccid and limp afterwards.
- Instruct the parents to administer acetaminophen to control fever (below 101°F) and prevent possibility of febrile seizure.
- Caution the parents of a child who has had one febrile seizure not to let the child develop a second high fever; provide instructions on measures to reduce fever, such as tepid sponge baths, cool cloths to forehead, and light clothing.
- Be aware that a child who has had two or more febrile seizures may be placed on a maintenance dose of phenobarbital.
- Teach the parents and child about anticonvulsant medications prescribed, including dosage, frequency, possible side effects, and need of compliance and follow-up.
- Instruct the parents and child about safety measures, especially if the seizures are not controlled by medications.
- If the child is receiving phenytoin (Dilantin), instruct the child in oral hygiene measures to minimize the effect of gum hypertrophy.
- During the seizure, remain calm and institute measures to protect the child from injury.
- Anticipate the need for oxygen if the child passes rapidly from one convulsion into another.
- Provide emotional support and guidance to the parents to help them deal with the chronicity of the disease.
- Provide instructions about the need for compliance with medication therapy and frequent follow-up, including blood studies to evaluate serum drug levels.

- Provide the parents with as much information as possible about their child's seizures to allow them to deal with a known disease rather than an unexplainable and unpredictable illness.
- Encourage the parents to treat the child as a normal member of the family; encourage the parents to let the child attend regular school and participate in active sports.
- Reassure the parents that occasional seizures are not harmful unless status epilepticus occurs and the child becomes anoxic.
- Be aware that in many children seizure activity increases during puberty.
- Advise the adolescent girl taking anticonvulsants that the medications are teratogenic to a fetus should she become pregnant.

## SEPARATION ANXIETY

### DESCRIPTION

- Separation anxiety is a normal phase of development in the toddler, usually beginning at about 6 months of age and persisting throughout the preschool period.
- It is considered a disorder when an older child shows excessive anxiety about separation or the possibility of separation from those to whom the child is attached.
- Separation anxiety in the older child may be a result of unresolved conflicts, uncertainty about one's caregiver, or parent-induced anxious attachment.
- It also may be present in the child who is hospitalized.

### NURSING IMPLICATIONS

- Advise the parents that separation anxiety is a normal phase of development in the toddler.
- Tell the parents that most toddlers react best to separation if a regular babysitter is employed and if the toddler can remain in his or her own home environment.
- Advise the parents that it is best to give the toddler fair warning that he or she will be left with a babysitter.
- Encourage the parents to say their good-byes firmly, repeating the explanation for their leaving and explaining that they will be there when the child awakens in the morning, and then leave.

- Provide emotional support and encouragement to the parents during this trying period.
- Anticipate the possibility of separation when a child is hospitalized; know that reducing the ill effects of separation should be a high priority.
- Attempt to limit hospital admissions by teaching the parents skills that may help them to care for their child at home, if possible and medically advisable.
- Promote open parent visitation to help reduce separation anxiety.
- Support sibling and grandparent visitation.
- Arrange staffing to provide a substitute parent and allow one nurse to give as much care to the same child as possible.
- Provide for adequate *play*; arrange for *play therapy* as needed.

## SERUM SICKNESS

### DESCRIPTION

- Serum sickness refers to a type III hypersensitivity response of the body to a foreign serum antigen or drug.
- Examples of foreign sera include *tetanus* antitoxin, *diptheria* antitoxin, and *rabies* antiserum, all of which are obtained from horse serum.
- Children may rarely have a serum sickness reaction to a drug, for example, penicillin.

**ASSESSMENT FINDINGS** (Symptoms begin 7 to 12 days after serum injection, sometimes as early as 1 to 5 days if the child has received the same type of foreign serum previously.)

- Itching, edema, and erythema at injection site
- Generalized *urticaria* with or without angioedema
- Pruritus
- Erythema multiforme (generalized macular eruption with dark red papules)
- Purpura
- Fever
- Arthralgia
- Lymphadenopathy (especially of the regional nodes near site of injection)
- Weight gain
- Nausea
- *Vomiting*
- Abdominal pain

*If extreme*
- Optic neuritis
- Stupor
- Coma
- Laryngeal edema

### NURSING IMPLICATIONS
- Obtain a thorough history and physical examination to establish a baseline.
- Ascertain if the child received any foreign sera recently or in the past and whether the child has experienced any similar reactions.
- Be aware that serum sickness lasts a matter of days or weeks and that treatment is symptomatic because the condition improves by itself with time.
- Administer antihistamines or epinephrine as prescribed to help alleviate the symptoms; administer salicylates to relieve fever and joint pain.
- Provide explanations to the parents and child about why the reaction occurred, that it was not anyone's fault, and that it did not occur from administration of the wrong compound.
- Provide support to the child and parents because serum sickness reactions can be frightening.
- Reassure the parents that the condition is not another disorder because serum sickness can mimic other diseases and that there will be no long-term effects from it.
- Instruct the parents and child to wear a bracelet or necklace stating the solutions to which the child is hypersensitive.
- Teach the parents that the child should not receive the foreign serum that was responsible for the primary occurrence again because the next time the manifestations of the reaction may be anaphylaxis.
- Encourage the parents to keep the child's *immunizations* and records current so that there is never a need to give sera such as *tetanus* or *diphtheria* antitoxins.

## SEXUALLY TRANSMITTED DISEASES (STDs)

### DESCRIPTION
- STDs refer to those diseases spread through sexual contact.
- They range in severity from easily treated infections, such as trichomoniasis, to life-threatening diseases, such as human immunodeficiency virus (HIV).

- STDs include *candidiasis* (a fungal infection), *trichomoniasis* (a single-cell protozoan infection), *bacterial vaginosis* (invasion of *Gardnerella* or *Haemophilus* organisms), *Chlamydia trachomatis* infection, *genital warts* (human papillomavirus infection), genital herpes (herpesvirus type 2 [HSV-2] infection), *hepatitis B*, *gonorrhea*, *syphilis*, and *HIV*.

ASSESSMENT FINDINGS (vary with the infection)
  *Candidiasis*
  - Vulvar reddening, burning, and itching
  - White patches on vaginal wall
  - Thick, cream cheese–like vaginal discharge
  - Pain on coitus or tampon insertion
  - Microscopic examination positive for organism
  *Trichomoniasis*
  - Frothy white or gray-green vaginal discharge
  - Vaginal irritation
  - Reddened upper vagina with pinpoint petechiae
  - Extreme vulvar itching
  - Asymptomatic (in males)
  - Microscopic examination positive for organism
  *Bacterial vaginosis*
  - Milk-white to gray vaginal discharge with fishy odor
  - Microscopic examination positive for gram-negative rods adhering to vaginal epithelial cells (clue cells)
  *Chlamydia trachomatis*
  - Heavy grayish white vaginal discharge
  - Vulvar itching
  - Culture positive for organism
  *Genital warts*
  - Rapidly growing lesions on vulva, vagina, or cervix
  *Genital Herpes*
  - Culture positive for HSV-2
  - Pinpoint vesicles on erythematous base progressing to ulceration, becoming moist, draining, open lesions
  - Accompanying flulike symptoms
  - Pain, increasing with contact with clothing or acid urine
  *Gonorrhea*
  - Urethritis (males)
  - Urethral discharge (males)

- Slight yellowing of vaginal discharge (females)
- Inflamed and painful Bartholin glands
- Culture positive for *Neisseria gonorrheae*

*Syphilis*
- Chancre (painless, deep ulcer) on genitalia, mouth, lips, or rectal area (from oral-genital or genital-anal contact)
- Lymphadenopathy
- Generalized macular copper-colored rash with low-grade fever and adenopathy (2 to 4 weeks after chancre disappears)
- Neurologic and cardiac destruction (in the final stage)
- Serologic serum test positive

*HIV*
- Poor resistance to infection
- Fever
- Swollen lymph nodes
- Respiratory tract infections
- Positive antibody tests (after age 15 months)
- Positive HIV culture (after age 15 months)
- *Failure to thrive*

### Nursing Implications

- Obtain a thorough history and physical examination to establish a baseline.
- Question the adolescent, in a nonjudgmental manner, about sexual activity.
- Provide health teaching regarding safe sex practices, including the use of condoms, and other measures, such as proper perineal hygiene, voiding immediately after coitus, and choosing sexual partners who are at low risk for infection.
- Educate adolescents that little immunity develops from STDs and that they can be contracted repeatedly.
- Instruct the adolescent in the need for adherence to treatment regimen and need for follow-up to prevent complications.
- Assure the client of absolute confidentiality in naming sexual contacts.
- For *candidiasis:*
    Administer vaginal suppositories or cream applications of antifungal preparations, such as miconazole (Monistat), nystatin, and clotrimazole, usually once a day for 7 days.

Instruct the adolescent about how to insert suppository or creams properly.

Encourage the adolescent girl to wear a sanitary napkin to avoid staining from vaginal discharge.

Keep in mind that although sexual contact is not the usual means of contracting the initial candidal infection, a reinfection cycle may occur through sexual activity.

Anticipate treating the male partner if the adolescent is sexually active.

If the girl has frequent candidal infections, test urine for glucose to rule out *diabetes mellitus* (often associated with candidal infections).

If the girl is using an oral contraceptive (commonly associated with frequent candidal infections), discuss the possibility of using another contraceptive method.

- For *trichomoniasis:*

  Administer oral metronidazole (Flagyl) as prescribed.

  Instruct the adolescent not to drink alcohol during the course of treatment to prevent acute nausea and *vomiting.*

  Obtain a pregnancy test before initiating drug therapy because metronidazole may be teratogenic to the fetus.

  Inform the adolescent that her partner also needs to receive drug treatment, and encourage her sexual partner to use condoms to prevent recurrence.

  Be aware that *Trichomonas* infection causes such inflammatory changes in the cervix or vagina that a Pap test taken during this time may be misinterpreted as showing abnormal tissue.

  If the adolescent is pregnant, treat with povidone-iodine or vinegar solution douche as prescribed.

- For *bacterial vaginosis:*

  Administer oral metronidazole or clindamycin as prescribed for 7 days.

  Inform the adolescent that her sexual partner also should be treated to prevent recurrence.

- For *Chlamydia trachomatis:*

  Administer oral doxycycline or tetracycline as prescribed for 7 days.

  If the adolescent is pregnant, treat with erythromycin.

- For *genital warts:*

  Prepare the client for excision of large growths by cautery or cryotherapy because they can lead to carcinoma.

  Anticipate using podophyllin to remove small growths.

- For *genital herpes:*

  Administer acyclovir as prescribed.

  When applying topically, use a finger cot to prevent contracting the virus or absorbing the drug.

  Instruct the client about how to apply the drug topically and about using sitz baths 3 times a day, keeping the lesions clean and dry and applying a soothing substance, such as cornstarch, to relieve discomfort.

  Advise the client to use ointments sparingly to keep the area dry and promote healing.

  Instruct the client to have a yearly Pap test (because of the increased association with cervical cancer) and to use condoms to prevent spread among sexual partners.

- For *gonorrhea:*

  Administer one intramuscular injection of ceftriaxone or oral amoxicillin plus oral doxycycline for 7 days.

  Inform the client that his or her sexual partner should receive the same treatment.

  Advise the client to return 7 days after treatment for a follow-up culture to verify that the disease has been completely eradicated.

  Be aware that a sexually active client should be given a serologic test for syphilis along with the gonorrheal culture; if the dose of ceftriaxone and doxycycline has effectively eliminated the gonorrhea, no further treatment for syphilis is necessary.

  Keep in mind that most states require that gonorrhea be reported to the health department and that adolescents are asked to name sexual contacts.

- For *syphilis:*

  Administer benzathine penicillin G intramuscularly in two sites as prescribed; if the client is allergic to penicillin, administer oral erythromycin or tetracycline for 10 to 15 days.

Inform the client that the sexual partner should
receive the same treatment.

Educate adolescents about the need for treatment;
many individuals are either unaware of it or
choose to ignore it.

Keep in mind that most states require that syphilis
be reported to the health department and that
adolescents are asked to name sexual contacts.

- For *HIV:*

Instruct the adolescent in safe sex practices.

Screen all infants of high-risk mothers for possible
HIV infection.

## SHIGELLOSIS

### DESCRIPTION

- Shigellosis, dysentery, is a bacterial infection that
causes *diarrhea* and *vomiting.*
- It is caused by organisms of the genus *Shigella.*
- The incubation period lasts from 1 to 7 days, with
the period of communicability ranging from approximately 1 to 4 weeks.
- *Shigella* is transmitted through contaminated food or
milk products.

### ASSESSMENT FINDINGS

- Severe *diarrhea*
- *Vomiting*
- Blood and mucus in stool

### NURSING IMPLICATIONS

- Obtain a thorough history and physical examination
to establish a baseline.
- Evaluate the child's intake for possible food or milk
contaminants.
- Assess the child's fluid and electrolyte status; institute
measures to restore balance, including intravenous
fluid and electrolyte replacements; monitor daily
weights and intake and output, and assess skin turgor
for signs of *dehydration* or possible *overhydration* resulting from therapy.
- Provide emotional support to the child and family to
alleviate fears and anxieties.
- Anticipate administering ampicillin or trimethoprim-
sulfamethoxazole as prescribed for treatment.

# SHOCK, ANAPHYLACTIC

### DESCRIPTION

- Anaphylactic shock is an immediate hypersensitivity reaction.
- Symptoms appear within minutes of antigen invasion.
- The antigen could be an insect bite or an injection of a drug to which a child had been sensitized.

### ASSESSMENT FINDINGS

- Nausea
- *Vomiting*
- *Diarrhea*
- Bronchospasm
- Cyanosis
- Dyspnea
- Hypotension
- Bradycardia
- Seizures
- Death

### NURSING IMPLICATIONS

- Teach the parent and child with a known sensitivity to insects or drugs that prevention is key.
- Encourage the use of allergy bracelets for known hypersensitivities.
- Know the history of allergies of your client and keep it on the medication card.
- Advocate hyposensitivity therapy to children who have hypersensitive reactions to insect stings.
- If anaphylaxis does occur:
  Intervene immediately to maintain an airway and possibly treat *cardiopulmonary arrest.*
  Administer epinephrine subcutaneously into the opposite arm of the insect sting or injection.
- Place a tourniquet proximal to the site of allergenic source to decrease absorption.
- Administer aminophylline intravenously or a bronchodilator to halt wheezing.
- Give oxygen as necessary if cyanosis is present.
- Position the child supine to counteract hypotension.
- Control *urticaria* with diphenhydramine (Benadryl).
- Administer phenobarbital or diazepam for seizures.
- Reassure and calm the child and the family.

- Decrease anxiety in the child because it can potentiate bronchospasm.
- Teach the parents of children with hypersensitivities proper procedures to follow:
    Place ice on the site of injection.
    Administer epinephrine medication or inhalant.
    Call for emergency help.
- Caution the parents not to give oral medication to a comatose child.
- Recommend that parents purchase an emergency kit (Ana-Kit) for insect bites, which contains two measured doses of epinephrine and an antihistamine.
- Inform the parents and children of the potential for related substances to cause the same anaphylactic reaction.

## SINUSITIS

### DESCRIPTION

- Sinusitis, an infection of the sinuses, is rare in children under 6 years of age because the frontal sinuses do not develop until age 6.
- It may develop as a secondary infection when streptococcal, staphylococcal, or *Haemophilus influenzae* organisms spread from the nasal cavity.
- Sinusitis, considered by many adults to be minor, can have serious complications if the infection spreads from the sinuses to invade the bone (*osteomyelitis*) or middle ear (*otitis media*).
- Chronic sinusitis can interfere with school and social performance because of the constant pain.

### ASSESSMENT FINDINGS

- Fever
- Purulent nasal discharge
- Headache
- Tenderness over affected sinus
- Nose and throat culture positive for organism

### NURSING IMPLICATIONS

- Administer medications as prescribed, including antipyretic for fever, analgesic for pain, and antibiotic for specific organism.
- Instruct the parents to complete the full antibiotic regimen to prevent recurrence and complications.

- Administer nose drops such as phenylephrine or oxymetazoline (Afrin) as prescribed to relieve nasal congestion and promote drainage.
- Instruct the parents in the proper method to administer nose drops; teach them that the prolonged use of nasal drops or sprays can lead to nasal polyps.
- Encourage the parents to use the nose drops or sprays for only 3 days to prevent a rebound effect (causing more nasal congestion than originally present).
- Encourage use of warm compresses to the sinus area to promote drainage and relieve pain.

## SKULL FRACTURE

### DESCRIPTION

- A skull fracture refers to a crack in the bone of the skull.
- In children, associated cerebral injury often occurs under the fracture.
- Many skull fractures are simple linear types, most often involving the parietal bones.
- In some children, the skull does not fracture, but the suture lines separate (more commonly occurs in the lambdoid suture line); a coronal suture separation is rare and, if present, indicates severe *head trauma*.

### ASSESSMENT FINDINGS

- Orbital or postauricular ecchymosis (fracture of base of skull)
- Rhinorrhea or otorrhea; drainage positive for glucose
- Skull x-ray positive for fracture
- Shock (rare with isolated head injury)

### NURSING IMPLICATIONS

- Obtain a thorough history to determine the strength of the blow to the head.
- Test escaping drainage from the nose with glucose reagent strip to identify the source of the drainage—tests positive if cerebrospinal fluid.
- If shock is present, check for bleeding points other than the *head trauma*.
- If the skull fracture is linear:
    Observe the child for changes in level of consciousness; administer mild analgesic as prescribed.

Instruct the parents in observations to note and the need to report any changes immediately.

Assist the parents with scheduling a follow-up x-ray film in approximately 3 weeks to confirm that healing has taken place; reassure them that a second x-ray this soon is not harmful but necessary.

- If the fracture is depressed (a bone fragment is pressing inward) or compounded (bone is broken into pieces):

  Prepare the child and parents for surgery.

  Provide physical and psychological support to the child and parents; include all aspects of preoperative and postoperative care.

- Allow the child and parents to verbalize their feelings and fears related to the injury and possible surgery.

## SLIPPED CAPITAL FEMORAL EPIPHYSIS

### DESCRIPTION

- Slipped capital femoral epiphysis refers to a slipping of the femur head in relation to the neck of the femur at the epiphyseal line.
- The cartilage covering the femur head may be destroyed by necrosis, resulting in permanent loss of motion of the femur head.
- An avascular necrosis similar to *Legg-Calvé-Perthes* disease may occur.
- Slipped capital femoral epiphysis occurs most frequently in preadolescence, being twice as frequent in African-Americans as in other races and twice as frequent in boys as in girls.
- It is seen more commonly in obese or rapidly growing children than others, suggesting an influence of the growth hormone in the preadolescent.
- Although this condition usually is unilateral, about 30% of affected children later develop the same condition in the opposite hip.

### ASSESSMENT FINDINGS (gradual onset of symptoms)

- Leg held externally rotated
- Complaints of pain in knee first (because of the way child favors hip joint putting stress on the knee)
- Pain in hip joint

- Difficult, painful internal hip rotation on physical examination
- X-ray film positive for slipped epiphysis at the femur head

### NURSING IMPLICATIONS
- Obtain a thorough history and physical examination to establish a baseline and help with early detection.
- Anticipate the need for surgical correction before the condition has progressed to epiphyseal destruction.
- Prepare the child physically and psychologically for surgical correction by internal fixation to stabilize the femoral head; include all aspects of preoperative and postoperative care.
- Instruct the adolescent about the need for being confined to bed; encourage continued contact with friends to promote *adolescent growth and development.*
- Teach the adolescent that this is a potentially serious condition so that, although the adolescent may not like being confined, he or she can accept it as necessary to maintain good healing and function of the hip joint, promoting compliance.
- Instruct the adolescent and parents about the need for follow-up care, with careful attention to the possibility of the condition developing in the opposite hip.

## SPINA BIFIDA OCCULTA

### DESCRIPTION
- Spina bifida occulta refers to a type of *neural tube defect.*
- It occurs when the posterior laminae of the vertebrae fail to fuse.
- Spina bifida occulta is most commonly seen at the 5th lumbar or 1st sacral level; it also may occur at any point along the spinal canal.

### ASSESSMENT FINDINGS
- Noticeable dimpling at the point of poor fusion
- Abnormal tufts of hair at the site

### NURSING IMPLICATIONS
- Obtain a thorough history and physical examination to establish a baseline.

- Be aware that simple spina bifida occulta is a benign defect occurring as frequently as in 1 of every 4 children.
- Inform the parents of its existence so that they are not surprised when someone points it out to them later on.
- Make sure to use the proper terminology when discussing the condition so that the parents do not interpret it to mean that the child has an extremely serious defect.
- Tell the parents that the child needs no immediate surgical correction; inform them that some children may eventually need surgery to prevent vertebral deterioration owing to the unbalanced spinal column.

## SPINAL CORD INJURY

### DESCRIPTION

- Spinal cord injuries result when the cord becomes compressed or severed by the vertebrae.
- Further cord damage can be caused by hemorrhage, edema, or inflammation at the injury site as the blood supply becomes impeded.
- Because of the resilience of their vertebrae, children have fewer spinal cord injuries than adults; however, because of the increase in motorcycle accidents involving adolescents, spinal cord injuries in this age group are becoming more common.
- Another major cause of spinal cord injury is diving into too-shallow water.
- Following the injury, children pass through three different recovery phases: first, second, and third.
- In the first recovery phase, occurring immediately after the injury, the child experiences spinal shock syndrome (or loss of autonomic nervous system function) leading to a loss of motor function, sensation, and reflex activity and flaccid paralysis in the body areas below the level of the injury. This phase lasts from 1 to 6 weeks (the shorter the phase, the better the final outcome).
- During the second phase of recovery, spastic paralysis caused by the loss of upper level control or transmission of meaningful innervation to the lower muscles replaces the flaccid paralysis of the first phase. During this phase, if the child's bladder is allowed to fill, the resultant sensory stimulation relayed to the

damaged cord initiates a powerful sympathetic reflex reaction (autonomic dysreflexia), which if not relieved can result in a cerebrovascular accident from severe hypertension.

- The third phase of recovery is the final outcome or permanent limitation of motor and sensory function. If the compression of the spinal cord is due to edema that is then relieved, no permanent motor or sensory disability occurs.

ASSESSMENT FINDINGS (vary with the level of the injury)
- Loss of respiratory function (with cervical injury)
- Difficulty maintaining effective respirations (with high thoracic lesions)
- Hypothermia or hyperthermia (with high thoracic lesions)
- Hypotension from blood pooling in the lower body (with high thoracic lesions)
- Loss of bladder control (with high thoracic lesions)
- Distended bowel with absent bowel sounds (with high thoracic lesions)
- Loss of motor function
- Loss of sensation
- Loss of reflex activity
- Flaccid paralysis followed by spastic paralysis

NURSING IMPLICATIONS
- Suspect a spinal cord injury whenever a child has sustained a forceful trauma of any kind.
- Do not move the child with a suspected spinal cord injury until the back and head can be supported in a straight line to prevent further injury; in the emergency room, do not move the child from the admission stretcher to an examining table until spinal x-ray films are done.
- Use a log-rolling technique when moving the child to prevent further injury.
- If resuscitation is necessary, keep the head in a neutral position; do not hyperextend.
- Perform a thorough neurologic assessment to determine the level of injury.
- Maintain spinal immobilization during all procedures.
- Assess the child's status frequently, including vital signs, level of consciousness, and neurologic function.
- Anticipate the need for *assisted ventilation, tracheotomy,* or phrenic nerve pacemaker, if the cervical level

of the cord is involved; anticipate periodic intermittent positive pressure breathing treatments to increase lung filling if a thoracic level injury is present.

- Position the child carefully to prevent compromising any chest movement.
- Monitor the child's temperature closely and apply or remove additional coverings to maintain body temperature and prevent hypothermia or hyperthermia.
- Carefully assess the child's skin frequently because with the loss of sensation, the child is unable to report skin irritation.
- Turn the child every 2 hours and use alternating pressure pad mattresses or sheepskin to prevent skin breakdown.
- During the first phase of recovery:

  Anticipate using cervical traction with Crutchfield tongs and traction belt or Halo traction.

  Provide emotional support and education to the child and parents to alleviate their fears and anxieties regarding the insertion of tongs into the skull.

  Administer corticosteroids as prescribed to relieve edema at the injury site.

  Perform full-range-of-motion exercises at least 3 times per day to promote circulation and prevent loss of calcium resulting from inactivity.

  Insert an indwelling urinary drainage catheter as prescribed to prevent urinary retention; be aware that the bladder can also be emptied by periodic suprapubic aspiration or Credé's maneuver.

  Assist with measures to promote bowel elimination, such as using a stool softener or daily suppository.

- During the second phase of recovery:

  Administer muscles relaxants as prescribed to prevent painful muscle spasms.

  Hold the legs and arms at the joints to help reduce the spasms.

  Perform exercises for muscle strengthening to preserve remaining mobility.

  Gradually increase the angle of the bed to help the child become acclimated to the upright position without experiencing vascular pooling.

Encourage the child to drink cranberry juice or
administer ascorbic acid tablets as prescribed to
acidify the urine and limit bacterial growth.

Begin teaching about bowel elimination measures
to aid in defecation and self-catheterization or
Credé's maneuver to empty the bladder.

Introduce the child to self-help methods for
activities of daily living; arrange for physical and
occupational therapy consultation.

- Provide counseling and support to the parents and
child, offering suggestions and practical examples
about how to deal with any remaining limitations.
- Allow the child and parents to grieve about the loss of
function and lifetime disability, and encourage them
to verbalize their feelings about the injury and its effect on their lives.

## SPLENIC RUPTURE

### DESCRIPTION
- The spleen is the organ most frequently injured in
  *abdominal trauma* because in children this is usually
  palpable under the lower rib.
- Splenic rupture is an emergency situation because severe blood loss can result.

### ASSESSMENT FINDINGS
- Tenderness in left upper quadrant, especially on
  deep inspirations
- Elevation of left shoulder to minimize pain of
  inspiration
- Radiated left shoulder pain when lying supine
  (Kehr's sign)
- Fractured rib on x-ray film (possibly suggesting the
  extent of trauma to that area)
- Fluid in abdomen
- Abdominal paracentesis positive for blood

### NURSING IMPLICATIONS
- Obtain a thorough history and physical examination
  to establish a baseline and identify the extent of the
  traumatic injury.
- Prepare the child and parents for diagnostic testing,
  including intravenous pyelogram to rule out damage

to left kidney, which because of its location probably also suffered trauma.
- Administer intravenous fluids to replace fluid losses.
- Obtain a complete blood count, as prescribed, to estimate extent of blood loss; obtain a type and cross-match to have replacement readily available.
- Be aware that a child is admitted to the hospital for observation if blood loss appears mild; anticipate immediate surgery if blood loss appears severe.
- Prepare the child and parents for possible splenectomy to halt bleeding and save the child's life; provide preoperative and postoperative teaching as appropriate.
- If the spleen is removed, instruct the parents and child about measures to prevent or minimize infections, especially pneumococci infection; most children are immunized with pneumococci vaccine to prevent this possibility.

## SPRENGEL'S DEFECT

### DESCRIPTION
- Sprengel's defect is a congenital skeletal deformity of the scapulae.
- With this deformity, one scapula is turned horizontally.

### ASSESSMENT FINDINGS
- Affected scapulae higher than the opposite bone
- Inability to raise arm on affected side above a right angle with the body
- Head held toward affected side
- *Scoliosis* (developing when approaching school age)

### NURSING IMPLICATIONS
- Obtain a thorough history and physical examination, comparing both sides of the body, to establish a baseline.
- Prepare the child and parents for surgical intervention.
- Keep in mind that the surgical intervention is extreme and may not be advised for solely cosmetic reasons.

## STATUS ASTHMATICUS

### DESCRIPTION
- Status asthmaticus refers to an *asthma* attack that does not readily respond to treatment.

- Status asthmaticus is often caused by pulmonary infection, which acts as the triggering mechanism for the prolonged attack.
- It is an emergency situation because if the attack cannot be relieved, the child will die from heart failure owing to exhaustion, *atelectasis*, or respiratory acidosis from bronchial plugging.

### ASSESSMENT FINDINGS
- Positive sputum culture
- Cyanosis
- Dyspnea
- Retractions
- Nasal flaring
- Wheezing

### NURSING IMPLICATIONS
- Obtain a thorough history and physical examination to establish a baseline.
- Ascerain what medications the child has already taken or received.
- Obtain a sputum for culture; ensure that the sputum is coughed from deep in the respiratory tract and not just from the back of the throat.
- Administer broad-spectrum antibiotic as prescribed.
- Administer humidified oxygen by face mask or nasal prongs to improve oxygen saturation.
- Keep in mind that oxygen is best administered at a concentration of 30% to 40%.
- Be aware that some children in severe status asthmaticus have such a carbon dioxide buildup from their inability to exhale properly that they develop carbon dioxide narcosis with no stimulation for inhalation.
- Obtain arterial blood gases as prescribed to evaluate oxygenation status; use pulse oximetry to monitor the child's status.
- Be aware that in severe attacks, *assisted ventilation* may be necessary to maintain effective respirations.
- Administer medications as prescribed, such as epinephrine subcutaneously or aminophylline intravenously.
- Continuously assess the child's respiratory rate and appearance, pulse rate, and blood pressure, and auscultate lungs for breath sounds and wheezing.
- If the child is becoming acidotic, administer sodium bicarbonate as prescribed.

- Anticipate using corticosteroids, especially in children who are on continuous steroid therapy or who have been on it in the past.
- Encourage the child to drink fluids to keep airway secretions moist; do not offer cold fluids because these tend to aggravate bronchospasm; administer intravenous fluids as prescribed to treat possible dehydration.
- Do not administer any cough suppressants; coughing helps prevent mucous plug formation leading to *pneumonia, atelectasis,* and acidosis.
- Monitor fluid intake and output and measure the specific gravity of urine; under stress, antidiuretic hormone is released, so that fluid retention and over-hydration may occur.
- Have the child rest in an upright position to improve ventilatory effort; encourage the child to rest as much as possible to eliminate fatigue.
- Provide emotional support to the child and parents to help minimize anxiety.
- Be aware that sedation may be prescribed for the child who is hysterical with anxiety; however, excessive sedation makes it difficult for the child to raise mucus.

## STRAINS AND SPRAINS

### DESCRIPTION
- Strains and sprains are common but difficult traumatic childhood injuries to an extremity.
- A strain is a muscle tendon injury; a sprain is a ligament injury.
- Because casting and complete immobilization are not used to treat a strain or sprain, they are often more painful than *fractures*, which are casted.

### ASSESSMENT FINDINGS
- Painful and swollen joint
- Bruising (possible)
- No fracture on x-ray film

### NURSING IMPLICATIONS
- Assess the child's extremity closely for signs of bruising and swelling.
- Question the child about how the injury occurred.
- Evaluate the child's complaints of pain, including onset, duration, severity, and type.

- Anticipate x-ray to rule out fracture.
- If the injury is recent, apply an ice pack to the injured area for 20 minutes to attempt to reduce the swelling at the site.
- Apply an elastic bandage to provide support.
- Help the child and parents to understand that strains and sprains are truly painful; administer analgesics as prescribed.
- Prepare the child and parents for the possibility of crutches to limit weight bearing for the next 3 to 4 days.
- Teach the parents and child how to apply the elastic bandage and how to check for circulation to prevent circulatory compromise from wrapping the bandage too tightly.
- Instruct the child and parents in the proper use of crutches.
- Encourage medical follow-up to evaluate healing.

## STURGE-WEBER SYNDROME

### DESCRIPTION

- Sturge-Weber syndrome involves a congenital port-wine stain of the skin of the face that extends to the meninges and choroid.
- The skin manifestation follows the distribution of the 5th cranial nerve (trigeminal nerve).
- The skin lesion is generally unilateral and sometimes is confined to the upper aspect of the face.

### ASSESSMENT FINDINGS (possible)

- Hemiparesis on side opposite the lesion
- Mental deficiency
- Intractable *seizures*
- Blindness
- Calcification in involved cerebral cortex on computed tomography or magnetic resonance imaging scanning; calcification following a diagnostic "railroad track" or double-groove pattern

### NURSING IMPLICATIONS

- Help parents accept the central nervous system component to this syndrome.
- Stress the importance of continued follow-up as the child grows, so symptoms can be identified and treated.

- Explain that surgery may be performed to relieve
  *seizures* in some children.

## SUBDURAL HEMATOMA

### DESCRIPTION

- Subdural hematoma is venous bleeding into the space
  between the dura and arachnoid membrane.
- It occurs when head trauma lacerates minute veins in
  this area.
- Subdural hematomas tend to occur in infants more
  than older children.
- Symptoms may occur within 3 days of trauma or as
  late as 20 days and generally reflect i*ncreased intracranial pressure* in infants.

### ASSESSMENT FINDINGS

- *Seizures*
- *Vomiting*
- Hyperirritability
- Head enlargement
- Anemia
- Extent of hematoma noted on angiocardiography
  or sonogram

### NURSING IMPLICATIONS

- Monitor for signs of *increased intracranial pressure.*
- Assist with subdural puncture to remove accumulated
  blood in infants.
- Make certain that the infant is held extremely still
  during the procedure.
- Anticipate daily subdural punctures until the space
  is empty.
- Prepare older children and infants with continued active bleeding following 2 weeks of subdural punctures
  for surgery.
- Explain the nature of the injury and the therapy and
  provide support to parents.

## SUICIDE

### DESCRIPTION

- Suicide is deliberate self-injury with the intent to end
  one's life.
- Successful suicide occurs more frequently in males than
  in females, although more females attempt suicide.
- Suicide ranks third as a cause of death in the 15- to
  19-year-old age group.

S

- Incest, increased chemical dependency, marital instability in the family, and poor problem-solving ability are reasons that may lead the adolescent to consider suicide.
- Loss is the trigger that most often precipitates suicide.
- Anger, trying to get even, and manipulation are other reasons that adolescents attempt suicide.
- If another member of the family, close friend, or another student has committed suicide, the chance that an adolescent will do so is greater.

**ASSESSMENT FINDINGS** (danger signs)
- Giving away prized possessions
- Organ donation questions
- Sudden, unexplained elevation in mood
- Accident proneness, carelessness, and death wishes
- Statements, such as "This is the last time you will see me"
- Decrease in verbal communication
- Withdrawal from peer activities
- Previous suicide attempts
- Preference for art, music, and literature with themes of death
- Recent increase in interpersonal conflict with significant others
- Running away from home
- Inquiring about the hereafter
- Asking for information (supposedly for a friend) about suicide prevention and intervention
- Almost any sustained deviation from the normal behavior pattern

**NURSING IMPLICATIONS**
- Watch for signs of depression during health maintenance visits.
- Follow-up on a history that the child is frequently absent from school, has failing grades, is a "loner," or is a "perfect" student and especially if the child has suffered a recent loss.
- Provide or obtain immediate crisis intervention for adolescents who are contemplating suicide, which includes trying to alleviate pain and depression and counseling them in an effort to help them change their perspective on the value of life.
- Encourage the adolescent to speak honestly about thoughts of suicide and the problems that have led them to thinking death is a solution.

- Help adolescents develop better problem-solving skills.
- Recommend a period of observation in a hospital adolescent unit after a suicide attempt.
- Refer the adolescent to a consultant well versed in suicide prevention for additional therapy and continuing evaluation.
- Explain that antidepressant medication alone may be of little value.
- Encourage family assessment and family counseling.

## SYNOVITIS

### DESCRIPTION

- Synovitis is an acute, nonpurulent inflammation of the synovial membrane of a joint, most commonly affecting the hip joint in children.
- Incidence peaks between 2 and 10 years of age.

### ASSESSMENT FINDINGS

- Pain in the groin, lower portion of thigh, knee, or buttocks
- Pain worse in morning on arising and later in the day
- Joint held flexed in a position of comfort
- Pain on examination with range-of-motion exercises
- Capsular swelling of involved joint on x-ray
- Feeling of well-being otherwise

### NURSING IMPLICATIONS

- Explain the need for bed rest until muscle spasm from pain has passed, usually in 3 days but possibly 10 to 14 days in some children.
- If flexion contractures occur, anticipate countertraction.
- Inform parents and children about the simple inflammatory process occurring, and reassure them that the disorder will heal without sequelae.

## SYSTEMIC LUPUS ERYTHEMATOSUS (SLE)

### DESCRIPTION

- SLE is an autoimmune disease in which autoantibodies and antigens cause deposit of complement in the kidney glomerulus.
- Approximately two-thirds of children with SLE develop symptoms of *acute* or *chronic glomerulonephritis.*
- This renal disease is the ultimate form of death in many adults with SLE.

### ASSESSMENT FINDINGS
- *Hypertension*
- Hematuria
- Decreased urine output
- Proteinuria
- Edema
- Elevated blood urea nitrogen and serum creatinine levels

### NURSING IMPLICATIONS
- Explain the disorder to the parents and child.
- Provide teaching about diagnostic testing procedures.
- Explain drug therapy, which may include corticosteroids or cytotoxic agents.

## TALIPES DEFORMITIES

### DESCRIPTION
- Talipes deformities are ankle-foot deformities, popularly called clubfoot.
- Talipes deformities occur more often in males than in females and are probably inherited as a polygenic pattern.
- The deformity usually occurs only as a unilateral problem.
- Pseudotalipes deformity from intrauterine position refers to the appearance of a turned-in foot that can be brought into good position by manipulation.
- The earlier a true talipes deformity is recognized and treated, the better the results.

### ASSESSMENT FINDINGS (one or a combination of the following)
- Plantar flexion—equinus or "horse-foot" position
- Dorsiflexion—heel held lower than the foot, or the anterior foot flexed toward the anterior leg
- Varus deviation—foot turns in
- Valgus deviation—foot turns out
- Equinovarus—foot points downward and inward and front of the foot curls toward heel
- Calcaneovalgus—walking on heel with foot everted

### NURSING IMPLICATIONS
- Straighten all newborn feet to the midline as part of initial assessment to detect this defect.

- Reassure parents, that in contrast to ineffective treatment years ago, correction with good orthopedic techniques available today should leave the child with no permanent foot deformity.
- Do not use the term "clubfoot" because it may imply permanent crippling to parents.
- Explain the casting procedure to parents of the newborn with this deformity and reassure them that the high cast extending over the knee does not imply an extensive problem.
- Teach related cast care; stress the need to change diapers frequently, to check circulation in toes, and to investigate all crying episodes.
- Explain the need for recasting every week or every other week because of infant's rapid growth.
- Stress the importance of performing passive foot exercises for several months following final removal of cast, at about 6 weeks.
- Explain the application of a Denis-Browne splint if prescribed for the child during sleep.
- If the child does not achieve correction by casting, prepare the parents and child for surgery to achieve a final correction.

## TAY-SACHS DISEASE

### DESCRIPTION

- Tay-Sachs disease is an autosomal recessive inherited disease in which the infant lacks hexosaminidase A, an enzyme necessary for lipid metabolism.
- Without this enzyme, lipid deposits accumulate on nerve cells, leading to *mental retardation* when deposits are on brain cells and blindness when deposits are on optic nerve cells.
- There is no cure for this disorder.
- Most children die of cachexia and *pneumonia* by 3 to 5 years of age.
- Carriers for the disease trait may be identified by hexosaminidase A assay.

### ASSESSMENT FINDINGS

- Ashkenazic Jewish heritage
- Extreme Moro reflex and mild hypotonia (early months of life)

- Loss of head control and inability to roll over or sit up without support (about 6 months of age)
- Cherry-red macula on ophthalmoscopic examination
- Spasticity symptoms (by 1 year of age)
- Inability to perform simple motor tasks (by 1 year of age)
- Generalized *seizures* and blindness (by 2 years of age)

#### Nursing Implications
- Provide intensive support for the child and parents.
- Be honest with the parents in discussing options.
- Explain that this disease may be detected in utero by amniocentesis.
- Recommend genetic counseling to parents.

## TETANUS

#### Description
- Tetanus (lockjaw) is a highly fatal disease caused by an anaerobic, spore-forming bacillus.
- The bacillus is found in soil and in the excrement of human animals, and it enters the body through a wound, such as a deep puncture wound or burn.
- As the bacilli grow in the body, they produce exotoxins that cause the disease symptoms by affecting the motor nuclei of the central nervous system.
- Death is usually due to asphyxiation; although survival is possible.

#### Assessment Findings
- Stiffness of the neck and jaw
- Muscular rigidity of the trunk and body (within 24 to 48 hours)
- Arched back (opisthotonus)
- Stiff, boardlike abdominal muscles
- Fever (ominous sign)
- Unusual facial appearance with wrinkling of the forehead and distortion of the corners of the mouth (sardonic grin)
- Painful, paroxysmal spasms on stimulation
- Clear sensorium
- Laryngospasm
- Airway obstruction

#### Nursing Implications
##### Prevention

- Help prevent tetanus by promoting active *immuniza- tion* as part of routine DPT *immunization* and suitable booster *immunization* at school age and every 10 years thereafter.
- Wash all wounds thoroughly with soap and water and a suitable antiseptic.
- If the child has a wound and you cannot locate the *immunization* record or if it has been more than 10 years since a booster injection, expect to administer a booster injection and tetanus immune globulin.
- If the child received basic *immunization* against tetanus (5 doses) and it has been fewer than 10 years since the last injection, anticipate that no booster or antitoxin management will be necessary at the time of the wound.

##### Treatment

- Provide care in a quiet, stimulation-free room.
- Provide tube feedings or total parenteral nutrition if prescribed.
- Administer prescribed medications, which may include tetanus immune globulin, parenteral penicillin G or a form of tetracycline, a sedative, and a muscle relaxant.
- If d-tubocurarine is to be administered, have intuba- tion and ventilation equipment available to maintain respiratory function because this drug produces sys- temic paralysis.
- Provide emotional support to the child and parents.

## THALASSEMIA

#### Description

- Thalassemia refers to an anemia involving problems with hemoglobin.
- There are two major types of thalassemia: *thalassemia major* and *thalassemia minor*.
- *Thalassemia major* (homozygous β-thalassemia) is an anemia in which the child is unable to produce nor- mal beta hemoglobim.

    This disorder is also called Cooley's anemia or Mediterranean anemia and is most prevalent in the Mediterranean population but also occurs in children of African and Asian heritage.

    Symptoms do not become apparent until the child's fetal hemoglobin has largely been replaced

by adult hemoglobin during the second half of
the first year.

Resulting hypertrophy of bone marrow,
hemosiderosis (excessive deposition of iron in
body tissues), and cardiac decompensation can
cause serious problems.

The prognosis is improving but still grave; most
children with the disease die from cardiac failure
during adolescense or as young adults.

- *Thalassemia minor* (heterozygous β-thalassemia) is an
anemia in which the child produces both defective
beta hemoglobin and normal hemoglobin.

This disorder is a minor form of anemia, requiring
no treatment.

This condition represents the heterozygous form of
the disorder or can be compared with children
having the sickle cell trait.

### ASSESSMENT FINDINGS
#### Thalassemia major

- Pallor
- Irritability
- Anorexia
- Increased facial-mandibular growth; slanted eyes;
broad, flattened base of nose; and malocclusion
- Jaundice possible
- Bone pain
- Hepatosplenomegaly possible
- *Epistaxis*
- Arrhythmias (possible)
- Cardiac murmur (possible)
- Hypochromic, microcytic red blood cells
- Hemoglobin level less than 5 g/100 ml
- High serum iron level; iron saturation at 100%

#### Thalassemia minor

- Pallor
- Normal red blood cell count
- Hemoglobin concentration level decreased 2 to
3 g/100 ml below normal levels
- Moderately hypochromic and microcytic red
blood cells

### NURSING IMPLICATIONS
#### Thalassemia major

- Help the child accept a permanently altered appearance, and promote interaction with peers.

- Encourage the parents to allow the child as much activity as possible and to permit attendance at regular school.
- Explain the benefits associated with hypertransfusion therapy: suppresses erythropoiesis; keeps facial alterations, osteoporosis, and cardiac dilatation to a minimum; and reduces possibility of splenectomy.
- Explain the risks associated with hypertransfusion therapy: *hepatitis B* and C, *acquired immunodeficiency syndrome,* and hemosiderosis.
- Provide teaching about measures to help prevent *congestive heart failure,* such as digitalis administration, diuretic therapy, and low-sodium diet.
- If splenectomy is planned, provide preoperative and postoperative care, and stress measures to prevent infection because the child will be more susceptible after this surgery.

### Thalassemia minor
- Provide information about the nature of the disorder.
- Provide reassurance that life expectancy is normal.
- Inform the parents that the child should not receive a routine iron supplement because the child's inability to incorporate it well into hemoglobin may cause him or her to accumulate too much iron.

## THYROIDITIS

### DESCRIPTION
- Thyroiditis (Hashimoto's disease) is the most common form of acquired hypothyroidism in childhood.
- The age of onset is 10 to 11 years.
- There may be a familial history of thyroid disease, occurring more often in females than in males.
- The decrease in thyroid secretion is caused by the development of an autoimmune phenomenon that interferes with thyroid production.
- Thyroid-stimulating hormone (TSH) stimulation from the pituitary gland increases when thyroid hormone production decreases in an attempt to cause the thyroid to be more effective.

### ASSESSMENT FINDINGS
- Hypertrophy of the thyroid (goiter)
- Nodular thyroid (possible)
- Impaired growth
- Obesity

- Lethargy
- Delayed sexual development
- Presence of antithyroid antibodies in serum
- Rapid radioactive iodine uptake with benign thyroid nodes (if no uptake, carcinoma is likely, a rare finding)

### NURSING IMPLICATIONS
- Report any suspected cases of thyroiditis promptly to permit diagnosis and early treatment before the epiphyseal lines close at puberty.
- Explain the disorder to the child and parents.
- Provide information about administration of synthetic thyroid hormone (sodium levothyroxine), the treatment for thyroiditis.
- Explain that with adequate dosage, the obesity should fade and growth will begin again.

## TIC DISORDERS

### DESCRIPTION
- Tic disorders are abnormalities of semi-involuntary movement thought to result from dysfunction in the basal ganglia.
- Tics are rapid, repetitive muscle movements, such as rapid eye blinking or facial twitching.
- Tics are more usually pronounced during periods of stress and usually diminish in sleep.
- These disorders tend to be familial, affecting males more frequently than females and usually occurring between the ages of 9 and 13.
- The tic disorders are classified into Tourette's syndrome, chronic motor or vocal tic disorder, and transient tic disorder.
- Tourette's syndrome is an inherited disorder in which the child suffers from a syndrome of facial and complex vocal tics.

### ASSESSMENT FINDINGS
#### *Motor tics (rapid, repetitive)*
- Eye blinking
- Neck jerking
- Facial grimacing
#### *Vocal tics (rapid, repetitive)*
- Coughing
- Throat clearing

- Snorting
- Barking

***Complex motor ticks (rapid, repetitive)***
- Facial gestures
- Grooming behaviors
- Jumping
- Touching an object
- Smelling an object

***Complex vocal ticks (Tourette's syndrome)***
- Coprolalia, the repeated use of socially unacceptable words, usually obscenities
- Palilalia, repeating one's own words
- Echolalia, repeating the last sound heard or the phrase of another person

### Nursing Implications
- Help the child and family reduce areas of stress in the child's life.
- Tell the parents not to point out the mannerisms to the child because this may intensify the manifestation.
- Provide emotional support and encouragement for the child with a tic disorder, especially Tourette's syndrome, which lasts a lifetime.
- Inform the parents and child about behavior modification programs, which may be successful in curing a particular tic.
- Explain that Tourette's syndrome responds to administration of dopamine receptor blockers, such as haloperidol or fluphenazine; provide drug information.

## TONSILLITIS

### Description
- Tonsillitis refers to infection and inflammation of the palatine tonsils, located on both sides of the pharynx.
- Tonsillar tissue is lymphoid tissue that acts to form antibodies and to filter pathogenic organisms from the head and neck area.
- Currently, tonsillectomy, removal of the palatine tonsils, is not recommended unless all other measures prove ineffective.

### Assessment Findings
- Drooling
- Sore throat
- High fever

- Lethargy
- Pus on or expelled from crypts of the tonsils
- Group A beta-hemolytic streptococcus common on throat culture

### NURSING IMPLICATIONS

- Instruct the parents about prescribed antipyretics and analgesics.
- Explain the need to complete the full 10-day course of antibiotic therapy, despite improved symptoms.
- If a tonsillectomy is planned, provide necessary teaching, including the reason why surgery cannot be performed while tonsils are infected.

    Before surgery, check to be certain that bleeding and clotting times, complete blood count, and urinalysis have been done and that the child does not have any loose teeth.

    Following tonsillectomy, position the child on the abdomen with a pillow under the chest to promote drainage from the child's mouth.

    Monitor vital signs frequently to check for signs of hemorrhage, and observe for other subtle signs, such as frequent swallowing, throat clearing, and a feeling of anxiety.

    If bleeding does occur, elevate the child's head and turn him or her on the side, and notify the physician.

    Anticipate a return to surgery if hemorrhage is extreme.

    If inspiratory stridor, increased respiratory rate, and cyanosis occur, suspect pharyngeal obstruction caused by local bleeding and clot formation, and notify the surgeon immediately.

    If appropriate, extend the child's head and neck over the edge of the bed and strike the back sharply to help dislodge the obstruction.

    Have suctioning equipment available to clear an obstruction but keep in mind that this procedure may initiate fresh bleeding.

    Offer frequent sips of clear liquid or ice chips as soon as the child has completely awakened from the anesthesia.

    Do not offer dairy products, carbonated beverages, or acid juices.

Tell the parents to progress to a soft diet in 24 to
48 hours and a selective diet by the second week.
Provide teaching to the parents, including danger
signs to watch for, need for activity restriction until after the 7th postoperative day, telephone number to use if they have a question, and need to keep
follow-up appointment in approximately 2 weeks.

## TORTICOLLIS

### DESCRIPTION
- Torticollis or wry neck occurs as a congenital anomaly
  when the sternocleidomastoid muscle is injured during birth.
- This tends to occur in infants with wide shoulders
  when pressure is exerted on the head to deliver the
  shoulder.
- The injury may not be noticeable at birth and may
  become evident when fibrous contraction occurs at
  1 to 2 months.
- Torticollis can lead to one shoulder continuing to
  be elevated with the potential to lead to scoliosis later
  in life.

### ASSESSMENT FINDINGS
- Head held tilted to the side of the muscle in-
  volved; head rotates to the opposite side
- Palpable mass

### NURSING IMPLICATIONS
- Teach the parents the importance of passive stretching
  exercises and encouraging the infant to look in the
  direction of the affected muscle.
- Explore with the parents ways in which daily activities
  can be carried out so that the infant looks in the desired direction.
- Explain that this therapy is usually effective, and further treatment is generally not necessary.
- If the exercises are not effective, however, and the
  condition still exists in a year, prepare the parents and
  child for surgery followed by a neck immobilizer.

## TOXIC SHOCK SYNDROME (TSS)

### DESCRIPTION
- TSS is an infection by toxin-producing strains of
  *Staphylococcus aureus* organisms.

- Organisms typically enter the body through vaginal walls damaged by the insertion of tampons at the time of a menstrual period.
- The risk of developing TSS is highest in young women.
- TSS reached its peak in 1980 and then incidence declined because women have become more cautious about heavy tampon usage.

## ASSESSMENT FINDINGS

- Temperature more than 38.9°C (102°F)
- *Vomiting*
- *Diarrhea*
- A macular (sunburnlike) rash that desquamates on palms and soles 1 to 2 weeks after illness
- Severe hypotension (systolic pressure less than 90 mm Hg)
- Shock, leading to poor organ perfusion
- Elevated blood urea nitrogen or creatinine level at least twice the upper limit of normal
- Severe muscle pain or creatine phosphokinase level at least twice the upper limit of normal
- Hyperemia of mucous membrane
- Impaired liver function with increased total bilirubin and increased glutamic-oxaloacetic transaminase levels at twice the upper limit of normal
- Decreased platelet count
- Central nervous system symptoms of disorientation, confusion, and severe headache

## NURSING IMPLICATIONS

- Explain the need for vaginal examination, removal of all tampon particles, and cervical and vaginal cultures for *S. aureus.*
- Administer penicillinase-resistant antibiotics, as prescribed.
- If warranted, administer prescribed intravenous fluids or vasopressors, such as dopamine.
- Administer diuretics if prescribed, and, if needed, implement measures to combat renal failure or cardiac failure.
- Explain that not using tampons helps prevent TSS, but if tampons are used, they should not be highly absorbent.

- Teach women to change tampons at least every 4 hours during use and to use sanitary pads at night instead of tampons.
- Tell women not to insert more than one tampon at a time, to avoid handling the portion of the tampon that will be inserted, and to avoid tampon use near the end of a menstrual flow.
- Also, discourage women from using deodorant tampons, deodorant sanitary pads, or feminine hygiene sprays.
- Instruct women to discontinue tampon use and immediately contact a health care provider if fever, *vomiting,* or *diarrhea* occur during a menstrual period.
- Discourage women who have had one episode of TSS from using tampons or at least not until two vaginal cultures for *S. aureus* are negative.

# TRACHEOESOPHAGEAL ATRESIA AND FISTULA

## DESCRIPTION

- Esophageal atresia (stricture) and fistulas (openings) are congenital anomalies resulting from some teratogen that does not allow the esophagus and trachea to separate normally.
- In the most frequent type of esophageal atresia, the esophagus ends in a blind pouch, and the trachea communicates by a fistula with the lower esophagus and stomach.
- The type occurring next in frequency is one in which both upper and lower segments end in blind pouches.
- The type occurring third in frequency is one in which both upper and lower segments of the esophagus communicate with the trachea.
- These are serious disorders because during a feeding, milk can fill the blind esophagus and overflow into the trachea, or a fistula can allow milk to enter the trachea, resulting in *aspiration.*
- Mortality rate is as high as 40% and is associated with presence of other congenital anomalies or low birth weight.

## ASSESSMENT FINDINGS

- Mucus accumulation in the mouth giving appearance of blowing bubbles
- Cough during first feeding

- Cyanosis with first feeding
- Obvious difficulty breathing associated with first feeding
- Catheter unable to be passed through the esophagus to the stomach and stomach contents aspirated
- Radiopaque catheter coiled in the blind end of the esophagus on x-ray film
- Possible stomach dilatation with air from trachea per flat plate of the abdomen
- Blind-end esophagus and fistula visualized per barium swallow or bronchial endoscopy

## Nursing Implications

- Prepare the parents and infant for emergency surgery essential to prevent *pneumonia, dehydration,* or electrolyte imbalance.
- Before surgery, keep the infant in an upright position and on the right side and perform oropharyngeal suction frequently to prevent aspiration of mucous.
- Check functioning of catheter if passed into the blind-end esophagus and connected to low suction; irrigate as needed.
- If surgery is to be delayed and a cervical esophagostomy is performed so mucus can drain, implement measures to protect the skin.
- Preoperatively, monitor drainage from gastrostomy, if performed to keep the stomach empty of secretions.
- Keep the infant in an isolette with high humidity to maintain body heat and liquefy bronchial secretions.
- Preoperatively, try to prevent crying, which causes air from the trachea to distend the stomach resulting in vomiting into the lungs.
- Administer antibiotics, if prescribed, to help prevent right upper lobe *pneumonia.*
- Administer prescribed intravenous fluids preoperatively and for a time postoperatively.
- Following surgery, provide care associated with chest tubes, and monitor for signs of respiratory distress.
- Keep an infant laryngoscope and endotracheal tube at bedside in case extreme edema develops causing airway obstruction.
- Continue to suction frequently but only shallowly to prevent catheter from touching esophageal suture line.
- Turn the child frequently and permit crying to help expand lung tissue following surgery.

- Administer gastrostomy feedings postoperatively when prescribed, making certain to introduce the feedings slowly and always allowing them to run by gravity.
- Offer a pacifier to provide sucking pleasure during feedings.
- Offer sips of clear fluid by mouth only when prescribed, and anticipate beginning a full oral fluid diet when the suture line is healed and the infant can tolerate it.
- Be especially vigilant during postoperative days 7 to 10, when sutures dissolve, because fluid and air may leak out into the chest cavity, and *pneumothorax* may occur.
- Teach the parents how to perform gastrostomy feedings only if the child is to return home with the tube in place awaiting a second-stage operation.
- Explain the need for esophageal dilatation at period intervals if stenosis or stricture at the anastomosis site occurs.

## TRACHEOTOMY

### DESCRIPTION

- A tracheotomy is a temporary opening into the trachea to relieve airway obstruction that has occurred above that point.
- Tracheotomy may also be used when accumulating mucus causes lower airway obstruction because accumulated fluid can be suctioned through the tracheotomy.
- Tracheotomy interferes with the cleansing action of the mucous membrane lining the airway and eliminates the warming and filtering action of the nose and pharynx.
- Therefore, *endotracheal intubation,* not tracheotomy, has become the method of choice to relieve airway obstruction except if the obstruction is in the pharynx because it is impossible to pass an endotracheal tube beyond this point.

### NURSING IMPLICATIONS

- Assist with emergency tracheotomy, as needed.
- Have suction equipment available for immediate use to clear blood from the incision and any obstructing mucus.

- Following tracheotomy, reassure the child, especially concerning inability to speak.
- Explain to the parents why the tracheotomy was necessary; assure them it is a temporary measure (provided that this is true).
- Suction frequently (perhaps as often as every 15 minutes), gently, yet thoroughly.
- Be certain you know how deeply you should suction.
- Administer oxygen or ventilate with Ambu bag for 5 minutes before the suctioning procedure.
- If prescribed, administer 1 or 2 ml of sterile saline into the tracheotomy tube before suctioning to loosen secretions; this is controversial, however, because it induces violent coughing.
- Apply elbow restraints to young children as needed during suctioning and possibly at all times when they are alone.
- Encourage the parents to support the child after suctioning rather than to learn the suctioning technique, unless the tracheotomy tube is to be left in place following discharge.
- Assess the child frequently to make certain he or she is not having respiratory difficulty.
- Spend time playing with or comforting the child so he or she thinks of you in other ways than just the person who comes to suction them.
- Check tracheotomy ties frequently to be sure they are secure.
- For preschoolers or younger children, consider covering the tracheotomy opening with a gauze square tied to the child's neck like a bib during eating to prevent crumbs or spilled liquids from entering the tracheotomy.
- Do not give children small toys that could possibly fit into the lumen of the tube and cause obstruction.
- If the child dislodges the tracheotomy tube, calmly and quickly slide the obdurator into the tube and gently replace it in the tracheal opening.
- If an inner cannula type is used, remove and clean the inner cannula using sterile technique, at least every 8 hours.
- Following cleaning, dry the inner cannula thoroughly before replacing it.

# TRACTION, SKELETAL

### DESCRIPTION

- Skeletal traction involves pulling on a body part in one direction against a counterpull (provided by bone) exerted in the opposite direction.
- Skeletal traction is used when a longer period of traction or greater strength of traction is needed.
- Skeletal traction involves the use of a Steinmann pin or a Kirschner wire passed through the skin into the end of a long bone.
- The area of insertion is shaved and prepared with an antiseptic.
- The pin is usually inserted under general anesthesia in the operating room.
- Ropes strung over pulleys and attached to weights exert a pull on the extremity at the pin site.

### NURSING IMPLICATIONS

- Observe the pin site daily for drainage, and perform pin site care as prescribed.
- Report signs of infection, such as excessive drainage or erythema at the pin site.
- Check the extremity in traction every 15 minutes during the first hour, hourly for 24 hours, and every 4 hours thereafter for signs of pallor, coldness, tingling, lack of peripheral pulses, edema, or pain.
- Assess for *hypertension* daily.
- Provide good skin care on the child's back, elbow, and heels.
- Encourage the child to use an overhead trapeze to help position himself or herself.
- Do not inadvertently move the weights or interfere with traction as you are administering care.
- Keep the child informed of his or her progress, especially because the child cannot see it.
- Provide activities appropriate to the child's age group.

# TRACTION, SKIN

### DESCRIPTION

- Skin traction involves pulling on a body part in one direction against a counterpull (provided by the skin) exerted in the opposite direction.

- Skin traction is used when only minimal traction is necessary; the child's skin must be in good condition.
- Bryant's traction, a form of skin traction, is used to treat fractured femurs in children under 2 years of age.
- Bryant's traction is also used as preparation for surgical repair of congenital developmental defects, such as developmental *hip dysplasia.*
- Buck's extension is an example of a skin traction used for immobilizing *fractures* in older children.

### Nursing Implications
- Assist in application of skin traction: Skin is coated with tincture of benzoin; moleskin or adhesive backed strips are molded to the extremity; the moleskin and a metal or wooden footplate are held in place by an elastic bandage wrap; ropes are attached to the wood or metal plate at the distal end of the extremity; ropes pass over pulleys attached to an orthopedic frame over the bed; weights attached to the end of the ropes exert traction or pull on the extremity.
- Check the extremity in traction every 15 minutes during the first hour, hourly for 24 hours, and every 4 hours thereafter for signs of pallor, coldness, tingling, lack of peripheral pulses, edema, or pain.
- Assess for *hypertension* daily.
- Provide good skin care on the child's back, elbows, and heels.
- Encourage the child to use an overhead trapeze to help position himself or herself.
- Do not inadvertently move the weights or interfere with traction as you are administering care; allow the weights to hang freely.
- Keep the child informed of his or her progress, especially because the child cannot see it.
- Provide activities appropriate to the child's age group.

## TRAUMA, HEAD

### Description
- Head injuries are serious not only because they cause an immediate life threat to the child, but also because a number of complications, such as *seizures,* memory deficits, minor personality changes, behavior manifes-

tations, headache, and postural vertigo, may follow head injury.
- Children receive head injuries during multiple trauma accidents, such as automobile accidents; falls, especially from bicycles; and when struck on the head by hard objects.

**ASSESSMENT FINDINGS** (with *increased intracranial pressure*)
- Pupils unable to react immediately
- Decreased level of consciousness
- Decreased motor ability
- Decreased pulse rate
- Decreased respiratory rate
- Increased temperature
- Increased pulse pressure (the difference between systolic and diastolic blood pressure)

**NURSING IMPLICATIONS**
- Stabilize the neck with a brace until cervical trauma has been ruled out.
- Monitor for signs of *increased intracranial pressure.*
- Anticipate insertion of central venous line and arterial line to monitor the child's hemodynamic status.
- Prepare the child and parents for computed tomography scan.
- If intracranial pressure monitoring is initiated, provide associated care and obtain pressure readings.
- Position the child with head slightly elevated to help decrease cerebral edema.
- If hypertonic solutions are infused to decrease brain edema, assess vital signs frequently, checking for intravascular fluid overload; monitor intake and output, and test urine specific gravity.
- Administer steroids if prescribed to decrease inflammation and edema.
- If *endotracheal intubation* and hyperventilation are prescribed to reduce intracranial pressure, keep in mind that the goal is to keep the $PCO_2$ below 25 mm Hg.
- Provide information as it is available to the parents, and urge them to help care for the child to increase their sense of control.
- To help prevent serious head injury, teach bicycle safety, especially the use of safety helmets, to school-age children, and encourage the use of child restraint seats and seat belts.

# TUBERCULOSIS

### DESCRIPTION

- Tuberculosis is a highly contagious pulmonary disease caused by the organism *Mycobacterium tuberculosis* (tubercle bacillus).
- The mode of transmission is inhalation of infected droplets.
- The incubation period is from 2 to 10 weeks.
- Nonwhite children are more susceptible than white children.
- Children with chronic illness or malnutrition are more susceptible than healthy children.
- The development of a primary focus, where the organism is walled off and permanently confined to a lung area, is the most common form of tuberculosis in children.
- If the child is in poor health or does not have adequate calcium intake to confine the infection, tuberculosis may spread to other lung areas or to other parts of the body (miliary tuberculosis).

### ASSESSMENT FINDINGS

- History of recent contact (suggestive finding)
- Slight cough (with primary inflammation)
- Anorexia (with miliary tuberculosis)
- Weight loss (with miliary tuberculosis)
- Night sweats (with miliary tuberculosis)
- Low-grade fever (with miliary tuberculosis)
- Positive tine test or Mantoux test (formation of one or more papules, 2 mm or larger in diameter)
- Positive sputum specimen by deep expectoration or gastric lavage
- Developing cloudiness and eventually calcification on chest film

### NURSING IMPLICATIONS

- If prescribed, administer para-aminosalicylic acid (PAS) after meals and never on an empty stomach.
- If isoniazid (INH), the drug of choice, is prescribed, administer it concurrently with pyridoxine (vitamin $B_6$) to help prevent peripheral neurologic symptoms.
- Do not expect to administer ethambutol to infants or long-term to young children because one side effect is optic neuritis, which is difficult to detect

because of inability to perform adequate eye examinations.

- If streptomycin is prescribed for the child with severe or progressive infection, teach the parents to monitor for signs of 8th cranial nerve deficit, such as pulling at an ear, cocking the head, or unsteady gait.
- Administer a diet high in protein, calcium, and pyridoxine.
- Inform the parents that drug therapy may continue for up to 18 months and that the child should have chest x-rays at yearly intervals for the rest of his or her life.
- Caution the parents about reactivation risks for the child during any chronic illness interfering with calcium intake, and stress the need to obtain regular childhood *immunizations,* especially against pertussis (*whooping cough*).
- Explain that women with a history of tuberculosis as a child should inform their obstetrician because lung changes in pregnancy may lead to tuberculosis reactivation.
- Although not routinely used with children, the bacille Calmette-Guérin (BCG) vaccine, if administered, always results in a positive skin test.
- Explain that the child with primary tuberculosis is not infectious because he or she has minimal pulmonary lesions and little or no cough; the child does not need isolation and can return to school following the start of chemotherapy and disappearance of symptoms.
- When any family member contracts tuberculosis, encourage all family members to have skin tests to screen for the disease.

## ULCERATIVE COLITIS

### DESCRIPTION

- Ulcerative colitis and *Crohn's disease* are categorized as inflammatory bowel diseases.
- Ulcerative colitis results in the development of ulceration of mucosa or submucosa layers of the entire lower bowel.
- Incidence is highest in the following groups: young adults and adolescents, Jewish children, families with a tendency toward *allergy,* and the white population.
- The cause is obscure, although there is a familial tendency; ulcerative colitis probably represents an

alteration in the immune system or an autoimmune process.
- Psychological factors and gastroenteritis appear to exacerbate the condition.
- There is an association between bowel carcinoma and ulcerative colitis.

## ASSESSMENT FINDINGS
- Abdominal pain
- *Diarrhea*
- Steatorrhea
- Blood in the stool
- Weight loss
- Growth failure in prepubescent children
- Recurring fever possible
- Sigmoidoscopy and barium enema positive for diagnosis

## NURSING IMPLICATIONS
- Obtain a thorough history and physical examination to identify bowel patterns and any possible contributing factors.
- Prepare the child for diagnostic testing, including bowel biopsy.
- Monitor vital signs and assess stool for blood following bowel biopsy.
- Monitor intake and output and weight.
- Explain the need for total parenteral nutrition to rest the bowel for a time and discuss necessary home care arrangements, if appropriate.
- When food is reintroduced, anticipate a high-protein, high-carbohydrate, high-vitamin diet to replace nutrients.
- Explain that the prescribed anti-inflammatory drug usually greatly improves symptoms.
- Caution the child about side effects of prednisone therapy, such as weight gain and a round facial appearance.
- If sulfasalazine (Azulfidine) is prescribed, caution the child that it turns urine an orange-yellow, so that the child does not mistake this color change as bleeding.
- If medical therapy is ineffective, prepare the child and family for possible bowel resection, colostomy, or continent ileostomy.
- Provide time to listen to the child talk about symptoms and family or stress problems.

- Refer the family for counseling if you sense there is difficulty expressing fear, anger, or aggression.

# URINARY TRACT INFECTION (UTI)

## DESCRIPTION
- UTI occurs most often as an ascending infection, most often caused by gram-negative rods, such as *Escherichia coli.*
- There is a high incidence of UTIs in preschool girls.
- Children with UTIs need vigorous treatment so that the infection does not spread to involve the kidneys (pyelonephritis).

## ASSESSMENT FINDINGS
### *Possible in young children with cystitis*
- Low-grade fever
- Abdominal pain
- *Enuresis* (bed-wetting)
- *Failure to thrive,* if child is under 2 years of age
### *Likely in young children with pyelonephritis*
- High fever
- Abdominal or flank pain
- *Vomiting*
- Malaise
### *Urine for culture*
- Any growth considered significant if obtained by suprapubic aspiration
- Bacterial colony count of more than 100,000/ml considered positive, if clean-catch specimen
- Bacterial colony count between 10,000 and 100,000/ml needs repeat test

## NURSING IMPLICATIONS
- Teach girls to wipe themselves from front to back after voiding and defecating to avoid contamination of the urethra.
- Discourage use of bubble bath and feminine hygiene sprays because they may cause vulvar and urethral irritation.
- Recommend drinking periodically during the day; wearing cotton, not synthetic underwear; and washing the vulva daily to help prevent a UTI.
- Encourage the child with a UTI to drink a large quantity of fluid to "flush" the infection out of the urinary tract.

- Explain the importance of completing the full course of prescribed antibiotic therapy for UTI, even though symptoms may disappear quickly.
- Explain that urine testing after completion of antibiotic therapy is important, as is follow-up during check-ups, to detect recurrence of infection.
- If more than one infection occurs, prepare the parents and child for more extensive diagnostic studies, to determine if the cause is due to congenital stricture or urethral reflux.

## URTICARIA

### DESCRIPTION

- Urticaria or hives refers to flat weals surrounded by erythema arising from the chorion layer of the skin.
- This is an immediate hypersensitivity reaction created by the release of histamine from an antibody-antigen reaction.
- The allergens that most frequently cause urticaria include drugs, foods, and insect stings.

### ASSESSMENT FINDINGS

- Flat wheals surrounded by erythema
- Coalescence of hives (possible)
- Intense pruritus

### NURSING IMPLICATIONS

- Administer prescribed subcutaneous epinephrine or oral antihistamine.
- Instruct the child and parents in skin care measures, if appropriate.
- Explain skin testing procedures, if they are planned.
- Educate the parents and child regarding known *allergies.*
- Encourage the child to play a role in the therapy.

## VARICOCELE

### DESCRIPTION

- A varicocele is abnormal dilatation of the veins of the spermatic cord.
- Identifying the presence of varicocele is important in adolescents because the increased heat and congestion in the testicles can lead to infertility.
- No treatment is necessary for a varicocele unless fertility becomes a problem, at which time the varicocele can be surgically removed.

- Asymptomatic
- Usually palpable on left side of scrotum

NURSING IMPLICATIONS
- If surgery is planned, prepare the adolescent, explaining that there may be some local tenderness for a few days after surgery.
- Apply ice for the first few hours postoperatively to keep edema to a minimum.
- Allow the adolescent to express his feelings and concerns related to the disorder, treatment, and effects.

# VENTILATION, ASSISTED

DESCRIPTION
- Assisted ventilation is necessary when oxygen saturation continues to deteriorate despite conservative interventions.
- Assisted ventilation is accomplished via positive or negative pressure.
- A negative pressure ventilator is a device that surrounds the chest; this device is less effective than positive pressure ventilation but has the advantage of not being connected to a ventilator by intubation; suctioning can be done without interrupting ventilation.
- Indications for use of a negative pressure ventilator include children with chronic respiratory disease, such as *cystic fibrosis,* or neuromuscular disease, such as *muscular dystrophy.*
- Pulse oximetry is used to ensure adequate oxygen saturation with negative pressure ventilation because of the lack of alarms on this ventilator.
- A positive pressure ventilator delivers humidified air or oxygen or both to the lungs under pressure, with appropriate timing for adequate inflation and deflation.
- Inspiration/expiration timed interval is determined by a volume or pressure limit, depending on the type of ventilator.
- Conventional mechanical ventilators supply high tidal volumes at a low frequency rate.
- Newer ventilation methods use low tidal volumes delivered at high frequencies.
- Medication administration, such as with pancuronium, may be necessary to abolish spontaneous respi-

rations and allow mechanical ventilation to be accomplished at lower pressures.

- If a child requires prolonged mechanical ventilation, a tracheotomy or endotracheal tube is necessary.
- Weaning from mechanical ventilation is sometimes difficult because of diminished respiratory muscle function loss and psychological dependence, especially with adolescents.
- Many potential complications exist with mechanical ventilation, such as tension *pneumothorax,* obstructed airway, *atelectasis,* detubation, oxygen toxicity, stress ulcer, and infection.

### NURSING IMPLICATIONS

- Perform a thorough assessment frequently, observing for signs of complications.
- Obtain arterial blood gases to determine oxygen saturation; make the necessary ventilator changes.
- Keep in mind that administration of paralytic agents, such as pancuronium, should be accompanied by sedation, and manual ventilation must be instituted in the case of power failure.
- Prepare and educate the parents and child during assisted ventilation to mitigate their fears.
- Maintain professionalism and confidence when caring for these patients so that they will feel confident that they are safe.
- Ensure that all the child's needs are addressed, including adequate nutrition, balanced intake and output, provision of rest and stimulation, and psychosocial needs.
- Institute consistent caregivers for any child on a ventilator so that the child is reassured and less anxious with familiar caregivers.
- Prepare for an immediate thoracentesis if a tension *pneumothorax* occurs.
- Suction the child regularly to avoid obstructed airways, and use normal saline to liquefy secretions.
- Perform postural drainage as indicated for *atelectasis.*
- Administer 100% oxygen by face mask if detubation occurs until the patient can be reintubated.
- Institute increased positive end-expiratory pressure if necessary to maintain nontoxic levels of oxygen.
- Administer an antacid or histamine ($H_2$) blocker to avoid stress ulcer.

- Monitor for signs of bleeding, and administer blood products if needed.
- Monitor for signs and symptoms of infection, send sputum cultures, and administer appropriate antibiotics as necessary.

# VENTILATION, LIQUID

### DESCRIPTION

- Liquid ventilation refers to the introduction of perfluorocarbons into lungs that inflate poorly because they are deficient in surfactant or in lungs damaged by trauma or disease.
- As the liquid moves into the lung, its weight, which is heavy when compressed with air, helps to distend the lung.
- Perfluorocarbons carry oxygen along into the lung, and as the liquid spreads over all lung surfaces, an exchange of gases occurs.
- The administration of liquid ventilation is being investigated in major research centers.

### NURSING IMPLICATIONS

- Follow established protocol if assisting with this therapy.
- Instruct the parents in all aspects of the treatment; allow them to verbalize their fears and anxieties related to the procedure and status of the child.

# VESICOURETERAL REFLUX

### DESCRIPTION

- Vesicoureteral reflux refers to retrograde flow of urine from the bladder into the ureters.
- The cause is a defective valve guarding the entrance to the bladder, which may be present at birth or result from scarring as a result of repeated *urinary tract infections,* bladder pressure that is stronger than normal, or ureters that are implanted at abnormal sites or angles.
- Reflux leads to bladder infection and is potentially serious because it can lead to back pressure on the kidneys, which destroys nephrons; it can lead to *hydronephrosis.*

### ASSESSMENT FINDINGS

- History of repeated *urinary tract infections*

- Voiding cystourethrogram, isotope scan, cystoscopy, or cystography with contrast material positive for urethral reflux.

## NURSING IMPLICATIONS

- Explain the need to treat *urinary tract infections* rigorously to decrease the possibility of glomerular scarring.
- Teach double voiding (having the child void, then in a few minutes attempt to void again) to help prevent recurring infection.
- If long-term antibiotic therapy is prescribed, provide health teaching, stressing its importance in reducing renal scarring.
- If the reflux is minimal and can be corrected by endoscopy, explain the procedure and related care to the child and parents.
- If laparoscopic surgery to correct placement of the ureters is planned, prepare the child and parents; especially explain the number and types of tubes that will be inserted.
- Provide opportunities for *play therapy*.
- Following reflux surgery, carefully check the amount and color of drainage from both ureteral catheters (stents) and the suprapubic catheter.
- Expect bloody drainage, which clears in 1 to 2 days; initial drainage of an equal amount from both stents for the first 3 days; and then drainage mainly from the suprapubic tube.
- Take special care to ensure that the ends of both the suprapubic tube and the stents drain to closed collecting bags and do not become contaminated because an infection can spread to the surgical area or kidneys.
- Administer prescribed antispasmotics to reduce bladder spasms and remind the child not to touch or move the tube because that could cause spasms.
- Following removal of the suprapubic tube (usually on day 7 postsurgery), keep a sterile dressing in place for 1 or 2 days to absorb the leaking urine.
- Provide discharge instructions to the child and parents, stressing that tub baths are not permitted until healing at the suprapubic tube site is complete and emphasizing that follow-up care is necessary to evaluate the effectiveness of surgery.

## VITAMIN A DEFICIENCY

### DESCRIPTION

- Vitamin A deficiency leads first to night blindness.
- As the condition becomes more severe, xerophthalmia occurs.
- Keratomalacia, characterized by necrosis of the cornea with perforation, is the final result of severe vitamin A deficiency.
- Keratomalacia occurs only in children with prolonged, severe vitamin A deficiency and is rarely seen in the United States.

### ASSESSMENT FINDINGS

- Inability to see well in dim light (night blindness)
- Dry, lusterless conjunctivae (xerophthalmia)
- Loss of ocular fluid (keratomalacia)
- Blindness (keratomalacia)

### NURSING IMPLICATIONS

- Obtain a thorough nutritional history.
- Administer prescribed supplementary vitamin A parenterally or orally.
- Counsel parents about the need to provide a diet rich in vitamin A, including dietary sources such as liver, carrots, and spinach.
- Explain that the effects of keratomalacia can be arrested at the point at which treatment occurs, but existing damage is irreversible.

## VITAMIN C DEFICIENCY

### DESCRIPTION

- Vitamin C deficiency may result in scurvy; however, the disorder is rare today.
- In scurvy, the walls of the capillaries become fragile, and hemorrhage of vessels results.
- Infantile scurvy occurs in infants 2 to 12 months of age, who are fed only milk.

### ASSESSMENT FINDINGS (for scurvy)

- Muscle tenderness
- Petechial hemorrhage of the skin
- Swollen gums that bleed easily
- Epistaxif

- Infant's legs held in froglike position
- Hemorrhagic areas on extremities of children

**NURSING IMPLICATIONS**
- Obtain a thorough nutritional history.
- Administer prescribed supplementary vitamin C parenterally or orally.
- Counsel the parents about the need to maintain the child on a diet rich in fresh fruits and vegetables.

## VITAMIN DEFICIENCY, FOLIC ACID

**DESCRIPTION**
- A deficiency of folic acid, combined with vitamin C deficiency, produces a macrocytic (megaloblastic) anemia, characterized by abnormally large erythrocytes with accompanying *neutropenia* and thrombocytopenia.
- Megaloblastic arrest may occur in the first year of life from the continued use of infant food containing too little folic acid.
- Goat's milk tends to be deficient in folic acid, so infants who are fed this are prone to megaloblastic anemia.
- The disorder is uncommon in the United States.

**ASSESSMENT FINDINGS**
- Increased mean corpuscular volume
- Increased mean corpuscular hemoglobin
- Normal mean corpuscular hemoglobin concentration
- Megaloblasts with bone marrow aspiration

**NURSING IMPLICATIONS**
- Obtain a thorough nutritional history.
- Administer prescribed oral administration of folic acid daily.
- Provide nutritional counseling to parents.

## VITAMIN DEFICIENCY, NIACIN

**DESCRIPTION**
- Deficiency of niacin, a B complex vitamin, may lead to the disease pellagra.
- Pellagra is seen most often in people who eat corn as their main dietary staple because corn is not a good source of niacin.

**ASSESSMENT FINDINGS** (for pellagra)
- Dermatitis, resembling sunburn in white children and marked by hyperpigmentation in black children (first stage)
- Scaly, dry, cracked lesions (following first stage)
- Sore, raw-looking tongue
- *Diarrhea*
- Dementia, marked by loss of memory and irritability

**NURSING IMPLICATIONS**
- Obtain a thorough nutritional history.
- Administer prescribed niacin parenterally or orally.
- Counsel the parents about the need to maintain the child on a niacin-rich diet, which includes dietary sources such as peanuts, rice bran, and liver.

# VITAMIN DEFICIENCY, THIAMINE

**DESCRIPTION**
- Thiamine (vitamin $B_1$) deficiency in children leads to the disease beriberi.
- Beriberi occurs primarily in people who eat polished rice as their dietary staple because the source of vitamin $B_1$ is removed.

**ASSESSMENT FINDINGS** (for beriberi)
- Tingling or numbness of extremities
- Occasional heart palpitation
- Exhaustion
- Thin, wasted appearance (may appear in infants)
- *Diarrhea* and *vomiting* (may occur in infants)
- Dyspnea and cyanosis (may occur in infants)
- Anesthesia of the feet
- Ataxic gait
- Aphonia (crying without making a sound)
- Edema (terminal stage or early sign in older children)
- Convulsions (terminal stage)

**NURSING IMPLICATIONS**
- Be certain to obtain a nutritional history for children with edema because beriberi may be confused with cardiac or renal disease.
- Administer prescribed thiamine parenterally and orally.

- Counsel parents about the need to maintain children with thiamine deficiency on a thiamine-rich diet, which includes dietary sources such as wheat germ, yeast, and pork.

## VOLVULUS

### DESCRIPTION

- A volvulus is a twisting of the intestine.
- Volvulus usually occurs owing to a fetal abnormality in which the mesentery does not attach to a normal position, so the bowel is left free to move and twist.
- The twisting leads to an obstruction of the passage of feces and compromises the blood supply to the loop of intestine involved.
- Symptoms usually occur during the first 6 months of life.

### ASSESSMENT FINDINGS

- Intense crying and pain
- Pulling up the legs
- Abdominal distention
- *Vomiting*
- Abdominal mass on palpation
- *Intestinal obstruction* noted on barium x-ray film

### NURSING IMPLICATIONS

- Anticipate immediate surgery to relieve the volvulus and reattach the bowel so it is no longer freely moving.
- Maintain the infant NPO (nothing by mouth) before surgery.
- Initiate prescribed intravenous infusion to prevent fluid and electrolyte imbalances.
- Following surgery, check functioning of nasogastric tube to ensure gastric decompression.
- Monitor intravenous fluid therapy to prevent fluid and electrolyte imbalances.
- Introduce the infant to oral feeding on a gradual schedule.
- Encourage the parents to feed and hold the infant postoperatively to regain confidence.

## VOMITING

### DESCRIPTION

- Vomiting is a common and frightening symptom of illness in children.

- The symptom is usually caused by a viral or bacterial organism resulting in a mild gastroenteritis.
- The condition is always potentially serious because *metabolic alkalosis* may result.

### NURSING IMPLICATIONS

- Withhold food and fluid for a time, depending on the age of the child, usually 3 to 6 hours.
- In the older child, following a period of fasting, offer a few ice chips, then sips of water, then progress gradually to a regular diet by the 4th day.
- In the infant, introduce fluid such as glucose water or a commercial electrolyte solution, such as Pedialyte, in the same slow manner following fasting period of 3 hours. Begin with 1 tbsp every 15 minutes for 2 hours, then 1 oz every 2 hours for the next 12 to 18 hours.
- Progress diet gradually in infants as well.
- Teach the parents the importance of following these slow routines of increasing fluids at intervals.
- Instruct the parents to avoid using over-the-counter antiemetics for children.

## VON WILLEBRAND'S DISEASE

### DESCRIPTION

- Von Willebrand's disease is often referred to as angiohemophilia because there is not only a factor VIII defect, but also an inability of the platelets to aggregate and of blood vessels to constrict.
- It is an autosomal dominant disorder affecting both sexes.

### ASSESSMENT FINDINGS

- Hemorrhage, mostly from the mucous membranes
- Prolonged bleeding time

### NURSING IMPLICATIONS

- Explain the long-term nature of the disorder and help parents set appropriate limits to protect the child from injury.
- Encourage the school-age child to monitor his or her own activities.
- Stress the importance of not picking at or rubbing the nose, because *epistaxis* is a major problem.
- Prepare the adolescent girl for heavy menstrual flow because staining may cause embarrassment.

- Teach the parents and child to apply pressure and cold compresses to bleeding sites.
- Explain that bleeding must be controlled with factor VIII replenishment or by administration of arginine desmopressin (DDAVP), a vasoconstricting agent.
- Explain the risks of childbirth to women with von Willebrand's disease.
- Refer parents for genetic counseling.

# VULVOVAGINITIS

### Description
- Vulvovaginitis is inflammation of the vulva or vagina.
- It may occur in a girl of any age but tends to be more frequent as a girl reaches puberty.
- Common causative agents for vulvovaginitis includes *Candida, Trichomonas, Gardnerella, Chlamydia trachomatis, Neisseria gonorrhoeae, Treponema pallidum, Enterobius vermicularis* (pinworm), herpesvirus type 2, and foreign body.
- Vaginal examination is required to locate a foreign object and to confirm full removal.

### Assessment Findings
- Pain
- Odor
- Pruritus
- Vaginal discharge

### Nursing Implications
- Recognize that bleeding before menarche is rare, and, if present, its cause must be investigated.
- Explain the need to avoid bubble bath and feminine hygiene sprays to prevent irritation.
- Encourage the use of cotton underwear to prevent a moist, warm environment for organisms to grow.
- Educate the girl about proper hygiene, including the need for daily washing and drying and wiping from front to back following voiding or bowel movements.
- For the adolescent, recommend frequent changing of tampons or sanitary napkins.
- Instruct the girl with vulvovaginitis to wash the vulva twice a day with mild, nonperfumed soap and water; pat dry front to back.
- To relieve discomfort of vulvovaginitis, recommend application of cornstarch (talc should be used sparingly because it may be associated with ovarian cancer).

- Explain that frequent sitz baths or use of warm compresses and acetaminophen every 4 hours may also increase comfort.
- Provide information concerning medications prescribed to treat the specific cause of vulvovaginitis.

## WHOOPING COUGH

### DESCRIPTION

- Whooping cough (pertussis), a serious bacterial infection of childhood, particularly in the infant period, is caused by *B. pertussis.*
- Transmission is by direct or indirect contact, with communicability greatest in the catarrhal stage.
- Contracting the disease offers lasting natural immunity.
- Pertussis vaccine given as part of DPT vaccine provides active artificial immunity and is recommended by the American Academy of Pediatrics for all children.
- Pertussis immune serum globulin provides passive artificial immunity.

### ASSESSMENT FINDINGS

#### *Catarrhal stage (lasting 1 to 2 weeks)*

- Coryza
- Sneezing
- Lacrimation
- Mild cough
- Low-grade fever
- Irritability and listlessness
- Increased white blood cell count, possibly as high as 20,000 to 30,000 mm$^3$
- Nasopharyngeal culture may detect *B. pertussis* bacillus

#### *Paroxysmal stage (lasting 4 to 6 weeks)*

- Paroxysmal cough tending to be more severe at night
- Characteristic "whoop," a high-pitched crowing sound following cough
- Cyanosis or red face
- Drainage of thick, tenacious mucus from nose
- *Vomiting* following paroxysm of coughing
- Exhaustion

#### *Convalescent stage*

- Gradual cessation of coughing and vomiting

**NURSING IMPLICATIONS**

- To prevent pertussis, encourage *immunization,* informing wary parents that the risk of complications from pertussis vaccine is less than the risk of complications from the illness.
- Maintain bed rest until coughing paroxysms subside.
- Seclude the child from cigarette smoke, dust, and strenuous exercise to minimize irritants.
- Administer frequent, small meals to maintain nutrition.
- Anticipate hospitalization for infants requiring airway suction for tenacious secretions.
- Consider using a mist tent to loosen secretions in infants.
- Explain the need to administer a full 10-day course of prescribed erythromycin or penicillin.
- Monitor for complications resulting from the illness.

*Section*
**5**

# Cross-Reference Index